Everyone's Everyday Guide to Practical Psychiatry

Everyone's Everyday Guide to Practical Psychiatry

A Handbook for Patients and Caregivers

W. Edison Houpt Jr., MD

With more than Ninety Diagrams, Charts, and Tables

iUniverse, Inc.
New York   Bloomington

Everyone's Everyday Guide to Practical Psychiatry
A Handbook for Patients and Caregivers

iUniverse books may be ordered through booksellers or by contacting:

iUniverse
1663 Liberty Drive
Bloomington, IN 47403
www.iuniverse.com
1-800-Authors (1-800-288-4677)

Because of the dynamic nature of the Internet, any Web addresses or links contained in this book may have changed since publication and may no longer be valid. The views expressed in this work are solely those of the author and do not necessarily reflect the views of the publisher, and the publisher hereby disclaims any responsibility for them.

ISBN: 978-0-595-52701-4 (sc)
ISBN: 978-0-595-62755-4 (ebk)

Library of Congress Control Number: 2010902207

Printed in the United States of America

iUniverse rev. date: 04/28/2010

Dedicated to all of my teachers

Wherever they are

Especially to those at the

Cleveland Clinic:

*A portion of
the net profits from
the sale of this book
will be donated to medical research
and to the training of young doctors*

Who Are Our Patients?

Our Patients live where we live.
They dwell amongst us.
We are our patients.
And they are a part of us.

Table of Contents

LIST of VISUAL AIDS:
CHARTS, TABLES, FLOWCHARTS, and GRAPHS

Chapter #	Title of Visual Aid	Comments
I-2	Information Resource on Diagnoses	
I-3-a	Psychiatry evolves from ancient medicine	
I-3-b	Holistic Psychiatry	
I-3-c	Comparison of Main Types of Doctors	
I-3-d	Treatment is not Cure (basic diagram)	
I-3-e	Treatment is not Cure (complex disease)	
I-4-a	Signs and Symptoms (S & Sx)	
I-4-b	Flowchart of the Evolution of Psychiatry	
I-4-c	Decades of Life	
I-6-a	Length of Treatment as a function of Diagnosis	
I-7-a	List of terms using "Pharm-"	
I-7-b	Drug Toxicities Appearing after FDA Approval	
I-7-c	Example of a "black-box" warning for a drug	
I-7-d	Pharmacologic Adaptation…	
I-7-e	Patient Reactions to Addicting Medicines	
II-1-a	Diagnostic tools-Treatment means	
II-1-b	Ever enlarging forebrain	
II-1-c	The brain and its schematic parts	
II-1-d	Schematic of brain and three cranial nerves	
II-2-a	Nerve to Nerve Communication	
II-2-d	Nerve function	
II-2-e	Three methods of nerve communication	
II-2-g	Direct electrical contact and relay	
II-4-a	Cytochromes are proteins	
II-4-b	Rapid and slow users of Paxil	The P_{450} system
II-4-c	Drug accumulates in a slow user of Paxil	

Section I
INTRODUCTIONS

Superscript numbers refer to references and citations at the back of the book

List of Common Abbreviations Used in this Book

	Description	Alternate Terms
ADHD	Attention Deficit-Hyperactivity Disorder	ADDH, ADD
APA	American Psychiatric Association	
CATS	CATScan = type of brain "X-ray" (see PETS)	CATS shows brain structure
CDC	Centers for Disease Control (Atlanta, GA)	rarely interacts with psychiatry
DA	Dopamine, a stimulating brain hormone	
DEA	Drug Enforcement Administration	Controls drugs: Valium, Xanax, ADDH drugs, sleeping pills
DO	Doctor of Osteopathy	Basically like an MD
DSM-IV-TR	The DSM-IV-TR is the official handbook of Psychiatry sponsored by the APA	This book shows us how to make A psychiatric diagnosis
ER	Emergency Room	ED—emergency Department
FDA	Food and Drug Administration	Approves drugs for sale in USA
FGA	First Generation Antipsychotic	
GABA	Gamma-amino-butyric acid	Natural relaxing hormone
5-HT	5-Hydroxy-Tryptamine = Serotonin	Other name for Serotonin
MAOI	Monoamine Oxidase Inhibitor	A type of antidepressant
MD	Medical Doctor, Doctor of Medicine	M.D. comes from *Medcinæ Doctor*
MRI	Magnetic Resonance Imagining	This is a type of X-ray
NE	Norepinephrine	NA—Noradrenaline
OTC	Over-the-counter pills (do not need Rx)	sold without prescription
PDR	Physician's Desk Reference	List of available Rx medicines
PETS	PETScan = type of brain "X-ray"(see CATS)	PETS shows brain function
PI	Package Insert = list of drug side effects	
PTSD	Post-Traumatic Stress Disorder	
Rx	Prescription medicine	
SGA	Second Generation Antipsychotic	
SNRI	Selective Norepinephrine Receptor Inhibitor	
SSRI	Selective Serotonin Receptor Inhibitor	
SSNRI	A drug with both SNRI and SSRI activity	
TCA	Tricyclic Antidepressant	

Format of the Book

This book is intended as a behind-the-scenes look at the workings of modern psychiatric practice. Some of it is also relevant to the general practice of medicine. I originally started this project in August 2007 envisioning it as a kind of public service to educate people about what psychiatrists do. Two years later, I now realize that it has become larger than first intended; however, I can honestly say that it has now technically become a public health measure, in the sense that I am trying to encourage people to attend more to their personal health issues by preventing disease. As we like to say in Medicine, "Prevention is the best form of Treatment". Each chapter or topic may include any or all of the following:

1. definition of the topic
2. introduction to the topic
3. characteristics of the topic which are specific to it
4. analysis of the significance of the topic
5. diagnosis
6. treatments available (medications are also listed in a special section)
7. forecast, outlook, or prediction
8. interspersion of typical patient questions: answers within the text: Q: A:

At the end of applicable chapters, I have tried to include a small section that outlines the usual, customary, and standard treatments available today.

I use the terms "medication", "drug", and "medicine" almost interchangeably.

▶*Superscript numbers* [11] *refer to cited references in the back of the book.*
▶*black triangles denote learning points and **Questions***
**Asterisks refer to chapter footnotes found at the end of the corresponding chapter*

Introduction to the Book

Superscript numbers refer to references and citations at the back of the book

First, this is *not* a textbook, but rather serves as a glimpse of how we practice psychiatry in the early part of the twenty-first century. This is not an erudite handbook, but is rather intended as a basic resource guide for patients and their families.

This book is a handbook and has been written with the intention that the reader can turn to certain pertinent subjects to retrieve pertinent information on that subject as needed. I do not necessarily expect that anyone will pick it up and read it through from the first page to the last page as if it were a novel. For example, if your loved one suddenly becomes very depressed, then you can turn to the following chapters for information: Chapters IV-2-3-4 and V-6-7-8-9. As a result, some of the same information has been repeated in different chapters. I have listed some of the most common problems that you the reader might encounter in the real world and have tabulated them with the most pertinent chapters to read followed by other chapters that might be applicable also:

Table I-2   Information Resource

If You Want information On this DIAGNOSIS ..._	then read these chapters:	these chapters may also be useful
DEPRESSION	IV-2-3-4 V-5-6-7-8-9	I-7 II-2-3 IV-6-7 V-18, VII-1
SEVERE DEPRESSION	IV-2-3-4-5-6-7, V-5-6-7-8-9-10-12-13-18	II-2-3 VII-1-3

SCHIZOPHRENIA	IV-1-5 V-4-16	IV-7 VII-2
ALCOHOLISM	VI-1-2-3	V-11-12-13-17 VI-7
ANXIETY	I-7 II-4 IV-8 V-11-12-17	
Psychiatry in general	I-4-5-6 III-1-2-3-4-5-6 V-3-19 VII-1-2-3	

▶Q: Who is Dr. Houpt?

A: Who I am:

This is an important question since it explains whether I have the requisite credentials to write such a handbook. I am a typical psychiatrist who has had background training in the Natural sciences and Humanities. I have worked in the Regional Psychiatric Emergency Room at St. Vincent's Hospital in Cleveland, Ohio; I have done in-patient and out-patient work and worked in the county and State systems as well as in private practice. Until recently, I was working for a large medical partnership in Southern California (where I had worked ten years).

I have not received any significant payments from any drug company and am thus neutral in my regards for the drugs and drug companies in general. I do have a slight amount of deserved cynicism about the whole American pharmaceutical system. Yes, of course, I tend to prefer certain drugs for certain conditions but do not intentionally hold any stocks in any one drug company. And I am not especially biased or prejudiced toward any one drug over another apart from its expected benefits to that particular patient.

▶Q: Why write such a book?

A: The usual in-office interactions with patients reveal that a lot of people have a lot of misconceptions or gaps in information about the workings of modern medical psychiatry. These small—and large—gaps suggested to me the need to write down some simple insights and instructions that I later expanded into this handbook. This is done with the hope that patients as well as their friends and families can learn about this psychiatric process before or while it is taking place. This book may serve to orient you so that you can follow the usual progression of treatment and find out whether you are on track and on which track, too!

Reading this book should also help you to partner with your doctor in a more meaningful and collaborative way and to enable you to have some participation in the decision-making process.

▶Q: How do you practice psychiatry?

A: At the end of the first major intake evaluation, I usually tell the patient what the working diagnosis is. Then I tell them the usual top two or three treatments (which they may have already looked up on the Internet, anyway). Then I try to involve them in the decision-making process. A number of patients just want me to make the decision, but at least they are given a sense of being involved in their own treatment that is important because you, the patient, are going to be putting these drugs into your body. I also tell patients to expect all the worst possible side effects from the drugs for two reasons:

1)-the pharmacy will probably detail these side effects plus a lot of other distressing additional information(see Chapter V-19); and,

2)-if patients expect the worst possible side effects (which is rare) but only have fleeting trivial side-effects (which is usual), then they will feel that they are doing better than expected—which is usually true anyway. In this way, patients can have a personal sense that all is going as scheduled.

This book will attempt to take you behind the scenes to find out how we think, why we make our decisions, and what those decisions might mean. This is not information that you would find readily on the Internet. I have not dwelled upon thousands of mere facts since these you can look up on the Internet. I try to present experience rather than facts. In this book, experience trumps data (hopefully). This book is based on my personal observations as I have witnessed in my office for a quarter of a century. I have not routinely quoted facts, figures, authorities, or statistics. The book is not intended to be a reference book. Some parts of this book represent my opinions and observations sometimes cynically—and hopefully intuitively—filtered through the lens of recent unwritten contemporary medical happenings.

The names of the pharmaceutical drugs are written using their patented trade names as proper nouns since these might be more familiar to the non-medical reading public. The name "Prozac" is used—not the word "fluoxetine"; "Thorazine" is used not "chlorpromazine". In this way, the drugs seem to have real names and sound familiar; moreover, it is a way of paying homage to the people who invented these beneficial treatments and brought them to market. Despite the many naysayers, these drugs have brought relief to hundreds of millions of patients over the last century. These patent names (e.g., "Thorazine", "Prozac") are usually the easiest to remember and to pronounce. Each one of these prescription drugs actually has three names and this is explained in Chapter I-8 on Pharmacology.

I have attempted to confine myself to psychiatric commentary except where I felt that a broader overview of American medicine in general was warranted in order to give more general background coverage of all events and how they come to bear on modern psychiatry. Public health concerns, the legal system, and the practice of [internal] medicine have exerted far more influence on psychiatry than vice versa.

I have devised a number of charts, graphs, and classifications that I present as visual learning aids. These are not really standardized and are based on experience instead of statistics. I hope they are useful.

W. Edison Houpt, Jr. MD
Pasadena
Los Angeles County
California

If all doctors live long enough, then we too will eventually end up being patients.

Introduction to Doctors in America
Classification of Physicians
Primum non nocere
(First, do no harm)

This chapter serves two purposes. Firstly, it shows how psychiatry came into existence, and how it came into existence as a type of medical specialty, medical psychiatry. Secondly, we draw upon the reader's probable familiarity with regular medicine and surgery to show how psychiatry is like regular medical practice and how it differs from regular medical practice. By showing the similarities to the practice of your family doctor, you will have an idea of how modern psychiatry is similar to the familiar.

In order to understand who psychiatrists are, the reader will need to know what we do. Modern psychiatry is an outgrowth of Western style Medicine.

In order to tell you who we are not, I am dividing doctors into Eastern style (Oriental) or Western style (Occidental) and telling you that psychiatrists are not directly descended from the Oriental tradition, but rather from the Western style. Western style doctors derive their treatment philosophies from the ancient Greeks and Romans (Latin), as well as from Arabs of the Middle Ages. Western style doctors are nowadays represented by European and American medicine (all the Americas). Western style doctors are the most numerous and include most of the doctors whom you might see—this would include your primary care doctor as well as specialists to whom he might refer you. Specialists, such as cardiologists or orthopedic surgeons.

Western doctors trace their origins back to the ancient Mediterranean world: Greece, Rome, Alexandria (Egypt), and Asia Minor (western Turkey). Hippocrates is honored as the "Father of Medicine" (according to Occidental tradition). He lived two and a half thousand years ago. Around the same time in India, there lived a famous physician, Susruta, equally honored in that region of the world. Galen lived two thousand years ago and was equally famous, as were other ancient doctors, such as Celsus. When Islam was in its ascendancy a thousand years ago, the Arabic world built up and established Baghdad as one of the greatest medical centers in the Mediterranean world. Then they imported some of the best physicians to come live and work in Baghdad, which became a renowned center for medicine and especially for ophthalmology. At that time, the great books on Medicine were translated into Arabic and kept in Baghdad. For the next few hundred years, while religious fanaticism raged through the Dark Ages and medieval Europe, Europeans burned all the great medical books from their ancient doctors. These works would have all been lost irretrievably except for the fact that the Arabic world prized these books and kept them safe until they could be back-translated into Latin at the beginning of the Renaissance.

Curiously, Western doctors who trace the origins of their style of medical practice back to Hippocrates tend to ignore the fact that he used only natural remedies for his treatments. Of course, those were the only remedies available back then. Nowadays, Hippocrates would be recognized as practicing a style of medicine that we often call alternative medicine, holistic medicine, or naturopathic medicine.

In the U.S., there are several types of licensed doctors, the two most common of which are M.D. and D.O.

This is an outline classification of the types of doctors based on their degrees (and requisite State licensure categories):

A—Occidental Medicine ("Western" Medicine)
    1—Allopathic medical doctor (M.D.)
    2—Osteopathic medical doctor (D.O.)
    3—Homeopathic practitioner (HHP, D.Hom. and others)
    4—Naturopathic Practitioner ("Doctor of Naturopathy", D.N.)

B—Oriental Medicine ("Eastern" Medicine: O.D.M., O.M.D.) of which there are several degreed titles depending upon the medical school and State of licensure
    1—Doctor of Acupuncture and Oriental Medicine (D.A.O.M.)
    2—Licensed Acupuncturist (L.Ac.), Master of Science in Acupuncture (M.S.A).
    3—Chinese Herbal Medicine

C—Surgeons: in antiquity, surgeons were a separate type of practitioner but nowadays they fall under the rubric of M.D./D.O. In some countries, they receive a Bachelor of Medicine Bachelor of Surgery degree (BMBS, MB BCh)

D—Doctors of the Nervous System: Neurologists, Neuropsychiatrists, Neuroscientists, and Psychiatrists
    1 Psychiatrists and Neuropsychiatrists are either MD or DO (A-1, A-2 above);
    2 classical Psychoanalysts typically hold an MD degree;
    3 Holistic Psychiatrists try to incorporate some of the principles of holistic medicine;
    4 Neurologists are MD or DO;

5   Neuroscientists usually hold a PhD degree—they are not licensed to practice human medicine.

E—Clinical psychologists (PhD, PsyD): see chapters I-5, I-6

F—There are also a number of other Western style clinicians who will not be discussed here (such as optometrists, O.D., podiatrists D.P.M., and chiropractors, D.Ch.).

These are the meanings of our professional classifications:

- Allopathy—Greek for *allo + pathos* meaning "opposite to" + " illness": in other words, the prescribed medicine produces the opposite effect as the symptoms of the disease
- Osteopathy—means "bone" + "disease". Osteopathic treatment originally relied on mechanical manipulations of the bones and muscles; osteopaths who are psychiatrists essentially practice allopathic medicine—or they could be holistic.
- Homeopathy—*homeos (homoios) + pathos* meaning "similar to" "the disease"; homeopaths prescribe medicines with the same side effects as the symptoms of the disease.
- Naturopathy—means "nature" "disease" and uses natural remedies and substances for treatments, which can include diet, rest, hydrotherapy, ozone, aromatherapy, botanical products, massage, and so on. Nowadays this is also called holistic or alternative medicine.
- Holistic—from *holo* means "wholeness": holistic refers to treating the patient as a whole person in whom many factors operate to create a balance of health; the focus is not on just one organ, cause, or symptom—but rather on the whole person.
- Physician—a "doctor of physic": in Greek, "physikos" means "natural"; later in history, the Europeans began to use "physic" to refer to a natural remedy (since synthetic drugs had not yet been discovered). A physician is literally a doctor of nature-sourced remedies. Over the last century, Western medicine has focused on synthetic (man-made) pharmaceuticals, and has thus practically abandoned the use of nature-sourced remedies. This is also true in psychiatry where almost all treatments are with synthetic drugs and not with "physic". Rare examples of natural sourced treatments in psychiatry would include Lithium, Valeriana, and St. John's Wort; the case could be made to include L-Tryptophan, Reserpine, and a few others.
- Doctor means "teacher" in Latin
- Psychiatrist is from Greek *psych + iatros* "doctor of the soul"
- In the USA we have recently popularized the terms "provider" and "clinician":

- The term "provider" focuses on money and reimbursement. A provider is any healthcare professional who holds a state license and renders direct clinical care to patients; typically—this is an important distinction—provider services can be billed to the government and insurance companies in expectation of reimbursement. Hence, a provider could be anyone licensed to bill for a professional medical, nursing, or health-related service: a psychotherapist, an art therapist, or a RN who gives injections of psychoactive drugs.
- The term "clinician" focuses on direct patient contact. (The Greek word *klinē* means "bed".) A clinician sees live patients ["at bedside"] as opposed to non-clinicians who do not; non-clinicians would typically include medical researchers, public health officers, coroners, pathologists, and administrators for the CDC, FDA, and so on. Opinions of clinicians are sought and valued in regards to patient treatment and diagnosis. Input from non-clinicians is important for medical theorizing, public health measures, preventive medicine, risk management (reducing medical malpractice risks), statistics, and the day-to-day running of the healthcare delivery system and of the physical plant of the hospital.

Background details on doctors and their treatment philosophies

Doctoring most assuredly had its origins in the mists of prehistory. Trephined skulls have been found: trephining refers to the deliberate surgical operation of opening a hole in the skull. Not only were these operations deliberate, but in a number of cases, the bone (skull) has healed, which means that the patient survived the operation long enough to heal. Psychoactive plant materials have presumably been used since those times, also. All these treatments would be classified as natural remedies. Thus, all doctors started out as naturopaths, technically speaking. Over many thousands of years, different specialties and treatment philosophies have evolved. These are some of them:

Occidental or Western-style Medicine is very common in Europe and the Americas.

The most commonly known Western-style doctors are the allopaths (MD medical doctors) who are also the most numerous (over a quarter of a million in the USA).

1—Allopaths (M.D.'s) treat existing symptoms and existing diseases with pharmaceuticals designed to have an opposite effect on the body. This is akin to adding acid and alkali and obtaining a neutral solution. Or adding a plus to a minus and ending up with both canceling out.

The dosing of allopathic treatment is usually proportional to the severity of the symptoms: for worse symptoms, take more pills. For example, anxiety would be treated with a drug that would calm the nervous system (Valium, in this case); hence, the patient would only take half a pill twice a day for mild anxiety but might be prescribed more pills for panic or agitation.

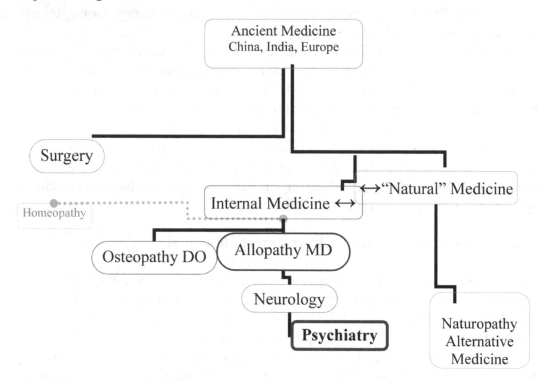

Diagram I-3-a showing how ancient medicine gave rise to Western Medicine (Allopathy). The arrows show the significant interplay between internal medicine and "natural" medicine. Internal Medicine has its roots in natural medicine. Psychiatry owes its very existence to this evolution of medicine. Neurologists and Psychiatrists might have MD or DO degree.

If the cause of disease is known, then allopathic treatment may be directed at correcting the underlying cause, but all too often the root cause may not be curable—only treatable (sometimes it may not even be treatable). Medical doctors are called physician because they are historically called doctors of "physic", a Greek expression suggesting nature or natural science, which was the original treatment that ancient physicians delivered. In ancient times physicians such as Hippocrates would usually prescribe natural substances, activity modification (bed rest or some physical therapy), physical therapy, diet, bodily manipulations (physical therapy), poultices, massages, and minor invasive procedures (bloodletting, leeches, incision and drainage, lancing and so on). In olden times, a typical physician was a type of naturopathic doctor in the sense that most of the treatments were sourced from nature, but other treatments were used too. Allopathic medical doctors look to Hippocrates as the Father of Medicine and allopathic M.D.'s take the Hippocratic Oath. In reality, Hippocrates was practicing naturopathy.

Some allopaths do invasive treatments such as sticking tubes into patients or inserting a "central line" into the cardiovascular system. Neurologists do lumbar puncture (sticking a needle into the spine). Some psychiatrists carry extra certification and liability insurance so that they can do "invasive" procedures such as sending electrical or magnetic waves into the brain.

2—Osteopathic treatment has a focus on healing the musculoskeletal system in the belief that secondary health benefits will accrue from mechanical manipulations of the body (bones and muscles).

3—Homeopathy was started by Samuel Hahnemann and is based on his casual observations that treatment benefits may result from using chemicals with the same side effects as the symptoms of the disease. He reasoned that such chemicals might supplant or replace the symptoms of the disease state. This resulted in his theory that "like heals like". For this reason, homeopaths prescribe chemicals with the same effects as the disease symptoms—but the chemicals are administered in tiny amounts. The active chemical is dissolved in water and then diluted many times so that only a tiny amount of the chemical treatment may remain dissolved in a bottle of treatment solution: the amount of medicine dissolved could be only a few molecules. There have been very few—if any—controlled clinical trials on homeopathic treatment. Hahnemann's beliefs no longer seem rational to a lot of allopaths; notwithstanding, Hahnemann Medical College in Philadelphia is named after him; and, it trains allopaths!

4—Naturopathy uses natural substances as remedies and treatments. These treatments can be diet, rest, hydrotherapy, ozone, aromatherapy, botanical products, massage, and so on. Naturopaths focus on eliminating the cause of the disease as opposed to allopaths who try to suppress the symptoms with drugs that produce an opposite effect to the symptoms. Naturopathy is also called holistic or alternative medicine.

Holistic practitioners may include any of the above practitioners, although allopaths are less likely to be holistic for the simple reason that they are kept on very tight schedules and are forced to focus on treating disease states and providing symptomatic relief. What makes a doctor holistic is the treatment philosophy.

Oriental Medical practitioners

Oriental medical practitioners have mostly been trained in both Chinese herbalism and in Acupuncture, but some practitioners specialize in only one of these two areas. Oriental Medicine focuses on the alignment of the *Qi* (the life force) and on the balance or harmony between the Yin and Yang. In Chinese herbalism an "herb" has a more extended definition, including any found item, such as plants, minerals, animal parts, marine life, and even dried rodent feces (for one gynecologic condition). Moxibustion is also used (burning of dried mugwort) as a therapy.

Acupuncture treatment requires knowledge of the meridians, which are parallel symmetrical segments of the human body. These meridians are considered as groupings of bodily functions that are grouped together in ways that are reminiscent of what Western Medicine calls "dermatomes" (which are derived from somites that also are parallel symmetric segments of bodily structure and function). Yet the meridians are a different pattern from that seen in Western Medicine. An Old European mummy (named Ötzi) was recently found and his remains were dated to around 3300 BCE. Curiously, he had odd tattoos on his body. After autopsy had revealed which diseases that he had suffered, researchers realized that his diseases and tattoos corresponded to the treatment meridians of Oriental Medicine! (The mummy had been found in the Alps on the border of Italy and Austria. It is doubtful that he had had any intercourse with the ancient Chinese. Did Old Europeans* invent acupuncture independently?)

Surgeons

Surgeons were originally considered to be a separate type of practitioner completely different from any of those listed above due to their treatment methods (wounds, cutting and amputations), but are now incorporated into M.D. / D.O. professional designation. As a matter of fact, European surgeons and barbers historically belonged to the same professional class (tonsorial), referencing their skill with cutting instruments. Surgeons in the United Kingdom may have a Bachelor of Surgery degree. Nowadays, neurosurgeons are in charge of any procedures involving psychosurgery.

When psychiatrists administer shock treatments of any kind (electric, magnetic, chemical, biochemical), they are technically practicing surgery and need extra malpractice coverage.

Doctors of the Nervous System

Neurologists typically treat functional problems that are [presumably] caused by permanent damage to the structure of the brain. Epilepsy is a good example: it can be due to visible or invisible damage of the brain. Visible damage would be such as a tumor, blood clot, or a "scar". Epilepsy can also occur without any apparent visible damage, but damage of some kind must be there, or else the patient would not be having epilepsy (seizures). Invisible damage can be very small or biochemical in nature. Signs of visible damage can be seen on MRI or CATScan; if it is invisible, it will usually show up on EEG, which is an electrical recording of brain activity. Neurologists do not perform surgery, but do insert needles into their patients ("spinal tap" and graphs of muscle electricity, EMG).

Neurosurgeons treat permanent physical damage to the structure of the brain. They deal with MRI, CATScan, and regular X-rays.

Neuropsychiatrists: have been trained both in neurology and in psychiatry

Neuroscientists have a Ph.D. degree and do important research in nerve functions. This would loosely include other specialists such as neuro-pharmacologists, and so on.

Psychiatrists treat behavioral alterations:
- alterations, which they believe to be due to biochemical changes in the brain: the changes can be temporary or permanent. In other words, this involves microscopic damage that can be seen only on PETScans (but not on CATScan or MRI). Examples could be mania, severe depression, brain damage from methamphetamines
- Other altered behaviors without apparent microscopic brain damage—such as personality styles
- Genetic psychiatric disorders
  a—families where many relatives have committed suicide,
  b—cases of neurological disorders that uniformly require neurological treatment and psychiatric treatment: such as Huntington's chorea, temporal lobe epilepsy, and others

Psychoanalysts are discussed in Chapter I-5.

Holistic Psychiatrists: this is how I tend to practice psychiatry. In psychiatry, holistic would mean looking at the whole person and all his needs: mental, spiritual, emotional, behavioral, and physical well-being. I would also include a criterion of reducing all stress levels, such as legal, marital, financial, and sociological. A person's physical health has a direct effect on his mental health and vice versa. Stress can also aggravate any existing mental or physical disease. A person's environment also has a great effect on his state of healthfulness.

I often make these treatment plans and suggestions for patients:

- seek causes of stress and try to correct them slowly
- if the stress cannot be corrected, then learn coping skills
- take prescribed medicines
- participate in individual or group therapy
- correct medical problems associated with poor physical health since this will adversely affect mental health
- exercise aerobically as this will release natural "feel-good" hormones
- stop eating junk food and fast food—these contain significant amounts of chemicals with unknown long-term health hazards
- consider using herbs, minerals, vitamins, and such
- Take a vacation
- Take time off from work (doctor's excuse)

Diagram I-3-b shows that our inner abstract self is our psyche that is related to the physical organ called the brain. The brain is the innermost and central part of the nervous system that uses brain hormones for internal communication. The nervous system communicates with the body using these and other chemicals. The human body is separated from the physical world by the largest organ in the body, the skin, which is very thin and porous to a certain degree, thus resulting in a constant interplay between our internal body and the outside world. The outside world contains beneficial chemicals (botanical remedies like St. John's Wort), beneficial physicals (sunlight to make vitamin D), as well as harmful chemicals (plant poisons) and harmful physicals (cosmic and solar radiation). The outside world is the Natural World. It is engulfed by the Cosmos (Outer Space), the workings of which are still being studied. This diagram shows the successive layers from psyche to Cosmos. Is there a more direct correlation between the two?

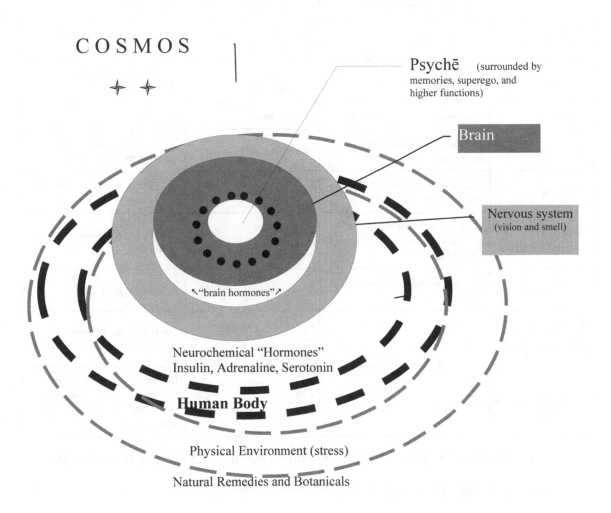

COSMOS

Psychē (surrounded by memories, superego, and higher functions)

Brain

Nervous system (vision and smell)

↖"brain hormones"↗

Neurochemical "Hormones"
Insulin, Adrenaline, Serotonin

Human Body

Physical Environment (stress)

Natural Remedies and Botanicals

Holistic Psychiatry
Diagram I-3-b

This is a chart showing comparison among these treatment philosophies:

Chart I-3-c Comparison of Doctors

Profession	Chemical Substances used	Physical Methods used	Treatment Philosophy
Allopath MD	Pharmaceuticals	Minimally invasive** moderately invasive***	Rx ⇌ Sx *
Osteopath DO	Pharmaceuticals	Mechanical manipulations	Treatment as per symptoms Rx ⇌ Sx
Homeopath	Micro-amounts of chemicals	Non-invasive	Rx = Sx
Naturopath (ND)	Botanicals, rest, aromas, hydrotherapy, ozone	Massage	Natural remedies treat the cause of the symptoms
Surgeons	Pain-killers, antibiotics, various Pharmaceuticals	Very invasive	Cut out (or into) the cause of symptoms
Doctor of Oriental Medicine	Herbs (which includes plant products, minerals, and "found" substances)	Acupuncture minimally** to moderately invasive	Chemical decoctions, thin fine needles
Psychiatrists	Pharmaceuticals, Lithium, rare herbs	Non-invasive	Behavioral modification
Psychologists Psychotherapists	~ ~ ~	~ ~ ~	Behavioral modification, analysis of "toxic" relationships
Psychoanalysts	~ ~ ~	~ ~ ~	Intensive in-depth analysis of how repressed behaviors and suppressed desires interfere with behavior

*Rx is "prescribed treatment"   Rx ⇌ Sx: prescription effect is opposite of symptom

*Sx is "Symptom" Rx=Sx: drug effects mimic symptoms of the disease

**minimally invasive procedures in medicine: injections, vaccines, blood drawing, "central lines", feeding tubes; and, arguably hypnosis in psychiatry;

***moderately invasive procedures in medicine: cardiac catheterization, colonoscopy, nuclear medicine; and, in psychiatry: ECT (shock treatments) and transcraneal magnetic resonance (passing magnetic waves into the brain)

IV—Treatment is not necessarily Cure

Dorland's Medical Dictionary defines "treatment" as *"management and care of a patient for the purpose of combating disease or disorder",* and "cure" as *"...successful treatment of a disease or wound...",* and "therapy/therapia" as *"service done to the sick...use of some chemical agent which will [treat/cure] patient without being seriously toxic for the patient"*

The learning point here is that treatment is not necessarily cure.

A person can lapse from a state of good health into sickness. At this point, the treatment may eradicate the sickness. At this point, he can lapse back into a state of good health. This is cure. If the disease cannot be eradicated, then the second choice is just to make it manageable. As far as symptoms in an uncured disease, the treatment may serve to make symptoms bearable—or the symptoms may be almost completely suppressed: so in this case, there is relief from treatment but no cure.

In psychiatry, we rarely use the word "cure". Some disorders can be well controlled (Depression or anxiety), moderately controlled (depression, anxiety, schizophrenia), poorly controlled (schizophrenia), and other disorders can "remit" after a period of treatment, usually a couple years (stress disorders). "Remit" or "remission" means that the symptoms of the disorder have disappeared—for a certain period of time. However, they may well return sometime in the future.

In figure *1-3-d,* we can see the basic cycle of disease, treatment, and possible cure. A person can be in a good state of health and experience an upsetting stress factor. This could be a cause of anxiety or could lead up to other events causing anxiety. Causes of anxiety can lead to anxiety symptoms that lead to a diagnosis of Anxiety. The anxiety itself can aggravate more anxiety symptoms (⇆). Likewise, first attempts at treatment may have no effect and just go back (⇆) into the Anxiety. Eventually the treatment will lead either to relief or to cure. A person can have treatment, go through one cycle of the disease, and feel better while the symptoms are in (allopathic) remission. The arrows show that treatment could lead to relief or cure. The disease might be cured altogether and the person could return to a state of good health. If not, then he will achieve relief in remission with the possibility that the underlying condition could flare up again.

Fig I-3-d Treatment is not Cure (simple case)

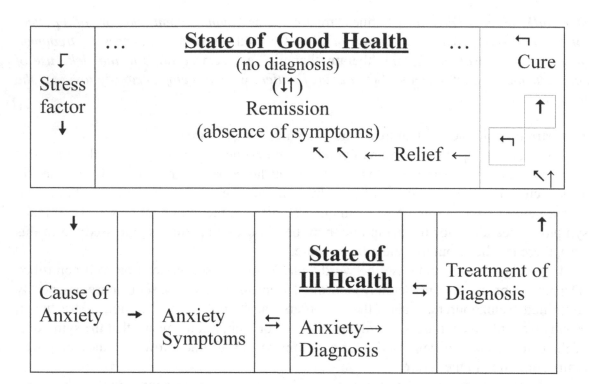

This next figure shows a complicated situation. In *figure 1-3-e,* we can see that

- (1) A child might start life in good health, then become depressed as a teenager (teen). He may receive treatment and then feel relief or cure. Stress factors might be grades, peer pressure, general coping skills, medical problems, or parental pressure to excel (at sports, academics, etc.).

- (2) If he starts to use street drugs and becomes agitated from the drugs, plus the original depression returns (D/D), then he will go through the whole cycle a second time. On the second pass through, he requires much more intensive treatment for the depression—plus the secondary problem of drug abuse. If his girlfriend is pregnant, then he will have two secondary problems plus the relapsed depression. Treatment will be more difficult and may last for [many] years. The dashed gray line shows that the remission state is more permeable or temporary than the state of good health. The light grey lines show weaker boundaries. Treatment can lead to cure. Cure can lead to good health.

- After one or two passes through treatment, the teenager might be cured or in remission from Depression and stay that way for years or decades. On the other hand, the teenager could recover from Depression and drug abuse and go into a state of good health.

- (3) A few years later, he could then develop a new illness, such as schizophrenia or mania (SM) and go through the treatment cycle for a third loop—unfortunately, these diseases are marginally treatable and never cured. Each time he goes through the loop the disease worsens, the mind sickens, and longer duration treatment with more medicine and higher doses will be required (as practiced in allopathic psychiatry).

- If he does not develop Schizophrenia or Mania, then he might become depressed again later in life.

This more complex case (I-3-e) is a good example of a real-life case. Also, in these types of cases, the patient may have seen one psychiatrist for episode (1) and then a new psychiatrist for episode (2). He may possibly end up seeing a third psychiatrist for episode (3). The third psychiatrist needs to reconstruct all this past history of the first two episodes. Background information from a manic or psychotic patient can be very scant or erratic. Background information from family is invaluable in reconstructing the past psychiatric history. Yes, real-life patients may have seen three separate psychiatrists. The first psychiatrist was seen while the child/teenager was on his parents' insurance. The second psychiatrist may have been consulted in a different city when the patient was in college. The third psychiatrist might have been seen after the patient began his first full-time job while on yet another insurance plan.

1-The first pass is written in normal font effect—he becomes depressed as a teenager

2-*The second pass is expressed in italics—he abuses drugs that make him depressed again and now he has a drug problem also.*

3-**The third pass is typed in bold font—he develops a severe and persistent psychiatric disorder** (possibly due to having stressed his brain with the first two passes; or the first two passes might have been the warning symptoms of the severe disorder to come, or the onset of severe disease was not related in anyway to the depression and drug abuse).

1—first depression (as child) 2—*second depression (as teen)* **3—third depression (as man)**

3	2	1	child	State of Good Health	Cure ↤	↰
↰	↱	↱	↵	↕ ↕		
				- - - - - Remission - - - - -		
3	2	1		- - - - - - (free of symptoms of Depression) - - - - - - Relief		↩ ↑

↳ (1) Stress factors lead to	Mild Depression →	Simple Treatment (1) ↲

			Result = two Depression Diagnoses	Complex Treatment	↑
↓	(2)				(2)
(3)	↓↳	↳ (2) drug abuse causes Drug Depression (DD) ↓ ↓	(i) Drug Depression	(i)Treatment of Drug Abuse	↲
	↓				
↓	(2) ↳	Drug Depression causes flare-up of Depression in Remission	(ii) Mild Depression	(ii) Treat Mild Depression	↲

↳ **Manic or**	New	**Treatment of**	(i)treat psychosis (ii)stop drug abuse	↲ 3 ↑
(3)Psychotic	**problems**	**NewProblems**	(iii)treat depression / mania	**No Cure**

Fig. 1-3-e Treatment is not Cure (complicated real-life case)

Sometimes psychiatric diseases are permanent. Despite being permanent, most of them are no longer disabling because we have a large selection of effective treatments available. In the past, anybody with a moderate or major psychiatric condition was automatically granted permanent disability. This need not be the norm any longer. The hope is that good treatment can rehabilitate a disorder so that is becomes a manageable chronic disorder. Patients need to adapt to this reality as do employers who often shy away from hiring individuals with these types of disabilities.

Parting Thoughts

The history of medicine is ancient. The various types of doctors have multiplied and branched off over time, giving these apparent contradictions:

1   Hippocrates is honored by allopaths, but he was actually a naturopath!
2   Hahenmann Medical College honors a homeopath, and yet the school trains allopaths!
3   "Modern" doctors originally practiced naturopathy but now look down on it.

Treatment goals in all branches of medicine are the same:
To relieve pain and suffering. The focus of treatment may vary.

---

* In using the term "Old Europe", I am referring to the anthropological tenets of Maria Gimbutas

Chapter I-4

Introduction to Medicine in General
and
a Very Brief History of Psychiatry

Modern psychiatry factually originated as a branch of neurology. The great early psychiatrists had been trained as neurologists. Neurological sciences were given a great deal of attention in the eighteenth and nineteenth centuries especially in Germany and France, two countries that seemed to have an unending rivalry in the sciences. Freud began to promulgate his new psychoanalytic theories based on and inspired by neurology. Do remember that neurology then was a lot less scientific than it is now. There were no exotic lab tests, no CATScan, etc. Even neurological underpinnings of our behaviors had not yet acquired the scientific veneer that is taken for granted today: neurological diagnosis—like medical diagnosis—relied more on intuition, clinical history, the doctor's experience, and physical examination.

Physical diagnosis (known also as Medical Semeiology) comprises the art of making medical diagnoses based solely on the clinical **signs** and **symptoms** without using high-tech testing Psychiatry can also employ similar means of diagnosis. The art of Physical diagnosis can be enhanced if the doctor can hear the HOPI "History of Present Illness". **HOPI** is an account of how the patient got sick, what he was doing before he got sick, how long he has been sick. If this sickness has happened before, then that is called **PMHx** (Past Medical History) which is also helpful. If other blood-relatives have had this same disease, then that too is helpful: this is called **FMHx** (Family Medical History). Additionally, these histories need not include any information obtained from high-tech testing methods. This is the art of practicing Medicine. Medicine has been practiced this way since prehistory and up until the present time when we have so much technology. This technology has added scientific input to the practice of medicine. Nowadays, medicine is still an art, but has also definitely become a science.

So, these are useful for making a diagnosis in medicine or psychiatry:
Physical Diagnosis
- **Symptoms**......(internal feelings and thoughts)
- **Signs**............(visible marks)
- **HOPI**
- **PMHx**
- **FMHx**

Most people have a general idea of what a symptom is, but may not be aware of the simple compartmentalization that doctors make in order to differentiate **signs** (visible bodily markers or defects) and **symptoms** (internal feelings).

A **sign** is some disease indicator that can be appreciated objectively: the doctor can see a sign, feel it, hear it, smell it, or taste it (yes, it seems disgusting, but doctors in olden times diagnosed sugar diabetes by tasting sweetness in the urine). Here are some signs in psychiatry: blood-shot eyes ("road-map sclerae" from marijuana), sweating (alcohol withdrawal), hoarseness (mania), "eye-darting" (auditory hallucinations), avoiding eye contact (hiding information), sweaty palms (anxiety disorders), dilated pupils (stimulant drugs), heavy eyelids (sedative-narcotic addiction), strange posturing (catatonia), limping (manic overexertion or aftermath of an antisocial escapade), healed wrist scars (probable bipolar-borderline), and many others.

Symptoms are based solely on information provided by the patient. That which the patient feels inside is a **symptom**; it is usually expressed, described, and related by the patient. In psychiatry these symptoms are feelings, ideas, thoughts, obsessions, and hallucinations. Even though these symptoms are apparently invisible, people might be able to see the patient physically reacting to the symptoms such as talking to voices. Such symptoms could include sadness, anxiety, fear, fixed false beliefs, or hearing voices. If psychiatric patients physically react to these kinds of symptoms, then those reactions can also be signs: if the patient is unmotivated, hyperactive, intrusive, threatening, reclusive, or trembling. He might be arguing with an invisible person or performing bizarre rituals. He might be setting fires or sharpening knives while muttering angrily under his breath. He may have lost a lot of weight. I call these "realized symptoms", symptoms that have been made real as signs.

Since ancient times, medical diagnoses have been made this way and have been based mainly on two main sources of information (and psychiatry uses its own version of this system):

1-- *History:* the disease's history and how the patient got sick [which we nowadays call "history of present illness", HOPI]. This is information gleaned from the patient himself and from family members, and is the story of when he got sick, how long it has lasted, and so on; if the patient is really ill, he may not be able to give a very good history;

2-- *Physical Diagnosis:* consists of noting the patient's disease markers which we call "**signs and symptoms**";

a)-"**signs** are physical characteristics detectable by the doctor such as agitation, vegetative behavior (apathy, loss of motivation), eye darting (eyes darting around the room), trembling, drooling, emaciation (obvious weight loss), hostility, downcast gaze, stooped shoulder, refusal to move or communicate, talking to invisible people, etc. Signs can be defined by how they are sensed by the doctor:

i)-signs which are heard (gasping, hoarseness, rapid speech);

ii)-signs which are seen (wrist scars, rashes, pupils, trembling, etc.);

iii)-signs that are felt (unusual in psychiatry: in medicine feeling a tumor);

iv)-signs which are tapped out or percussed (not in psychiatry; in medicine this could be a bloated stomach);

v)-signs which are smelled (acetone breath, alcohol breath, extreme body odor, etc.); and,

vi)-signs which are tasted (not in psychiatry; it is unpleasant, but yes medical doctors in olden times tasted urine for sweetness to diagnose sugar diabetes).

Psychiatrists have little need to touch patients directly; I only do this if checking pulse-blood pressure or doing quick "neuro checks".

b)-"**symptoms**" are experienced by the patient himself: sadness, anger, insomnia, euphoria, fear, hunger, etc.

Table I-4-a

If there is no one available to recite the HOPI (History of Present Illness), then the physician must rely solely on Physical Diagnosis. If there is no history and the patient is unable to give a list of symptoms, then the doctor would have to base the initial diagnosis on signs alone. In some cases where the patient is very impaired mentally, the patient's interpretation of the HOPI can be so skewed as to be more misleading than helpful; in general, if the doctor listens to the patient long enough, then the patient will eventually tell the physician what the diagnosis is. Since prehistory, Medicine has sometimes been practiced by relying upon semeiology alone without access to any meaningful clinical history—as it still is in very poor nations where modern testing may not be available or affordable.

Psychiatry—as a branch of medicine—relies mainly on this ancient technique of listening to the patient's story (as related by the patient and/or his accompanying family members); to a lesser degree psychiatry still relies on signs, too.

This may sound trivial to you, but signs and symptoms are very important in the practice of medicine: sometimes signs and symptoms may be all the information available if the patient is mentally impaired. The combination of signs and symptoms can guide the doctor in making a probable diagnosis.

One of the main reasons that Psychiatry is looked down upon by the modern High-Tech Bio-Medial practitioners is our lack of sophisticated laboratory tests and expensive diagnostic machinery. Hence—in a sense—the rest of medical practitioners reject their own history by the act of belittling the process of psychiatric care.

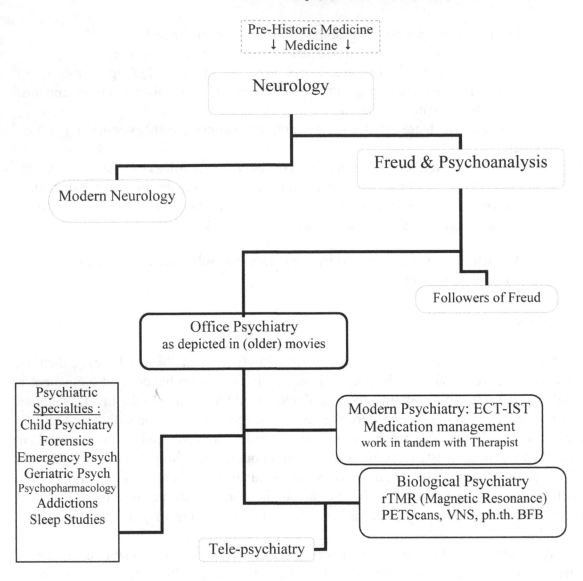

I-4-b   Flowchart of the Evolution of Psychiatry

VNS=vagal nerve stimulation (using an implanted electrical "pacemaker")
rTMR=Transcraneal magnetic resonance treatment (stimulating the brain with powerful magnetic fields)
ph.th=phototherapy with bright lights
BFB=biofeedback
ECT and IST are Electro-Shock Treatments and Insulin Shock Therapy:

Beginning at the top of the flowchart, primitive medicine evolves into modern medicine and then into Neurology. In the nineteenth century, Freud started psychoanalysis. In the twentieth century, psychoanalysis evolved into "Office Psychiatry" which is how it is depicted in older (and some newer) movies when patients spend an hour receiving psychotherapy from the psychiatrist on a weekly basis. In the twenty-first century, psychiatry is going to biological psychiatry, due in large part to learning about the biochemical underpinnings of psychiatry (BFB, ECT, IST VNS, TMR, et al). Tele-psychiatry may be the next step: patients can have appointments in their own homes; they can put their wrists into a device that can measure blood levels of medications; the psychiatrist can tell the patient if a dosage adjustment is necessary and the change of dosage can be faxed to the pharmacy. The machine may measure vital signs and physical signs of drug side effects (tremors).

So psychiatry had its origins in nineteenth century European neurology, which was a branch of general medicine at a time when both neurology and general medicine still relied a lot on Physical Diagnosis and not on high technology machines. Psychoanalysis was the beginning of Psychiatry. Psychoanalysis does not typically rely on the traditional tools of physical diagnosis, symptomatology, and history of present illness—or relies upon these in a very abstract way. Psychoanalysis attempts to find out what is going on inside that particular patient's mind that causes him to react in such a way or to think in such a way. Psychoanalysis reveals how the patient has suppressed past emotions and memories; it also relies on dream interpretation that would qualify as subjective information provided by the patient, hence, dreams are a kind of symptom.

In the meantime, the mainstream medical disciplines acquired new technologies that came into use. This new modernized medicine served to separate psychoanalysis further from general medicine. By the 1950s and 1960's, modern medicine had made many advances, but psychoanalysis remained an esoteric discipline with questionable reproducibility regarding treatment strategies; analysis was also very expensive and time-consuming (three days per week for an hour or more each day). Psychoanalysis typically required between three and seven years of treatment. It was expensive due to office visit charges and the cost of training an analyst, which can take up to nine years or more. It is not usually covered by health insurance. The world of modern medicine had meanwhile moved forward and was dancing to a faster tempo. Psychiatry needed to popularize itself and help millions—not just thousands—of patients. The world seemed to be craving a kind of "Psychiatry à-go-go". Psychiatry needed to reinvent itself for the late twentieth century and to give faster results for millions of patients. But how to do this? Psychoanalysis cannot be accelerated by one or two orders of magnitude.

The window of opportunity opened with the discovery of Thorazine by the French [Navy].[1] This was followed soon by the creation of Imipramine, Elavil, and other similar "tricyclic" antidepressants (the chemical structure has three carbon rings). This opened the gates to a new flood of psychiatric drugs, which then, of course, had to be studied in order to see exactly how they helped depression and schizophrenia. These studies were important so that we could learn to understand a drug's possible toxicities and also—back to the bottom line!—to have the chance to create new improved drugs by starting with a known drug and modifying it slightly to enhance other desirable therapeutic effects or to make it less toxic.

Since that time a few decades ago, Psychiatry has become biologically-oriented and "medicalized" and has started to re-align itself with General Medicine and Neurology—in a sense coming back into the huddle—up to the point of adopting and even using a number of "neurological medicines" as psychiatric treatments. At this current rate, Psychiatry will [again] become "neurologized" and the pendulum will have swung back—at least for a while. Psychiatry is now embracing new electronic treatment devices such as rTMR (repetitive transcraneal magnetic resonance) and VNS (left Vagus Nerve Stimulator). rTMR offers new treatment options as an advance over shock treatments. VNS offers long-term treatment of psychiatric symptoms by using an implanted battery-driven device similar in fabrication to that of a cardiac pacemaker. As a result of these new electronic devices and techniques, Psychiatry may be on the path to mainstreaming itself again and coming into alignment with modern medical and neurological practices.

The modern psychiatrist in the usual urban practice is involved with psychiatric urgencies and emergencies and with the bio-pharmacologic side of patient care. This includes prescribing medications, ordering appropriate lab tests, and interfacing with the primary care doctors and/or neurologists.

Patients may be chronologically classified by notating their decade of life. Also, we can refer to diseases and classify them by "a disease that often starts in such-and-such decade of life".

Decades of Life (general age classifier) are:

Decade Of Life	Corresponds to ages	Age-Typical Psychiatric Disorder (Adjustment Disorders, Anxiety at any age)	Unlikely Age of Onset Of such a Disorder*
I	0-9 years old	Autism, Attention Deficit	Alzheimer's
II	10-19 years old	Anorexia, Drug Abuse, Dysthymia	Jealous Delusions
III	20-29 years old	Schizophrenia, Bipolar, Panic-Anxiety, PTSD, Drugs, Stress	
IV	30-39	Depression, Bipolar, Panic-Anxiety	Tourette's
V	40-49	Alcoholism, Stress Disorders	Attention Deficit
VI	50-59	Paranoia, Prescription pill addiction	Anorexia
VII	60-69	Depression↔Bereavement, Memory problems,	Schizophrenia, Mania, "Multiple Personality"
VIII	70-79	Alzheimer's, Delusions, Depression	Personality Disorder

Table I-4-c Decades of Life   (*but there may be very rare cases of such*)

These decades are often used in describing the age at which an illness begins: in other words, we could say that Schizophrenia usually begins in the third decade of life for females and slightly earlier for males. This is another general way of thinking about psychiatric diagnosis. For example, a diagnosis of schizophrenia with onset in the sixth-seventh decades of life is unlikely. Any such schizophrenia-like symptoms should prompt a medical search for other diseases that are commoner at that age and that might have early symptoms similar to those of schizophrenia (like "glandular" disorders, brain tumors, alcoholism, etc.).

General medicine forms a backbone for the practice of modern "biological" psychiatry. Some psychotropic medicines are useful in general medicine and some general medical medications are useful in psychiatry. I prescribe general medical medications only if I am using these medications to correct some side effect occasioned by the psychoactive medications that I am prescribing and hence for which I am primarily responsible, too.

If the current trends in biological psychiatry continue, then most psychiatrists in the future will be even more involved with biological, pharmacological, genetic, and biochemical aspects of behavioral disturbances and will likely leave the "talk therapy" to those who already do most of it and do it quite well.

1--ref. 1, p.400

Chapter I-5

Introduction to Psychiatric Practice

This chapter serves as a guide for persons without a medical background who are seeking psychiatric treatment for themselves or for their loved ones. Psychiatry is a new branch of Medicine, having started less than a century and a half ago. In such a short time, the practice has gone from "soft" neurology (treatment of hysteria) to abstract treatment philosophy and dream interpretation (Freud and psychoanalysis) to once-weekly one-hour therapy sessions (as shown in movies) to modern biological psychiatry (pills and lab tests). That is much more change than the rest of Medicine has experienced throughout its last three thousand years.

People who watch movies—especially old black and white movies—might be surprised on their first visit to a psychiatrist. They might expect to see a couch and might expect a one-hour session, neither of which is likely if seeing a psychiatrist in the HMO system. There are still a few psychiatrists who practice in this manner, but they may also be in private practice and charge higher rates for this enhanced service. A patient can usually get what he needs today by going through the usual and customary modern practice style. If he is still not satisfied, then he could discuss this with his HMO or mental health professional. Apart from that, this chapter points out how to begin seeking treatment.

Getting Started:

- Professional Designations: who we are, what we do
- Finding a mental health professional
- Initial visit
- Doctor-Patient (contractual) relationship
- Ongoing therapy sessions
- Termination of Therapy

- *Professional designations:* You will need to know who we are and what our licenses allow us to do. This might help you in determining which professional you need to see. For relationship problems, see a therapist or psychologist. For medications, see a psychiatrist. For specialized services, see the list below.

- The two commonest ways to *find a professional* are by word of mouth or by referral from the patient's health insurance plan. Occasionally patients may see ads in a publication or may choose somebody who is geographically close or has evening hours, etc. The next step is to call the office and make an appointment. Prospective patients are allowed to ask about fee structures over the telephone—or to ask about anything they wish—before coming in for the initial evaluation. Remember that you are technically a potential "consumer" of psychiatric services. (Psychiatrists hate to have their patients referred to as "consumers", but some of the non-medical personnel do use this terminology.) as such, you are allowed to ask consumer type questions.

- Then comes the *initial visit* with the mental health professional at which time the patient/client can reach a preliminary opinion as to whether she wants to come back for a second appointment. If definitely no, then the patient might leave by stating that she needs to look at her schedule and then will call back to make her next appointment. If maybe, the patient may make the appointment then but call back later to cancel it. If definitely yes, then the patient will probably make the next appointment at the end of the first appointment.

- *Doctor-patient relationship* is essentially a legal contract whereby the doctor agrees to give the patient "usual and customary" treatment and whereby the patient agrees to pay the doctor for his services. This contractual relationship begins when the doctor has initial contact with the patient—typically in person. (see also Chapter VII-1) Interpersonal reactions will occur between the patient and the treatment provider. The real reactions are the obvious and socially appropriate reactions. There is also a set of not so obvious reactions called transference and counter-transference. Transference is a term that refers to the patient's reaction to the doctor (or therapist) for some [subconscious] reason. Transference can be a positive comfort level or a negative sense of discomfort. Counter-transference takes place if the therapist (or doctor) feels uncomfortable about the client. Therapists have been trained to deal with counter-transference and may or may not elect to continue seeing the patient. Oftentimes the counter-transference is quite brief and may dissipate once the therapist can focus on the work at hand. Patients are allowed to try different therapists—this is like shopping for a new car. If the patient does not want to continue with that therapist, then there is little reason that she should be forced to do so. Of course, this would be an excellent opportunity for the patient to investigate the source of these transference issues and maybe get rid of them once and for all. However, most clients who are paying good money do not want to be challenged in this way.

- *Ongoing treatment:* If the patient/client feels comfortable with the therapist, then therapy will begin and continue until a future time when there will be a mutual decision to phase out therapy or decrease the frequency of visits.

- *Termination:* Therapy finally comes to an end as per mutual agreement. This is the time for the client to try to "leave the nest and fly on her own". She is always welcome to come back and continue therapy if too many unresolved issues are weighing her down.

Professional Designations: what we do and who does it

Psychiatrists

M.D. and D.O. psychiatrists usually refer to people in treatment with them as "patients"; The other professions listed below usually refer to their cases as "clients".

A psychiatrist is an M.D. or D.O. who specializes in psychiatric medicine and as such the psychiatrist holds an unrestricted (hopefully) State license to practice medicine and surgery. The medical aspects of psychiatric treatment include prescribing medications in the form of pills, liquids, skin patches and giving injections. Psychiatrists also order lab tests (blood tests), request CATScan and MRI of the head, and ask the primary doctor to do heart wave testing (EKG). Psychiatrists will interface with the family doctor at times—with the patient's permission. The psychiatric aspect of treatment includes interviews and short talk therapy sessions (unless the psychiatrist will also be doing one-hour therapy sessions). The surgical aspects of psychiatric practice are limited to shock treatments and transcraneal magnetic resonance; both of these treatments send waves across the skull and into the brain and are classified as invasive procedures, hence classified as surgery, and thus carry an extra malpractice insurance burden. In a given community there will usually be one psychiatrist who carries the extra malpractice insurance needed for shock treatment, and he receives referrals from the rest of the nearby psychiatrists and becomes the treatment source for shock treatments. Shock treatment is so uncommon nowadays that it would occupy only a small part of the daily practice of even this one specialist psychiatrist. Much of modern day practice involves prescribing medications: psychiatrists prescribe medicine—sometimes too much, perhaps! Thus, psychiatrists are concerned directly with the practice of Medicine because they do the following:

a.) prescribe drugs/chemicals/salts/herbs;

b.) order blood tests and other medically relevant tests (such as CATScan or MRI of he head) and request EKG (electrical testing of the heart); and,

c.) interface with other doctors—mainly your primary physician.

The average psychiatrist has usually received a minimum of twelve years of education:

4 years of college
4 years of medical school
<u>4 years of residency</u>
12 years minimum

Psychologists

Psychologists hold Ph.D. degrees or Psy.D. degrees. A professional with the Psy.D. degree (Doctor of Psychology) is a *clinical psychologist* who will typically see clients for one hour a week for talk therapy. A professional with a Ph.D. degree in psychology who is in private practice will typically offer the same service as the Psy.D., in other words, clinical psychology services, seeing clients for one hour a week. However, the Ph.D. has also been trained to teach psychology, do research, and administer psychological testing. Psychological testing is an extremely valuable service for clinical practice. Psychiatrists who would like a battery of psychological tests will typically send their patients to a psychologist for testing since psychiatrists are not trained to administer these types of tests. Readers who are interested in finding a psychologist for talk therapy can start with a clinical psychologist with either degree, PhD or PsyD.

Some psychologists are specialized and limit themselves to special patient groups. Examples would be neuro-psychologists (they assist neurologists in assessing extent of brain damage), child psychologists, or forensic psychologists (working in the criminal justice system).

PhD clinical psychologists are not [yet] permitted to prescribe medicines in most jurisdictions.

Other professionals with allied doctorates may also do counseling: Ed.D. (Doctorate of Education) and licensed educational psychologists.

Therapists hold degrees which permit them to do "talk therapy"

(Some of them may have secondary degrees such as in Art Therapy). Therapists—also known as psychotherapists—are numerous and usually do not hold any doctorate degrees; thus their office visits might cost less.

Psychoanalysts are MD doctors who have received the classical Freudian training and analyze a patient's behaviors in great detail. They are keenly interested in your transference issues. Chances are good that you will never see or even meet an analyst as there are comparatively few of them in the USA. They provide a highly specialized treatment which is not covered by insurance and is very costly usually requiring the patient to come in at least twice a week. Furthermore, this treatment can continue for up to seven years.

Counselors for drug and alcohol abuse also hold State certification.

Psychiatric Specialties

Just like surgeons or internal medicine doctors, psychiatrists also have job specialization in regard to certain patient populations:

- *general psychiatrists* see patients of all ages and prescribe in a general way in the sense that your family doctor does also. The general psychiatrist sees everybody, but refers the more difficult cases to a psychiatric specialist.
- *Emergency psychiatrists* work in emergency rooms in large hospitals and are involved with urgent and "emergent" psychiatric disorders. They may also be on 24-hour call to hospitals and locked nursing homes where patients may have severe mood disorders (mania and depression) and severe thought disorders (psychosis and schizophrenia).
- *Child/adolescent psychiatry* specializes in children and teenagers. Some children can have serious disabilities. Autism and related disorders are among these serious disabilities. Problems specific to teenagers include depression, drug abuse, and early onset of serious adult psychiatric conditions. Child psychiatrists may be treating both children and teenagers for ADHD.
- *Geriatric psychiatry* specializes in the treatment of late-life psychiatric problems, dementia commonly. Since dementia eventually affects the whole brain, other secondary psychiatric problems can co-occur with dementia, such as depression and psychosis.
- *Psychopharmacology* is the art of prescribing, complicated drug regimens to patients who have very complicated medication schedules or severe psychiatric conditions;
- *Consultation-liaison psychiatry ("C-L" psychiatry)*: This involves hospital work on general medical and surgical wards. These psychiatrists work in large general hospitals where they address the urgent needs of medical or surgical patients who are temporarily hospitalized. C·L psychiatrists see these basic types of patients: (a) people who are already in treatment for a pre-existing psychiatric condition and need to have their psychoactive medications managed or coordinated with the medical and surgical medications while hospitalized; (b) medical and surgical patients who develop psychological problems while in the hospital; and, (c) people who had recovered from a previous psychiatric condition before the hospital stay but have now been in the hospital so long that the psychiatric problem is starting up again due to a prolonged and stressful hospitalization. The C·L psychiatrist needs to be

very knowledgeable about internal medicine and its treatments as well as all the medical and psychiatric medications available.

- *Addiction psychiatry* focuses on treatment of alcoholism and drug addiction.
- *Forensic psychiatry* evaluates people in the criminal justice system. The main types of patients are: (a) ordinary criminals who try to "beat the rap" by pretending to act "insane"; (b) inmates who have already had long-standing psychiatric problems before incarceration and who need to have their medications adjusted while they are in jail, no matter how or why they ended up in jail—the fact that they had quit taking their medicines and had become really psychotic is another issue; and, (c) people who have "suddenly snapped" and now really are criminally insane—these are the ones who have committed highly publicized heinous crimes that attract the attention of the news media. Forensic psychiatrists may take on product liability cases where the plaintiff alleges mental suffering (for example, a woman who is suing the company that sells a shampoo that allegedly left her permanently bald)— these are private forensic patients.
- *Sleep lab*: some sleep laboratories are staffed by psychiatrists, but neurologists and pulmonary specialists usually run sleep labs nowadays.

Subspecialty training as outlined above typically requires an extra two years minimum of training beyond the four years of general psychiatric residency.

Finding a Mental Health Professional

When some people feel so bad as to seek out professional help, they are usually in an emotionally compromised state already and have diminished decision-making capacity. A person may feel that he has reached such a low bottom in his life, that life has little meaning or importance. Friends or family may urge him to seek treatment. Sometimes, employers insist upon it. Despite feeling this way, you will need to make a decision about finding and then choosing some one to help you.

Slamming the Doors and Kicking the Tires

Choosing any mental health professional should be approached as if buying a car (this would not apply to patients who are doing one-time psychological testing or going for second opinions).

It is perfectly legitimate to announce at the first session that you are in the process of seeking a provider. Pick someone with whom you feel comfortable and with whom you feel able to communicate when articulating your feelings. Also important is choosing someone who is appropriate to your circumstances with whom you can work on a long-term basis. Find a provider with whom you feel engaged. Treatment should be whatever you need.

In some cases, you might be stuck with your assigned provider and will not have many options to change. This might happen if your employer has forced you into therapy ("see some one or we will terminate you"). Or if you have an HMO plan. Some mental health professionals—mainly, HMO providers—insist that you should continue seeing a provider with whom you do not click since this is supposed to be a controlled example of why you do not get along well with most people in the real world. This insistence is often linked to the restrictive mechanics of an HMO, as well as to the difficulty and expense that the HMO might incur if it had to refer its patients "out of network".

Some of these HMO providers may be nurturing, confrontational, or middle of the road ("objective"). Sometimes confrontation can be too intimidating for emotionally fragile patients who are in early recovery or who still have low self-esteem. If you are seeing a therapist and doctor for combined services, the doctor may be providing only prescriptions, so that his attitude may be less important than that of the therapist. However, confrontational medication psychiatrists may allow their clinical style to affect rescribing practices: they may refuse to prescribe very limited amounts of medicine or may refuse to give you medicine you want or seem to need. They may also be stubborn about changing medications—this may have a medical rationale. A first-time patient should probably try to find providers who seem caring and nurturing, and then if this treatment seems too soft or too slow, that can be discussed.

Choosing a Psychiatrist (MD/DO)

Freud and his followers set up a precedent a century ago of seeing patients for hourly sessions, perhaps at least twice a week. At that time the training period was for many years and all psychiatrists were psychoanalysts—there were no modern psychiatrists as we know them now. As time went on, universities started to train "office" psychiatrists in three or four year training programs. If they wanted to become psychoanalysts, then they had to do the extra years. This new cadre of "office psychiatrists" gave birth to the modern system and its "avant-garde" treatments consisted of seeing patients less frequently, for forty or fifty minutes on a weekly, biweekly, or even monthly basis (which would never work for traditional psychoanalysis). In the meantime, psychoanalysts have become living dinosaurs. Thus, "office psychiatrists" had become the new "traditional" psychiatrists by the middle part of the twentieth century. This practice style works well in movies so that is mainly where you will see it nowadays. These doctors are in private practice and charge very high fees, usually having offices in affluent neighborhoods. Some of these doctors may offer "medication management" for patients who do not need ongoing talk therapy or hourly sessions on a weekly basis. These medication-only patients may come in for half an hour once every two to six weeks (monthly is average). These are private practices, and they do not do business with any HMO. In some cases, the psychiatrist accepts fee-for-service only and does not do insurance billing. The patient will pay the psychiatrist with cash or a credit card and if the patient has health insurance, then it is up to the patient to try to obtain direct reimbursement from her health insurance company. If you can afford these psychiatrists, then you are quite lucky.

Some elderly psychiatrists who do accept modern HMO referrals, may still retain a traditional practice style that harks back to a time when the psychiatrist provided both therapy and medication management. These doctors may still be seeing patients for one-hour sessions weekly, biweekly, or monthly. This type of practice is no longer so common in the fast-paced world of modern biological psychiatry (and managed care). This one-hour session is sometimes still depicted in movies, but is no longer typical or representative of modern practice. In such a movie depiction, it is likely that the movie plot flows better with this (contrived) scenario. Elderly psychiatrists continue to do this because it is rational medical practice and is their habit, but do so at their own financial disadvantage. They may be on the road to extinction.

Most modern psychiatrists will spend forty to sixty minutes on the initial visit. However, follow-up appointments will be shorter, in the range of fifteen to thirty minutes (average of about twenty minutes) during which time the focus of the visit will be on medication dosages, side-effects, lab tests, and the medical aspects of your treatment. If you need therapy sessions, then you will likely obtain a referral to see a professional who specializes in talk therapy, probably a psychologist or therapist. It is usual and customary practice for psychiatrists to work closely with therapists and vice versa. These relationships allow a patient to receive "medical management" while simultaneously receiving psychological management. In a sense, that patient is already receiving individualized care from two specialists.

In our office practice, the first visit is with the therapist who opens the chart and does an extensive all-inclusive interview gleaning a great deal of background information on the patient—this is when the therapist would typically instruct the patient about our split system of therapy sessions and medication visits. The initial session with the therapist centers around gleaning important information concerning: the patient's past history; past issues, whether they might be resolved or still unresolved; and, other possible therapy issues. This is done so that the patient's needs can be assessed, and if it seems that therapy is indicated, then the patient will be scheduled for a second session with the therapist.

My first visit is usually forty-five to ninety minutes, depending upon complexity of the case (past history, diagnosis, and treatment). I prefer to handle the medical aspects of the treatment while having the patient see a therapist for psychotherapy sessions. This seems to work out well because the patient may need specialized therapy as well as specialized psychiatric treatment. Some patients still come to my second visit expecting a long drawn out session of forty-five to ninety minutes. They sometimes are surprised to find that there is no therapy part to the session; however, there had not been a therapy session during the initial "medicalized" intake. Some of these patients do not wish to pay twice for what they consider to be one service: they do not see medical management as a separate treatment from talk therapy. Some of them try to circumvent this system by trying to squeeze in a talk therapy session with me during their regularly scheduled medication management appointment and then may cancel the real therapy appointment. Many patients come in merely for the doctor visit in order to receive prescription medicine. They do not plan on having long follow-up visits. Nevertheless, there will still be a few patients who assume that their second session with me will be a one-hour therapy session. This usually occurs in either of two cases: if they have not "clicked" with their intake therapist or if they truly are in need of therapy from any and all sources available. The appropriate response is to have them discuss their therapy needs with the intake therapist or to choose a different therapist.

Nowadays most insured Americans will be directed by their HMO to see a psychiatrist who has an agreement with that HMO. The nature of these visits can be variable. In some cases, they may have very brief medication-oriented visits (ten to fifteen minutes) on an infrequent basis (every few weeks).

I often tell my patients that in about half the cases it is not unrealistic to expect an 80-85% overall improvement—provided that they follow the treatment plan! Some patients just want pills and have no desire to follow a comprehensive treatment plan—except for their own treatment plan, apparently. The treatment plan might also involve attending spiritual groups or organized gatherings, especially Alanon, Overeaters Anonymous, Emotions Anonymous, etc. Many patients are loath to attend any Twelve Step program or any appropriate support groups. This usually compromises the quality of recovery. This automatically nixes the optimistic estimate of 85% overall improvement. They may end up with only a partial recovery and feel surprised that they do not feel better. If an alcoholic husband stresses a patient so much that she ends up in therapy, then dealing with that primary problem should be a good starting point. This would require attendance at Alanon, a self-help program for spouses of alcoholics. I cannot make wives better with pills alone if they need collateral treatments. She needs to address the primary problem (how her husband's drinking affects her). It is curious that people seek advice from a specialist and then refuse to avail themselves of that advice.

We can only lead a horse to water—we cannot make it drink.

Choosing a psychiatrist is almost as important as choosing an effective therapist or psychologist for talk therapy. Most general psychiatrists would be able to give you reasonable pharmacologic treatment. If your general psychiatrist feels that you need specialized care, your general psychiatrist might refer you to a specialty psychiatrist.

Choosing a Therapist or Psychologist

I have included these together since they both involve talk therapy. I would choose a psychologist for more severe situations, especially those that might require interfacing with the legal system where a doctorate would carry more weight. Psychologists are also uniquely qualified to administer specialized psychological testing. Therapists are an excellent choice for interpersonal relationship problems.

Choosing a therapist for "talk therapy" is perhaps an even more exacting choice for some people because they may need or want a specific kind of therapy. Furthermore, there are many types of therapy and of therapists available nowadays. Patients should avail themselves of this cornucopia of choices in order to find a therapy tailored to their needs. There are a few reasons for making a comfortable choice. Firstly, the patient should find a personality with whom he can work. Another important reason is that therapy can be long-term and costly so each session needs to be as productive as possible so that the patient can feel that he is making reasonable progress in therapy. Patients should not feel that they are just being tossed into a whirlpool of endless open-ended therapy sessions (unless he implies a need for this kind of supportive therapy).

In the case of therapists, especially, some may seem nurturing, supportive, and maternalistic, whereas some may seem more confrontational. Supportive and nurturing professionals provide a sense of stability to patients who feel extremely fragile and vulnerable. This supportive type of therapy tends to go very slowly—for years, perhaps. Confrontational therapists will force you to face up to any of your contribution to the current crisis in your life. Confrontational therapists will strive to get you well sooner and will try to prod you into making detectable progress month by month. If you sense a positive rapport with a confrontational therapist, you might want to keep her for a while. If she annoys you too much, then you should probably go shop for another "new car". You will need to decide how much of a balance you want between nurturing and confrontation. In general, therapists in private practice are more nurturing, and those in HMO practice are more confrontational. (The HMO wants its patients to get better faster.)

Some of the HMO therapists may ascribe to some notion like that of Twelve-Step programs: namely, that "that which does not kill us, makes us stronger". If you do not want to have "strengthening" sessions, then you should discuss this with the therapist. In opposite cases, if a nurturing therapist might need to pick up the pace and be more direct with you, then you could discuss this with her. Or you could attend some sort of therapy group. Therapy groups are notorious for giving out a lot of collective "strengthening" feedback. However, this confrontation can be too intimidating for emotionally fragile patients who are in early recovery or who still have low self-esteem. A first-time patient should probably find a provider who seems caring and nurturing, and then if this treatment seems to be moving too slowly, this situation can be discussed with that therapist regarding any need for more confrontation.

Therapy should have a stated purpose (which issues to work out), a process and procedure, a goal, and a definable end-point at which the patient could be released onto his own recognizance. Truly some people with horrific multiple therapy issues and long history of abuses may need to feel consoled and supported in therapy for a number of years. Most patients do not require therapy of this duration or intensity. It is important that the patient and therapist try to formulate a reasonable treatment plan on the first or second session so that the patient might have a sense of how he is progressing in therapy and what his goals of success might be.

Initial Visits

Getting started may be a little scary, but it need not be. Think of it as the beginning of a new and unique relationship.

After finding a mental health professional, you are now ready for the first appointment. This visit need not be frightening or anxiety-provoking. In a very large group practice, there will be many forms to fill out and sign. Typically, you will be asked about medical history, family history, personal psychiatric problems, allergies, and so on. The receptionist will give a brief explanation to any issue that you might have. In a small private practice, there might not be very much paperwork.

Fee Schedules

A lot of patients are shocked to find out how much a visit to one of these mental health professionals might cost (in the case that the patient has no insurance coverage). Our main expenses are office overhead and malpractice insurance (although psychiatrists do have some of the lowest malpractice rates and relatively low incidence of malpractice cases, too). In keeping with the fact that therapists do not [usually] hold doctorates they will usually charge somewhat less than the professionals with doctorates (psychologists and psychiatrists). I believe that our fees are not that different from those charged by lawyers or CPA's. The only doctors who might make slightly less salary than psychiatrists are the pediatricians and some family practice doctors. Some people are horrified that we charge (so much) "just for talking to people"; however, many studies have shown that patients who have a good therapy session can feel as good for the rest of the day as if they had taken a pill. To those people averse to pill-taking this might be a possible treatment tack.

Medication Management

In some cases, research has shown that talk therapy can result in positive alterations in the brain hormones—just like taking a pill. The common wisdom is that patients can feel about 50% better using psychotherapy alone or about 50% better just taking pills; or, they can get at least 75% better using both therapy and pills. I believe that many patients can feel 85% better if receiving proper treatment and are willing to accept proper treatment—even those who have been deemed "treatment refractory" (practically incurable). I personally strive for this result at all times. The goal of 85% is possibly achievable. The exceptions to this 85% rule would include severe personality disorders and patients who might have two or three serious diagnoses ("dual diagnosis" or even "triple diagnosis")

Some patients just want to come for one visit and get a prescription "that works" and then have their family doctor dole out all the refills of the same medication. These patients are missing the point that seeing a specialist is always going to be more effective than doing it their way.

The doctor should have an unrestricted license to practice Medicine in that jurisdiction (this can be checked on-line at the State Medical Board website or on the National Practitioner Data Bank website). These websites might alert you to any unusual circumstances surrounding the doctor you are going to choose. This background check should certify that the doctor possesses the requisite amount of expertise in his stated specialty to practice medicine within the limits of "usual and customary practice" in that area. However, this status and licensure does not prevent the doctor from using less common treatments (used by "the respectable minority" of doctors) or unusual treatments (sometimes called "off-label" prescribing) as long as these would be acceptable treatments under those situations and with those kinds of patients as adjudged by a group of peers (other doctors in that area). Some patients look forward to a more "personalized" experience—and some do not. The new patient can clarify these wishes on the first visit. At any rate, the doctor should make a diagnosis and prescribe a treatment that is acceptable under normative medical practice.

Doctor-Patient Relationship

This is an implied-in-fact legal relationship.

The doctor-patient relationship is a contractual situation wherein the doctor performs the role of healer and is subject to certain legal and ethical requirements and restrictions. The patient for his part agrees to pay the doctor for professional services. This relationship is established when the patient makes contact with the doctor and asks for treatment. (A brief telephone conversation may or may not qualify.) If the doctor makes a diagnosis and prescribes treatment, then this contractual situation exists from that time forward, as it indicates his willingness to take on your case. If, however, upon first encounter, the doctor would tell the patient that he is not able to treat her, then there is no legal contract. (Examples are that a morbidly obese teenager goes to a geriatric psychiatrist to get diet pills, which is not really part of geriatric psychiatry; or a wife brings in the patient who clearly has an untreated Parkinsonism, whereupon they are referred to see a neurologist).

The patient, for his part of the contractual relationship, is supposed to take his treatment as prescribed; if he does not, then this is called medical non-compliance or medical non-adherence (not complying with or not adhering to the treatment plans). If this becomes a serious problem, then the patient's behavior must be discussed, as his non-adherence might be a symptom of his serious psychological problem(s). He may feel self-destructive, hopeless, or oppositional (to authority figures). It is unlikely that the patient will get better unless he follows doctor's orders. Psychiatrists—unlike most non-psychiatric doctors and surgeons—will continue to see non-adherent patients, but even psychiatrists will eventually state that the patient's non-adherence is undermining the treatment plan. Perhaps the patient is not willing to work on his recovery but would prefer to put it off until some future time. If the patient dislikes the treatment offered, then he is free to seek treatment elsewhere. He is not obligated to stay with any one doctor or therapist. In these cases of non-adherent patients, perhaps the patient should seek out a different doctor, therapy, or treatment facility. Find someone who can help him.

I have had cases like these. One young man was in the early stages of alcoholism. Every time that he drank, he felt depressed the next day. I told him to go to AA, which he adamantly refused to do. I also prescribed him various antidepressants which he would take for a couple days and then proclaim the pills to be treatment failures. Eventually, he was drinking every night and feeling depressed every day. He would not go to AA and would not stay on any one antidepressant. His motivation levels did not seem very high, and there was a question of whether he was coming to see a doctor because he wanted to do so or because someone else was mandating it. This question was partly clarified when his sister later called and rebuked me for not curing him. (Analysis: if alcohol causes unpleasant depression, then the first step is to quit drinking—if you cannot quit drinking on your own, then go to AA. Secondly, neither I nor anyone can make the alcoholic quit drinking—only he can do that to himself. Thirdly, it is not wise to medicate alcoholics with psychiatric medicines until they have been dry (or sober) for a few months, otherwise the psychiatrist will just end up reacting to all the early withdrawal symptoms for which there is no one specific treatment—except for tincture of time. Finally, the sister needs to be educated about alcoholism and consider attending Alanon herself—she may be quite co-dependent or controlling).

In another case, a young man with medication-controlled depression came in to see me every month for years. At each appointment, he complained about his alcoholic girlfriend who would not quit drinking. At each appointment I told him that he should go to Alanon—

but he never did! He preferred to pay me for an office visit (twenty or thirty dollars) instead of going for the specific Alanon treatment, which only costs one dollar!

I had a patient with serious anxiety who came in for anxiety treatment. She had previously been addicted to Valium, so could not take any addicting medications like that. I gave her an appropriate medication. On the second visit, she said that she did not fill the prescription for the anti-anxiety medication because the pharmacist had made some negative statement about the new medicine. I encouraged her to try the new non-addictive medicine. On the third visit, she brought the full pill bottle to the appointment. But she had not taken any of the pills because she was terrified by the package insert (PI see Chapter V-19). On the fourth visit, she stated that she was taking her husband's Xanax prescription (from a different doctor). Xanax is in the same family as Valium and is even more addicting than Valium!

When there is a contractual situation, the legal system will deal with doctors who commit a legal wrong. The illegal act could be forbidden by the federal government (Medicare fraud), State law, or local law. A doctor who is convicted of committing an illegal behavior might pay a fine (civil wrong), go to jail (criminal wrong), or receive probation. On the other hand, unethical behavior may not be illegal, but the State Medical Board has the right to sanction (punish) unethical behavior; examples: accepting a lavish or special gift from a wealthy patient might be unethical but not illegal; also, trading treatment sessions for haircuts from a barber patient; or, allowing himself to be named as executor in a patient's will (these have all happened). Rules, laws, and ethical guidelines are fairly uniform, but may vary slightly in different jurisdictions.

The doctor has a *duty* to maintain *confidentiality* and not talk about the patient's case to people outside the doctor-patient relationship—this includes strangers as well as spouses and family members. Unless the patient had legally given such permission. The rules of confidentiality are strict and intolerant of breaches. As in all contractual situations, the patient—as well as the doctor—also has obligations and privileges protected by ethics and laws.

Apart from a right to privacy, the patient has "privilege", a medico-legal term. Privilege means that the patient can control or restrict any information released by the doctor to third parties.

Sensitive information or extraneous information unrelated to the case can also be subjected to patient privilege at the patient's request. This information is never released unless the patient requests that the iformation be released—often in cases where the patient is involved in a lawsuit and information is exchanged between the attorneys. For example:

- a woman suing a realtor for construction defects that allegedly caused her emotional suffering can request that the doctor not release the information that she had had an abortion three years prior;

- a married man may ask to omit all details about his mistress; however, this might create so many gaps in his information as to render it weak. Nonetheless, the patient may need to release some of the privileged information if it forms the basis for a legal complaint (where the patient is plaintiff). Of course, privilege and confidentiality may take a backseat in two cases:

1—if the sensitive information is essential to understanding the case; and,

2—in forensic (criminal) cases there is no patient privilege, but it is still appropriate for the forensic psychiatrist to tell this fact to the patient before the interview begins.

Absence of Confidentiality

Any information supplied to a doctor, therapist, or group is confidential and cannot be discussed with any third party or outside party.

Exceptions would include: a patient who is actively homicidal or has confessed to murder.

Another exception would include any legitimate reason to suspect child abuse or any one who admits to child abuse in therapy.

Absence of Doctor-Patient Relationship

The doctor should avoid prescribing for friends, in-laws, family members, and friends of friends because there is no real contractual relationship and no legal documentation (medical chart notes). This kind of prescribing truly leaves the doctor without medico-legal defense—especially since we have all been schooled to know that this is wrong and yet we still retain that urge to help. What if the non-patient dies or has a serious drug reaction? Will the doctor feel guilt and remorse? How much? And for how long? If the non-patient has resulting catastrophic medical bills, then who will pay them? There is no malpractice insurance available since this took place outside the doctor-patient relationship. Furthermore, third-party insurance will not pay for the prescriptions unless prescribed by a doctor on the "panel".

Intimacy

It is illegal in all State jurisdictions for any licensed health professional of any kind to go out on dates or sleep with his/her clients/patients. If this has happened to you, then you should call the Licensing Board of the State where this happened. This would apply to all licensees: psychiatrists, psychotherapists, psychologists, and other providers of medical/dental services

Ongoing Therapy

This is the period of time (weeks, months, years) that you spend seeing your doctor on a regular basis.

Therapeutic Alliance

This will hopefully materialize in the first few sessions of therapy (typically with a therapist or psychologist). This is a condition in which both the therapist and the client/patient feel that the relationship is workable and can be therapeutic. This relationship will hopefully continue until the patient feels better.

The length of time in treatment will depend upon several factors. If a person has a persistent and serious psychiatric illness (Schizophrenia), then the length of treatment may be for life. For severe bipolar disorder, treatment may also be for decades, at least. Patients with less serious problems may require shorter treatment times, maybe six months or a couple years. Some people may stay until they feel better, then quit therapy until sometime in the future when they feel the need to return to therapy for several months or more. Duration of treatment can be discussed in the first or second appointment.

The doctor cannot decide unilaterally that he does not want to see the patient any more—if he did, then this would legally be called "abandonment". However, the doctor may terminate the relationship unilaterally if he can refer his patient to his partner or to another colleague—in a timely manner. This may arise in situations where the doctor feels that he is being asked to operate outside his medical expertise or outside his "comfort zone" (such as being requested to continue prescribing amphetamines for drug-addicted adults who have a very questionable "ADHD" diagnosis). The doctor might phase out the therapy if the doctor inadvertently develops a new relationship with somebody who is somehow connected to the patient—although, in some of these cases, the doctor should probably not be involved in such an outside relationship. The most serious situation is that in which the doctor starts to feel sexually attracted to the patient and wisely decides to refer the patient out before any misconduct will have a chance to arise. Or the doctor may come to learn that the patient's beliefs or acts are so morally repugnant that the doctor does not think that he can work with that patient anymore (a dog-lover therapist who finds out her male patient has sex with his dog on a regular basis or a devout Christian therapist who learns that her patient is a Satanist, etc.). There may be other "boundary" issues or personal reasons (an Elvis Presley fan club president who soon discovers that her patient is an Elvis impersonator); these are all valid—just as long as the patient is appropriately referred. The patient does not need to know the exact reason. In some cases, it would be helpful to apprise the patient about these circumstances and in others, it may not be; that usually depends upon the doctor-patient rapport. (Read the paragraph on counter-transference at the end of this chapter.) These types of problems are usually more of an issue when patients are in regular one-hour therapy sessions with the therapist as opposed to brief occasional in-and-out medication visits with the doctor, where the focus is on medicines and biology.

Treatment

"Talk Therapy" is called Psychotherapy and is an important part of the treatment process. Numerous studies have documented that some patients experience 50% relief from psychotherapy alone, and that some patients derive 50% benefit from medications alone. The possibility of feeling really good again is often achievable by combining an appropriate amount of psychotherapy sessions along with the judicious use of psychiatric medicines.

These are the main treatment modalities
- Primary treatments are medications and therapy
- Secondary treatment modalities are bio-physical and spiritual—these include Twelve Steps
- Supportive interactions may be found in socially-based support groups.

Primary

The doctor will prescribe and monitor any needed medications. Individual psychotherapy (talk therapy) with a therapist or psychologist serves a twofold purpose of being both confessional and stress-lowering, both of which have been demonstrated by changes in levels of biochemical markers in the body. Also helpful are marital therapy, couples therapy, and sex therapy. Group therapy is also valuable for many people for many reasons. This would be traditional group therapy run by a mental health practitioner. The extra therapeutic effect of these may reside in the fact that they may offer an entrée to problem-specific groups such as A.A. or A.C.A (Adult Children of Alcoholics). These latter groups provide a sense of hope by providing exposure to other people who are on the same path, so that apparent pain can be shared and not borne alone.

Secondary

Bio-physical includes biological treatments such as biofeedback as well as physical exercise (yoga, aerobics, etc.).

Spirituality training can include a range of activities from active religious affiliation to insight meditation as well as grief group at church, or regular attendance at Twelve Step Programs.

There are many different types of non-traditional group therapy such as: groups with medical focus, (Weight Watchers), or specialized groups with psychological support (such as men's groups). Some groups may be legally mandated (anger management, DUI school).

Supportive

Other socially-based support groups may be helpful in that they provide support to the patient or to the patient's caregivers. Examples would be Alzheimer Support Groups or Autism support groups.

If you are just embarking on a course of treatment and have a lot of doubts, remember that if you drop out your misery will come back again. You may take one step forward and half a step backward and may feel very frustrated and unhappy. You are in this for the full treatment, you should not quite mid-way. Remember the old saying "quitters never win, and winners never quit". And most importantly, as you go along, try to remember that

"Pain may be necessary, but suffering is optional."

Everybody wants to get better, but some patients are so disorganized that they cannot focus on treatment and may appear to sabotage their own treatment by not following through with treatment goals. If they can stay in treatment until the fog lifts, then they can get on track and "make a flight into health".

Derek is a young man who knows that he has serious overwhelming psychotherapy issues yet refuses to avail himself of any of these combined treatment modalities. He does not wish to attend individual therapy, group therapy, family therapy, or marital therapy. He declines psychological testing, involvement in a spiritual program, aerobic exercise, or attendance of formalized groups such as Twelve Step Programs. He continues to come to medication visits, but medications alone will not substitute for all these other treatments that are needed. This is unfortunate, since Twelve Step programs are essentially free or available for the nominal cost of only one dollar per meeting. Patients like Derek often have a less successful outcome. Some people want instantaneous recovery through pills alone, and figure they can go see another psychiatrist who will cure them immediately. One of the most common issues is that their only ambition is to find the one right pill that will make them feel completely functional. They will invest a lot of energy into seeing one psychiatrist after another in order to try to find the magic bullet pill that will strike them sane. They end up doing a lot of treatments halfway and in the process, they spend more time and money and energy than they would have if they had just stayed with the first psychiatrist and his original recommendations. In some cases, they are not convinced that they need anything besides pills.

In Derek's case, he was "forced" to come to therapy by his fiancée, but most of his close friends and family accept him the way he is, and hence he has little motivation to improve. His close friends continue to tolerate his behavioral "quirks". Friends are used to his behavior and even find it interesting or amusing. "Never a dull moment with Derek!" The most insidious problem might be his desire for a "quick cure" or escaping reality and seeking solace in a chemical (prescription medicine). This may inform of a possible early chemical dependence problem. Certainly, if his fiancée is already noting problems in his youth, then the behaviors will worsen with age—close friends will distance themselves and casual friends will drop him. Middle-aged men with these behaviors are no longer interesting or amusing, and may fall into the category of "hangers-on".

Fred is a middle-aged man who comes to the psychiatrist to get a first-time prescription but does not want to pay to see the psychiatrist again, hoping instead to have it refilled "for free" by his family doctor (providing that his doctor is even willing to do this). Fred may have limited   financial constraints or have control issues in that he does not want to see a psychiatrist because he thinks this is useless or valueless. He may have serious concerns that psychiatric visits imply that he is really "crazy" (social stigma) or that he might soon be. Another fear is that friends and neighbors will learn of Fred's embarrassing and potentially stigmatizing secret. (as per his perceptions).

Patient Concerns about Treatment

As therapy goes on, other issues will surface for the patient, such as telling his secrets to a stranger and the issues of "transference/counter-transference". Transference and Counter-transference issues involve some sixth sense feeling that the doctor or the patient or both feel toward each other based on subtle body language or subconscious associations. In other words, if these were two strangers meeting for the first time at a social event, they might feel awkward together. They would both have some unperceived negative or positive feelings about each other based on some childhood experience, which is totally unconnected to the current situation. Transference is the term used when the patient feels this. Counter-transference refers to the way that the doctor responds to subtle cues from the patient. Extremely negative feelings might require changing doctors; extremely positive (romantic) feelings would also require a change. Psychiatrists are aware of this possibility. These are some of the other concerns:

- confidentiality issue: patient is supposed to tell a stranger some of his secret problems that nobody else knows
- control issue: patient feels that he is not in control of his situation
- trust issue: patient wonders if he can trust this stranger
- fear of unknown: patient may learn of a catastrophic diagnosis

- embarrassment or shame concerning the office visit or concern about being seen going into or coming out of the office.

The patient will need to reach the conclusion that he feels so bad that he needs this treatment or nurtures the hope that he can feel much better with it.

Termination of Therapy

This refers to that time when you would like to stop having regular appointments with the doctor or therapist.

Mutual Decision

There are different schools of therapy, but in all of them the client/patient will eventually arrive at a point where the therapy is not anticipated to provide much more immediate benefit. This can be mutually decided and discussed. Usually the therapy will not be terminated abruptly, but will slowly be phased out and then there will come the last session. At this point, the client/patient will start to rely upon himself, being armed with what he has learned about himself in therapy. He will learn to use community resources and other sources of benefit and solace. The patient is free to leave the relationship whenever he chooses to dismiss the psychiatrist, but it should be announced in advance in case the therapist or doctor wishes to give cautionary feedback.

Involuntary Termination

Patients can be unilaterally terminated by the doctor or medical group if they are assaultive to medical staff. They can also be disenrolled for sabotaging their own treatment and malingering.

Firstly, any patient who is assaultive to medical staff is automatically terminated on the spot.

Secondly, large medical groups can terminate a medical patient's contract due to medical non-compliance of such a degree that it is actually sabotaging their recovery. This type of administrative termination is called "disenrollment". In reality, any medical or surgical patient who insists repeatedly upon sabotaging his treatment is jeopardizing his health. This can cause grave medical injury to the patient because of his omission to follow through: this is a risky behavior. This behavior also makes the doctor medically—if not legally—liable for any bad consequences of this self-sabotage. At the very least, it reflects badly upon the patient's treatment as perceived in the court of public opinion. In these cases, the medical group will suggest that the patient go elsewhere and find some treatment that he likes. This is easier to do with "commercial plans" (employer-based health insurance) and harder to do with "senior plans" (any person who is legally disabled or elderly). This is not "abandonment" because patients' health insurance plans offer them other choices of medical group—especially Medicare patients. In the case that the patient's only choice is that one medical group, then disenrollment would be very difficult indeed and highly improbable.

Under a third set of conditions, medical groups may also opt to terminate (disenroll) patients for showing clear signs of Factitious Disorder, Malingering, and Münchhausen Syndrome. Factitious patients deliberately and intentionally make themselves sick due to severe subconscious emotional illness. Medical doctors and surgeons are very annoyed when they find out what is going on; psychiatrists will willingly see these patients, because their issues can be treated. Malingerers are trying to manipulate the system in order to access entitlements—this is deception and can also be fraud if they are trying to get on SSD when they know that they are not really disabled. All doctors—including psychiatrists—have negative reactions to this sociopathic manipulation. Münchhausen patients deliberately and intentionally make themselves ill because they crave constant medical treatment.

These three types of patients can be very ingratiating with their new doctors who often arrange for all sorts of extra medical care and attention. Eventually the doctors find out what is going on and suggest (demand) a visit to a psychiatrist. The second tactic of the doctor is to call a psychiatrist and discuss this case at which time the whole fiasco starts to come into focus. Non-psychiatric doctors usually have mixed reactions (mainly anger) at these kinds of apparent deceptions and may insist that the patient see a psychiatrist, which rarely happens. Factitious patients and malingerers are usually least resistant to seeing a psychiatrist. The Munchausen patients uniformly disappear when psychiatry is mentioned. (Read more in chapter on Pain.)

Psychiatrists would not usually disenroll patients for not following primary doctors' orders because this is seen as a psychological issue that needs to be addressed and may be an entrée into some of the patient's "emotional baggage" (psychiatry even has a diagnostic code for this behavior, V15.81). Psychiatrists are likelier to be accustomed to dealing with these kinds of inappropriate, disruptive, and "quirky" behavior: factitious cases need talk therapy, malingerers are reported if possible, and Münchhausen patients disappear suddenly when they sense that their doctors have discovered that their illnesses are all self-induced. Munchausen patients are very resistant to seeing psychiatrists and usually disappear when they are ordered to go see a psychiatrist. It is presumed that they go to some other region of the country and start all over again there…Munchausen patients constantly seek out needless treatments. Some of them do have a real medical diagnosis, but it may not be the focus of the needless treatments. Thus, they expose themselves to a lot of testing and treatments on their bodies. They also run up a huge medical bill for physical symptoms—when in fact most of their problem is psychological.

Summary

Talk Therapy

The whole treatment process can be somewhat complicated but only for a minority of people. Most people will have a very unremarkable experience. Anything that seems remarkable at first will have been—in hindsight—probably due to your anxiety. This is how it will work for most people with therapy issues who have health insurance. You call your insurance company and they give you a list of mental health professionals. You call around and find someone who has openings. You make an appointment. You show up for intake (first appointment) and meet your therapist/doctor. If you like that person, then you continue; otherwise, cancel the next appointment and start calling around all over again. If you are self-pay, try to find out who is good in your area, call and make an appointment, etc.

And when this whole talk therapy process is finished and you are able to have a mutual termination, then your are ready to make a "flight into health" to see how well you can "fly" on your own. If not well, then you can always come back to the "nest" for more therapy sessions.

Reality Orientation Therapy

People who have chronic conditions should not withdraw from therapy. Ever. This includes major mood disorders and major thought disorders. Examples are: Schizophrenia and Bipolar conditions. People with chronic PTSD and chronic depression may be able to take (long) breaks from treatment, but they should not delude themselves into thinking that they will never again need to see a psychiatrist. They may not need talk therapy, but they do need medcines and do need to face this fact as a reality of their conditions. No one wants to be sick with a life-long disorder requiring chronic treatment. The only thing worse is being sick with an *untreatable* chronic disorder.

Just remember that the doctor is licensed to do and know all these issues of concern, so you, the patient, must rely on trust to override fear at the earliest visits.

▶Remember: You can do a basic background check on your doctor:

at the State Medical Board website
or on
the National Practitioner Data Bank (NPDB) website

▶ QUESTIONS

Q: How will I know when I am better?

A: That should be obvious both to you and to the therapist. It can be discussed often. There will be times when the therapist will review your progress.

Q: What happens if the patient does not want to be referred to see any other doctor?

A: The doctor will usually say something to the effect that he feels that he cannot provide adequate treatment for the patient's condition. The doctor should try to see the patient at the usual regular treatment times until the patient is connected to the new doctor.

Q: What should I do if the doctor is often rescheduling my appointments?

Q: What should I do if the doctor charges me for a one hour visit (usually fifty minutes in reality) but sees me for a half hour or less?

A: This is disrespectful of your part of the contractual relationship: that you will pay (for what you get). I would consider changing doctors if it were a habitual problem. You will start have resentments (negative transference issues) that may make therapy strained. This is tantamount to overcharging, which insurance companies technically consider to be fraud (illegal). It is unethical by violating my definition of "ethical", which is "how I would like to be treated".

Q: What if my doctor's practice is not like the treatments on the "Oprah" show or on the Internet?

A: He may be customizing it for you—or not. Ask him.

Q: What happens if the patient objects to the particular doctor of referral?

A: Other referrals can be given also.

Chapter I-6

Introduction to Visiting the Psychiatrist
What to expect and the mechanics of how it works

This should be a process in thirteen steps I-XIII:

I   The first encounter will be the same as visiting any other doctor's office. You will be asked to fill out financial responsibility papers, health insurance forms, intake forms, and confidentiality forms some of which are governmentally mandated.

II You will be given the patient forms to fill out in which you disclose your living situation and some basic information about yourself. This will usually include a list of feelings and symptoms which you are experiencing. You will be asked to list your current medications (plus all of the prescriptions from other doctors).

III Then you will have an hour intake in person with the therapist who will ask in-depth questions about your childhood, civil status, drug-alcohol history, traumatic experiences, family history of psychiatric disorders, and perhaps what you would like to accomplish during your visits to the psychiatric office.

IV If family members have accompanied you, they probably will not go with you for your intake with the therapist unless you are so impaired that you are not sure why you have an appointment. In this case, the family should come into the office to give the background history. If you are able to give a good account of yourself, it is usually desirable to see you alone as there may be sensitive questions about your relationships with your family members, sexual problems, symptoms, or other personal and private information. Indeed maybe the person who brought you to your first psychiatric visit is the imagined or real souce of much of your emotional turmoil. You, the patient retain the legal right to determine who accompanies you into the confidential session with the therapist and doctor.

V   Then you will have an appointment with the psychiatrist either on the same day or soon thereafter. During this visit, the same guidelines pertain about family members coming into the office with you and the psychiatrist: as the patient, you have the right to decide who comes into the office with you. You may choose to come in alone. Certain patients need to have the family present

51

in order to provide important background information especially in cases of memory failure or certain types of delusions. In a typical delusional case, the patient believes the delusion to be completely true and reality-based—hence, it is not a symptom or a problem from his viewpoint; it is not of interest to him to remark on this anymore than you might mention some reality-based fact. The most difficult delusions are the jealous delusions, because these are really a subjective experience and hard to prove or disprove. However, the family believes that the delusional jealousy is ludicrous and thus has brought the patient (most usually the husband, sometimes the wife). The delusionally jealous spouse will never voluntarily refer himself to see a psychiatrist since he "knows" that it is "true" that his seventy-six year old wife of fifty years is sleeping with the neighbors and the gardeners. Other patients may not be able to give an account of them selves because they have poor memory or selective memory. This occurs in cases of dementia or traumatic brain injury or after strokes. Some stroke patients remember their medical history but have lost the vocabulary necessary to express it.

VI   The type of psychiatric visit depends upon the type of health insurance and venue. If you are seeing a psychiatrist privately and he is the only person in the office, then he will actually do everything himself from steps I-V. If you are in a county or government psychiatric office or seeing someone in a large medical group practice then this procedure outlined here will pertain to you. The visit with the psychiatrist (the doctor) will last from about 40-75 minutes*, depending upon how complex the case is. Very psychotic patients will be seeing the psychiatrist as the primary treatment source; those who are mildly anxious may focus mainly on therapy appointments with the therapist.

VII   The psychiatrist will talk to you and gather information to determine which problems you have and how best to address the problems. This will all be reflected in a report which he will typically dictate after your visit. The basic format of his dictation will be something like this: First he will write the **Identification** which identifies you, for example "This is a 65 year old widow who has a three year history of prolonged grief and depression." (An example of a psychiatric evaluation is presented at the end of this chapter**). Then the next part of the dictation will be **HOPI (History of Present Illness)** which will describe what you have been doing recently and what happened to make you decide to come in to seek psychiatric consultation. Next, will come a list of your **Symptoms** (insomnia, weight loss), also called Psychiatric review of systems (**ROS).** This is followed by a detailed personal **Past Psychiatric History**—if any: have you ever been in a psychiatric hospital? any suicide attempts? any psychiatric medication prescribed in the past? alcohol and drug history? Then we will review your

Medical History (high blood pressure, low thyroid function), any **Lab tests and X-Rays & Imaging Studies of Head (CATScan, MRI etc),** and then a list of all your current **Medications** prescribed to you by all your current doctors.

VIII   After this information is collected (however long it takes, depends upon how much medical and psychiatric history you have). Then the psychiatrist formulates a "diagnostic impression" which becomes a "tentative diagnosis" (a preliminary diagnosis) and this is the diagnosis that is reported to the billing office. In psychiatry, we may modify the diagnosis somewhat as treatment continues and more background information comes to light with each new doctor visit.

IX   At this juncture, I usually announce the best or most usual and standardized treatments for this problem and try to get the patient involved in the process. I have found that this approach is helpful because it lets our patients try to make informed decisions as treatment consumers. Most of the time, the patients decide to let me decide—remember that the patient is coming in because his mind is not well, so a number of patients feel overwhelmed in trying to analyze the choices. Others will dialog about the choices then make a choice for this condition—that is, if there is more than one treatment available (usually there are a few). I usually outline the advantages and disadvantages of the possible treatment(s). This works out better when the patients can be told a short list of usual and customary choices and then let them choose. I do guide them in the right direction, also— especially if they have questions about pharmaceutical advertisements seen in magazines and on TV. This also gives me a chance to tell patients the major risks involved instead of just sending them to the pharmacy where they will feel overwhelmed when they read that the drug is dangerous and has so many side effects. Then they will not take the drug at all and will later call me with great concern about the drug side effects. Having these discussions before the patient goes to the pharmacy is useful for patient, doctor, and pharmacist. Rarely a patient may have a somewhat unorthodox idea about treatment that might or might not be feasible but subject to discussion. A few patients do not want any chemical treatment. In these cases, there is always the possibility of herbs, sunlight (phototherapy), psychotherapy alone, or other somatic (bodily) treatments. Pregnant patients are not good candidates for synthetic drugs or herbs.

X   Some patients are already stabilized on a certain medicine and decide to continue it. This is certainly possible. If this medicine begins to lose effect, there are others on the market. Occasionally I will need to order some lab tests that are relevant to the treatment medication.

XI   If we have samples of the new treatment drug then some of them will be dispensed to the patient. As far as samples are concerned, you should know: (1) yes, the supply of samples left in a medical office by "drug reps." can sometimes affect treatment decisions; (2) it is considered unethical to maintain patients on samples indefinitely in cases where the patients do not have insurance coverage—it makes people dependent on something which is not guaranteed to be readily available; (3) doctors can not remove sample pills from factory packages and re-package them—this is called "shucking" and carries penalties.

XII   At this point you will be given a second psychiatrist appointment if you are planning on taking prescription medicines or need a follow-up with the psychiatrist for any reason. This might also include a visit to talk about your response to tapering off of a former drug or other issues. In cases where the patient has been on a certain medication for a long time from another doctor and has decided to taper off the drug, then that person will be given a schedule to wean himself slowly off the drug. In such cases, the drug will likely disappear from his body within a couple days, but the therapeutic effects of the drug can last for weeks after it is out of the body (the drug may no longer be in the urine, but the effects on the brain can last longer than that). This is the result of having altered brain chemistry from the previous prescription. After a few days or weeks drug-free, the brain should revert to "default" status. If the patient is still feeling good three months after stopping the drug, then he has probably healed. He might be able to forego the drug and live without it indefinitely, unless he has a relapse. The possibility of relapse has been estimated to occur in about one third of first-time cases of anxiety and depression. In cases of such a relapse, oftentimes the same drug at the same dosage may be useful. However, there are cases in which that drug is no longer beneficial: this is one reason why patients should not stop and start their drugs based on their judgment and initiative alone. Some patients will start to feel bad after only one or two weeks of stopping the drug and should be given instructions to resume the medicine at the first sign of a relapse/recurrence of symptoms and to call and make an immediate appointment. When patients are tapering off drugs, they are given a schedule of when to change the dose and when to call or come back for the next appointment—the schedule differs significantly depending upon the drug that is being tapered.

XIII   If you need to see the therapist for a second visit then this will be scheduled at the end of the first visit. Patients with therapy issues will schedule another appointment with the therapist. Patients needing only medication visits may continue seeing only the psychiatrist. Some may see both the therapist and the psychiatrist. In rare cases, the patient may have come in for a once-only visit, for example for a second opinion (or even a third opinion).

Diagnosis	Estimated duration of treatment
Mild anxiety, mild depression	about a year
Moderate anxiety, panic, moderate depression	about two to four years
Schizophrenia, dementia, most psychotic disorders	for the rest of your life probably
Borderline syndrome	seven to thirty years
Typical therapy issues	varies depending upon many factors

I-6-a Length of Therapy as a function of Diagnosis (meant only as general guidelines)

---

*some practices charge more for longer interviews but charge less for shorter sessions—realize two basic facts: (1)-the psychiatrist is not only the doctor but is also the treatment(!); and, (2)-time is what we offer so it is directly related to fee structure

** *This is a brief example of a typical* psychiatric evaluation *(see section VII above)*

ID: This is a 65-year-old widow without prior psychiatric history who is complaining of "depression". (Use of quotation marks refers to patient's exact words—this is not a diagnosis by the doctor.)

HOPI (History of Present Illness): Three years ago she lost her husband of forty years to heart failure after caring for him at home in a bed-ridden state for three years. She had intense grief and had to go stay with her eldest daughter for three months. She developed severe insomnia and started to receive nightly "visits" from her deceased husband who appeared to her but did not talk. Then she started to feel tingling on her skin as if somebody were in bed with her. After she went home to live alone, she started to see him at night and in the daytime too.

ROS (Review of Systems): loss of appetite and forty-pound weight loss, can not fall asleep, sees dead husband at night along with her own deceased grandfather, feels tired all day too.

PΨHx (Past Psychiatric History): no formal history; she became very depressed after her second child was born but never saw a psychiatrist: her mother came to live with them for a year.

Substance Hx: denies herbs, cigarettes, coffee, and alcohol

PMHx (Past Medical History) high blood pressure, history of left mastectomy in 1999 for breast CA (cancer)

FΨHx (Family Psych. History): her only brother has been on Stelazine for thirty years for presumed Psychotic Diagnosis, grandmother had "Alzheimer's", grandfather died from alcoholism

FMHx (Family medical History) dementia, alcoholism, as well as stroke (father)

Medications: Femara, Atenolol, Dyazide

Psychological testing: memory testing normal (29/30) for age and educational level; geriatric short-form depression scale was 12/15 (very depressed)

Lab tests: thyroid test slightly abnormal, low red blood corpuscle indices, slight decrease in kidney filtration rate, cholesterol levels low, fasting blood sugar normal

MSE (mental status exam): this would be at least a paragraph that describes her behaviors during the interview; this is but a brief example: "she arrived half an hour early for the appointment and seemed so confused that Rosemary had to do some of the paperwork with her and her daughter did the rest of it. She walked slowly and appeared tired, looking older than her stated age. She had a flat affect, downcast gaze, sad mood. She did not have any eye darting or trembling and did not appear to be internally stimulated..." (and so on)

Dx (or diagnostic impression): Pathologic Grief and Severe Depression with some genetic loading and an undocumented episode of probable moderate post-partum depression

Rx: (1) Zyprexa 5mg in the p.m. (2) weekly grief therapy at church (3) weekly therapy sessions with the therapist or psychologist (4) return to see doctor in ten days. ,

Chapter I-7

Introduction to Pharmacology

Caveat #1: Every prescription drug is poison taken in small amounts.
Caveat #2: For every ongoing psychoactive drug prescription,
we should ask ourselves whether the benefits
outweigh the risk.

In the previous chapters in this first section, we discussed medicine in general and how modern psychiatry evolved out of modern medicine. We also looked at doctors in general and how psychiatrists are related to other doctors. This chapter is about pharmacology in general. Later in the book, we will look into the discovery and uses of psychoactive medicines.

Pharmacology in General Medicine basically means drugs, pills, injections, and other chemicals. Pharmacology in psychiatry is also just pharmacology, but it has a special name, psychopharmacology. We have this special term because the drugs that we prescribe have special qualities of being mind-altering and mood-altering chemicals. This seems to set them apart from mere "blood pressure pills" or insulin. If we consider that biochemical changes in the heart and blood pressure are no odder than biochemical changes in the brain and nervous system, then psychiatry might not need to have this special term, "psychopharmacology". But we have it anyway, because human behavior is important and any odd behavior can quickly become not only a medical issue, but also a social and legal issue. Oddness of blood pressure is only a medical issue or medical emergency and would not involve the police in the way that an emergency psychiatric problem would. Any substance that controls behavior needs special oversight.

This chapter looks at general pharmacology with references to psychopharmacology. There is more on psychopharmacology in chapters V-1 and V-2. This is the outline of this chapter:

I—This chapter starts off with all the "pharm-" professions—this is for your own special interest; it can be skipped over.
II—The next pages describe how drugs are discovered and brought to market.
III—The rest of the chapter is devoted to explanations of what drugs do to us.

I–This section can be skipped over:

List I-7-a (terms using "Pharm-)

In classical Greek, *pharmakon (φάρμακον)* meant "drug, remedy, medicine, poison, enchanted potion, dye, color".[27]

In modern medicine, "pharmaco", is used to refer to medicinal chemicals used for healing purposes.

These are some medical terms using "pharm-":

1- "Pharmacology" involves knowledge of how drugs act and what they do to the body.

2- "Pharmacognosy" teaches how to find and fabricate drug substances from a variety of sources, including "natural" sources (plants, minerals, and animals); however, some of these medications inspired by nature or discovered in nature may need to be mass-produced in a factory since the natural extraction process could be quite costly (galantamine, for example). Pharmacognosy may involve discovering new species of animals and plants with novel medicinal applications (such as those in the endangered rain forests).

3- "Pharmacy" refers to compounding, preparing, and dispensing medications to the patients. "Pharmacy" is also the name of the place where patients pick up prescription medicines. Retail pharmacies sell to the public and are usually either corporate "chains" or stand-alone "mom & pop" local neighborhood pharmacies. The profits of chain drug stores depend upon volume, so they are usually very rushed and busy; the local neighborhood drugstores often provide better and more attentive service but with shorter business hours. Wholesale pharmacies may provide better prices.

4- "Pharmaceutics" is the whole process of Pharmacy;

5- Pharmaceutical industry refers to research and development of new drugs, marketing the drugs, the process of synthesizing new drugs and bringing them to market and post-marketing activities.

6- Pharmacists may have a "Pharm.D." degree (doctor of Pharmacy) or R.Ph. degree (registered pharmacist);

7- "Pharm. techs" (pharmacy technicians) have completed an approved training course of about one year's length, followed by an internship. Pharm techs help the pharmacists and as such are pharmacist "extenders".

8- Pharmacy students are enrolled in a formal program at a College of Pharmacy which itself is typically associated with a larger university. The pharmacy students spend four to six years studying to become registered pharmacists. Pharmacy students may also work behind the counter helping degreed pharmacists. This is a normal part of their training.

9- Doctorate of Pharmacology is not a pharmacist. This is distinct from Pharm.D. who is a pharmacist with an advanced degree. Doctorate of Pharmacology is usually a Ph.D. degree earned in graduate school: it is usually an academic degree and does not confer to the licensee any privilege of prescribing drugs to human patients, unless the doctor of pharmacology also has a medical license.

10- Psycho-pharmacologists are usually fully trained psychiatrists who do a two-year special fellowship in clinics and hospitals where they prescribe for psychiatric patients with very advanced and complicated regimens of psychiatric medications.

11- Pharmacology involves the intellectual aspect of medications whereas Pharmacy is the practical side of providing medications. Pharmacognosy would be useful for research and development. Pharmaceutics nowadays centers on pharmacy activities and the marketing of medications. These are all necessary for current pharmaceutical practice.

II—How Drugs are Discovered and Brought to Market

Drug companies must meet high standards in order to get approval to sell a drug in this country. The drug must pass through three tiers of testing in order to be sold legally as a drug intended for the *general* public:

A—Animal Testing

B—Controlled testing in human patients which involves three phases
   (Phases I, II, and III)

C—Aftermarket surveillance

These are special uses for special populations:

D—Compassionate use of a drug

E—Orphan drugs

F—"Black box" drugs used in Psychiatry (these are dangerous drugs available on prescription)

A—Firstly, the drug company must demonstrate the effects of the drugs on animals (typically rats and mice*, and this study involves all aspects of the drug activity on rodents such as:

    1- pregnancy outcome data for both the mother rat and her pups;

    2- analyzing drug effects on all organs of the body; and, additionally—in testing new potential psychiatric medicines—analyzing a number of behavioral changes in the rat:

        a-) undesirable behavioral manifestations indicative of unpleasant side-effects or clear-cut toxicity, in other words, if the rats behave very strangely or violently; and/or,

        b-) desirable, beneficial, and sought-after effects, such as increased activity or improved motivation and stamina in rodents.

B—Secondly, after the tier of animal studies, then the drug must go through three phases of human testing:

1-phase one is totally experimental and involves giving the drug to several human volunteers who are aware of the potential risk. Occasionally, these volunteers have a fatal reaction. If they all survive, then there will be:

2-phase two studies involving experimentation on a limited number (hundreds) of humans who are very ill and desperate for any new medicine to treat their disease. If that testing goes well, then:

3-phase three testing will be done in major medical centers: this is the expanded experimental testing on humans euphemistically called "clinical trials". These patients are sick also but less desperate—or more cautious—than those in phase two are. Phase three involves many more volunteers (several hundred or even thousands) carefully selected from a pool of patients who are suffering from the disease that the new medicine is supposed to treat. This will hopefully provide definitive results that will be acceptable to the FDA.

4-If the FDA remains somewhat unconvinced, then the FDA will ask the drug company to do some more testing or provide some additional information on the new drug. This will require the drug company to spend millions of dollars more—this is the financial risk for the drug companies: the drug might run the risk of never coming to market, having its debut date delayed, or never coming to market in the USA (but being available in some other countries).

5-Other countries around the world may be convinced by all three FDA phases up to that date and may not request further testing. At that point, the drug company may eschew further attempts to enter the North American market. In some of these cases, the drug companies may abandon hopes of marketing the drug in the USA or become reluctant to do so because:

a-) A drug which has been rejected once by the FDA, may earn a bad reputation. Even if it is later approved on its second pass through the FDA approval process, the drug could then become an easy mark for litigation in the future

b-) The drug company might feel obligated to charge a much higher retail price in the USA so as to contribute to amassing financial reserves to put into the future litigation kitty.

6-In some cases (Wellbutrin, for example) the drug company may be aware of a possible serious side effect (seizures) and withhold the drug from the American market pending further clarification of this serious side effect. In the case of Wellbutrin's possible link to seizures, further public market exposure overseas revealed that it is a reasonably safe drug as long as it is not prescribed to known epileptics or bulimics. So, Wellbutrin finally came to market in the USA and went on to earn profits over the ensuing years. Part of this success was due to the fact that Wellbutrin is biochemically unique and competing drug companies did not market any "me-too" drugs (slightly modified versions that would be eligible for a separate patent).

C—Thirdly, after the drug is FDA-approved for sale to the general public, there will be post-market surveillance which has as its primary purpose to monitor for serious side effects that had gone undetected in human testing ("clinical trials"). Post-market surveillance often reveals a serious undetected side effect: this happens with some frequency. Some of these serious side effects can be quite toxic or life-threatening. Some of these side effects appear soon after the drug is released to the general market. Some of these serious side effects appear early in treatment within a few weeks or months of the patient's starting the drug; other serious side effects appear quite late in treatment, perhaps after the patient has been taking the medicine for year(s). Examples of these kinds of side effects are:

1-*Uncommon, early, and serious side effects*: These are uncommon side effects that can occur commonly soon after a patient starts taking the medication. This has happened with some medications such as Merital (Nomifensine) which could cause internal bleeding in a few patients within a few weeks or months of starting the medication. The sponsoring drug company voluntarily withdrew Nomifensine from the US market; other examples are the ability of Halcion, Ambien, and Quaalude to cause nocturnal disruptions (Halcion is now banned in the UK, and Quaalude is banned in the USA after being elevated to the status of a dangerous Schedule I drug);

2-*Common and early (or of early-intermediate onset)*: If this happens too commonly to too many people, then the FDA may withdraw the drug from market, or the drug company might voluntarily withdraw the drug from market (high legal risk). If the drug stays on the market, then the FDA may issue warnings or severe warnings (called "black box" warnings because they appear printed inside a black box in the text of the PDR, Physician's Desk Reference). In the case of a few drugs, this serious side effect could occur commonly and frequently but these kinds of drugs are so urgently needed to relieve suffering that special arrangements have been made for them to stay on the market despite their serious side effects. This is the case of Clozaril used as a last resort for treating very severe schizophrenia. (It can cause fatal infections.) "Orphan drugs", such as Orap, also fit into this category—see section "D" on the next page.

3-*Common and early but manageable*. Some drugs turn out to have very common serious side effects but only under certain uncommon circumstances. These drugs went on to be marketed with the caveat that the patients be told to avoid these certain and known circumstances that could be life threatening. In the case of Nardil, patients were given dietary restrictions (to avoid stroke). In the case of Lamictal, the dosage is increased very, very slowly (to avoid serious rash). Thalidomide was no problem for men and non-pregnant women, but could not be given to pregnant women (and was withdrawn from the market—its only use now is in Leprosy). In the case of Wellbutrin, as long as epileptic and bulimic patients are screened out, then the rest of the population may continue taking the drug.

4-*Common and late*: Halcion (somnambulism) and Mellaril (heart side effects); the antipsychotics can cause diabetes or trembling (Parkinsonism);

5-*Uncommon and late*: The other purpose of post market surveillance is to track the possibility of a delayed, very rare, and very serious side effect that might occur but only if the patient takes the drug for a long time (usually). After enjoying years of modest market success, Serzone started to be linked to liver failure. Serzone is still on the market in the USA, but new prescriptions are not being generated and most former Serzone patients have been switched over to other medications. Another example would be that of the addictive potential of Klonopin. When Klonopin debuted on the market, we were all assured that it is not addicting "because of its long half-life". Klonopin is like long-lasting Xanax, and Xanax is quite addicting. Both Xanax and Klonopin are in the Valium family of drugs, which are all habit-forming and addicting.

6—*Questionable and Ambiguous effects:* recently, the FDA has "black-boxed" some of the antidepressants if used in teenagers and children for fear that these antidepressants cause depressed teenagers to commit suicide. The warning may apply to young adults, too: this could possibly include any one under the age of twenty-five in this higher risk group. This FDA move seems to be erring on the side of caution. Unfortunately, suicide is one of the biggest risks in all depressed people of all ages. Suicide is one of the leading causes of teenage deaths (and young adult deaths) whether the teens are taking antidepressants or not. Prozac is the only SSRI antidepressant approved for use in children. Both Prozac and Lexapro are approved for use in teenagers.

Imipramine (and possibly other tricyclic antidepressants) may be associated each year with sudden cardiac deaths in athletic teenage boys. These medications had been used in the past for bedwetting (enuresis) and ADD (Attention Deficit Disorder).

Pseudo-ephedrine also has an association with teenage cardiac deaths. It is available without a prescription (available OTC, over the counter). The problem with pseudo-ephedrine abuse by teenage athletes (heart attacks) became so bad in the mid 1990's, that the Ohio Legislature was going to make this a prescription-only medication. (Pseudo-ephedrine can increase endurance—see chapters V-2, V-4, V-6.)

Effexor can cause high blood pressure, and in my middle-aged and older patients, this condition persisted even after the Effexor was stopped—more unbiased research is needed.

Chantix is used to quit smoking—it may cause depression.

Chart I-7-b   Drug Toxicities appearing after FDA Approval (during post-Surveillance period)

Drugs of main concern are in bold print

	Toxicity appears early in treatment	Toxicity can Appear at anytime	Toxicity appears later
Serious side effect	**Lamictal** (rash) Rashes* caused by any drug	Antidepressants (?? causing suicide in young people??) Chantix (depression)	**Mellaril,**(heart) Ambien and Halcion**, (confusion/amnesia) Klonopin (addiction) **Xanax** (much addiction)
Serious/ lethal but Manageable Side effect	**Clozaril**—special program is needed **Nardil, Parnate**— special diet needed		**Serzone** (liver failure) Anti-psychotics (Diabetes and Parkinsonism)
Life- threatening side effect	(Nomifensine—off market in USA)	Ephedrine, Imipramine, Pseudo-ephedrine (heart)	

*any rash that appears soon after starting a drug is a cause of concern; any drug can cause this reaction; the most common in my practice have been: Paxil, Vivactil, Effexor, Prozac
** this can also occur with Quaalude, barbiturates, and any other addicting sleeping pills

There are still toxic drugs that are on the market in the USA such as Xyrem and Clozaril. Since these drugs are unique and invaluable, they have remained available, but the burden is on the prescriber to manage any toxicities. These decisions sometimes seem odd when we consider that there are less toxic drugs that have been withdrawn from the market either at the request of the FDA or voluntarily by the drug company.

D—"Compassionate Use" is another form of access to certain medications which tends to bypass some of the above steps. Usually, these drugs may only be in early phases of human testing. Compassionate use is what its name describes: these are for patients with terminal illness with little or no hope of surviving unless a miracle drug appears. These conditions may typically be AIDS or cancer.

E—"Orphan drugs" are typically already FDA-approved for other purposes or are drugs well known in Europe which are allowed to be marketed here without all the FDA testing requirements based on safety studies in Europe. This is a similar situation to that of compassionate use drugs in the sense that these drugs are destined for a tiny amount of the population, but differing in the fact that orphan drugs have a track record of safety—or if they have any toxicities, these toxicities are known. (Orap can cause heart rhythm problems.) The term "orphan" refers to the fact that no American drug company wants to go through all the cost of marketing a rare drug for a very rare purpose. Our government will then step in to make special arrangements, trade-offs, and agreements with one drug company to handle this drug. (Orap for Tourette's Disorder, for example).

G—Black box drugs used in Psychiatry (this is what a black box warning looks like)
These drugs are all known to be addicting or dangerous and should be used cautiously. If you look inside the Physician's Desk Reference (PDR), the most toxic drugs (that are still on the market) are framed inside an attention-getting and ominous-looking "black-box".

I-7-c   Example of a "black-box" warning for Mellaril (Thioridazine)
        (referencing its effects on the heart) source: PDR[13]

> **WARNING**
> **THIORIDAZINE HAS BEEN SHOWN TO PROLONG THE QTc INTERVAL IN A DOSE RELATED MANNER AND DRUGS WITH THIS POTENTIAL, INCLUDING THIORIDAZINE, HAVE BEEN ASSOCIATED WITH TORSADE DE POINTES-TYPE ARRHYTHMIAS AND SUDDEN DEATH. DUE TO ITS POTENTIAL FOR SIGNIFICANT LIFE THREATENING PROARRHYTHMIC EFFECTS, THIORIDAZINE SHOULD BE RESERVED FOR USE IN THE TREATMENT OF SCHIZOPHRENIC PATIENTS WHO FAIL TO SHOW AN ACCEPTABLE RESPONSE TO ADEQUATE COURSES OF TREATMENT WITH OTHER ANTIPSYCHOTIC DRUGS, EITHER BECAUSE OF INSUFFICIENT EFFECTIVENESS OR THE INABILITY TO ACHIEVE AN EFFECTIVE DOSE TO INTOLERABLE ADVERSE EFFECTS FROM THOSE DRUGS.**

Also of interest, please note that:

All these forms of Ritalin and Dexedrine (and Cylert) are also black-boxed!!
Metadate, Concerta, Focalin, Vyvanse, Adderall,
Dexedrine, DextroStat, Ritalin LA,
and
Desoxyn a/k/a/"crystal meth"

Depakote also carries a black box warning about liver and pancreas problems. Common practice suggests that these problems are likelier in children. I have used this drug for a quarter century in all of its available preparations and so far, my patients have not had a problem.

▶▶ QUESTIONS

Q: Why is there so much testing for so many years?

A-1: The Food & Drug Administration (FDA) wants the drug to be as safe as possible under the circumstances.

A-2: Probably because the USA is a wealthy country and can afford the whole process which does generate a lot of clinical and financial activity.

Q: How much does it cost nowadays to bring a new drug to market?

A: Upwards of a billion dollars; the cost of bringing a new drug to market is extremely high. This stems in part from complying with all FDA testing requirements. Many countries do not have the financial resources to do this kind of in-depth testing. Some countries will allow the sale of these medications in their homelands based solely upon approval by the FDA in the USA. This tends to be a common practice. Sometimes we Americans end up shouldering the costs of drug research and development for the whole world.

III—What Drugs Do To Us

Pharmacology consists of studying the chemical properties of a medicine and its toxicity and its actions on the human body. Prescription drugs are all poisons which we ingest in small controlled doses so that the drug's toxicity will be minimized while the beneficial effects are maximized. This is often a precarious balancing act. Either our bodies adapt to the pharmaceuticals or they do not, in which case the pharmaceutical can be stopped or changed. This is a significant part of modern psychiatric practice. The following chart I-7-c illustrates the different phases of starting and continuing on a prescription medicine. Chart I-7-c also shows the marked differences between using addicting and non-addicting drugs.

Treatment Phases	*Non-Addicting Medicines*	**Addicting Medicines**
Induction Phase (starting the drug)	*Odd side effects*	**Immediate relief**
Short-term issues (first few weeks)	*Give ongoing encouragement to continue the medication*	**Still having a good immediate response**
Accommodation (adjusting to the drug)	*Benefit of medicine appears*	**Patient becomes accustomed to drug**
Intermediate Phase	*Address minor but annoying side effects*	**Check for habituation (when drug becomes habit-forming**
Later phase	*Continue drug and see doctor every 3-6 months*	**Encourage to taper medicine Monitor for addiction**
Stabilization	*Sense of well-being and Normalcy*	**Odd side effects appear? Mild discomfort?**
Risks of long-term use	*Any long-term toxicity? Cardiac? Liver? Renal? Parkinsonism?*	**Addiction**

Chart I-7-d   Pharmacologic Adaptation

Pharmacologic "Adaptation"

There are different ways to specify the reaction of the body to the introduction and ongoing use of medications. The two main ways of visualizing this really depend upon the addictive nature of the prescription medication. Use of a non-addicting medicine is typically going to be a long-term undertaking that needs more medical management in the early stages but not in later stages. Quite the opposite, use of an addicting medicine requires less early oversight but requires careful scrutiny later in regards to the risks and benefits of long-term use (addiction).

Non-Addicting prescription medications

These drugs are difficult in the first few weeks to months when they cause side effects. Patients often take one pill and refuse to take a second pill. This is the rule rather than the exception for people who have been taking addicting pills and are switched to non-addicting pills: they almost all uniformly detest the non-addicting pills! The doctor's role at this time is to function like a "pill coach". The trouble is worth it, because we know that the patient will not become addicted. Once the patient has adapted to the non-addicitng drug, he can do spectacularly well—unless he has already decided that he wants—or craves—an addicting drug.

1—Induction phase: this is when a person is starting the medicine and going through the following sub-phases:
    a)- first few days of very early side effects
    b)- first and second weeks of other early side effects; some patients may report feeling much better now: we call this the week of "placebo effects" this is when patients may feel the drug is helping, but scientists insist that that is not possible and that the drugs take around six weeks to become effective; whether it is one or eight weeks, in clinical practice, what really matters is that our patients feel better as soon as possible—maybe rats' brains do require six or eight weeks. "Placebo" effect means that people could be given a sugar pill to treat depression and if they believe strongly enough, then they will believe that depression is getting better with a sugar pill. Placebo pills were actually on the market at one time and were available as orange, red, or blue "Cebo-caps".
    c)- onset of beneficial therapeutic effects in the next few weeks
2—Accommodation phase
    d)- further adjustment to beneficial therapeutic effects in the following weeks
    e)- management of any new side effects;
3—Stabilization phase: this is when the patient reaches stability and is completely adjusted to the medication and continues to receive the same daily effect from it—unless new problems appear. These might destabilize the patient who will then need to be restabilized. Examples would be new medical problems requiring additional medications.

4—Post-stabilization phase

f- the patient feels completely recovered and wants to try to taper off the medicine; or,

g- patient's body starts to "reject" the drug; or,

h- the patient has become "refractory" (resistant) to the drug: this means that the patient is not receiving so much benefit from the drug anymore or has become resistant to its effect.

5—Alteration phase involves:

i- tapering off the medicine to see if patient is well now; or,

j- changing to a different medicine if the patient does not yet feel recovered.

k- changing to a different medicine if patient is showing signs that the drug is becoming psychologically habit-forming to him or making him too psychologically dependent on it.

Addicting Prescription Medications

This description includes drugs that are outright *addicting*. The next description discusses medicines that cause lesser degrees of *physical or psychological dependence.*

This is the terminology that I like to use:

–Psychological Dependence—a person needs the medication to feel emotionally balanced; if left without the medicine, the person might turn to food, sex, gambling, smoking, or shopping (symptoms of possible mental or emotional withdrawal)

–Physical Dependence—a person needs the medicine to avoid unpleasant bodily sensations; if left without the medicine the person might over-exercise, oversleep, or start drinking (signs of possible physical withdrawal)

–Habituation—a person needs the same dose each day to feel stable

–Addiction—a person needs to increase the dose to feel stable

–Cross-addiction—if a person becomes addicted to drug X, then he will also be addicted to all the drugs in that family, even though he has never tried them (for example, Xanax belongs to the Valium family which is a large group of habit-forming drugs, so all those drugs become addicting too)

–Drug Misuse is taking someone else's prescription medications in the manner of drug abuse   (as described below).

–Drug Abuse occurs when a patient takes his own prescribed medication in an unintended or erratic manner because he thinks it will make him feel, act, think, or look better. Examples include:

- taking three or four [of his own prescribed] Valium pills if really upset;
- taking extra pills[of his own prescribed] amphetamines in order to dance all night at a rave.

Addicting drugs are usually controlled by a federal agency, the DEA (Drug Enforcement Administration), whereas non-addicting drugs are controlled by State laws. DEA has the right to control every step in the manufacture, distribution (shipping and handling), prescribing (doctors' prescribing patterns), selling and dispensing of controlled drugs (by the pharmacy), and misuse of the drugs (individual consumption of that drug without having a valid prescription for it). The DEA also has jurisdiction in case of the theft of the doctor's prescription pad. The DEA has six rankings for addicting drugs. These rankings are called "Schedules". "Schedule I" drugs are the most addicting. These are examples of scheduled drugs used in psychiatry:

Schedule I includes drugs that are not only addicting but *very dangerous*, such as LSD, heroin, and GHB (the "date-rape drug").

Schedule II is the most addicting class to which doctors have prescription rights: Ritalin and amphetamines, for example—as well as Methadone and Morphine. This also includes Desoxyn (a/k/a "crystal meth")

Schedule III drugs are less addicting include male hormones, Suboxone (for narcotic addicts), barbiturates, and Marinol (synthetic marijuana for "nausea")

Schedule IV includes the usual assortment of modern and old-time sleeping pills and tranquilizers (valium family drugs, Ambien, Sonata), as well as a few diet pills and stimulants (Provigil, Nuvigil, and Cylert)

Schedule V: Lyrica

"Behind the Counter": Pseudo-ephedrine is mildly stimulating and is also used to make "crystal meth", a dangerous Schedule II amphetamine.

A few drugs which are arguably addicting (they can cause dependence) have recently been changed to addictive status: male hormones, Midrin (for headaches), and Soma (our bodies turn Soma into Miltown which is definitely addicting). The FDA has recently assigned Lyrica to the lowest level of addictiveness (called "Schedule V"). Amyl nitrite, an old heart medication used as a euphoriant, may be classed even lower than that, at "Schedule VI", which is a ranking for drugs that defy any specific definition but might be in need of government oversight.

Drugs which are not controlled but can cause dependence include: Ultram (for chronic pain).

Some of the antidepressants can cause psychological dependence; it is quite difficult for a small percentage of patients to quit these drugs, because they will have "flu"-like symptoms for a week, followed by depression or anxiety. These patients might have psychological dependence or they may simply have chronic depression and anxiety that will need additional treatment. I prefer the latter explanation. Some older people are simply unable to stop these drugs. They have been on these drugs so long, it almost seems that their brains are treating the drug as some kind of "micro-nutrient". Also curiously, if one of these long-term patients is taken off one drug such as Doxepin and given a very similar drug such as Pamelor, the patient may not feel well until given the Doxepin again.

Sometimes patients may need addicting medicines because they need immediate relief: using Xanax for panic attacks is a good example (or using Vicodin short-term for pain control). With addicting drugs, the early treatment phases start out very smoothly, but long-term use of these medications brings a risk of habituation (needing the pill every day) or addiction (needing higher doses of the pill). The risk is greatest for Xanax, a cousin of the Valium family of drugs. The risk is significant for other Valium family drugs, including Ativan. However, Ativan is preferred because it is not long-acting, less likely to interact with other medications, ant not associated with liver problems.

This is the usual course of treatment with addicting drugs: we get off to a quick and easy start but later on have the possibility of addiction. Once addicted to these drugs, the addiction is for life.

1—Induction phase: patient feels much relief —this brief time is probably the best that the patient will ever feel from this medicine. First dose may seem best.

2—Accommodation phase: patient is still feeling good

3—Stabilization phase: the effects of the medicine seem weaker

4—Post-stabilization phase: patient needs more medicine to try to feel better: this is habituation.

5—Alteration phase: the drug is no longer working well and patient feels that he needs more of it: this usually means addiciton.

Prescription-grade amphetamines and psycho-stimulants involve different addiction problems from the tranquilizers (and sleeping pills), and I know of no "emergency" or "urgent need" for amphetamines.

Degrees of Addictiveness:

- Narcotic painkillers are considered the *most addicting*—and among them Fentanyl is the most highly addicting, followed immediately by heroin, methadone, and then morphine:

- Cocaine is quite addicting as are the amphetamines

- *Nicotine* (cigarette) is considered about *as addictive as cocaine.*

- Xanax is next in addicting potential

- The old sedative-hypnotics are addicting and intoxicating They can be fatal in small overdoses (i.e., a one-month supply). You may never hear of these drugs again: Placidyl, Seconal, Noludar, Doriden, et al.

- Halcion was removed from the market in Britain for causing nocturnal confusion. Ambien also seems to cause a similar problem.

- The addicting sleeping pills, minor barbiturates, minor narcotics, and sedatives are somewhat addicting and should be used with respect! This includes Sonata, ProSom, Lunesta, Restoril, Fioricet, Vicodin, et al.

Intermediate Medicines causing psychological dependence to various degrees but little physical dependence (not classified as addictive)

Drugs in this category are highly effective and are *not* addictive but are capable of causing Discontinuation Syndrome. Sometimes a patient has become so well-adjusted to a non-addicting medicine that he has problems stopping it suddenly. This results in what we call "discontinuation syndrome" which is not a real withdrawal since it does not cause physical harm just some physical discomfort for a while. There is no psychic craving for the drug; but patient may feel psychologically symptomatic for many days. Patients can resume these drugs at a later time without problem or take other drugs in the same chemical family without problem—although they will very likely experience discontinuation symptoms again if they stop that medicine again. This discontinuation syndrome may feel like the "flu"; such drugs include:

- Paxil

- Zoloft

- Effexor

- Elavil

- Celexa / Lexapro

- and a few other psychiatric drugs

One patient may experience discontinuation with one drug, e.g. Zoloft but not with Paxil or Effexor, or vice versa. The chances that one patient will get discontinuation symptoms with every drug is unlikely. Unfortunately, we still cannot predict who will get this side effect.

Sometimes, the patient's reasons for wanting to stop the medicine are unfounded, and sometimes the patient stops these medications without talking first to the doctor. Discontinuation syndrome is not so profound that it could drive patients to commit crimes in order to get money to buy more of the drug on the street (which is the case with addicting drugs). If patients are feeling uncomfortable, then I give them some days off work. This whole discontinuation syndrome should be thought of as temporary "flu"-like symptoms. In some cases, the underlying anxiety or depression is still present and the patient may not yet have healed, in which case she should simply resume or continue taking the medicine.

Mechanics of Treatment

Let's take the example of a young woman Stacey who has her first ever episode of anxious depression and is taking Zoloft. She needs to come in for appointments when the doctor indicates. She also needs to remember that treatment is usually individualized for each patient. The mechanics of the actual treatment can be subtle and often vary from doctor to doctor and from patient to patient. Doctors will want to change doses, change medicines, add a new medicine, or change the manner or timing of doses and so on. Sometimes medication treatment can be subtle, and progress may be measured in weeks and months. If eighty-five percent of patients stay in treatment, then approximately eighty-five percent of them should eventually feel better (based on personal observation, my rule of "85%").

Some psychiatric drugs are safe and well tolerated: patients with minor psychological problems typically need only minor benign medicines and not for long time periods, either. Stacey rarely experience serious problems with medications. However, patients with major psychiatric illnesses require major medications to control major psychiatric symptoms. Major medications may be immediately toxic for some patients. In other patients, the drug effects may slowly accumulate and become overtly toxic after many months or years have passed. Immediate side effects and long-term side effects of medications are listed on the package inserts. Package inserts are the printed information that retail pharmacies dispense along with the pills (see chapter V-19). This listing often contains a dizzying array of possible side effects most of which are highly improbable or quite vague and many of the warnings are about as generic as the drugs are. Sometimes the lists are very long. These lists are based on patients' self-reporting of symptoms. If a patient breaks a leg or gets the "flu" while on the medicine, and if any patient reports this during clinical trials, then "broken leg" and "flu" will appear on the package insert as possible side effects. Some of the psychiatric drugs are safer than aspirin and Tylenol. It is important for Stacey to learn about the basic uses of the medicine and a few of the commonest short-term and long-term toxicities (if any). I would discuss this with Stacey before writing her new prescription.

I usually suggest that patients discard these package inserts and talk to me about any concerns.

A typical patient like Stacey will experience trivial side effects and lack of benefit for the first week or two when starting on a new [non-addicting] prescription medicine. After that, she will usually start to feel gradual improvement and then will feel better and better as time goes on—hopefully. Surprisingly, some patients start to feel really good in the first couple days of treatment and then a few days later they report feeling worse and worse. Commonly received wisdom suggests that this latter type of patient is just having "placebo effect" (imagined improvement). However, it may be a real and valid report. It is also plausible that Stacey's body uses the drug very slowly and that it accumulates very quickly in her body, quickly producing very high drug levels which then cause toxic side effects (even though a few drugs have available blood level testing, most do not). It is entirely possible that some patients need only tiny amounts of a drug in order to feel better. (see Chapter II-4)

Danny is a young man who has severe panic-anxiety and started Xanax, which helped him on the first day. Xanax use needs monitoring by both the doctor and the patient. The best way for Danny to monitor the Xanax is to receive feedback from the prescriber at every office visit. Danny should also try to feel what his body is telling him about the Xanax. If not, he might fall into Xanax addiction. This is how the progression works: once Danny crosses over into addiction, he can never make himself un-addicted. He can never "come back" from the addiction or undo the addiction. If he stops before he crosses that threshold, then he will not suffer addiction at that time. Once arrived at the threshold, however, all bets are off.

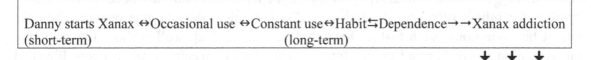

Danny starts Xanax ↔Occasional use ↔Constant use↔Habit⇆Dependence→→Xanax addiction
(short-term)   (long-term)

Xanax addiction will now result in cross-addiction with all the drugs in the Valium family (Klonopin)

Flow-chart I-7-e Patient Reactions to Addicting Medicines

Flow-chart I-7-e Patient Reactions to Addicting Medicines

Herbs

Some patients believe that herbal remedies are better. Sometimes I do recommend herbs for a certain person (St. John's Wort). Resorting to the use of herbs is really no better at all since each herbal dose contains dozens or hundreds of plant chemicals which are even less familiar and have not even been extensively or scientifically studied. And have not been vetted by the FDA. The herbal plant's growing conditions (soil, sunshine, rain, air, fertilizer) can alter the herbal contents quite a bit, too. Herbs usually receive recommendation by word of mouth and from millennia of usage without any significant toxicity. Some herbs should not be mixed with certain pharmaceuticals. Herbs lack rigorous scientific background studies since they are mostly sold without a prescription. Valeriana is a habit-forming herb. Kava kava and khatt can be habit-forming, also. Herbs come from plants. Certain plant products are addicting, such as tobacco, cocaine, opium, and coffee.

The Law and Pharmacology

All Prescription medications have a legal classification as well as a chemical classification. The addicting and habit-forming drugs require a written prescription. At issue is the propensity of the medicine to promote violence or lead to illegal behaviors. This has little to do with the physical chemistry of the medication. Medical scientists have a different take on these medications from that of legalists.

Summary

Among the addicting medicines, narcotics are usually considered most addicting. Nicotine also falls into this category. Sedatives and sleeping pills can become somewhat habit-forming for some patients (psychological dependence) and may become very habit-forming for others (physical dependence). Psychological dependence occurs when the patient has symptoms such that he feels that he cannot sleep well without the medicine but otherwise is not harmed except for a couple days or weeks of poor sleep. Physical dependence is more serious and means that his body has uncomfortable physical signs of withdrawal such as tremors or impending seizures. We cannot yet predict who will become addicted. Once a person has become addicted to that drug, he will remain addicted to it forever—and probably to all the drugs in the same chemical family as that of the addicting drug.

▶▶QUESTION

Q: How do I know if a drug is addictive or habit-forming?

A: Addictive drugs are all classed legally as controlled substances: "C-II", "C-III', "C-IV", or "C-V". The "C–" designation means that the drug is controlled (addicting). The

Roman numeral ranks it as to how highly desirable (addicting) it is and, hence, how much it is controlled. Access to controlled drugs is controlled by doctors and the government. (C-I drugs are not available to the general public and include LSD, Quaaludes, ecstasy, marijuana, heroin, et al). Non-addicting drugs are signaled by the symbol "Rx".

Q: Are certain people addiction prone while others are not?
A: This is not clear. And studies would be impossible to conduct. Perhaps anyone can become addicted to addicting drugs if taking enough medicine for long periods. In 19th Century America when narcotics were available without a prescription, estimates of habituation and addiction ran as high as two-thirds of the population.

---

* animals other than mice may be used depending upon their anatomic and/or physiologic similarities to Man: dogs for narcolepsy and vascular studies, pigs for heart valves, rabbits for dermatology, etc. The importance of humane treatment cannot be over-emphasized.

Section II
The Brain and its Chemistry

Superscript numbers refer to references and citations at the back of the book

Chapter II-1

BRAIN and its STRUCTURE

This chapter provides background information on the physical aspects of the brain: its size and appearance. This is anatomy. Neurologists and neurosurgeons are concerned with brain anatomy.

Psychiatry focuses on the electrochemical activity of the brain (see Chapter II-2).

Basic Terminology:

Brain	Cerebro- Cerebello- (this means "little cerebro-") Encephalo- (this means "in the cephalo-")
Nerve	Neuro-
Head Skull	Cephalo- Cranio-

These have the same meaning Brain "structure" = anatomy	Abnormalities Abnormal structure = physical disorder (tumor, blood clot)
	lesion, defect, injury*
Brain "function" = physiology	Abnormal function = electrochemical disorder ("short circuit")

* the terms "lesion, defect, injury" can be either physical or electrochemical

Human brain / Animal brain

Our brains (and nervous system) are similar to the brains of the "higher mammals" such as dogs, pigs, cats, raccoons, dolphins, and monkeys. Our brain works like theirs as far as walking, running, vocalizing, feeding, mating, socializing, and balancing. This is not surprising since we are all "higher mammals". However, we humans seem to excel at more sophisticated and complicated brain exercises. As far as memory, cleverness, social cues, and responses, some animal researchers note that dogs and pigs operate at the level of a small child and that some chimpanzees can communicate with their trainers by learning a few hundred "words". Dogs can be very astute time-keepers—how do they do that? Cats outrank us by having a relatively larger cerebellum (brain center of acrobatic grace). Some animals may show artistic tendencies such as dolphins who blow air-rings, not air bubbles (youtube.com/watch?v=bT.fctr32pE). Yet we do seem to share with mammals the same basic wiring plan for the brain and nervous system. This can be seen by dissecting cadavers of humans and animals. Undergraduate anatomy students may verify that a cat brain is quite similar to ours. Two differences are apparent, however, in the human brain. Firstly, humans have brains larger in proportion to body size than do animals. Secondly, our cerebrum is relatively larger: these relative enlargements correlate to language control and to the front of the brain, the latter of which appears to house the centers of decision-making, planning, self-control, and judgment (although any superiority of these latter two functions often seems debatable in humans). Like us, animals clearly have emotions, do love their offspring, and have awareness. Animals have sleep cycles like ours complete with REM sleep (Chapter V-13). Some reports suggest that REM sleep extends down through all mammals and that even chickens have very primitive REM sleep. Dogs show shame and happiness and—like us—suffer from epilepsy and narcolepsy (suddenly falling asleep) as well as other neurological disorders. Whether animals have human-type self-awareness is still under study. I tend to view animals as if they were feral children instead of beasts who—if given enough time, support, and opportunity—might perhaps one day amaze us all with their fully realized potential. Conversely, it sometimes seems as if we are little more than big beasts (read about bonobos). We are all just one part of the biological continuum, and that applies to the nervous systems that we all hold in common.

Brain Basics

The brain is made up of billions of nerve cells all of which need to contact each other in order to interact. They are like very short wires and micro-circuits in a wiring diagram. They have direct and indirect interconnections among themselves. With direct interconnection, they actually touch each other; with indirect, they have a tiny gap between themselves, as in a sparkplug. Electrical and chemical information can be sent from nerve to nerve across this gap. Thus the nerves relay information to the brain, the brain makes decisions, and then the nerves send return messages in the form of muscular activity (speech and action). All this information exchange is done thanks to our internal electrical wiring. The nerves act like our internal Information Technology system. The nervous system receives important information from the "outside world" but also receives messages from inside our bodies. It also manages information from different areas inside the brain itself. After receiving information, the brain then processes the information and actualizes a plan of response—or of delayed response or even of non-response, depending upon the circumstances.

The brain is the main control center for the whole nervous system. The activity of the brain is due to electrochemical activity inside the nerve cells. The brain never really stops working (does not turn itself off) but is able to "relax" as demonstrated by its decreased electrical activity while in slow-wave sleep or watching television (see next chapter).

a—stimulation from outside the body} ⬎ .. .. .. ↪ {	reactive response
b—messages from inside the body} → . . . ↗⬨ . . ⇉ {	delayed response
c—messages from inside the brain} ↗ . . . brain . . ↳ {	no response

In this diagram, the nerves are relaying information back and forth, to and from the brain ↗⬨. For example, the sense of sight starts behind the eyeballs in the front of the head at the optic nerve (which is really an outgrowth of the brain and not a separate nerve); however, the processing of the sensation of sight actually occurs at the back of the head in a part of the brain furthest removed from the eyes. The brain decides how it wants to handle the new information: to respond, to wait and see, or ignore the information totally. A more complete picture is this one showing actualized results:

a—stimulation from outside the body} ⬎ . . . . ↪ {inside to body (swallow)
. . . . . .(kissing)
b—messages from inside the body } → . ↗⬨ sends ⇉ {inside brain (think/recall)
. . . .(light-headedness)
c—messages from inside the brain } ↗ . . brain . . . . ↳ {outside body (move, act)
. . . .(joy)

Brain Structure

Structurally, the brain is a large lumpy organ which contains a lot of fatty substance. It does not move—unlike the heart. The size of the brain does not necessarily control intelligence. Large brain size might correspond more or less to intelligence, musicality, and greater musculature. However, Einstein's brain was relatively small. Neanderthals had brains larger than ours. Of course, Neanderthals had double or triple our muscle mass. The extra large brain size probably represents more brain area needed to control this greater amount of muscle mass and may not shed any light at all on their intellectual capabilities. Birds are notorious for having really small brains, yet parrots and crows are smart, and migratory birds possess a special magnetic alignment sense that enables them to find their winter havens and summer nests (this is a whole sense that we lack).

Primary psychiatric illness by its very definition is not a structural illness. In other words, Schizophrenia, Panic-anxiety, and Bipolar do not show up as anatomical abnormalities on CATScans or skull X-rays. Modern psychiatry does not typically diagnose structural diseases of the brain. In other words, we do not typically interpret CATScans or skull X-rays to make any psychiatric diagnosis. However, there are many structural diseases of the brain that have a set of well-known psychiatric disturbances that appear as a direct cause of the structural defect. These are anatomically abnormal conditions with secondary psychiatric symptoms. Examples are the psychiatric symptoms that result from strokes, closed head injury, and diseases such as lupus or multiple sclerosis. Neurologists and neuroradiologists read the CATScans and X-Rays and that tells us which structural disease exists, and thus which set of psychiatric symptoms to expect.

Our brain is such an important organ that it is protected by several kinds of complete coverings to keep out germs and protect it from physical injury. The outermost layer is the skin of the scalp and its underlying tendons ("galea") that cover the hard bone of the skull. Inside the skull are three more enveloping layers called the meninges, which surround the brain to keep out germs and large chemicals. Thus, surgical invasion of the brain requires a lot of hard work done very carefully. Fortunately, this kind of invasion occurs rarely and hopefully through the easiest access points so as to cause the least damage. Apart from emergencies or disabling diseases, surgery on the brain structure is rare.These are examples of such invasion:

    a.) "Psychosurgery" for functional disorders: Cutting the front part of the brain has a calming effect on very agitated or violent patients. This is the infamous lobotomy which is no longer used. Another rare surgical treatment involves cutting the thalamus.

    b.) Brain surgery (Neurosurgery) for surgical conditions such as brain tumors;

    c.) Treatment-Diagnosis of Neurological disorders:

        (i) Removing a tiny piece of the brain is called brain biopsy and may be used to establish a diagnosis in serious rare brain diseases.

        (ii) Implanting healthy nerve cells into the brains of Parkinsonian patients is being studied.

        (iii) Removing diseased parts of the brain to regulate epileptic seizures—done only under special circumstances and in highly skilled neurosurgical centers.

        (iv)Spinal tap to diagnose neurological conditions (this does not impinge on the brain but does cut through the meninges and thus makes direct contact with the fluid that bathes the brain)

The only way of correcting structural brain problems is to cut the brain or remove part of it—this is part of brain surgery (neurosurgery) and not of psychiatry. Modern psychiatry does not include any of these above circumstances. Modern psychiatry does take structural injury into account when making diagnoses.

Brain Functioning and Activity

This topic has much relevance to psychiatric diagnosis and treatment as we understand it. The brain's abnormal electrochemical activity can be detected and used to make a diagnosis. The brain's electrochemical activity is frequently the focus of treatment in psychiatry. Most psychiatric diagnoses are based on the history of the illness as well as symptoms. Most of these diagnoses do not require specialized testing; however, some or many of them may show abnormal results on CATScan, MRI, PETScan, blood tests, or PSG (see below). We still do not have a reliable standardized system for making a specific psychiatric diagnosis, but this will probably become the standard practice in the near future. PETScan shows us the electrochemical activity level of the brain, specifically if the brain is functioning at a normal rate, slowly, or not at all. PETScan will probably become our primary imaging study, but its use is still restricted to university researchers who have obtained amazing images of the electrochemical defects of Alzheimers, schizophrenia, mania, and amphetamine addiction.

Electrical activity can also be used for diagnostic purposes in sleep disorders. In order to diagnose sleep disorders we have the patient spend the night in the sleep lab. During the night, we make a complicated electrical tracing of the brain's abnormal functioning. This tracing is the PSG (polysomnogram). The PSG may help diagnose abnormal sleep. Neurologists diagnose epilepsy by recording electrical waves called EEG (electroencephalogram).

For the average case, psychiatric diagnosis does not much rely on such high-tech backup, and current psychiatric diagnosis presumes that there is a known (or knowable through PETScan) electrochemical defect. Thus modern treatments represent attempts to normalize abnormal functional activity by using electrochemical means. We use electricity in the form of shock treatments, and we have chemicals in the form medications and herbs. Both of these are primary treatments and have direct effects on the brain's electrochemical activities. Apart from these primary treatments, secondary treatments can have indirect effects on electrochemical activity. This would include such treatments as aerobic exercise, biofeedback, and talk therapy (see Chapter II-2).

Magnetism is a physical force that is becoming a new type of treatment. Magnetism is already available as a diagnostic tool, Magnetic Resonance Imaging (MRI).

II-1-a	Functional		Physical-Structural	
	Electrical	Chemical		Magnetism

Diagnostic tools	PSG*	PETScan	CATScan	MRI
Treatment means	ECT	Medication	**	Transcranial MR

*PSG is an electric wave sleep test; ** no such treatment is routinely available

Primary psychiatric illness by its very definition is a functional illness and not a structural illness. Schizophrenia, Panic-anxiety, and Bipolar do not show up as highly specific abnormalities on CATScans or skull X-rays. For the time being, we shall continue to make diagnoses in our traditional low-tech manner while eagerly awaiting new standardized high-tech testing methods.

Brain Layout

Our brain—like the brain of most mammals—has the same basic layout:
   1—the *forebrain* which contains the:
      a—cerebrum, the area where planning, decision-making, and conscious intellectual activity occurs; and,
      b—the "between" brain, i.e. the part that connects the forebrain to the midbrain and acts as a major relay center to coordinate incoming messages to and outgoing messages from the cerebrum; this is the location of the thalamus that has certain "activating" functions;
   2—the *midbrain*, a central receiving and dispatch area for nerve signals
   3—the *hindbrain* which is involved in basic functions of living and also it houses the cerebellum (meaning "little brain" in Latin) which is involved in balance, locomotion, mechanical grace, and coordination. The hindbrain connects the whole brain to the spinal chord which in turn connects the whole body to the brain.

As far as special senses:
   1—the forebrain processes the sense of smell detected by Cranial Nerve I
   2—The midbrain receives visual input from the eyes, Cranial Nerve II
   3—The hindbrain receives sound and voices from the ear via Cranial Nerve VIII
(Cranial nerves I & II are actually modified extensions of the brain substance itself, whereas C.N. VIII is one real nerve, but it has two parts:)

The forebrain (cerebrum) of primitive animals is very simple or rudimentary to the point that it is only a few layers of tiny nerves: this is the case in fish and amphibians. Reptiles have a more substantial cerebrum. In land mammals, the cerebrum can be large depending upon the type of animal. Humans, of course, have the largest forebrain relative to body size. So too, do intelligent animals such as dogs, pigs, cats, dolphins, chimpanzees, orangutans, and bonobos. Size, however, may not matter so much when we consider that certain breeds of dogs are more trainable than others. Furthermore, some birds are considered to be quite clever despite having brains relatively smaller than those of the mammals listed above: corvids (crow family) and psittacids (parrot family).

The following schematic representation shows the ever enlarging forebrain of various animals from that of small primitive creatures up to that of man. In higher animals, the cerebrum increases in size relative to intelligence and agility.

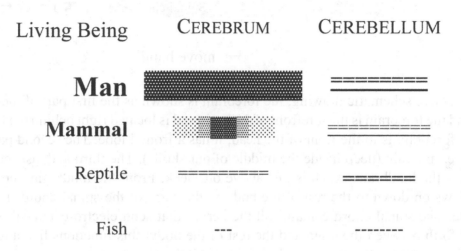

Table II-1-b   ever-enlarging forebrain

In the fishes, the cerebrum of the forebrain is shown as a dotted line suggesting that the cerebrum and cerebellum are hardly even present. Reptiles do have a tangible cerebrum and cerebellum, but their craftiness is limited mainly to improved and clever food gathering techniques. In the mammals we see that they have the same amount of cerebrum and cerebellum as do the fish and reptiles but it is also expanded to include special intelligence lacking in reptiles and fish. Mammals have all the brain power of reptiles plus a lot more. What is said of the cerebrum can also be said of the cerebellum: it is simple in fish, medium-sized in birds and most complex in mammals (especially in graceful animals such as cats). The cerebellum enables Man to do gymnastics, for example. Man, of course, has all the cerebrum and cerebellum and intelligence of mammals plus additional human attributes.

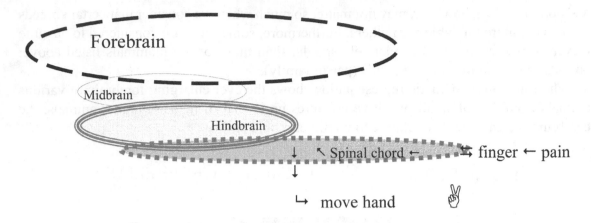

In the above schematic drawing, the forebrain is shown as the first part of the nervous system and the forebrain is the forefront of the brain and is located right behind the forehead. Since the forebrain is in the front of the head, it has a frontal lobe. The second part of the brain is the midbrain (deep inside the middle of our skulls). The third and last segment of the brain is the hindbrain which is just above our neck. From the hindbrain, the nervous system flows on down to the rest of the body in the form of the spinal chord inside our back bone. The spinal chord contains all the nerves that send electro-chemical messages back and forth between the brain and the rest of the body: this functions like a telephone line sending messages to and fro, back and forth. All the messages from the brain that flow back down to the body will tell the body what to do in response to the messages that the body has sent up to the brain to be processed. The brain is giving directions or expressing its response. The brain may choose no response as a response.

Some messages stay inside the nervous system and interconnect the parts of the nervous system to itself (⇆). The messages going up to the brain (shown by arrow ←) are usually sensory messages involving one of the senses: smell, taste, vision, touch or hearing; but may also involve information about equilibrium, vibration, position sense, or other sensations such as stomach acidity. The brain will process these incoming data and make a decision plan and then send that message back down the spinal chord (shown by arrow →) to tell the body how to respond to the message that the body had just sent up to the brain. If you burn your finger then a pain signal goes up the nerves to the spinal chord and then up into the brain which will (hopefully) send a signal back down the spinal chord to tell the hand to remove the finger from the hot object. Drugs that slow the up-going pain signals (belladonna) or drugs that slow the down-going response messages (anesthetic drugs, muscle relaxers) can result in the finger being exposed for a longer time to the heat, resulting in a burnt finger. Drugs that slow the brain in processing this information can also result in a burnt finger (for example: narcotics, marijuana, major tranquilizers).

A diseased brain might make the wrong choices—this is what happens in neurological and psychiatric disorders. The brain makes the wrong decision for some reason: either its "wires are crossed" or a small part of it has deteriorated (caused by street drugs, Parkinsonism, stroke, untreated schizophrenia, and so on). This is a cardinal feature of nervous disorders.

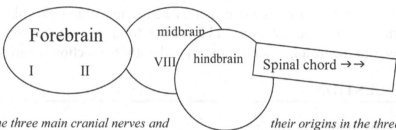

Figure II-1-d   This depicts the three main cranial nerves and their origins in the three parts of the brain: I—Olfactory (for smell)   II—Optic (visual)   VIII—acoustic (for hearing and balance). The part of the brain that extends into the body is the spinal chord (nerves II and VIII are more complicated than shown.)
Anatomically, the cranial nerves are numbered from I to XII; however, functionally, some of them represent a merging of two or more of the original cranial nerves.

Figure II-1-d   This depicts the three main cranial nerves and their origins in the three parts of the brain: I—Olfactory (for smell)   II—Optic (visual)   VIII—acoustic (for hearing and balance). The part of the brain that extends into the body is the spinal chord (nerves II and VIII are more complicated than shown.)
Anatomically, the cranial nerves are numbered from I to XII; however, functionally, some of them represent a merging of two or more of the original cranial nerves.

Figure II-1-d shows three of the important cranial nerves. These three nerves correspond to the senses of smell, vision, and hearing, respectively. Each of these three nerves has its own central receiving area in a part of the brain. Visions coming in via Nerve II go to the "Optical Center" (visual cortex) where the brain interprets that vision. The same happens with other cranial nerves. Real stimuli from the real world travel into the brain via these nerves. However, hallucinations of taste, vision, and hearing do not travel into the psychotic brain from the external world, but they do affect the brain centers exactly as if they were coming from the outside world. A psychotic person cannot distinguish if the source of the hallucinations is inside his brain or traveling in from the external world via cranial nerves I, II, or VIII. Hallucinations of touch would be perceived in the brain as if they were entering the brain as a real stimulus as shown in figure II-1-b.

Psychiatry and the Brain

Psychiatrists study the treatment of altered behaviors, which we tend to treat as if they are rooted in the physical organ of the brain. We believe that the altered behaviors are coming from an alteration in the electro-chemical activity of the brain, but we also believe that this altered electro-chemical activity is linked to microscopic alterations of the structure of nerve cells. Unlike neurologists, we are also very concerned about how negative environments, ugly memories, and childhood traumas can influence the electrochemical activity and thus permanently change the status of brain functioning. All evidence so far shows that the brain is the center of neurological and psychiatric events. The brain has both structure and function, and there are different branches of medicine that deal with its structure (neurology, brain surgery) and with its function (neurology and psychiatry).

▶QUESTION

Q: Who studies the brain?
A: Both psychiatrists and neurologists study the brain.

Psychiatry was once a branch or subspecialty of neurology. Sigmund Freud had been trained as a neurologist and was in contact with the famous European neurologists of that time. His studies of psychoanalysis divided the brain into three abstract parts: id, ego, and superego; however, these three parts did not really correspond to the anatomy of the brain, but rather to its mental activities. Neurologists study alterations in the physical structure of the brain. They also study how these alterations can affect the measurable electrical activity of the brain and how that can result in poor functioning of the brain, whereas psychiatrists are concerned more with the presumed effects of biochemical brain alterations that produce extremes of behavior. Nonetheless, the two specialties of neurology and psychiatry still share much in common. There are a number of medications that are shared and used equally by both professions.

Q: Why did Neanderthals have brains larger than ours?
A: The extra brain area was probably devoted to centers of muscle control: they had much larger muscles than do we.

Chapter II-2

The Brain and its Electro-Chemical Functioning
ECT (Shock Treatments)
(this material is presented with simplifications)

Material presented in this chapter is optional information.

The structure (anatomy) of the nervous system was presented in the preceding chapter II-1. This chapter concerns the function of the nervous system. The nervous system is just like every other organ system of our body in that the nervous system has structure and function that have both adapted to each other. Every organ in our body has a specific structure associated with its specific function. The heart is in charge of pumping blood around the body; the liver detoxifies environmental poisons that get into our bodies; and, the nervous system and brain are in charge of keeping us aware of our environment, helping us to react to needs, promoting our well-being, and of course, expressing emotions and thoughts. This chapter concerns the way that nerves function to keep us in a relatively normal state of mental health. By understanding normal brain structure and function, we can learn about all the things that can go wrong. Although abnormal structure can cause secondary psychiatric symptoms, psychiatry is primarily interested in abnormal function of the brain which causes primary symptoms.

The nervous system functions as the Information Technology center of our body. This function is facilitated by an enormous number of nerves and nervous networks, and these are braided together to shape the very complex "wiring diagram" of our body that transmits messages to and from the brain. Nerve function is electrochemically based. Chemical changes in nerves cause transmission of electrical activity that in turn causes further chemical changes to alter the electric potential of nerves. Under normal circumstances, the electric potential flows normally, but in abnormal states, it may not. Under normal circumstances, there are certain biochemicals that act mainly on the surface of nerves and a different set of biochemicals that act mainly inside the nerves. The surface biochemicals (○○○) are made inside our bodies for the purpose of affecting the surface of our nerves. The biochemicals inside the nerve (⌇) help the nerves to be ready for information transmission. Altogether, the surface biochemicals, inside biochemicals, and electrical activity work together to transmit information through the nervous system up to the brain, inside the brain, or down from the brain.

(The surface biochemicals (○○○) help promote rapid electrochemical transmission. These biochemicals are usually hormones or neurotransmitters. Hormones can be of many general types. However, the neurotransmitters are usually purpose-made for this special nerve function; there are a few main neurotransmitters such as serotonin, norepinephrine, dopamine, GABA, glutamate, and others that will be covered in Section IV.)

Information may be relayed electrochemically from one nerve to a second nerve downstream, then to a third nerve and so on. A second way to transfer information is chemically only, such as letting the surface biochemicals "leak" to various nearby nerves resulting in a cascade of information transmission spreading out like a pool of liquid biochemical. These are two methods of sending messages by relay and cascade.

In psychiatry, the nerves of the brain are not functioning normally. There may be excess electrical activity leading to a "brown-out" or "short-circuit", or there may be too little electrical activity, resulting in depression. Likewise, there may often be shortages of surface biochemicals or of inside biochemicals. Sometimes there are excesses of some of these biochemicals. In other cases, an outside biochemical (●●●) may upset normal nerve function. These outside biochemicals are then called "poisons"—or toxins or venoms. There are so many opportunities for electrochemical disturbances in the nerves that it is amazing they can function at all.

these are the Terms and Symbols used in this Chapter

●●● chemicals from outside the body (drugs, poisons, venom, toxins)
⁄⁄ electrical activity of the nervous system
○○○ surface biochemicals (hormones, neurotransmitters)

⌁ inside biochemicals made inside the nerve
════╧════ first nerve   ⫴────── second nerve

The nerves have two ways of contacting each other: direct or indirect. With direct contact [A], the nerves touch each other directly ⁄⁄ like wires connected directly to each other. The second type of contact is indirect [B]. In the case of indirect contact, two nerves do not lie in direct contact with each other; instead, the nerves are separated by microscopically small gaps that cannot be bridged by electrical activity. These gaps must be bridged by biochemical messengers ○○○, which are usually neurotransmitters (or hormones). The neurotransmitters are released by electrochemical messages from inside the nerve.

direct _**electrical**_ contact between two nerves	With indirect _**electrochemical**_ contact, there is a small gap between the two nerves: first nerve can squirt chemicals into the gap in order to complete contact with second nerve
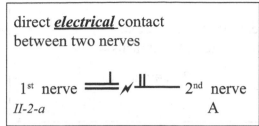 *II-2-a* A	1st nerve ═══ooo══ 2nd nerve B

For the rest of this chapter, I will not differentiate whether the contact is direct electrical or indirect electrochemical, since the outcome is the same: namely that of activating the second nerve. I shall show this general nerve-to-nerve contact as:

II-2-b	1st nerve ═══𝒩 ooo═══ 2nd nerve

First nerves often respond to an internal message 〰 which is what really orders them to pass on electrical activity 𝒩 or to release a chemical neurotransmitter message (nt) ooo

1st nerve has its own internal chemical orders
1st nerve ══〰══𝒩 ooo═══ 2nd nerve

Furthermore, first nerves may receive electrical 𝒩 or biochemical impulses ooo coming from further upstream. It may also be activated by an outside chemical such as a poison or a drug ●●●. Any of these impulses may release first nerves' own internal chemical commands 〰, which result in first nerves' release of neurotransmitters or transmission of electrical activity, thereby causing electrochemical effects on the second nerves.

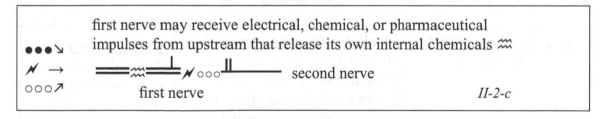

first nerve may receive electrical, chemical, or pharmaceutical impulses from upstream that release its own internal chemicals 〰

●●●↘
𝒩 →   ══〰══𝒩 ooo═══ second nerve
ooo↗   first nerve   *II-2-c*

As a result of first nerves' activities, the second nerves can experience their own internal chemical orders and go on to release their own neurotransmitters ooo or electrical 𝒩 impulses that pass further downstream to third or fourth nerves.

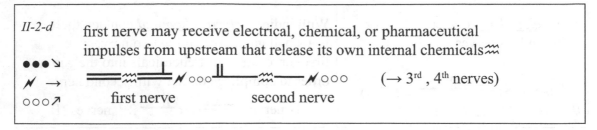

II-2-d   first nerve may receive electrical, chemical, or pharmaceutical
impulses from upstream that release its own internal chemicals〰

first nerve   second nerve   (→ 3rd , 4th nerves)

Thus, we can see that electrical activity can trigger chemical activity and vice versa. The nerves function as a result of a complicated electrochemical interplay.

Expanded explanation for those who are especially interested
(the casual reader can skip down to the next section, if so desired)

The brain and nervous system operate by electro-chemical activity that basically consists of impulses jumping from nerve to nerve. When the electrical impulse goes from a first nerve to a second nerve, the impulse can cause any or all of three possible responses in the second nerve. The second nerve can release biochemicals inside itself. It can release chemicals outside itself in the form of neurotransmitters (nt). The second nerve also has the option of passing the electrical message on to a third nerve. Electrical activity ultimately consists of interacting with each other by changing electrical charges.

Direct electrical contact between two nerves can be by direct nerve-to-nerve contact [A], like two bare wires crossing each other.

Electrochemical relay refers to the fact that the first nerve recives an impulse that prompts the first nerve to squirt chemicals into a tiny gap or boundary between themselves (like a spark-plug gap).

II-2-e   three methods of nerve-to-nerve communication

direct electrical contact between two nerves	with ***electrochemical relay***, there is a small gap between the two nerves: first nerve can squirt chemicals into the gap in order to complete contact with second nerve	***chemical cascade*** chemicals come from elsewhere
first nerve second nerve A	1st nerve ⚊○○○⚊ 2nd nerve B	○○○ C ○○○ 1st nerve 2nd nerve

1st nerve = first nerve   _2nd nerve = second nerve_   _(X= inactive)_
represents direct nerve-to-nerve contact   _represents electrical activity of any kind_
represents surface biochemicals (neurotransmitter,"nt") represents biochemicals inside nerve the second nerves could react to by activating a third nerve

With chemical cascade [C], the chemicals come from elsewhere—maybe even from outside the brain—and act directly on second nerve; the first nerve is not involved in any way.

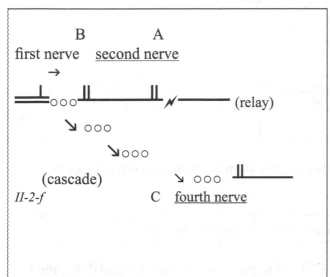

In this diagram we can see all three types of nerve contact:
[B] Electrochemical Relay where 1st nerve spurts chemicals into gap → to activate 2nd nerve

[A] Direct electrical contact: The 2nd nerve makes direct contact with

[C] Chemical Cascade: some chemicals from 1st nerve leak ↘ to activate a nearby 4th nerve

figure II-2-f

Any of these events can change the chemicals inside or on the surface of the second nerve. Second nerve can go even further by producing its own suite of chemicals that it then sends out to a third nerve. The nervous system also has ways to control all this electrochemical activity, otherwise the nerves might constantly be activating each other like a short-circuit: we would feel "wired" and then frayed and then browned-out!

Electrical Effects

These are the effects of nerves touching each other directly. The first nerve has been stimulated to emit an electrical signal to the second nerve. The second nerve can pass on the electrical contact directly to a third nerve.

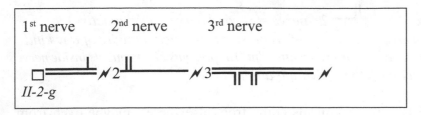

The next diagram shows more detail. Each one of the nerves has its own internal chemicals ∿ that propagate the electrical signal ⚡ on down the line. These inside chemicals may also trigger the release of outside chemicals ○○○.

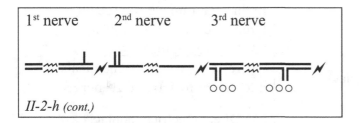

Thus, we can see that electrical signals can pass along nerves as electrical impulses that can also release internal chemicals.

Electrochemical Relays and Chemical Cascades

The electrochemical effects can be a RELAY to pass one chemical signal down the line from first nerve to second nerve to third nerve.

RELAY Function

Chemicals from 1ˢᵗ nerve○○○ go to
II-2-j

2ⁿᵈ nerve is activated∿to send○○○

to

Or the chemical effect can be a cascade that leaks out chemicals to nearby nerves.

```
Chemicals from 1st nerve
Leak out to
  ○○○
          ○○○  to
          ○○○  to
          ○○○  to
```

Researchers believe that surface biochemicals ○○○ (neurotransmitters, also called "brain hormones") control moods, anxiety-panic, and thoughts. To this end the pharmaceutical companies have invested trillions of dollars in trying to develop drugs that act on these "brain hormones", some of which are:

- dopamine (DA) promotes euphoria, motivation, pleasure, and sense of well-being

- noradrenalin (NA) produces energy, activity, and readiness

- GABA, a derivative of butyric acid that exerts anti-anxiety properties

- Glutamic acid/glutamate

- serotonin (5-HT) decreases depressive ruminating and obsessing

Serotonin is an important brain chemical that is made from the amino-acid Tryptophan which is part of the food we eat. For unknown reasons, the brain may lose some of its ability to manufacture Tryptophan, and the levels of serotonin may decrease. Although turkey and milk are well-known to contain Tryptophan, increasing the intake of these foods will not correct clinical depression. Nonetheless, intake of Tryptophan should not be discouraged.

Brain Functioning, Activity, and Treatments

(also see chart II-1-a) relevance to psychiatric diagnosis and treatment:

Functionally, the brain acts somewhat like a car battery: it operates by electro-chemical processes, which is to say that the brain has electrical activity and chemical activity (biochemical activity). Changes in the brain function can be slow or fast. Non-addicting drugs (antidepressants) can take weeks or months to effect noticeable changes in the brain's chemical activity—which may be long-lasting or only temporary changes. However, if a person takes a highly addicting drug such as methamphetamine, then we can see immediate changes in his brain—the P.E.T.Scan image will show alterations in functional activity, but no apparent change in brain structure (anatomy). This is an outline of the brain's electrochemical activity:

- Chemical function
  1—used for diagnosis (PETScan)
  2—used for treatment (pills, chemicals, medications, drugs)
- Electrical function
  1—used in diagnosis (PSG for sleep disorders; EEG in epilepsy)
  2—used in Treatment (ECT, Electro-Convulsive Therapy)

Diagnosis by chemical brain function is rather limited and is still being researched. It is available in large medical research centers in the form of "PETScan". It can be useful for analyzing Alzheimer's Dementia .Hopefully PETScan can be popularized soon.

Treatment of chemical dysfunction consists of the therapeutic consumption of outside chemicals (●●●), in other words: herbs, drugs, and minerals. These outside chemicals presumably correct functional brain abnormalities. This is the primary treatment for brain disorders nowadays and apparently acts like the addition of recharging chemicals (medications) to the brain. There are more than a hundred medicines available now for neurological and psychiatric disorders. These medicines have many different purposes and sometimes some of them will help some people with some conditions but not others. Sometimes a patient will need to try a variety of medicines before finding the ideal medication or the effective combination of medicines. Patients who have received a PETScan before and after medication treatment demonstrate significant functional chemical changes as a result of taking outside chemicals (medications). The patients report feeling much better, so it seems that chemicals are helpful for treatment of some psychiatric patients with biochemical irregularities.

Diagnsosis by electrical activity ↗ of the brain uses a machine called an EEG. This is a way of detecting abnormal brain wave electricity. EEG is painless and has no side effects. The technique of EEG consists of putting little electrical sensors all over the head and then measuring the origins and flow and pathways of electrical activity in the brain. These sensors can also be left in place all night and used to study normal or abnormal sleep patterns. The overnight recordings plus other electrical data result in a tracing called the PSG used to diagnose sleep disorders.

Treatment of electrical (electrochemical) dysfunction is of interest to psychiatry. It is believed that depression occurs when the "brain-battery" has lost a lot of its charge and needs to be "recharged". This can be accomplished by passing charged waves of electricity through the brain, which is called ECT (electroconvulsive therapy), also known as "shock treatment". ECT usually can be quite therapeutic but may result in some memory loss. In the past, ECT had received a lot of negative publicity, but like all other mechanical devices, it has been steadily upgraded and refined so that it is now an excellent treatment for a tiny number of appropriately chosen patients. It is reserved for use in cases that have failed trials of many medications. Such cases would include severe depression, mania, or psychotic depression (anecdotally, ECT will also suppress the symptomatic trembling of Parkinson's disease for a while, possibly by releasing a surge of stored Dopamine). The ECT delivery device has advanced in the last fifty years, as have other machines. Because of all the negative publicity, ECT is no longer readily available to most of the chronic mentally ill, and is not covered by Medicaid. This strange turn of events means that ECT is now available only to the wealthy who have superlative health insurance.

Addendum on SHOCK TREATMENTS: technique and rationale

It has been known since the sixteenth century that psychotic behavior is improved after an epileptic seizures [ref.3-p.2129] , but it has only been since the 1930's that we have been able to deliver electrical shock treatments to the brain (Drs. Cerletti and Bini). The electrical discharge causes a convulsion, similar to a convulsion seen in epilepsy. Shock treatment is now called Electro-Convulsive Therapy (ECT). Any substance that is capable of delivering a controllable convulsion is therapeutic. Originally, camphor was used, but was not adequately controlled. Insulin has also been used to lower blood sugar to the point of causing a convulsion. Electricity is the current method. Original ECT caused violent muscle contractions, which could often lead to broken bones, which is no longer a problem due to new modernized techniques. As a result, modern ECT can be stronger than a true epileptic seizure, and in this way can enhance treatment outcome.

This is how it works: Gwen is a sixty year old woman who has recurrent psychotic depressions and has become so ill that she is delusional; she has dropped from 160 pounds to 105. Over the last twenty years, she has tried most antidepressants, including a couple that were mailed in from Europe. This is her third episode and she is having all the same symptoms as before. The symptoms are getting worse with each depression. She wants ECT again, which had helped her a lot after the second episode a few years ago. Gwen will receive an electrical shock to her brain that will cause the brain to have its own electrical discharges. Nowadays Gwen will be given drugs to paralyze her muscles briefly so that she does not have muscle contractions that would otherwise cause fractured bones. ECT will also impair her breathing muscles temporarily, so she is given breathing assistance. Also, a short-acting anesthesia medicine is given. It is desirable to have both an anesthetist and a psychiatrist do ECT together. The main risks now are from the anesthetic medicines—and the possibility of some mild memory loss. The typical patient is already old or elderly. It is rare for young depressives to be incapacitated to this degree. Obviously, ECT is a treatment of last resort, but it can save lives where all drugs have failed.

Gwen is outfitted with a non-conducting "diadem" around her head. Two electrodes spaced somewhat apart are connected to the diadem. The electricity will flow through her brain between the two electrodes since that is the most direct route to complete the electrical circuit. The button is pushed and the electrical discharge is very brief (one millisecond). The ECT machine gives a read-out of electrical discharge to inform the treating psychiatrist. And, that is the whole psychiatric treatment. After an hour she will regain control of her muscle function, be able to breathe, and her documented brain electrical activity will return to her baseline electrical activity.

So, what happens during the seizure? She experiences a loss of consciousness for a minute and a half in her brain, but the seizure affects only the brain and nervous system. We do not know how ECT makes psychiatric patients well, but it is known that ECT releases a surge of dopamine, the "pleasure hormone". This dopamine surge can make depressed patients feel better—and can also help mobilize patients with Parkinson's Disease. Curiously, the dopamine surge makes manic patients calmer instead of more stimulated. Other biochemical changes occur in other "brain hormones" as a result of the artificial seizure.

ECT is useful for very severe mood disorders: severe mania and psychotic depression. Most people need at least eight treatments. Does it work? Yes, for those who have severe mood disorders. One of my supervising psychiatrists (head of the department) often said that if he got depressed he wanted us to give him ECT. Some chronic psychiatric patients come in once a month for a "booster dose" of ECT which acts as treatment and as prevention. If Gwen had been doing this, she probably would not have gotten ill again. This may be a good option for her.

Memory loss is not such a problem now with improved techniques. Bone fractures are a thing of the past.

Transcranial magnetic resonance therapy is a new treatment that sends powerful magnetic waves into the brain instead of electricity. This does not require pre-medication with muscle relaxants and anesthesia. This seems a hopeful treatment for the future.

Chapter II-3

Brain Chemistry and Well-being

Everyone wants to feel "normal", but some people have trouble achieving this. Some people are unflappable in any circumstances. Some people can maintain balance unless they are exposed to a barrage of environmental stressors at which time they may show agitation, anxiety, depression, and other signs and symptoms of psychological disturbance. And a small minority of people has significant vacillations of behavior that are almost constant, environmental factors notwithstanding. Psychiatry believes that their instability is due to involuntary internal biochemical disturbances. Their conditions may be present since birth, or may begin at certain age "milestones" soon after puberty, after pregnancy, in midlife, or in the elder years. For other people, the onset can be sporadic (occurring at any time in life). The people who are born with psychiatric illness cannot be brought under control unless they take medications. Fortunately, medications are available; unfortunately, understanding from the majority population is unavailable. "Normal" people suppose that psychiatric patients are failing to exercise self-control, which is part of the stigmatization of psychiatric conditions. The truth is that no one wants to be abnormal or out of control.

For the groups of people who have onset at "milestone" ages, medications are usually very helpful and necessary, but the medications may not be continuously necessary for the rest of their lives. People who have sporadic onset are usually adjusting to a stress factor. They might not need medicine at all. They might take medicine for a year or so and not need it again. These three groups highlight the differences in case severity:

- People born with psychiatric illness often have severe cases
- People with onset at "milestone" ages often have a range of disease from mildly-moderate to severe
- Sporadic cases are usually the mildest

As far as the symptoms and feeling-states themselves, the general groupings are: thought disorders, anxiety disorders, obsessions-compulsions, and mood disorders. People with thought disorders generally have the severest psychiatric illness, followed immediately by mania, and then by all mood disorders. Anxiety and panic can be a hindrance to enjoying life, and certainly, PTSD can be so; PTSD is sometimes an incapacitating anxiety disorder. The same may be said of comupulsive disorders as of anxiety disorders.

Thought Disorders

People with thought disorders can run the range from over-trusting to paranoid:

Trusting	"Normal"	Suspicious ↔ Paranoid

Anxiety Disorders

People with anxiety disorders can run the gamut from serenely unexcitable to "pan-anxious" (constantly intensely anxious):

Serene	"normal"	Anxious ↔ Panicky ↔ "Pan-anxious"

Compulsive Disorders

Compulsions revolve around feelings of responsibility. People can have a normal level of responsibility that can range from abject slothfulness to extreme compulsivity ("schizo-obsessive disorder"). The relation of Obsessive-Compulsive Disorder (OCD) to schizo-obsessive disorder is not clear, and this latter term may be more of a clinical description than a formalized diagnosis:

Slothful	Undisciplined	Responsible	Compulsive	OCD	Schizo-obsessive?

Mood Disorders

Most people can experience a reasonably "normal" range of moods as shown in the next table.

Suicidal thoughts	Depression	Dysphoria	Sense of well-being	Euphoria	Ecstasy	Mania
			← Typical person →			
		←	Mood Disorder	→		
	←		Bipolar		→	
←			Manic-Depression			→

Alexithymia

The average person who does not need to see a psychiatrist has a "limited" repertoire of moods and moodiness. He has probably not known the extremely pleasant sensations of ecstasy or exaltation, but has also been spared the depths of depression. There are some people who exceed this normal range. People with mood disorders can experience a wider variation in moods as well as a wider departure from the center point of well-being. If mood swings are extreme, they can result in death by suicide or reckless behaviors. On the other hand, there are a few people who have little moodiness. Otherwise, we can all experience the spectrum of feelings ranging from depression to euphoria—and some of us can experience an even broader spectrum.

One condition seems to be exempt from moods and moodiness, Alexithymia. This refers to an unusual condition in which people lack any range of emotion. Some people are apparently born with alexithymia and are not aware of their mood and do not have apparent mood reactions. Additionally, patients with certain damage to temporal lobes and thalamus do not have feelings and can appear "flat". When people have no range of mood, we call this "flat affect". Schizophrenics can present with a flat affect, but it is not permanent and can change to volatile if they become psychotic again.

Everyone wants to have a sense of well-being, but for many psychiatric patients, well-being can be a life-long quest with an elusive goal. Our nature and nurture make us who we are, which in turn crafts our destinies—we can not escape that fact. Our greatest triumph in life indeed may be the ability to rise above this basal destiny by imposing self-willed control over our behaviors wherever possible—and when that is not sufficient, then taking the courage to admit that there is a personal problem by beginning to seek professional mental health help.

Chapter II-4

Genetics and Psychiatry

Genetics is becoming more and more important for understanding ourselves, both structurally and functionally. Genetics controls how our nervous system forms and how the chemicals in our bodies are made. Genetics controls timing of activities and aging of our bodies: puberty, for example. Genetics affects psychiatry in two very important ways. Genetics increases the chances of getting a psychiatric disorder that runs in the family. Genetics also affects the way that psychiatric drugs are processed inside the body. Thus, genetics has a direct link to the diagnosis (cause) and a somewhat less direct link to treatment (individual responses to individual medications).

Genetics of Psychiatric Illnesses that run in Families (genetic effects on diagnosis)

(For the genetic underpinnings of alcoholism, see chapter VI-1)

Common wisdom and casual observation suggest that some families are likelier to have emotional, psychiatric, and/or alcoholic disorders. Research statistics supports some of this common wisdom and casual observation. Many studies have yielded similar results: namely, that certain diseases are more pervasive in certain families. Studies in the Ohio Amish have demonstrated their genetic predisposition to inherit manic-depressive illness (they are more vulnerable since their gene pool is rather limited). Likewise, alcoholism seems to run in certain families. The percentage of risk increases with consanguinity ("blood-relatedness"). Consanguinity refers to having very close blood lines to another individual. The closer the relationship, the higher the percentage of risk of being affected. Your chances of becoming schizophrenic increase if one of your blood relatives is schizophrenic. The risk is higher, the closer the relation. Taking Schizophrenia as an example, these are general approximations of the chances of your becoming schizophrenic[3] if you are or you have:

Genetic Risk of Schizophrenia

Identical twins ....33-78% risk ←(This is your risk if your twin has it.)

Both parents schizophrenic...............35% risk ←(This is your risk if both parents have it.)

Fraternal twins ....8-28% risk   "   "

Siblings and first-degree relatives...5-10% risk   "   "

No schizophrenic relatives............0.06-1.1%

(These percentages vary depending upon the sources and various studies[3].)

Mood disorders, anxiety, panic, and alcoholism tend to run in some families. In other families, minor mental illness can be prevalent from generation to generation, for example minor depression. In still other families, not everyone is affected, but the predisposition or chance of getting any mental disability can run in families, also. This mental disability may then manifest once in every generation or once in every other generation. In some cases, it may be difficult to separate out the effects of nurture (childhood) and nature (genetics) on a family problem. Researchers believe that traumatic childhood events and chaotic family environments can have a huge impact on a child who otherwise might have grown up to be unaffected ("normal"). On the other hand, these environments may have been created by parents who either suffer from genetic mental illness or are themselves recipients of traumatic childhoods from previous generations. It becomes a which-came-first-chicken-or-egg conundrum. Not infrequently, genetics and childhood both may have some hand in causing minor or major psychiatric conditions.

Role of Medical Genetics in Drug Reactions (genetic effects on treatment)

Our ability to tolerate psychiatric medications is rooted in our genetics. If we have depression, we may be intolerant of a number of antidepressants: this is not a figment of your imagination. This is your genetics at work behind the scenes (in your liver and brain). You may also need very high or only very low doses of the antidepressants, sometimes to the consternation of your prescribing doctor. This also is a real effect due also to genetics.

Our bodies contain many kinds of biochemicals necessary to maintain life. One large biochemical group consists of proteins. Within the proteins are many types of chemicals, some of which are enzymes. There are many kinds of enzymes. (see figure II-4-a) We are going to focus on one special family of enzymes called Cytochromes P_{450}, simply called "cytochromes", which are special kinds of protective proteins that recognize poisons and deactivate them so that we will not be harmed. Cytochromes reside in our bodies—especially, our livers—and try to "neutralize" any poisons that get into our bodies. There are thousands of types of cytochromes and they all belong to their own families. Out of this huge family, there is a handful that is important for human health. They have names such as: 2D6, 3A4, 2C9, 2C19.

In the distant past, these cytochromes mainly had to deal with various plant poisons that we had eaten; now they have to contend with all the synthetic drugs and chemical pollutants, too. Although our forebears had subjectively divided plant products into (1)-poisonous, (2)-nutritional, and (3)-medicinal, the cytochromes consider many from all three types to be alien toxic chemicals that needed to be detoxified. The cytochromes prevented our ancestors from getting ill throughout the long history of humankind on earth. That is why we are still here and still have cytochromes to protect us.

In modern times, cytochromes are more necessary than ever before, because they also process modern drugs (environmental poisons and noxious chemicals). They may not always succeed in processing all these modern drugs, but at least they try to do so. Our bodies recognize most pharmaceuticals as poisons and will quickly set about processing them into smaller chemicals until the body no longer considers them dangerous or until they are processed enough to be eliminated. The following illustrates how Valium is generally processed by our body.

Valium pill in mouth$\rightarrow\rightarrow$*Cytochrome P$_{450}$*$\rightarrow\rightarrow$ *nor-Valium*

The liver has processed the Valium into nor-Valium: this is the first step in our body's attempt to get rid of the Valium. Nor-Valium actually has sedative properties like its parent drug, Valium.

The liver does not know this but it is putting the Valium into the system in this first step in attempting to detoxify the Valium. Without a cytochrome system, poisons and drugs would spend more time inside our bodies, probably causing more harm (and death) since the amount of contact time between toxins and

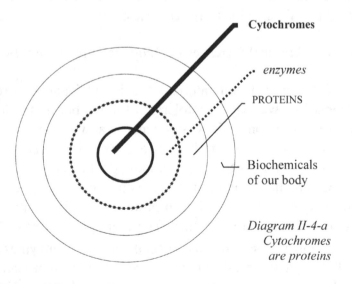

Cytochromes

enzymes

PROTEINS

Biochemicals of our body

Diagram II-4-a
Cytochromes
are proteins

body would be increased: our only choice might be to take much less of the medicine—or get quite ill. Without cytochromes, we might overdose on just one Valium pill.

Each person is [hopefully] endowed with a complete set of these vital proteins; however, they are genetically encoded which means that different people can end up having too many, not enough, or a "normal" amount of cytochrome enzymes. The quantity and quality of cytochromes that we each have is ordained in our genes. You might end up with a normal amount of genes to help you get rid of Valium, but your neighbor could have a deficiency. This is just like having genes for tallness, baldness, cystic fibrosis, HIV resistance and so forth. The result is that some people might have an extra amount of cytochrome-2D6 for example and somebody else might have very little. These genetic endowments are extremely important because they dictate how quickly and easily—or how slowly and arduously—our body can dispose of the drugs and chemicals. In the worst-case scenario, your neighbor might not be able to get rid of Valium in the usual way so that one Valium pill would seem five times stronger for him than it would for you. Under normal circumstances, this cytochrome system is like a wary guard dog always on the look-out for potential threats; without this system we would not have health—maybe not even life. Fortunately, there are tests available that can give general guidelines and information about our individual genetic abilities to process drugs.

The handful of cytochromes that act as sentinels for human health have names such as: 2D6, 3A4, 2C9, 2C19. Cytochrome 2D6 is in charge of neutralizing a number of psychiatric drugs. By way of example, Paxil is degraded in the 2D6 system. So, let's take patient Rory who has a lot of 2D6 enzyme. Rory can rapidly process Paxil (and probably other 2D6 drugs). Rory is called a rapid user (rapid "metabolizer" or even "ultra-rapid-metabolizer"): he will use up a dose of Paxil quickly. On the other hand, let's take someone like Sally has very little 2D6 enzyme in her body. She will need a long time to degrade one dose of Paxil. Sally is a slow user (slow "metabolizer").

By way of analogy: your yard will get cleaned up quickly with a crew of four, but slowly with just one gardener. Or, a rapid user of Paxil has extra "machinery" to process one dose of the drug. This is as if Rory were Xeroxing 400 pages by using four copy machines simultaneously—the work will finish four times faster than in a slow user like Sally who uses only one copier to copy 400 pages. Or, imagine that each copy of the 2D6 is like one animal at a feeding trough: if four animals are given two pounds of fodder (Paxil, in this case, is the fodder) then, the fodder will all be chewed up rapidly; now, assume that one animal has two pounds of fodder, then the fodder will be consumed much more slowly and will last much longer, lasting perhaps four times as long.

🌑 Since Rory is a rapid user of Paxil, his once daily dose might not last for 24 hours— he might need a larger dose or even to take the Paxil twice a day to maintain an acceptable blood level of Paxil in his body. (Another practical solution is Paxil-CR, 24-hour controlled release pills). Rory might need to take two of the largest Paxil-CR pills each day. If he has HMO medical coverage, it will often initially refuse to pay for sixty of these pills per month for him—unless the psychiatrist can prove such a need. The HMO will prefer that he take generic Paxil.

🗣 On the other hand, Sally is a slow user of Paxil. Her body may require 36 hours to dispose of the Paxil. The result of this is that she needs less Paxil. If her dosage is not adjusted downward, then she will start to develop annoying side effects from the Paxil, due to fact that her Paxil blood levels will continue to go up and up. She may feel ill as if overdosed on Paxil (nausea, headache, raciness, poor sleep).

This is one reason that I am always skeptical when Sally tells me that her neighbor takes Paxil and feels great: this does not show me anything about Sally's biochemistry and genetics. However, if she states that her mother and sister are doing really well on Paxil, then that is useful genetic information. Patients more often than not will do well if other family members are taking the same medicine. Nonetheless, she could have inherited a genetic deficiency from her father, but it is less likely. Despite genetics and heredity, we are all slightly different regarding how we process environmental "poisons".

In *Diagram II-2-b,* we see Rory with his extra copies of 2D6. Thus, he will use 20 mg of Paxil rapidly: within twelve hours or less, maybe even nine or ten hours: the one dose may last only from 6 a.m. to 6 p.m. His blood level of Paxil might drop to zero by midnight; hence, the Paxil may not be helping him for twenty-four hours until the next morning dose. He will need more than 20 mg a day: maybe 40-60 mg a day or 30 mg twice a day. Some rapid users may need even 80 mg a day. Once again, the HMO will refuse to pay for 80 mg a day, unless the psychiatrist can provide proof of such need. The definitive proof is the cytochrome genetic blood test—but, the HMO will not pay for that blood test, either.

Diagram II-2-b also shows Sally, a very slow user of Paxil. A 20 mg dose is too much and feels almost like an overdose to her: the drug will start to build up in her body and cause annoying side effects such as headache, nausea, poor sleep, and possible sexual dysfunction. She needs much less Paxil than Rory. She may need thirty hours to clear an average dose of 20 mg. If she continues taking 20 mg a day, she will accumulate so much Paxil in her body that within a couple weeks she will feel ill from all the side effects. Ultimately, she may need only 10-15 mg Paxil a day. People like Sally who seem to be exquisitely sensitive to drugs may just be very slow users: they need to have customized treatment, take tiny doses, and have blood levels monitored—if available (Paxil has no routine blood level tests available—just the cytochrome genotyping lab test).

Diagram II-4-b   a rapid user and a slow user: smaller font corresponds to lower blood levels: Rory's one dose of Paxil does not last for 24 hours

Sally's one dose lasts for a day and a half

Patient	Dosage	— Blood	levels	of	paxil		—
	They both take 20 mg Paxil at 6AM	6 AM	NOON	6PM	Midnight	6AM	noon
Rory	rapid user: He has many 2D6 receptors ℧℧℧ ℧℧℧ ℧℧℧	Paxil ☺	Paxil ☺	Paxil 😐	PAXIL ☹		
Sally	Slow user: She has few 2D6 receptors ℧℧℧	Paxil ☺	**Paxil** 😐	**Paxil** ☺	Paxil ☺	Paxil ☺	Paxil 😐

Diagram II-4-c   drug levels continue to rise to unpleasant levels in a slow user: Sally's once a day dose last for a day and a half; after three doses, she has as much medicine in her as a normal person would have in four and a half days: larger font corresponds to more unpleasant side effects; higher blood levels are shown by arrows going up continuously day by day

Sally	Slow user: She has few 2D6 receptors ℧℧℧	6 AM Day#1 Dose#1	NOON	9PM	6AM Day#2 Dose#2	NOON	9PM	6AM Day#3 Dose#3
blood level	Ø	↓	→	↑	↑↑	↑↑↑	↑↑↑↑	↑↑↑↑↑
Sally	Paxil 20 mg on day #1	Paxil ☺	**Paxil** 😐	**Paxil** ☺				
Sally	Dose #2 Paxil 20 mg on day #2				Paxil 😐	Paxil ☹	😐 side effects *PAXIL*	
Sally	Dose#3 Day#3							☹

All of this information is very interesting; however, at a much more practical level, you should be aware that there is a blood test that reveals how we process drugs. This test has been available for several years. In light of the fact that over 110,000 patients die every year as a direct result of drug reactions, one would think that everybody should be tested. The testing has advantages and disadvantages.

On the positive side, testing would probably save lives. Another advantage is that each person only need be tested once in his life, since our genetics are reasonably stable throughout our lifetimes—as far as we now know.

However, among the disadvantages there are some expenses, limitations, and possible risks. The blood test is still expensive (over a thousand dollars). It is quite likely that the Managed Healthcare plans do not wish to pay so much for this testing. They simply may be waiting for the price to come down—which it already has done in the last few years (down from $1600 at the turn of the century). If the HMO's tested every patient, then couldn't the price of the test be deeply discounted? The limitation is that the test results do not indicate how each patient would respond to each specific drug—the test informs only about the amount of cytochrome genes present in the patient. If Sally wants to know in advance if she will tolerate Paxil well, she can pay for the testing. The result will estimate if she is a slow, very slow, normal, rapid, or ultra-rapid user (metabolizer) in the 2D6 family of cytochromes. Since Paxil is in the 2D6 family, this provides some general and useful information, but it still does not predict her exact reaction to Paxil specifically.

A major disadvantage of the testing concerns the possibility that the health insurance companies could discover the results and use this information to establish pre-existing conditions and thus reject health insurance applicants based on the results of the genetic testing (just one more reason that we need a nationally uniform health care delivery system with elimination of "pre-existing disease" clauses). Yet another possibility is that an astute insurance company might authorize only tiny doses for the slow metabolizers, thereby denying them access to higher doses. Wouldn't cost issues be balanced by the fact that slow metabolizers would need fewer doses of costly medicines, thus saving money at the cash register? Of course the money saved on slow metabolizers would be spent on the rapid metabolizers who would need higher doses of costly medicine These two extremes should balance out at the end of the day. Hopefully, by the time you read this handbook, the HMO's will have started to undertake this kind of testing.

Our genes make us who we are, thereby shaping our fates—we can not at this time escape these facts. Our greatest triumph might lie in the likelihood that we rise above this state by capitalizing our genetic strengths and willfully suppressing our weaknesses.

(Also see Chapter V-16, last topic)

Section III
DIAGNOSIS and EXPECTATIONS

Superscript numbers refer to references and citations at the back of the book

Chapter III-1

The Mechanics of Psychiatric Diagnosis

"If you listen to the Patient long enough, Edison, he will tell you his diagnosis"
—one of the favorite aphorisms of Richard Krause, MD, Cincinnati, Ohio, a great teacher–

Whenever I have trouble reaching a satisfactory initial diagnosis, I always remember Dr. Krause's words. Eventually, a satisfactory and workable diagnosis presents itself.

What is Diagnosis? In Greek, *"dia"* means "…with a view to/as a means to…[27]" and *"gnosis"* means "knowledge". So, basically it means "in order to know". To know what? We use "diagnosis" as "to know which disease that is". This is what modern doctors mean when we say "diagnosis". However, *Dorland's Medical Dictionary* adds a second connotation: "the art of distinguishing one disease from another". This second connotation we call "differential diagnosis"—for the sake of clarity. So how do we make a diagnosis?

The first step is to realize that a first-time diagnosis on a first-time patient is going to be a "preliminary diagnosis" (also called tentative diagnosis). If I proceed to treat the patient based on the preliminary diagnosis, then I call it a "working diagnosis" since I am now "working" with it. We are allowed to amplify or change the working diagnosis with time. The diagnosis in medicine, surgery, and psychiatry is based on the history of the disease, the signs and symptoms, and lab tests. Other important factors might be if the patient already had this disease in the past (past history) or if anyone in his family had this disease (family history). The combination of these histories, signs, symptoms, and labs are analyzed intellectually, and the doctor will reach a preliminary/working diagnosis. The accuracy of diagnosis is very important because it points the way to effective treatment. If a treatment goes horribly wrong, then there might have been a "failure to diagnose"—although, there are sundry reasons that that treatment might have failed. There is a certain comfort in knowing that we are allowed to modify or change a preliminary/working diagnosis. Half-way through treatment, the working diagnosis should be the correct diagnosis, otherwise we are going down the wrong path. If the disease is not getting better, then we should revise or change the working diagnosis—we might need to consider that there are other diagnoses involved, in which case, these secondary diagnoses need to be factored into the treatment. By the end of the treatment, the patient should have a final diagnosis (in medicine and psychiatry).

How do psychiatrists think about diagnosis? How do they make a diagnosis?

Psychiatrists approach their patients in exactly the same way that internists or surgeons do—as outlined above in chapter I-4. In any branch of medicine—be it psychiatry, surgery, or internal medicine—these are the bases of diagnosis:

General Medical Diagnosis

People who are born with a serious psychiatric condition already have a diagnosis. However the mild and moderate cases with onset in adolescence and adulthood are probably going to go see their family doctor before seeing a psychiatrist. They often present with a collection of vague symptoms that the family doctor must diagnose as medical or psychological. If psychological, then he refers his patient to a mental health professional. These are some of the symptoms that he might encounter. Keep in mind that his patients may not know that they are depressed and may think that they have a true medical problem. Patients with panic and anxiety usually know that they have anxiety and panic. Sometimes the family doctor's patients come to see him because they have both a psychological and medical problem at the same time. The family doctors must often rely on their instincts—they have a hard job!

History of Present Illness (HOPI): let's take the case of a young man named Toby for example, who got to the point of feeling so bad as to need to see a doctor. HOPI is the story of how he came to feel this way. Perhaps he was unexpectedly jilted by his fiancée. Perhaps he is susceptible to certain types of medical illness (asthma) that can cause him to have high anxiety. Perhaps he is becoming depressed just like his father and at that very same age. It is likely that he will tell his family doctor that he feels lousy, no motivation. Women may think that they have anemia, men may complain that their "male hormones must be low or something". Both genders often have an odd assortment of vague aches, poor sleep, appetite disturbance, frustration, and vague sense of uneasiness: "Hey, doc, maybe it's my sinuses acting up again?" And so on.

Disease Markers with emphasis on what we call signs and symptoms:
- —Symptoms (shorthand "Sx") which consist of Toby's self-report and reflects how he feels. Symptoms can not be measured by any man-made device. Doctors must rely solely on what Toby says that he feels. Examples are aches, poor sleep, nausea, fatigue, guilt, frustration with life in general, lightheadedness, lack of motivation, and so on.

- —Signs which are physical alterations of the body that anybody can see, and a trained doctor can use these visible signs to make the diagnosis. Examples are scarred wrists, bloodshot eyes, hand trembling, dilated pupils, and so on. This is the basis of the Art of Physical Diagnosis (also called Semeiology) which is a way of diagnosing a patient's illness by merely examining his body. This is how all diagnoses were made throughout history before the invention of biochemical blood tests and X-rays. This may also be the main way of diagnosing patients in impoverished and technology-deficient countries even today. Physical diagnosis in Medicine relies on inspection (looking at), palpation(feeling and kneading), percussion (thumping on the body,) and auscultation (listening to body sounds) and rare use of the chemical senses (smell and taste).

- —Biochemical and laboratory analysis of bodily floods: urine test, thryroid test, liver and kidney function tests, blood count, syphilis (and HIV) tests, and so on.

- —X-rays and other electronic imaging techniques (CATScan, MRI, etc)

- —Measures and metrics of bodily function and status: change of weight, rapid pulse.

Psychiatric Diagnosis

Psychiatric diagnosis relies mainly on history of the present illness (HOPI) and symptoms.

History of Present Illness (HOPI): usually the psychiatrist has to piece this together by interpreting fragments of information that Toby provides. This does not mean that Toby is dishonest—he simply tosses out various events in a random pattern. The psychiatrist must arrange the jumble in order to forge it into a coherent HOPI. This is an abbreviated version of the HOPI as retold to the psychiatrist:

Toby is a young man who likes to drink on the weekends, and recently he has started bingeing on the weekends. His fiancée is going to break up with him if he does not stop. He says that he can not quit because he feels stress coming from "somewhere". His asthma is not so well controlled as before. A patient such as Toby can sometimes tell us the *history of the present illness* unless he is so disorganized, confused, or slowed own that he can not remember or cannot focus.

Disease Markers

- —Symptoms are Toby's feelings, which he can usually retell fairly well: feeling sad, seeing strange people, hearing strange things, feeling afraid to go out alone and so on.

- —Signs: In some cases, we rely on signs as disease markers: this is physical diagnosis. Physical diagnosis in psychiatry is more superficial and consists of inspection, listening and smelling: wrist scars, bloodshot eyes, trembling hands, dilated pupils, the smell of alcohol or of poor hygiene, slow speech, fast speech, slurred speech, angry tirades, threatening behaviors, rapid pacing about the room, hyperactivity-restlessness, arguing with invisible (disembodied) voices, extreme amounts of poorly applied makeup, confusion of clothing (mismatched buttonholes, shirt on backward or inside out, barefoot), and so on. Examples: Toby is actively hallucinating or is very slowed down; he has hand tremors, really large pupils (eyes), scars on the wrist, levels of grooming and hygiene, slovenly attire, inability to walk, stooped shoulders, mumbling incoherently, downcast gaze, and in women, lack of makeup or excessive make-up, and so on;

- ▪ —lab tests might include measures of blood test for alcohol and street drugs, blood tests for prescription medications, urine test, thryroid test, liver and kidney function tests, blood count, syphilis (and HIV) tests, urine drug tests, measures of cortisol levels, and so on.

- ▪ —Imaging studies could include CT Scan of the brain, MRI of the brain, and/or brain wave mapping (EEG).

- ▪ —Biometric measures: psychological testing, such as the TOVA test (a computer based test for ADHD) or psychological testing such as the Minnesota Personality Test ("MMPI") and other types of emotional inventories/tests.

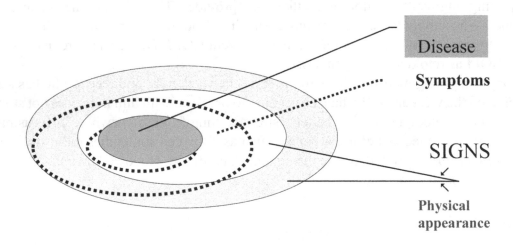

Diagram III-1-a   Relationship of signs and symptoms

- • Inner core—In this diagram we can see that the innermost core of Toby is his diseased biological functioning which may be more or less normal or abnormal. Since this is his source of functioning, it will affect signs, symptoms, and appearance.

- Symptoms are internal and are perceived by Toby. He relates his inner symptoms. Sometimes the symptoms cause signs: sadness (symptom) causes crying (sign). The symptom dashed-ring touches the edge of signs to signify this fact in the diagram.

- Signs are external markers of illness: dilated pupils, sweating, cowering, hoarseness.

- The outermost ring represents his outermost appearance—the way that people perceive his anatomy and overall functioning (thin, obese, strained, drained, tense and so on)

After the psychiatrist reviews all the data available, he will make a tentative diagnosis (a working diagnosis) which usually is based on the DSM-IV-TR, the standard source book for making psychiatric diagnoses. Of course, you must realize that the use of this book to make the correct diagnosis relies upon years of personal experience. Toby would probably not be able to open the book and correctly diagnose himself, his friends, or family members.

The "Axial" diagnosis

Psychiatric diagnosis relies on five sets of "axes", the first three of which are the most important to the psychiatrist (from a doctor's viewpoint). These are arbitrarily called Axis I, Axis II, and Axis III. (Axis IV refers to qualitative listings of stress factors in the patient's life. Axis V then assigns a numerical "score" that describes how well the patient is doing when saddled with the stress factors listed in Axes I-IV).

Axis I refers to all the main psychiatric diagnoses (these may be permanent conditions, such as schizophrenia, or may be temporary conditions; most Axis I conditions can be favorably altered or improved by using medications.)

Axis II refers to personality style that will likely not change very much throughout our lifetime. Some people have personality styles that interfere with their levels of happiness in life or with their acceptance by others. This might soften with age (the opposite of physical problems, which worsen with age). Personality style is hard to change and has no real cure. The only way to treat it is to bring it under some level of conscious control by identifying it and then by learning in therapy how to manage it as best as possible. If this personality style is extreme then it can cause a lot of unhappiness in the life of the patient and those near him. It can bring him into the cross hairs of the legal system. The only real treatment is to begin therapy with a therapist or psychologist.

Axis III refers to Toby's medical problems, such as diabetes, asthma…

Axis IV consists of listing stress factors, such as engagement, bankruptcy, bingeing, unemployment, homelessness…

Axis V is an arbitrarily assigned number that is supposed to correlate to the patient's functional level: this can be any number from 0 to 100, but is usually in mid-range. Rankings are usually in units of ten's or five's: a ranking of 70% indicates mild symptoms; 60% corresponds to moderate symptoms; 65% would be mild-moderate symptoms.

This is an example of how we make a working diagnosis for Toby on his first visit.

Axis I—Adjustment Disorder with Anxiety, Alcohol Abuse
Axis II—mixed personality traits
Axis III—Asthma
Axis IV—recently broke up with his fiancée, still working full time
Axis V—78

We write these five axes in his confidential chart.
It might also be helpful to visualize the Axial system in this way:

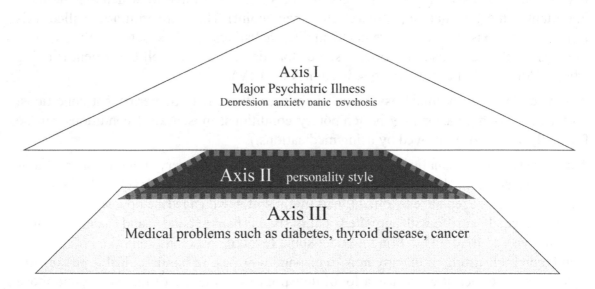

Figure III-1-b   The "Axial" System of Diagnosis

Figure III-1-b demonstrates that Axis III and Axis II conditions are foundational, in the sense that they will not change a lot. Axis III is larger, suggesting that it is major and will probably increase in complexity with time. Axis II is usually unbudging and "indelible". Axes I and III can impact each other. Axis I problems can change, worsen, improve, diminish, expand, depending upon physical health. Poor physical health can have a negative impact on Axis I conditions. Axis II personality style can shape the way in which Axis I illness appears. Axis I problems will not change pre-existing Axis II conditions, but might cause them to aggravate. As Axis I illness increases in severity or in number, it can "inflame" Axis II. This psychic "inflammation" can affect the way that Toby presents his symptoms and signs to other people. Axis II can distort how Toby asks for help—it can make him seem helpless and childlike, angry and entitled, sulky and brooding, aggressive and intrusive, agitated and anxious, or apathetic and sullen.

Everyone has a personality style, which is their Axis II diagnosis. Most people are lucky and fall somewhere in the "normal" range, which means that their personality is "acceptable" to most people. However, our Axis II behaviors seem to have a "default position" which I believe is part of the unique "hard-wiring" of every person. I believe that—given extremely severe Axis I conditions—anyone can revert to an off-putting Axis II default presentation. The greater the number of Axis I conditions at any one time, the more extreme will be the Axis II regressions and perturbations. As Axis I problems improve, then the Axis II symptoms should no longer be "inflamed" and should gradually subside.

The real litmus test comes with recovery from the Axis I conditions. If the Axis I condition is treated, then the Axis II symptoms should abate. If the Axis II symptoms do not abate, then that is the person's baseline personality style. If the baseline personality style is distressing, then it is an Axis II condition that might warrant further attention.

As times goes by, Toby may acquire more psychiatric and medical problems so that by middle age, the axial assessment (diagnoses) might enlarge and become:

I—	Depression, Insomnia (poor sleep), Nicotine Addiction (cigarettes), Alcoholism
II—	Passive-dependent personality style
III—	Diabetes, asthma, obesity, sleep apnea (sleep disorder)
IV—	Stressors: daughter in car accident, change of jobs
V—	General functional level 65

As time goes by, we may add new diagnoses with age. This is especially true for Axis III medical problems. Note that Axis II conditions do not change. These are possible diagnoses for an elderly Toby listed along with their proper numerical codes:

AXIS I— MajorDepression,singleepisode,mild296.21,BereavementV62.82,Adjustment Disorder with mixed emotional features 309.28, possible early Dementia 780.9

AXIS II— passive-dependent personality style

AXIS III—Emphysema, asthma, gastric cancer, obesity, high blood pressure, diabetes, early dementia

AXIS IV—stressors (lawsuit, bankruptcy, death in the family, etc.)

AXIS V— general level of functioning 45

"Prevention is the best treatment."
If you cannot prevent a condition, then take care of it as early as possible,
If not early, then attend to it before other worse conditions accumulate.

Toby should have quit drinking before he started smoking. The smoking aggravated the asthma that he already had, and all that led to emphysema. He gained weight from the alcohol, which led to the obesity that then caused diabetes. Hypertension is a predictable outcome of the accumulation of all these medical problems. If Toby had attended to preventing these medical problems by exercising regularly, then his main psychiatric condition might have been depression and anxiety which can improve with current medications. Stomach cancer is likely related to nicotine and alcohol. People who quit drinking, show better judgment and might not end up with so many social and legal problems. With disease management in youth, elderly Toby might have had far fewer problems and hence better quality of life. This scenario is now very common.

These above examples also show that treatment of the psychiatric diagnosis is still variable and relies a lot on the doctor's experience and philosophy and upon a patient's willingness to continue in treatment until changes can make him feel healthy. An obese middle-agent diabetic might receive a very different treatment plan from that of an athletic diabetic college student. The psychiatric diagnosis manual, DSM-IV TR, does not give any suggestions for treatment. There are many treatments available and may differ somewhat from site to site, region to region, and country to country. There are many treatments available nowadays. Psychiatry is in the process of establishing "treatment algorithms" which are like a decision-tree informing on step-by-step treatment options; of course, this can be modified to individual needs.

Advisements regarding the so-called Axis II Disorders.

The Axis II conditions are properly called "Personality Disorder". Perhaps "Personality Style" would be a more politically correct diagnostic term. The term "Personality Disorder" sounds harsh and judgmental. Psychiatrists do have the option to refer to Axis II conditions as "personality traits". Personality style only becomes a treatment issue when it assumes massive proportions that cause the patient significant stress and distress. Personality style can also cause the patient to sabotage his own treatment whether he is aware of it or not. This condition can also be helpful for reminding us that it needs attention and adjustment to improve the outcomes of the other prescribed therapies for the primary Axis I condition, which is a treatment focus that will get better with treatment even though the personality style may not.

The origins and causes of personalities is a much-debated topic, especially whether nature (genetics) and nurture (childhood) have the same effects or if nurture (happy childhood experiences as well as childhood trauma) is the predominant shaper of personality.

Under extreme stress, everybody has a breaking point—or threshold—at which he will start to manifest a pronounced underlying personality style; apparently, some people have higher thresholds and some, lower.

If you listen to the Patient long enough, he will tell you his diagnosis…

Introduction to the
Process of Psychiatric Diagnosis and Treatment
Five essays on Psychiatric Diagnosis and Treatment are in Chapters III-2 through III-6

This chapter begins a series of five chapters. Each chapter is devoted to a particular aspect of treatment of the patient. Part III-2 provides the origins and bases for modern psychiatric treatment. Part III-3 discusses the diagnosis and treatment from the doctor's viewpoint. Part III-3 is the most important of all five parts because the successful outcome of diagnosis and treatment ultimately relies on the doctor's involvement. He can "make or break" the whole process. Part III-3 tries to show some of the complexity involved in treatment planning. Part III-4 discusses what the patient feels during his own treatment process. We always strive to make treatment feel better than the original condition. Part III-5 takes into account that sometimes one or more family members may want to have a say-so in this whole process. The last part, Part III-6, discusses aspects of treatment.

The process of diagnosis and treatment is so important that I have divided it into these parts:

(III-2) Introduction
(III-3) Diagnosis from psychiatrist viewpoint (the "five phases") (III-4) Diagnosis from patient viewpoint (the "nine stages") (III-5) Diagnosis from family viewpoint
(III-6) Treatment from the viewpoint of doctor and patient

Definition of a Psychiatric Disorder

Since many psychiatric disorders lack hard evidence such as fever or bleeding, then how do we know if a person even has a psychiatric disorder? Bleeding is obviously abnormal. What about certain beliefs? Delusions are "fixed false beliefs". Who decides which beliefs are false or not? If a person shares the same fixed false beliefs (delusions) with his tribe, and if the whole tribe believes these are not false, then do they all share the same "delusion". Do they all have a delusional disorder? Do any of them have a disorder?

If they all have the same fixed false beliefs, then must this be classified as a disorder that has a diagnosis? These are interesting philosophical issues. Nonetheless, in the USA at this time, we recognize many disorders and many corresponding diagnoses at a practical level. This is why it is important to consider beliefs within the context of that culture and civilization. "Delusions" in Los Angeles in 2010 might have been "normal" beliefs three thousand years ago (although perhaps superstitious).

How do we deal with this baffling issue? In current psychiatry, the real litmus test for any psychiatric disorder is whether a person's behavior is seriously affecting one or more areas of his life, areas such as interpersonal, occupational, social, legal, or financial functioning. If so, then these areas of his life are out of order, hence in disorder, hence a disorder. So, a "strange" thought needs to be considered as such by (a majority of) his "tribe". It is possible that the patient on his own feels that this is a "strange" thought, or maybe he does not, in which case the majority of friends, family, employers, doctors, and society will voice their opinion about his strange beliefs. The majority usually decides the outcome regarding the need for psychiatric treatment. However, a court might cite his First Amendment Rights (to be left alone) and overrule the majority opinion. Psychiatric diagnosis and treatment are obviously different from diagnosis and treatment of fever and bleeding, although in these medical cases, patients also (almost always) retain their First Amedment Rights as well: they can leave a hospital AMA (Against Medical Advice).

Introduction to Psychiatric Diagnosis and Treatment

The process of diagnosis and treatment starts with the diagnosis. On the first visit to the doctor, he will make a working diagnosis. He will then discuss treatment tactics and strategy with the patient. The short-term goal is to relieve some of the patient's suffering; however, there are also long-term goals for which the doctor must plan. He will be in charge of overseeing this outcome. He alone has the unique vision for coordinating short-term tactics so that they will dovetail into a palatable long-term treatment strategy where the ultimate goal is that of recovery. The doctor should have alternate plans to change tactics in case the treatment strategy might change: the main reason for a change is the appearance of new symptoms, stress factors, or diagnoses.

History of Psychiatric Diagnosis

In prehistoirc times, there was no known effective treatment for mental illness. Treatment might have been rendered by the local shaman or by priests in early civilizations. Traditionally, the heart was often perceived as the center of emotions and as the most important organ. The ancients apparently had a lesser opinion of the brain. Nevertheless, anthropologists have found prehistoric human skulls with healed "surgical" holes, the reasons for which are unclear. Modern humans presume this to be some kind of ancient neuro-psychiatric treatment, but that remains to be proven. We can, however, make two presumptions in the cases where the holes had time to heal: that the patients apparently survived a while and that they were presumably nursed back to health.

In historic times, we have some records from some civilizations regarding their responses to mental illness. In those olden times, psychiatric illness was labeled according to cultural norms such as: ill-starred fate, neurological illness, demonic possession, and witchcraft. Astrologers and soothsayers were consulted. In Europe, the mentally ill were chained up in dank institutions resembling jails. The Hospital of St. Mary of Bethlehem (pronounced "Bedlam") in England was notorious. As recently as eighty years ago, patients received hydrotherapy—hot and cold immersions. Since then, psychiatric care has gone through these transitions:

- Before Freud, the diagnoses were descriptive and were based on groups of descriptive symptoms fabricated out of Greek and Latin words (for example: involutional melancholia, dementia præcox, hysteroid dysphoria, hebephrenia, dipsomania, and so on)
- In the nineteenth and twentieth centuries, Freudian psychiatrists (psychoanalysts) detailed symptoms that were interpreted by resorting to analyzing possible subconscious factors including dream interpretation—this was an interesting time period in which psychiatric diseases were analyzed from a theoretical viewpoint
- Modern American system (twentieth and early twenty-first century) came into play in an attempt to try to list diseases together depending upon symptoms and classify them by rational diagnosis. This was a method for linking seemingly similar conditions to other seemingly similar conditions. Standardized naming went into effect; the use of descriptive disease labels gave way to a standardized naming system for the diseases. Nowadays the diagnosis of these disorders relies upon the reference book called DSM (Diagnostic and Statistical Manual of the American Psychiatric Association, APA). The DSM has been evolving also, and is now going into its fifth revision.

Each era has its own best-intentioned attempt to understand mental illness. Contemporary approaches will eventually show themselves to be inadequate in a future age (perhaps no more enlightened than now but certainly more confident in its righteousness). And that will become the basis for providing future mental healthcare. One can only hope that contemporary prejudice and economics play the smallest part possible in whatever new schema is proposed.

This book relies on the DSM system.

I also use the term "mechanics" of treatment in referring to the process of diagnosis and treatment. This process occurs in sequential stages (unless the patient drops out of treatment prematurely). This table shows the general correlation between progress as seen from the doctor's viewpoint and also from the patient's feeling state. In the left column are nine stages of patient illness from the patient's subjective experience. In the right column are five phases of patient illness from the doctor's viewpoint:

Table III-2 *from the Patient's Viewpoint..........................from the Doctor's viewpoint*	Diagnosis and Treatment *
From the Patient's viewpoint Nine Phases of Treatment	**From the Doctor's viewpoint** **Five Stages of Treatment**
0—there may occur an external or internal stressor acting upon the patient's genetic factors 1—very early onset ("prodrome") 2—early onset 3—symptomatic stage (sum of stages 1, 2, & 3)	**the doctor has not yet seen the patient**
4—patient comes to first visit with the doctor and receives a working diagnosis; patient is given a first prescription or free samples and then, patient comes back for first follow-up visit (2nd visit)	**I)) First phase: diagnosis of the patient: doctor formulates a working diagnosis** **II)) Second phase: early treatment (this is patient stage 4): start pills**
5—early treatment (next few doctor visits)	**II)) Second phase: early treatment** **Deal with side effects from pills**
6—mid-treatment (next few months of doctor visits)	**III)) Third phase: entering stability treatment: dealing with side effects, symptoms, and situations**
7—remission (feeling 70% better)	**IV)) Fourth phase: dealing with any other side effects, symptoms, and situations unique to that patient that might lead to impending decompensation or relapse**
8—recuperation (feeling 85% better)	**V)) Fifth phase: continue effective treatment with little or no change**
9—recovery (more or less back to baseline behavior and feelings)	**V)) Fifth phase continued: make any medication adjustments as needed (if patient develops a new medical disease or starts new pills from primary doctor)**
Patient might be able to stop the treatment at some time in the future	- - - - - - -
Patient's symptoms might come back: Stages 0, 1, 2, 3, and/or 4	**First phase repeats**

Coming to see a psychiatrist is a big event for most people and they can come voluntarily, semi-voluntarily, or involuntarily.

After presenting to the psychiatrist's office there will be an initial interview. The doctor will assign a working diagnosis and will proceed with treatment plans. In reality, the treatment will be geared toward improvement of the symptoms themselves regardless of the diagnostic label. In other words, we will preferentially treat the specific symptoms within the general context of that formalized diagnosis. The prescribed medicines may or may not be indicated for that diagnosis, but the medications will be indicated for the symptoms that the patient is having. This is due to the fact that a lot of symptoms may overlap each diagnosis. Often patients find information on the Internet and try to second-guess the doctor. This could actually jeopardize treatment plans. Patients approach psychiatric diagnosis too rigidly and forget that many drugs help many conditions that are not on the Internet. Initially it is important to give the patient some symptomatic relief or else he will drop out of treatment.

▶▶QUESTIONS

Q: How do patients become patients? In other words, what happens to people to make them seek psychiatric treatment?

A: What this really is asking is "what is the source or cause of psychiatric illness?" The source tends to be a genetic vulnerability ("genetic predisposition") which can be set off by stress factors—a tiny percentage of people are so sensitive that almost any stressor can bring on these symptoms, whereas in many people, a bigger stress factor is required. Some people seem to be resistant to any stress factor. The most highly sensitive people usually start suffering in their teens or before and go on to have life-long psychiatric disabilities. Most people have variable responses to stressors and variable responses to medications and varied outcomes, which by any account are not permanent disabilities. A certain rather large percentage of people seem to be immune to these supervening stress factors and will never have occasion to see a psychiatrist.

Q: Is each psychiatric diagnosis self-exclusive to the point that a patient has only one specific diagnosis?

A: No. There are many overlapping symptoms and overlapping disease states. Every patient is different and also will have differing symptoms. In reality, we can have six schizophrenic patients with six sets of symptoms which may be similar but not the same. They will all probably have six ways of responding to anti-schizophrenia medicines. Each patient seems to have somewhat unique symptoms so that a hundred patients represent a hundred distinct cases.

* these are terms that I have devised

Diagnosis from the psychiatrist's viewpoint
Five Phases of Treatment

This chapter is the second in a series of five chapters. Each chapter is devoted to a particular aspect of treatment of the patient. Chapter III-2 provides the origins and bases for modern psychiatric treatment. This Chapter III-3 discusses the diagnosis and treatment from the doctor's viewpoint. This is probably the most important of all five parts because the successful outcome of diagnosis and treatment ultimately relies on the doctor's involvement. He can "make or break" the whole process. Chapter III-3 tries to show some of the complexity involved in treatment planning. Chapter III-4 will discuss what the patient feels during his own treatment process. We always strive to make treatment feel better than the original condition. Chapter III-5 takes into account that sometimes one or more family members may want to have a say-so in this whole process. The last Chapter III-6 we shall discuss aspects of treatment.

Working Diagnosis

The process of diagnosis and treatment starts with the diagnosis. On the first visit to the doctor, he will make a working diagnosis. He will then discuss treatment tactics and strategy with the patient. The short-term goal is to relieve some of the patient's suffering; however, there are also long-term goals for which the doctor must plan. He will be in charge of overseeing this outcome. He alone has the unique vision for coordinating short-term goals so that they will dovetail into a palatable long-term treatment strategy. The doctor should have alternate plans in case the treatment strategy might change: the main reason for a change of strategy is if new symptoms or new diagnoses appear.

Chapter Outline

- We focus on whether the patient is even **willing** to see a doctor for treatment.
- **Referral patterns** are related to willingness
- We **collect information** on how the patient came to be this way—this is the patient's "history".

- Patient states his **symptoms**.

- We try to understand what might be the **cause** of these symptoms.

- We collect and add up all the symptoms to make a working (tentative) **diagnosis**. This diagnosis is based on the patient's "history" and symptoms (the number and severity of symptoms).

- The patient may have **more than one diagnosis**—the worst one is treated first.

- Start treatment plan

Willingness (from doctor's point of view)

"Willingness" refers to whether the patients have a cooperative attitude about diagnosis and treatment plans. Willingness is very important. Willing patients look forward to treatment. Unwilling patients cannot be treated legally unless permission is granted by the patient, the patient's guardian, or a judge. Someone has to determine if an unwilling patient needs to be treated against his will.

"Referral" concerns the way that patients are recommended to find their way into a doctor's office (see below).

Summary on the degrees of "Willingness"

Voluntary patients recognize their symptoms: these patients have "**insight**" or "observing ego", their internal self (ego) can "observe" that the patients are ill. They may want psychiatric treatment or some alternative treatment, such as religion or a non-traditional program of spirituality.

Voluntary patients will usually be cooperative with most or all of the prescribed treatment.

Patients who are aware that they have a disorder needing treatment will usually fare far better than involuntary patients. Patient awareness enhances a patient's ability to work with the psychiatrist instead of resisting treatment. Self-awareness characterizes self-referred (voluntary) patients.

Semi-voluntary patients have partial insight and some "**resistance**" to psychiatric intervention (or a lot of resistance). "Resistance" means that they do not want to see a psychiatrist.

Semi-voluntary patients may come back later and state that they have perceived that the original prescription was tolerable but not great and so they took it willy-nilly. This patient often comes in to "visit" the psychiatrist because she has gained a sense that there may be other treatment choices or she is getting a lot of peer pressure to behave. Sometimes she comes in because she has nowhere else to go (i.e. the family doctor has nothing else to offer). Friends and family may decide to withhold support until she comes back to treatment. Patients who have already had this disease may experience a flare-up and try to ignore it. They will eventually recognize it as a relapse, but may balk at restarting psychiatric treatment and may hope that it just goes away. As it gets worse, they will remember that it was treated with some success in the past. So, they come in after the disease is getting worse.

Involuntary patients may have three presentations. There are usually three somewhat distinct groups, each represented in about equal proportions. The first group may deny they have any problems ("**denial**"). The second group might know they have a problem but feel that they are beyond medical help. This is usually because they are delusional, help-rejecting, or feeling "hapless, hopeless, helpless". The third group is aware of all their problems and symptoms, but just want to be left alone (personal right to privacy: it is not illegal to be insane as long as a person does not harm himself or endanger others). In this third category, you will also find a subset of long-term psychiatric patients who have taken medicine in the past, and—whether or not it stopped the symptoms—the medicine felt worse than the original disease. Each group needs a different treatment approach.

A sizable fraction of members of the first group will often remain in denial for years or decades. In their case, denial appears to be part of their personality style: self-admission of psychiatric illness causes unbearable suffering to their self-esteem. Certain degrees of narcissism may be operative. Since this type of denial is linked to personality (Axis II), we should anticipate that *"it will not change much with the rising and setting of a few suns"* (Tolkien).

Persons in the second group have a prominent depressive component and sense of utter futility with all aspects of life and of the world in general (including psychiatry). They imagine that they are well beyond help from mere human intervention. These thoughts seem to range somewhere between depression and temporary delusions. I have stated earlier that delusions are "fixed false beliefs" that are usually not negotiable by logic, but the delusional depression of this second category of person is amenable to improvement to human intervention. Once they have been taking appropriate treatment for a period of weeks, the treatment usually starts to make them feel better and they gain "insight" into the fact that they had been ill, but are now better thanks to modern medicine. Medicating them in the first week or two may require coercion or coaxing, and some cases might require a court order to get them to take their medicines, but as a group, their overall outlook for recovery is good.

People in the third group like to do as they please and do not enjoy having other people scrutinize their lifestyle choices, including any kind of medical treatment. They may have partially valid reasons for refusing treatment. Often they have had little success with medicines. Perhaps most medicines tried have been useless, and the useful medicines either caused true allergic reactions (rash) or toxic reactions (abnormal heartbeat, diabetes, eyes-rolling, or severe infection). They choose to remain unmedicated and modify their lives accordingly, even if it means living in a transient hotel in downtown LA. They are content to be taken to the psychiatric hospital when they are really out of control: this is their idea of a personalized treatment plan.

From our viewpoint, the involuntary patient shows up in the office with a rather significant number of flagrant signs and symptoms and usually comes in when the disease process is already in full force. He may be so disorganized that he does not even have the wherewithal to know what is wrong with him. In this case, a few of the concerned family members bring him in to our offices. Oftentimes a number of family members have decided to shun him, believing that all of this is under his voluntary control. In some cases, his friends—if any are left—might bring him in. Employers and bosses might send him to our office or drop him off in the waiting room and then go back to work, but they usually do not accompany him to the office. (If police bring psychiatric patients to treatment, it is usually directly to the hospital.) Psychiatrists are completely accustomed to dealing with all these types of patients and have something to offer them all.

Also, some patients who are involuntarily brought in for a first visit by family, will later become more voluntary when they start to recover and can understand their disease.

But others who are unaware that they have a disease, rarely take pills as prescribed—if at all. This is usually due to two issues: (1) the disease is telling him that he has no disease; and/or, (2) the first doses of pills produce only side-effects and no benefit, so the pills are discarded as useless.

These are the commonest willingness scenarios of patients who might come in for a visit:

1—those who already had this disease in the past and now know that they are in relapse (*voluntary* self-referral);

2—those who have never had this disorder but begin to understand how ill they are and agree to full cooperation with the treatment plan (*involuntary patient becomes voluntary*);

3—those who deny having any really significant disease but may show up periodically off and on when their symptoms really flare up for various reasons: pressure from job or family. Occasionally, they just want to keep some tenuous connection to their "psychiatrist of record" (the treating psychiatrist whose name appears on any of their paperwork, such as SSD forms or workplace forms from their EAP, Employees Assistance Programs). They stop and start medications on their own and have no regular follow-through (*erratically semi-voluntary*);

4—those who are aware of some minor vague sensations which need treatment (the symptoms may be worse than the patient senses: a conditional semi-voluntary patient who may also accept only conditional "semi-treatment"—but only if he "approves" of the treatment. Their reasons for "approval" often seem capricious), *"conditional semi-voluntary"*; and,

5—those who are so ill that they deny that anything is wrong and refuse to come in for any visits (*involuntary*); or,

6—those who are hallucinating and delusional and unable to process reality in any meaningful way (they are so mentally impaired that they can not summon the will to make any kind of [voluntary] choices: this patient is legally involuntary. Since he has no idea what is going on, I classify him as *"non-voluntary"*). If these so-called "non-voluntary" patients receive some medicine, then after several days, they may pink up and state that they have had this condition before, and that they definitely want the same treatment again. Some of these "non-voluntary" may end up being resistant, aggressive, and involuntary, whereas others may become semi-voluntary or conditional semi-voluntary.

Referral patterns

Referral concerns the way that patients are recommended to find their way into a doctor's office. There are self-referrals, professional referrals, casual referrals, and "police referrals".

Self-referral usually means that the patient has decided that he might have a problem that needs treatment—in suburban practice, this is often not a major psychiatric illness, but rather problems with relationships and job stress. A self-referral may be made for more serious problems, also, such as serious "baby blues" (post-partum depression). These will be voluntary patients.

Professional referrals might come from another health professional, such as the family doctor. Psychotherapists can also refer their "talk therapy" clients to see a psychiatrist for prescriptions. These will be voluntary patients (or semi-voluntary—sometimes the therapist's clients are leery of pills—after all they started with talk therapy first! That is a first clue that medication is not likely to be their top treatment preference).

Casual referrals originate with trusted friends or family members. One could probably also include advertisements in select local or regional monthly publications (such as found in the "Pasadena Magazine", the L.A. chapter of the Sierra Club, local Christian sources, and so on). These will be voluntary also.

The *police* are also a source of referrals—these are usually psychiatric emergencies. Most of them will be involuntary or "non-voluntary", but some will be semi-voluntary or voluntary, as in the case of people who call 9-1-1, stating that they need help or else they might commit suicide.

Collecting background information (the history of the present illness)

Next we talk to the patient and family members and find out the story of what led up to the first visit. We will inquire if other family members have had these symptoms, if patient ever had these symptoms or any psychiatric symptoms in the past, if there are drugs and alcohol involved, if he is taking other medicines for major medical disorders, and so on.

Symptoms and Signs (disease markers)

These have been covered in Chapter III-1.

Trying to find **Causes**—if any

The whole process begins with developing psychiatric symptoms. What might cause these symptoms? The main causes are genetics, environment, internal biochemistry, or unknown factors. Environmental symptoms can arise in relation to some external stressful event in Toby's life. An internal stress refers to something within the body that is not apparently genetic. Of course, the psychiatric disturbance can be set off by a combination of some [external] stress factor acting upon the patient's genetic make-up.

External stressors

This can be a sudden catastrophic event (natural disaster or extreme stress), long-standing chronic stress, or a smaller stressor or series of stressors:

1—sudden catastrophic events can be natural disasters or man-made stressful events such as war, horrendous car-crash, or witnessing murders;

2—longstanding chronic stress that slowly erodes away at a person's natural defenses or gradually strips away his support system;

3—a series of smaller events all occurring around the same time in a person's life. Taken individually, any one of these stressors might not have been enough to set off a psychiatric response. But when grouped together the factors can be stressful. An example of such a clustering of events would be: divorce finalized in early March, loss of job due to outsourcing in late March, and a new cancer diagnosis in a close friend in April.

Drs. Thomas Holmes and Richard Rahe compiled an excellent table of life events[3(a)], wherein each stressful event is assigned a numerical value that can suggest susceptibility to stress-induced illness. The higher the score, the greater the likelihood of suffering a stress-related medical illness.

4—there may not be any one obvious or major external stressor in which case the stress is of debatable origin;

5—the only apparent stressor may be so trivial that it is not a usual candidate cause; or,

6—some as-yet unknown external force.

Internal Stressors

In the alternative, there may be internal sources at work. Examples of internal stressors:

1 sudden catastrophic internal events would famously be strokes which can suddenly result in massive psychological changes and upheavals. In some cases, suppressed psychological urges come to the fore—such as being sexually inappropriate. At times, this patient may exhibit totally new and bizarre symptoms that have never occurred in him before—or at least not to the recollection of family and close friends;

2 Theory suggests that the age of the (previously sane) patient may "release", suppress, or activate a "timing gene" (in the patient's DNA). This timing gene could activate other genes that could cause a mental illness. He has received these genes from one of his parents. It is not uncommon to see fifty-something patients who have come down with the same mood disorder that their parent had had at the same age. Depression can appear this way.

3 Aging can result in stereotyped behavioral changes that are possibly due to a mixture of causes. Examples of these well-known changes occur at certain times of life, such as those associated with puberty, "seven year itch", "midlife crisis", or "grouchy old man syndrome". Male schizophrenics often start to get ill around or after puberty[3(b)], whereas the peak age in female schizophrenics is in their mid-twenties.

4 There may be a series of chronic internal stressor or just one internal stressor perhaps of an endocrine nature.

5 There may be as yet unidentified internal processes.

Internal-External (Stressors)

Sometimes a psychiatric condition can be set off by an internal-external combination. We all inherit different genes to code certain proteins in differing quantities at different times and at different stages of life; the way that these proteins are handled in our nerve cells can lead to cascades of biochemical events that can make us susceptible to having certain symptoms. Being susceptible, however, does not necessarily create the psychiatric illness automatically. Oftentimes an external agent or event needs to supervene in order to set off the psychiatric disturbance. Examples of external agents can be a virus, toxic chemicals, or inflammation; examples of events can be anything traumatic such as impending death, massive trauma, loss of a loved one, etc. In many cases, this external agent or event adds the final straw to the camel's back to set off chemical changes in our brains to create an officially recognized psychiatric disorder.

Personality style can be partly inborn, but it can also be modulated by nurture (environment), which in its turn can effect changes in personality style. This variability is indicated by ↗ and ↙. Intense chaos of personality is shown by loops ∪∪. Personality style is present in every person and rarely changes in quality, but its intensity may modulate during various phases of life.

(1) Thad   *figure III-3-a genetic predispositions*

DNA→ "normal"→	Childhood "normal"→	Teen Years→	*	Adulthood
↳Personality style→	↓↑Personality↗	↘↗Personality↓↑	→	↳Personality style→

In (1) we see Thad who has no real genetic disorder and is not affected by his childhood, apart from some typical teenage tumult. His personality goes through fluctuations before adulthood but eventually straightens out (*) and the rest of his life normalizes and stabilizes. Thad is probably going to have a "normal" life (not needing to see a psychiatrist).

(2) Jake

DNA→→	Childhood "normal"→	Teen Years→	*	Adulthood
↳genetic possibility for depression might shape personality style → ↓↑Personality withdrawn↗	↓↑ few depression symptoms	Depression drug abuse ∪ ↓↑ ∪ ↘personality erratic	⇄	depression ↘Personality↘

In (2) we see Jake who has a genetic tendency for depression. His childhood does not affect him too much, but he has tumultuous teen years that leave him (*) with a mild depression diagnosis by adulthood. The arrows ↓↑ indicate the eventuality of the disorder.

(3) Nellie

DNA→(genetic loading)	Childhood→	Teen Years→	*	Adulthood
↳ childhood trauma ϟϟϟϟϟ Personality style→	1-massive trauma 2-abuses 3—virus, toxins, lead ↓↑Personality↓↑	Permanent brain Changes ∩∩ Psychiatric symptoms ℧℧ ℧℧ Personality	‡ ‡	Major psychiatric disorder ℧℧ ℧℧ Personality

In (3) we see Nellie who has a genetic tendency plus a traumatic childhood—she will be badly affected. Her disorder can feed the symptoms ∩ thus aggravating the disorder. She will have trouble with her young adult coming-of-age activities, since she may still be chained to specters of bad childhood memories and abuses (*). She will have problems throughout adulthood.

*this refers to young adult coming-of-age activities such as college, military service, peace corps, au pair service, etc.

The definition of "massive trauma" varies from person to person—even between identical twins. In severe disorders, these sudden chemical changes can cause permanent chemical changes, which can not be reversed with current technology. Examples of such serious disorders are manic-depression, schizophrenia, post-traumatic disorder, and the truly classic case of alcoholism. Alcoholism really seems to be the most cogent argument for this irreversible chemical change; all alcoholics in AA know that "a pickle can not be turned back into a cucumber". The build-up of all these stressors can eventually lead to decompensation (falling apart).

Working Diagnosis

Next we make a working diagnosis at the time of the first visit, and this diagnosis becomes the point of departure for understanding the patient's situation in life. This diagnosis is based on all the information that we glean from the patient and from any of her friends and family whom she permits in the office at the time of the first visit. (We cannot legally call your friends or family to request background information.) The information which is taken into account includes: current stressors, signs and symptoms, medical history, psychiatric history, current medicines, recreational drugs and alcohol abuse, family psychiatric history, job situation, civil status, and whether the patient came in alone or with a troupe of concerned relatives. The whole person and her situation need to be taken into account also and this is what leads to individual treatment plans. This working diagnosis is important because it will inform and guide the first prescription. (Working diagnosis is also called preliminary or tentative diagnosis—although there are slight differences in nuance in these terms.)

As an example of a working diagnosis, let's look at Asperger's Disorder [1(a)] a childhood psychiatric disorder in the same group as Autism.. Asperger's Disorder is mainly seen by child psychiatrists, but there has been a growing trend for adult psychiatrists to seek out undiagnosed cases in their adult patient case load. It is becoming a more recognized diagnosis. (I chose Asperger's mainly because it has very convenient A1-4 B1-4 criteria for demonstration purposes).

First, we can look at the signs and symptoms required for diagnosis of Asperger's Disorder in a child. Then we listen to and observe the signs/symptoms that the patient's parents are mentioning and the symptoms/signs that they are reporting. We tend to group the same kinds of symptoms/signs together. This is from the DSM-IV-TR textbook[1]. These are the kinds of required symptoms to make a real working diagnosis of Asperger's Disorder (in this disorder, the DSM-IV-TR refers to both signs and symptoms as "symptoms"):

Asperger's Diagnosis requires   *table III-3-b* two (or more) symptoms from Group 'A' *and* one (or more) symptoms from group 'B'

Group 'A' symptoms of social impairment
Patient must have a least two of these Group A symptoms:
   1- symptom #1 nonverbal behavior impairment
   2- symptom #2 no peer group
   3- symptom #3 lack of spontaneous joy sharing
   4- symptom #4 lack of social reciprocity

-plus-

Group B symptoms of repetitive activities
He must have at least one of these :
   1- symptom #1 abnormal preoccupation with restricted interests
   2- symptom #2 inflexibility to change
   3- symptom #3 constant repetitive movements
   4- symptom #4 preoccupied with parts of objects

(Criteria C, D ,E, F not listed) DSM-IV-TR: Pervasive Developmental Disorders
(without this minimum number of symptoms, the Disorder can not be diagnosed)

A formal diagnosis requires only two symptoms/signs from "A" and one from "B". Obviously, a patient with all four symptoms/signs in "A" and all four symptoms/signs in "B" will have a more severe case. The more symptoms, the worse the disease state. (These groupings and symptoms are just examples of a conceptual disease and merely demonstrate the general approach that we take to make a DSM-based diagnosis.) These symptoms may or may not really be interrelated at all, but because we deal with them every day, we come to recognize them as if they were similar or the same and thus assume them to be originating from the same region of the brain. Research is beginning to reveal more. Symptoms #1-4 may have nothing in common other than the fact that we traditionally find them together in severe cases of Asperger's and thus we list them together. This is how we make a diagnosis based on past history, present history, and symptoms. This system seems fairly uniform but has a few flaws—as we shall soon read.

If the symptoms change enough, then the patient might acquire a new diagnosis, or the former diagnosis can be revised in the case that new history comes to light. An example would be that of a young woman who comes in with enough symptoms to qualify as a mild major depression. If it later turns out that she is alcoholic, then the diagnosis could change to "depression due to alcoholism". If she has a disease and must take prednisone which makes her manic, then she might be considered as a "mood disorder, due to prednisone". Or, the whole diagnosis might be changed to "depression due to disease-related inflammation of the brain". She might remember that she had had a mild depression in high school, in which case she might qualify for a diagnosis of mild recurrent major depression. Diagnoses adapt to symptoms and also to patients' responses to treatments. A diagnosis can be changed or modified as treatment continues.

This part of diagnosis is somewhat of a judgment call; however, the treatments are usually based on symptoms not just on diagnosis, so that even if a diagnosis is later changed, it is not likely that the treatment will change much. This is when we remind you of our mantra "Medicine is an art not a science". And this certainly applies to psychiatric medicine as well. A hundred psychiatrists examining the same patient will all probably diagnose a similar condition and prescribe similar medications, so there is no need for alarm regarding any minor alterations in the working diagnosis.

Each patient's case is unique and each patient's symptoms are somewhat different. Psychiatrists assign a diagnosis to each patient. In very rare cases where there is no significant psychiatric diagnosis, we still code a "place-holder" diagnosis of 799.0—this is a diagnosis of "no diagnosis".

MORE THAN ONE Diagnosis: In case of more than one Diagnosis, the worse or worst diagnosis is treated first.

Main concept: the diagnosis suggests a treatment approach, but there may be more than one diagnosis needing treatment. Usually only one diagnosis (or one set of symptoms) will be the focus of treatment initially. The psychiatrist might periodically update the diagnosis or even make some modifications in the primary diagnosis. The doctor may detect other diagnoses that were not the initial focus of concern (such as gambling addiction or hoarding). The real goal of diagnosis is to guide prescription patterns in order to alleviate suffering. Diagnosis is not just an academic exercise since it points us toward effective treatments. Diagnosis is the map for taking the person to relief—medications and psychotherapy are the vehicle.

Sometimes the new patient might have more than one diagnosis in which case the most salient and most critical diagnosis will usually be treated first. The patient may request to treat a secondary condition first and this request should be discussed because she obviously has different priorities: if the apparently appropriate treatment is not to her liking then she probably will not be able to engage in a mutual treatment plan. These requests should be taken seriously since her real-life experience may encompass more discomfort from the secondary diagnosis than from the primary [text-book] case. These requests, however, cannot be honored if the patient is having a psychiatric emergency (suicidal, homicidal, or actively hallucinating). In case of psychiatric emergency, the patient will likely need to be sent to a hospital. Apart from that happenstance, we will begin treating each diagnosis one at a time, or treating each symptom one pill at a time until there is symptomatic improvement.

Treatment begins (see chapter III-6). Diagnosis may depend upon certain factors, but the symptoms are always going to be the same and will still require very similar treatment regardless of any diagnosis.

▶▶QUESTIONS

Q: It seems that diagnosis is arbitrary (as well as the treatment for that diagnosis), so how do psychiatrists know what to do next?

A: The practice of medicine (as it pertains to any specialty including psychiatry) is an art not a science. At least this system seems to represent an improvement over the older systems. And this current system provides quick relief as opposed to psychoanalysis which can take years.

This seemingly arbitrary system is now in the process of significant review thanks to new understanding of genetic underpinnings. The most recent theory is that we all inherit different genes to code certain proteins in differing quantities at different times and at different stages of life; the way that these proteins are handled in our nerve cells can lead to cascades of biochemical events which can make us susceptible to having certain symptoms at certain ages. Being susceptible, however, does not necessarily create the psychiatric illness automatically.

Q: Why make more than one diagnosis?

A: There are several reasons:

    1—psychiatrists—like most doctors—focus on details and want all of the data to be as complete as possible;

    2—In modern psychiatry the government still requires listing these arbitrary diagnoses in order for psychiatrists to be reimbursed for seeing patients. And as a matter of fact, the more diagnoses we can assign to a patient, then the more payment we might receive (for example, from Medicare);

    3—It is quite likely that the patient has more than one diagnosis; and,

    4—The presence of two or more diagnoses may often support the use of two or more medications and especially may justify using one of the medicines "off-label".

Q: But are some of the psychiatric disorders reversible?

A: Reversible is not the term that we would use. Sometimes some of the so-called "minor" psychiatric disorders can be a temporary and one-time event; however, these disorders may crop up again in the near or distant future and can often take on a more grotesque and pernicious character at that time. If you have had one minor psychiatric disorder for a year followed by a prolonged and complete recovery and never had a recurrence of this disorder for the rest of your life, then you are doing well. It is estimated that about 10-15% new patients will continue to have a diagnosis that is hard to bring under control; about one third will recover completely from the first episode but will have a recurrence later in their lives. And perhaps half of patients will not have a major recurrence.

Q: What about identical twins?

A: By definition, identical twins are supposed to be exact copies of each other; however, oftentimes identical twins do not have the exact same psychiatric disorders. They might both become depressed; they might both do well with Paxil. The course of the depression may last about the same; but, in many cases the psychiatric disorders are not shared identically and mutually between them. It is well known that if one identical twin has schizophrenia, then the other twin has usually a 40-75% chance of becoming frankly schizophrenic—not 100% as one might think. In some cases one twin might be frankly schizophrenic and the other might just be a little strange or reclusive or mistrustful but not to the full-blown extent of the frankly ill twin. Ditto for alcoholism: one identical twin might become an alcoholic while the other does not. There are various attempts to group together certain well-known symptoms and then label that particular grouping as a psychiatric disorder. In reality, this system is rather arbitrary because the trend is to look at each patient separately.

3-a-(reference 3), p.1547

3-b-(reference 3), p.890

Psychiatric Diagnosis from the patient's viewpoint
Nine Stages of Treatment

This chapter continues a series of five chapters. Each chapter is devoted to a particular aspect of treatment of the patient. Chapter III-2 provides the origins and bases for modern psychiatric treatment. Part III-3 discusses the diagnosis and treatment from the doctor's viewpoint. This part, Chapter III-4, discusses what the patient feels during his own treatment process. Patient participation is about as important as the part played by the doctor. If a patient does not like the diagnosis or the treatment, he might drop out and continue to suffer. We try to make treatment as user-friendly as possible. I am aware that first visits to a psychiatrist can be very anxiety provoking. We always strive to make treatment feel more comfortable than the original condition. Chapter III-5 takes into account that sometimes one or more family members may want to have a say-so in this whole process. The last part, Chapter III-6, discusses aspects of treatment.

The process of diagnosis and treatment starts with the diagnosis. On the first visit to the doctor, he will make a working diagnosis. He will then discuss treatment tactics and strategy with the patient. The short-term goal is to relieve some of the patient's suffering; however, there are also long-term goals for which the doctor must plan. He will be in charge of overseeing this outcome. He alone has the unique vision for coordinating short-term goals so that they will dovetail into a palatable long-term treatment strategy. The doctor should have alternate plans in case the treatment strategy might change: the main reason for a change of strategy is if new symptoms or new diagnoses appear.

Treatability

Treatability can refer to the disorder or to the patient. Most psychiatric conditions are treatable in the sense that a known therapy is available, but some conditions are very hard to treat, such as severe personality disorders or paranoia. Any patient who does not want treatment, is not very treatable. On the other hand, if he desires treatment, then he is certainly willing and probably treatable, too. The surest path to success depends upon the patient's willingness to engage in treatment.

Patient "Willingness"(from doctor's viewpoint—see Chapter III-3)

Voluntary patients recognize their symptoms and they usually want psychiatric treatment or some alternative treatment, such as religion or a non-traditional program of spirituality.

Semi-voluntary patients want to get better, but are leery of seeing a psychiatrist for any number of reasons (social stigma, cost, inconvenience, and so on). Some prospective semi-voluntary patients have some "**resistance**" to psychiatric intervention (or a lot of resistance). "Resistance" means that they do not want to have a psychiatric treatment.

Involuntary patients do not want to see a psychiatrist and do not want psychiatric treatment. (In the traditional sense, the psychiatrist is both the doctor and the treatment, so these are the same concept).

Willingness from patient's viewpoint

Nowadays Americans are more psychologically sophisticated and will often refer themselves for treatment. Let's consider a theoretical patient, Mary. If Mary is not having an emergency and comes in of her own accord to engage in meaningful treatment, then she is basically a voluntary patient. However, a surprising number of patients will not come (voluntarily) and will not obtain treatment until some third person brings them in for assessment: this can be friends, family, police, etc. In any case, these patients are coming on a semi-voluntary or perhaps a weakly involuntary basis. People who come in early are usually able to recover well since they came in before the disease "festered"; the converse is usually true of the involuntary patients; and, the semi-voluntary patients fall in middle ground.

In some cases, a patient like Mary may be completely unaware of her symptoms for a long time. However, eventually she will feel so bad that she (voluntarily) seeks out a psychiatrist for her emotional suffering. In other cases, she will not be aware of her symptoms but her friends, family, and primary care doctor are aware. She is often visiting the primary doctor for various symptoms, which end up being psychological and not medical. At this point, her primary doctor will either give Mary a prescription (Lexapro, for example) or insist that she go to see a psychiatrist. This is a semi-voluntary (or quasi-voluntary) patient who arrives skeptically, reluctantly, or even defiantly at the psychiatrist's office.

In still other cases, the family members bring in an unwilling (involuntary) patient, such as Brad who is having a psychotic depression. Involuntary patients like Brad usually do not believe that they have any problem at all. Hence, they reason that there is nothing that needs fixing. Brad denies that there is anything wrong. Another type of involuntary patient Ken knows that he is depressed but believes that no medical intervention can help him perhaps because no doctor can understand him (he is delusional or help-rejecting). In some of these cases, involuntary patients like Ken believe that they are sick but with the stipulation that only a divine power can cure them and they resort to religion for healing.

Treatment Stages

Patients will go through these several treatment stages—unless they drop out of treatment:

0—possible internal or external stressors—or both. Brad is usually aware of the stressors, but may ignore them or shrug them off—unfortunately, these little molehills can grow into small mountains sometimes, and this growth process may be sudden or gradual. If it is sudden, Brad might recognize it. If it is gradual, month by month, then it may go unperceived.

1—prodrome (the beginning of the beginning)—Brad is showing a few changes in behavior; subtle changes in his "normal" behavior; he is rarely aware of this, but others may comment. (Why aren't you playing soccer on Saturday mornings any more?")

2—onset—he is becoming symptomatic; paradoxically, as symptoms get worse he may feel that they are not significant or that he is not "worthy" of psychiatric treatment, or, in other cases he may come to the conclusion that all his symptoms are due to some stress factor. Men may start having a few beers. Women may start "nervous nibbling".

3—Symptoms progress and worsen if left untreated. He may start having a few more beers—or a few too many. Or he may drive recklessly or buy a new truck for no real reason. Women may seek solace in "retail therapy".

These first three stages may evolve quickly over days, weeks, months (usually), or even years: disease with fast onset is more obvious; but, the slower the progression, the less likely to be noticed and more likely to be "discounted" by friends as a mere "personality" problem or as a stress-related occurrence. "Oh, he's just going through a phase." (That is true: a depressive phase);

4—psychiatric visits finally begin; Brad is missing work, sleeping all weekend, up late at night watching old re-runs and using beer to asleep; Mary may become emotionally overwrought over small things;

4a—intake information is collected as well as signs and symptoms of disorder;

4b—a working diagnosis is assigned;

4c—treatment goals and options are outlined and the patient is involved in the decision-making process; Brad and Mary will possibly forget much of this, but forgetfulness or distractibility can be normal;

4d—treatment begins with oversight (by doctor—and by family, if any are involved). Call doctor with any concerns about medication or side effects. ALWAYS call doctor if a rash appears after starting medicines.

5—early stage of treatment might be accompanied by a lot of uneasiness and side-effects; once again, do not hesitate to call doctor.

6—mid-stage treatment is when he begins to feel better; the medication routine is established, life is coming back into focus; there is better job performance, as well as less emotionality;

7—remission occurs when the patient is up and about doing his business as usual. Although he might not feel normal, he will feel propelled gently forward and will take up most of the usual activities; friends and family may comment approvingly on this positive step forward; he is now able to stand up and walk around on the earth;

8a—(relapse will likely occur if he quits taking the medicines prematurely, usually resulting in a return to step 3 above;);

8b—if he does not stop medicines and does not relapse then he will move into the recuperation phase;

8c—recuperation phase: the patient feels normal and others see him as normal;

9—recovery phase: after a variable time span, some or many people will taper off their medicines (hopefully under psychiatric supervision) and be able to go back to a normal life; this is recovery.

No one should give up on Brad or Mary as long as they continue to take the treatment and appear at least to be "going through the motions"—eventually they will merge back into normalcy. Outsiders may be the first to opine that Brad or Mary have recovered; insiders such as family will note some improvement but still detect some minor problems; Brad and Mary themselves may not feel recovered until much later; they may feel "medicated" during many of these phases—this is not to say that they feel bad. They may feel that there is something inside themselves doing for them what they cannot yet do for themselves. This is a depiction of how the "return to normalcy" will look to outsiders, then to insiders, and then to the patients themselves:

Table III-4-a   *Patient looks better before he feels better*

Stages	0, 1	2, 3	4, 5	6	7	8, 9
Outsiders see	normal	*change*	*abnormal*	better	normal	normal
Insiders see	*change*	*abnormal*	*worse*	*change*	better	normal
Patient feels	empty	*change*	*abnormal*	medicated		better

Unfortunately, a sizable fraction will never quite go back to 100% better or "normal" baseline. This might be due to the time duration of the illness. Someone who has been taking depression medications for four years may be able to taper off his medicines and feel that he is 90-95% better after treatment. Who is to say that the 5-10% is due to the disease, or the treatment, or simply the natural fact of aging—we all experience a very slow mental and physical decline while aging.

Some people will continue to need psychiatric medicines off and on—or continuously—for the rest of their lives. Many people are discouraged to reach this realization (needing medicines for life), but please remember that we have only had these significant pharmacologic options for the last century—assuming that all the herbs used for thousands of years are not so significant. If a patient can stay with the treatment plan and collaborate meaningfully with his doctor, then he should get better—quite a bit better. I often cite my 85% rule: 85% of patients should get 85% better at least. The two main problems are that people want instantaneous treatment that will rapidly result in a total cure, and that they are not willing to follow a prolonged treatment plan.

Chart III-4-b	Nine stages of Treatment … from the Patient's viewpoint
0—there may occur an external or internal stressor acting upon the patient's genetic factors
1—very early onset (prodrome)
2—early onset (prodrome)

3—symptomatic stage (sum of stages 1, 2, & 3)

4—patient comes to first visit with the doctor and receives a working diagnosis patient is given a first prescription or free samples as starters and then, patient comes back for first follow-up visit

5—early treatment (next few doctor visits)

6—mid-treatment (further months of doctor visits)

7—remission (feeling 70% better)

8—recuperation (feeling 85% better)

9—recovery (more or less back to baseline behavior and feelings)

Patient might be able to stop the treatment at some time in the future

Patient's symptoms might come back: Stages 0, 1, 2, 3,and/or 4 repeat

If a person has spent the last few years stewing over these problems as they gradually worsen, then I cannot cure him in a week. In these cases, the process will be significantly more involved. If he stays the course and follows instructions, then he will begin to recover—and that is a lot better than psychiatric treatment was one hundred years ago.

Chapter III-5

Diagnosis from the family's viewpoint

This chapter continues a series of five chapters. Each chapter is devoted to a particular aspect of treatment of the patient. Chapter III-2 provides the origins and bases for modern psychiatric treatment. Chapter III-3 discusses the diagnosis and treatment from the doctor's viewpoint. Chapters III-3 and III-4 are the most important of all five parts because the successful outcome of diagnosis and treatment ultimately relies on the mutual engagement between doctor and patient. Chapter III-5 takes into account that sometimes one or more family members may want to have a say-so in this whole process. The last of the five parts, Chapter III-6, discusses aspects of treatment.

Legal Issues

The number-one issue that usually arises within the family is their desire to have the doctor keep them informed about all aspects of the patient's ongoing treatment process. Unfortunately,the law states that as long as the patient is a competent adult, he can dictate if he wants any family members involved. He can request that the doctor avoid contact with any family members or with only certain ones. Concerned family members can call the psychiatrist and offer him information, but the doctor's responses to or involvement with that family member can be limited by the patient's request. The patient can outright forbid the doctor to have any contact with the family, but this is extreme. These laws apply to all "competent" adults. Additionally, these laws also apply to "emancipated minors"; these are teenagers whom the courts consider to be the same as an adult.

One dilemma occurs in demented elderly patients who have been brought in for their first psychiatry visit and receive their first-time dementia diagnosis. Technically speaking, these patients are not incompetent when they arrive at my office, but they are "incompetent" when they leave. These patients have not been officially and legally declared incompetent. If the psychiatrist finds that the person does have probable dementia, then the doctor should make medico-legal documentation that the person now has the medical diagnosis of dementia. This dilemma can become a big problem where the adult children all want to be involved, but they all have their own versions of the family history and—to make matters worse—they want to try to forbid the psychiatrist from paying attention to one of the other adult children. The psychiatrist needs to learn how to filter their information (and agenda) and put it into balance, which in some cases, may mean partially discounting large parts of the history.

This dilemma does not apply to a child or the ward of a guardian, where it is clear that the child or ward is not legally "competent". The parents and guardians make all the treatment choices. Parents of children have a legal right to information, unless the child is an "emancipated" teenager. Certain States have laws regarding how doctors deal with teen pregnancy or adolescent venereal disease.

Elderly patients who are clearly demented are not considered competent adults; the legal system will appoint some family member or other responsible person to be the guardian (conservator) of that elderly person. This designated person has legal rights to discuss the case with the doctor. That person can dictate which family members have access to the elderly person's medical records. Anyone who has legal standing of being a parent, guardian, or a conservator of a patient, is usually the person with whom the psychiatrist must communicate regarding treatment issues.

In case of true life-and-death emergencies, patient safety may override any confidentiality issues.

Patients cannot legally restrain the family from giving information to the doctor: this is a family matter. However, the patient does have the legal right to control information flow from the doctor to the family. If the family wants to tell the doctor information, then he is allowed to listen—unless a competent adult patient has forbidden this too. Any family "secrets" divulged to the doctor might be taken into account as far as treatmen plans. If any adult patient permits the family to accompany him into the doctor's office, then that is the same as giving the doctor the freedom to have free interchange with the attendant family members. At any time during the interview, the patient can order any or all family members to leave the room and stop telling tales to the doctor (however, the family can go home and call the doctor and give him more information on the telephone). At the end of the first interview, the doctor will then discuss treatment tactics and strategy with the patient—and with concerned family members as per patient's wishes.

Family Contribution

Based partly on any family history, the process of diagnosis and treatment starts with the diagnosis. On the first visit to the doctor, he will make a working diagnosis of the patient—oftentimes, background information from the family is extremely important for understanding how the patient became ill. In this situation, the psychiatrist is allowed to hear everything that famly and friends have to say about the patient's history. This history can be important, because patients in crisis often have poor recollection of the past. Usually, patients will not report some psychotic symptoms because they cannot tell the difference between reality and psychosis—that's usually why they end up in the doctor's office in the first place.

Treatment is almost always better if the patient allows his doctor to communicate freely with family members. Families sometimes call in when they remember important facts about patient's background history, alcohol-drug use, or other family secrets. Remembering where patient keeps his firearms is really important, since a patient should not have access to firearms when he is having a psychiatric crisis.

The short-term goal is to relieve some of the patient's suffering; however, the family may see that the patient is having side effects but not calling the doctor about them. The reason is that the patient feels less bad from the side effects than the original illness. When the side effects get worse than that, then the patient will call, or his family member might call. The family—if involved—needs to be aware that there are also long-term goals for which the doctor must plan. Doctor will be in charge of overseeing this outcome. He alone has the unique vision for coordinating short-term goals so that they will dovetail into a palatable long-term treatment strategy. The family should be encouraged to call in any important information that happens during treatment (DUI or rage attacks, for example).

Family Observations

In the *early (prodromal) stages*, the family may or may not be aware that anything is amiss and casual observers and acquaintances will not note it at all. Spouses, however, are the first to detect the earliest "herald symptoms". The patient is often not aware of these.

The *second patient-s*tage is the onset stage in which a patient feels that something might be happening, but dismisses it. In this stage his friends and family, however, will notice "eccentric" behavior or other alterations in the patient.

In the *third patient-stage*, a patient starts to experience uncomfortable symptoms, and he partly understands why friends and family are concerned. The symptoms are like those of any chronic or long-term illness in the sense that they will slowly worsen until treated. However, the family will still note more symptoms than he does. The commonest cases are: mania, psychosis, "slowed-down" depression, or irritable depression.

In cases of slowed-down *depression*, the family may notice that the patient has sadness, stays in bed too much, avoids socializing, gains weight, and has no interest in his usual hobbies.

Patient's basic message to the world is: *"I'm too tired!"*

In cases of *irritable depression*, the family will notice that patient snaps at everybody, is busy "spinning his wheels" but not going anywhere, expends a lot of energy without doing much work, has poor sleep and appetite, and may be losing weight.

Patient's basic message to the world is: *"I'm too stressed out!"*

In cases of *mania*, patient is awake all day and night, feels intensely happy for no apparent reason, has many new projects going on but does not finish any of them, and loses weight because he is hyperactive and forgets to eat.

Patient's basic message to the world is: *"I'm too busy: I've got a million projects!"*

In cases of *psychosis (or schizophrenia)*, the patient stays up all night, sleeps all day, is sullen and suspicious, mumbles to himself, talks to invisible people, and may lose weight because he thinks his food is poisoned

Patient's basic message to the world is: *"I don't trust you!"*

The family can relax somewhat after the patient starts formalized treatment, but they will still send feedback that the patient is better with treatment but still not back to his "old self"—returning to "old self" might never occur depending on a number of clinical factors such as patient's age, medical history, psychiatric history, and family history.

Visualizing all these disease symptoms as part of one spectrum is quite helpful since in many cases there may be overlap symptoms e.g., severely depressed patients might imagine that food is poisoned for some irrational reason, and some psychotics could have depressive symptoms, etc.

If left untreated, the third patient-stage will last a long time—perhaps, until it gets so bad that others acknowledge it. This duration is variable. Some patients are brought in almost immediately and some may wait many years to come to psychiatric attention. It is amazing how long some people have tolerated significantly symptoms before coming in for treatment.

The *fourth patient-stage* begins when patient comes to the psychiatrist's office. In our office, the intake and evaluation can be fairly lengthy—usually two hours or more, depending upon the complexity of the case. The simplest case would be that of a youngish person, Brad for example, with no previous psychiatric problems, no major medical problems, no alcoholism/drug addiction, no serious psychiatric disorders on either side of the family, and no usage of herbs or prescription medicines (or not a lot of prescription medicines—psychiatric or otherwise). The opposite situation would, of course be a complex case.

After the intake process I usually tell Brad and the family members what the working diagnosis is and which treatments are available [in this country]. The only exception would be in the case of a severe "personality disorder" in which case the diagnosis could be alluded to without specifically naming it. The focus of treatment would be on the list of symptoms in need of immediate attention. In truth of fact, psychiatric diagnosis may seem imprecise but the fact speaks for itself: if we give Brad our version of the appropriate treatment, then Brad will probably get better. This kind of outcome suggests that the disease-specific treatment was effective and hence the original diagnosis was on target. Of course, in some cases we modify the diagnosis as time goes on or add diagnoses as more information comes to light (such as gambling, sexual disorders, etc).

▶▶**QUESTIONS**

Q: How could somebody allow all these symptoms to accumulate?

A: There may be more than one reason:

1)- a diseased mind lacks full capacity to realize what its current state of mind is (or is not); and,

2)- these symptoms often accumulate so slowly that the disorder creeps up on the patient. These two reasons apply to severe depressive states; and for psychotic states, there are two more reasons:

3)- the patient is also totally out of contact with reality;

4)- the patient may also have severe paranoia and thinks that everything is involved in some sort of a plot against him by everybody.

Chapter III-6

Treatment from the viewpoint of the doctor and patient
Doctor-Patient Cooperation

This chapter ends a series of five chapters. Each chapter is devoted to a particular aspect of treatment of the patient. Chapter III-2 provides the origins and bases for modern psychiatric treatment. Part III-3 discusses the diagnosis and treatment from the doctor's viewpoint. Chapter III-3 is the most important of all five parts because the successful outcome of diagnosis and treatment ultimately relies on the doctor's involvement. He can "make or break" the whole process. Part III-3 tries to show some of the complexity involved in treatment planning. Chapter III-4 discusses what the patient feels during his own treatment process. Part III-5 takes into account that sometimes one or more family members may want to have a say-so in this whole process. This last part, Chapter III-6, discusses aspects of treatment.

The process of treatment started with the diagnosis, which guides us toward reasonable treatment choices. On the first visit, the doctor will make a working diagnosis that in its turn suggest a treatment plan. Treatment prescribed by a doctor is almost always going to involve pills, and frequently a few non-pharmaceutical suggestions too (aerobic exercise, talk therapy, Twelve Step programs, and so on). The doctor will then discuss treatment tactics and strategy with the patient. The short-term goal is to relieve some of the patient's suffering; however, there are also long-term goals for which the doctor must plan. He will be in charge of overseeing this outcome. He alone has the unique vision for coordinating short-term goals so that they will dovetail into a palatable long-term treatment strategy. The doctor should have alternate treatment plans in case the treatment strategy might change: the main reason for a change of strategy is if new symptoms or new conditions appear.

From Brad's perspective , he is now at *stage four*, the beginning of formalized treatment (see above in Chapters III-4 or III-5). After a working diagnosis is assigned on the first visit, we will discuss the treatment options. These will include the most currently appropriate treatments (which the family probably already knows if they have been on the Internet). I try to get Brad involved in this process, but some patients are so mentally clouded that they have trouble making a decision and just prefer that I start them on some medication. Others will suggest that my experience is the only guidance that they want initially. I will

149

offer this option to make patients and family feel involved in the treatment process. I prefer to have patients who partner with me so that they will have more of a sense of control—it works out better if Brad does not feel that he is being railroaded into some choices.

The *fifth patient-stage* of treatment revolves around physiological adjustment to the new medication. This is the stage at which the first group of side effects may crop up. Side effects which appear in the first week or two will usually resolve and disappear; if they persist for three weeks or more then they will not get better and the patient will need to change medications. Patients often come in for their second visit (their first check-up visit) within one to three weeks, depending upon the medication. For drugs like Paxil and Zoloft (prescribed for depression) the patient will usually come back in two weeks. If I prescribe Paxil or Zoloft for panic attacks without Ativan, a person might need to come back within a week. If he responds well to Ativan and is starting very low-dose Paxil or Zoloft, a return visit of two weeks is acceptable. The timing of the return visit varies a great deal depending upon the stage of treatment, the diagnosis, the medications in use, and other factors.

In the *sixth patient-stage*, Brad has been on the new medicines for weeks and should begin to feel better. The sense of improvement varies a lot depending upon him, the medicine, and the condition under treatment. This newfound sense of improvement is welcome and he feels somewhat improved. This is the good news. The bad news is that the well-being is due to the medicine. The disorder is still down there writhing around in turmoil but the medication is starting to suppress it and keep it in check. If he stops the medicine prematurely then a relapse is likely. A relapse early in treatment is not desirable. Usually the symptoms will flare up again quite quickly and will usually—but not always—abate when the medication is resumed.

In the *seventh patient-stage* Brad will usually be back to his usual self or sometimes even feeling better than that—perhaps feeling better than in years. This is a dangerous stage for two reasons. First reason: Brad may declare himself cured and erroneously stop taking the medicine.

In one scenario, he forgets that the medicine made him better and stops taking the medicine without medical supervision. Other patients feel so normal that they see no reason to continue on the medicine. Still other patients feel a persistent twinge of symptoms on a daily basis but feel that that twinge is tolerable, yet also decide to stop the medicine since they feel better, not realizing that the original symptoms are still lurking down there just waiting for a chance to flare up again. Another group of patients may dislike taking synthetic chemicals and, thus they decide to stop the medicine. They may even rationalize that they are becoming dependent on the drug and do not want to depend on any drug in order to feel better (even though they have been told that their prescription is not addicting). Second reason: a new set of "long-term" side effects may appear which prompt patients to [want to] change medicines because of an annoying side effect. In any case, stopping the medicines suddenly is usually a bad turn of events since the original symptoms will usually flare up and sometimes are much harder to bring under control again—as if the body had developed a certain resistance to the medicine because of stopping it prematurely. Patients with this issue should make an appointment and come in for an office consultation (do not just stop the medicine suddenly). For these and other reasons, the course of treatment may be long and last for months or years.

In the *eighth patient-stage,* Brad should continue the medicine as prescribed. New side effects are not likely to appear. There is usually one set of side effects that appear very early in treatment and another separate set that appears after a few months.

In the *ninth patient-stage,* Brad's need for ongoing medicines will be re-evaluated. If this was a first time episode and was not very severe, then he can be slowly weaned off the medicine. If he has a severe psychiatric disorder, then the ninth stage of treatment may last for a long time. If he has been through this before and always got sick again after stopping the medicine, then the medicine should probably be continued much longer. The course of treatment in the ninth stage is subject to review by both the doctor and the patient. In some cases, the future of Brad's disorder may be in the gray zone. Some people are chagrined by the fact that this can not be reliably predicted. More bad news: some people may recover after a variable time and some may not. Good news: at least, nowadays we have such treatments available. Compare to this analogy: surgical patients may heal their bones completely and go on jogging for twenty more years; and, some may have a permanent arthritis. The same may be true of psychiatric conditions and psychoactive medicine.

Types of Treatments Available

Treatment will usually involve a combination of medication plus non-medication therapy. I will prescribe medicines for the biochemical problems in the form of written prescriptions. For the other part of the treatment, I will recommend non-pharmacologic resources.

Chemical Treatments*: Medications and Herbs* (see the chapters on Treatment in Section V).

Biological Physical Treatments might be necessary in severe cases: treatment with electro-shock or magnetic waves. Not infrequently, some of our patients can feel better with non-pharmacological treatment and might not need medications.

Non-Chemical Treatments

The other part of the prescription for recovery will include an array *of **activities:***

individual psychotherapy, group therapy, spirituality and other activities:

individual psychotherapy takes place with the therapist. Many people do not want to do this because therapy is perceived as imprecise, slow, costly (up to $35 per session with insurance and up to $100 without), and lacking in "high-tech" appeal. The people who resist this the most are usually the ones who need it most. Truly, it is a corollary of modern psychiatric practice that people who want a lot of drugs probably don't need them, and people who don't want to take drugs, really ought to. Studies have shown, over and over, that the combination of therapy plus medicines is superior to either treatment alone. Psychotherapy sessions done under electrical brain imaging have shown that talk therapy can produce the same effect as a mild medication—the only problem is that this therapy effect lasts for just one day. (Technically speaking, most pills usually only last for one day also.) That is still no reason to shirk the responsibility of taking charge of your overall healthfulness. Some people want only pills: their recovery might be incomplete since pills alone do not solve all problems. Some patients adhere to the treatment plan for a couple sessions and then when they are stabilized on the psychoactive prescription they decide to have their family doctor give them refills (this can have a variable outcome also). These people are not getting such good treatment because the patient who treats himself has a fool for a doctor. (the opposite is also true, by the way)

group therapy can be very useful for everyone no matter the problem:
- —AA for alcoholics
- —Al-anon for alcoholics' family members
- —Emotionals Anonymous for other psychiatric problems
- —Overeaters Anonymous or Weight Watchers for obesity;
- —Day Treatment for Schizophrenics
- —Senior centers for Dementia patients
- —A large array of other Twelve Steps Programs and groups

*program of spirituality***:** take your pick of Church, Yoga, Meditation, etc.

aerobic exercise on a regular basis is important for mind and body health: exercise also causes releases of important brain hormones that enhance our senses of well-being, verve, and happiness (dopamine, enkephalins, and endorphins which are natural internal narcotic-like substances, etc.)

Other treatments might include *Phototherapy* with "natural" sunlight; biological treatments such as *Biofeedback*; or, therapeutic hobbies such as volunteerism, making pottery or gardening;

When patients come into the office, the psychiatrist will [hopefully] approach each case as unique and will prescribe standardized FDA-approved medication for the core symptoms. The primary anti-schizophrenia drugs are all approved for the primary symptoms of schizophrenia. Oftentimes we need to add a second or even a third medicine to the primary anti-schizophrenia medicine in order to help the schizophrenic patient feel better. Some of these secondary medications may be FDA-approved for this specific diagnosis and some may not. In some cases, these secondary drugs are prescribed to control certain symptoms that may not be helped by the primary drug. Prescribing according to symptom instead of by diagnostic category is called "off-label" prescribing which means that the FDA has not specifically authorized use of the secondary drug for that diagnosis because the drug company never did that kind of testing on schizophrenic patients; off-label use is usual practice in psychiatry. The secondary drugs are approved by FDA for other uses which is why they are available in our country.

For example in table III-6, we can see that (#1) Risperdal is FDA-approved for treatment of Schizophrenia. Once the schizophrenia is under control with Risperdal, Brad may develop new problems, such as insomnia and trembling. Since he feels good on Risperdal and since his primary problem of schizophrenia is stabilized, we will want to continue the Risperdal and treat any secondary problems or side effects with secondary medications and side effect medications.

Brad has insomnia as part of the schizophrenia, and the Risperdal dose is not high enough to make him sleepy by bedtime so we will need to give him a sleeping pill that is not addicting. We choose a non-addicting drug because we know that he will be taking this medication for a long time into the future, and we do not want him to become addicted to a sleeping pill because that will make his situation worse. So we choose (#2)Vistaril, which is a non-addicting sedative originally marketed for anxiety, but this medicine can be used effectively in low or high doses to help sleeping. Although Vistaril is FDA-approved for anxiety and itching, and is not technically a sleeping pill, it helps people relax at bedtime and sleep better. In women, we often use low-dose Trazodone at bedtime for sleeping: this is an old sedating antidepressant that helps induce sleep. At low doses, it lacks much antidepressant effect, but most women do feel better the next morning, partly because they have slept well. These are examples of off-label use of Vistaril and Trazodone. (Most men do not want to try Trazodone after I tell them of its worst possible sexual side effect.)

Cogentin is approved for a trembling disease called Parkinson's Disease, a disorder that is treated by neurologists. Cogentin is FDA-approved for neurological Parkinsonism, which is also called "Primary Parkinsonism". Cogentin was a somewhat helpful neurological treatment in the past, but it is now considered to be an old medication that most modern neurologists no longer use; however, psychiatrists use it a lot. Some psychiatric drugs can cause trembling that looks like Parkinson's Disease. If medicines are causing this type of Parkinson's Disease, then we call it "Secondary Parkinsonism". Cogentin is the number one drug that psychiatrists use to treat the shaking of Secondary Parkinsonism. This is a technical example of using Cogentin off-label.

Symptoms and **Signs**	Diagnosis Schizophrenia	**R$_x$**	
Symptom **sign**	Patient is *hearing voices* and **talking** to himself	#1	**1st drug is Risperdal**—it is FDA-approved for hearing voices in Schizophrenia
Symptom	then he develops *insomnia* but can not take addicting sleeping pills	#2 #2	2nd drug: **Vistaril,** an anti-anxiety medication Or 2nd drug: **Trazodone**, a non-addicting sedating anti-depressant used for sleeping
sign	then he develops **hand tremors and shaky knees** ("secondary Parkinsonism")	#3	Rx 3rd drug **Cogentin** approved for tremors in "Primary" Parkinson's Disease

Figure III-6 　　*Off-label prescribing in Schizophrenia*

Almost all of the prescriptions written by psychiatrists are for either primary psychiatric medicines or for secondary drugs to help the main drug work better and make the patient feel better.

▶▶ QUESTIONS

Q: What are the possible treatment outcomes?
A: My 85% rule: I hope to attain at least 85% symptom improvement in at least 85% of patients.

Q: Should Manic-depressives and Schizophrenics take stimulating antidepressants when they are in a depressed mood?
A: I try to avoid doing this since antidepressants can trigger a new psychotic or manic episode. These conditions may not necessarily need a standardized course of traditional antidepressants in the usual doses. Sometimes short-term use of low dose Desyrel at bedtime or very low dose Wellbutrin (37 ½ milligrams) in the morning can be helpful.

Take-home Message—especially for those who want only pills and no psychotherapy: If pills and chemicals alone were the cure-all for emotional problems then the Government would probably be putting them into the public water supply.

Section IV
PSYCHIATRIC DISORDERS

Superscript numbers refer to references and citations at the back of the book

Introduction to Section IV

This section concerns the most important psychiatric diagnoses: thought disorders, mood disorders, anxiety disorders, Borderline syndrome, and suicide. Borderline and suicide follow the chapters on mood disorders, since they are closely linked. All of these important psychiatric conditions are major psychiatric conditions (anxiety, less so).

It might not seem that they have much in common, but they do—in some respects. People with thought disorders can have moodiness. People with mood disorders can also have disordered thinking. People with anxiety can have mixed emotions. Axis II (personality styles) influence how we interact with other people, and as a result, personality style acts as a lens in the presence of any mood, thought, or anxiety disorders. Here is a brief chart showing some of their shared ranged of symptoms.

This will all be explained in this section. This is merely presented as a brief introduction.

Symptoms	Minor depression	Bipolar	Schizoaffective Man-mix-schiz	Psychosis Schizophrenia	Borderline personality	Anxiety Disorder	Axis II
Moods	+ / ++	++++	+++ / ++ / +	-/+	++ /+++	-/+	varied
Thought	-0-	- /+ /++	+ / ++ / +++	++++++	+ / ++	-/+	Varied
Anxiety	- / +	++	+	+	++/ +++	+++++	+
Axis II	+	+	+	+	++++++	+ / -	++++

Table IV-8 symptoms and disease   (These are classifications that I have devised.)

This chart shows four of the basic symptoms in the left column (mood, thought, anxiety, and Axis II) and their varying contributions to named diseases along the top horizontal row. "Axis II" refers to components from personality style.

For example, we can see that, in general, bipolar has serious amounts of mood symptoms (++++), lesser amounts of thought disorder symptoms, a moderate amount of anxiety (++), and some possible mild "lensing" of personality traits (+).

In psychiatry, the real litmus test for any psychiatric disorder is whether a person's behavior is seriously affecting one or more areas of the patient's life, areas such as interpersonal, occupational, social, legal, or financial functioning.

Thought Disorders

(Psychosis, Psychotic Disorders, and Schizophrenia)
In Greek, "Psychosis" means soul-disease and
"Schizophrenia" means split-mind or cleft brain.

Thought disorders are characterized by psychosis and schizophrenia.

1—*Psychosis* is a noun and is the general term for all psychiatric disorders where the patient is out of touch with reality to an extent that it is negatively impacting his ability to live.

2—*Psychoses* is the plural of Psychosis: one Psychosis but two Psychoses. Thought Disorders are all Psychoses.

3—*Schizophrenia* is the most severe form of psychosis, hence schizophrenics are the psychiatric patients who are most out of contact with reality.

4—*Psychotic* is an adjective which means "out of touch with reality".

We can say that a patient, Brad, is psychotic if he is misinterpreting reality so badly that it interferes with his basic ability to function. He might be unable to function at work or at home because he has beliefs so peculiar as to be out of the realm of possibility. The important test is if these peculiar beliefs bring Brad into conflict with friends, family, employers, and society (police). If so, then his thought disorder probably needs to be brought into alignment with the thoughts of his friends, family, and society. If all of them are out of touch also, then that is a different situation.

Brad might believe in something that is obviously bizarre, such as the neighbors are pumping poisoned gas into his house. A psychotic patient might have only one main psychotic symptom. If he has a number of psychotic symptoms, then he qualifies as schizophrenic.

Also in psychiatry, the real litmus test for any psychiatric disorder is whether a person's behavior is seriously affecting one or more areas of his life, areas such as interpersonal, occupational, social, legal, marital, or financial functioning. Thought disorders usually satisfy this criterion, although there are people who walk around with one psychotic thought but never talk about it or act on it. In this case, the thought appears not to have too much effect on the areas of his life. For example, he may refuse to eat food grown in a certain region due to a certain delusion. He may refuse to fly on planes due to some paranoid delusion. He may have unfounded jealous delusions about his wife and the poolboy. He can refuse to eat those foods citing "allergy; he can travel on trains, boats, and cars; he may have stopped sleeping with his elderly wife when the jealous delusions began. The extra time spent brooding about a delusion, however, redirects otherwise productive brain activity to unproductive ends. As long as he never mentions his delusions, no one may know of them. If he acts on the delusions, then they will start to have obvious interfere with areas of his life.

About Thought Disorders

Thought disorders—or disordered thinking—are mental conditions in which the patient's thinking does not agree with the thinking of most people (assume that "most people" make up around 98% of the population). It is true that "normal" people have differences in opinions and differences in thinking about these different opinions, but we are talking here about thinking that is so disordered that its abnormality is obvious to most of the population, assuming that the normal population has "orderly" thinking. Making this kind of diagnosis can become somewhat subjective depending upon the viewpoint of the listener.

Thought disorders present as unrealistic, improbable, or incredible concepts and are usually obvious to "normal" people as abnormal. Thought disorders vary from person to person, from epoch to epoch, from culture to culture, and from country to country. Men in Southeast Asia have a common thought disorder that tells them that their external genitals are being pulled back up into their abdomen—but this condition does not occur in Europe. Eskimos can have severe Vitamin-A psychosis from eating too much polar mammal liver. Hysterical fainting was common in Europe in the 1700's and 1800's but not nowadays. We rarely see [classic] catatonia any more in the USA—but it was commoner in centuries past. An Iranian psychiatrist told me that Muslims who hear voices do not claim to hear the voice of Allah because even in their state of psychosis, they know that this would be an extreme sacrilege (with possibly severe legal punishment), whereas hearing the voice of God is a common hallucination in the USA. Even between two patients who are age and gender matched, living in the same town at the same time, disordered thoughts may be quite different. An athletic young man and former high school football player from a western Cleveland suburb, Brad, can have intense paranoid thoughts that differ from those of another young Caucasian male from a neighboring suburb. Bob, the football player trusts no one, refuses all medication, and has intense driven urges that propel to him wander the streets mumbling angrily to himself. The other young man, Ken—who had received scholastic awards in high school—also hears voices but likes to self-isolate in his parents' basement, usually takes his medication dutifully, and occasionally throws furniture out the window. Both these young men have the same/similar Axis I diagnosis (schizophrenia) but it presents itself quite differently when filtered through the lens of Axis II personality style. Both young men will continue to have the similar thought disorder, but their interactions with the rest of the world will always be dissimilar because they have different personality styles. There is one very rare condition called *folie-à-deux* ("crazy-by-two") when two close companions share the exact same thought disorder—and, no, *folie-à-deux* is not just a whirlwind romantic fling!

Every "normal" person has a slightly different opinion on various topics and this applies to patients with thought disorders, also: each psychotic patient endorses his own variations in the content of his disordered thoughts.

Causes

Psychiatrists approach the question of causes of psychosis with as few assumptions as possible; as such, they recognize that the cause of a psychosis may be known or unknown. (I am aware that this sounds as if we are trying to cover all bases, but read on…). These are some of the known causes: a) diseases of the nervous system and brain—including dementia, strokes, brain tumors, other neurological diseases; b) street drugs and prescription drugs, environmental poisons, and alcohol; c) extreme stress, including maternal psychosis after a baby is born; d) lack of sleep (temporary psychosis). These conditions commonly produce visual hallucinations or illusions (rarely, hallucinations or illusions of smell or touch). Delusions and hearing voices may occur. The unknown causes are the true psychiatric disorders and commonly include schizophrenia and the delusional disorders. Delusions are "fixed false beliefs". Stroke patients can develop a delusion after a stroke. This delusion will remain the same usually for many years and can be treated somewhat successfully with anti-psychotics.

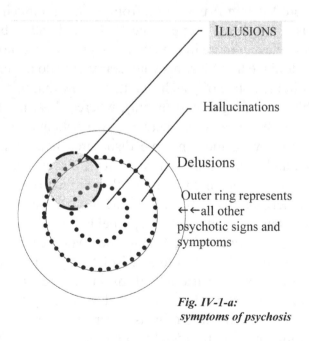

ILLUSIONS

Hallucinations

Delusions

Outer ring represents
←←all other
psychotic signs and
symptoms

Fig. IV-1-a:
symptoms of psychosis

Symptoms of Thought Disorders

There are a number of symptoms. The three most dramatic symptoms are: delusions, illusions, and hallucinations. In diagram *IV-1-a,* we can see that the core symptoms are hallucinations and delusions. Illusions are less important, usually. Oftentimes, the delusions and hallucinations play off each other. (The outermost ring represents all other psychotic manifestations, such as denial, projection, and so on—which are not covered in this book).

1—*Illusions* are mistaken interpretations of a real event: overhearing casual conversations of real people but over-interpreting their comments as having some sinister meaning; seeing flashes of light but thinking it is an alien laser beam; believing that the wafting smell of barbecue from next door is poisonous gas;

2—*Hallucinations* occur when Brad perceives something where there is nothing in reality: these sensations seem real to him. The classic example is that of hearing voices that are not real—called auditory hallucinations. This can be a very common symptom in Schizophrenia. The next most common hallucination is visual which consists of seeing things that are not there. For example, an elderly person may see children dancing in the dining room, a purple elephant in the living room, and dead people in the bedroom at night. These are some of the main causes of visual hallucinations. Visual hallucinations can be caused by street drugs, certain prescription drugs, brain tumors, dementia, any psychosis, and alcoholism. It is also possible to have hallucinations of smell (olfactory hallucinations), touch (tactile or haptic hallucinations), taste (gustatory), or crossed sensory hallucinations (synesthesias).

3—*Delusions* are "fixed false beliefs": Brad has made up his own interpretation of reality. When telephone solicitors call, the jealous husband Brad "knows" that they are really the secret lover of his wife and he rages at her. These are delusions of jealousy and can destroy a marriage. Other delusions are the fixed false belief that the government is spying on us. (Maybe this is not a delusion.) There are many delusions: the problems occur when a patient proceeds to behave as if the fixed false beliefs were reality-based. When he does so, then he will experience problems in at least one aspect of his life, which fulfills the requirement for a psychiatric diagnosis (dysfunction in one or more areas of life).

Delusional patients like Brad will make false statements based on personalized fixed false beliefs. Brad believes his delusions to be true. Thus, he believes his false statements are true because they are based on false beliefs that he also believes to be true. The issue is how much he believes and how much he believes to be true. There is usually more than a 51% likelihood ("reasonable medical probability") that he believes in his delusions. How do we know this? Because he will act on these beliefs no matter what the personal consequences are to himself. There might be some lingering doubts in his mind, but his delusional convictions are stronger than any lingering doubts. After Brad takes treatment for the fixed false beliefs, he may likely recant his delusions and be able to give a better account of his mindset during the psychotic period—or, he may remember little, if anything. Oftentimes, psychotic patients do not form clear memories of their psychotic episodes. False statements based on delusions are not deliberate attempts to dissimulate or deceive. In contrast, sociopaths and personality-disordered people will tell lies to get what they want. This is not a thought disorder, it is just plain chicanery, grifting, and swindling, which is premeditated and intended to extract undeserved goods from others.

Delusions come in many "flavors". There are all sorts of delusions (fixed false beliefs). Some of the more famous kinds of delusions are:

- —paranoid delusions: the fixed false belief that some one is plotting against Brad or that some agency is plotting to harm him in some way or other: the methods are as varied as the patients themselves: maybe they think that the police are tracking their every move;

- —grandiose delusions: fixed false belief that the patient is truly some major celebrity, or the head of vast enterprises, (a "person of substance to be reckoned with"), and so on;

- —sex-obsessed (erotomanic) delusions: the false belief that a certain celebrity desires the patient and is accumulating celebrity status in order to be worthy of the patient's friendship or love. This includes the fixed false belief that the celebrity is singing directly for the patient's entertainment but that nobody else knows about this secret relationship. In some cases, there really is a love interest on the part of the patient; but, in many cases, these are attempts at companionship: I had a female patient who was obsessed with Buffy Springfield.

- —persecution delusions (persecutory delusions): fixed false beliefs that somebody is following the patient everywhere and is tracking patient's activities—perhaps some secret government agency;

- —Bodily delusions (somatic delusions): the fixed false belief that something absurd or impossible is happening to the patient's body. (See below in topic V-Delusional disorders.)

The characteristics of thought disorders are*:

◆ Longevity: the same disordered thoughts can last for decades as permanent thoughts or they can last for days or weeks as temporary thoughts (psychotic husband is convinced that his wife has had a long-time love affair with the gay neighbor man);

◆ Rigidity-Flexibility: some patients can change their thoughts somewhat by talking to authority figures and become less rigid (more flexible), whereas some patients are rigid and stubbornly refuse to change any thinking. Delusional people can rarely be reasoned out of their odd thoughts but some can be partially reasoned (a priest might help Brad to see things differently but probably not—nor can the presence of the gay neighbor's live-in lover convince the psychotic husband otherwise); some people might be willing to exchange or modify one of their delusions;

◆ Factuality: Thoughts can have a factual origin based in reality of something that happened or that patient thought that he saw really happen whereas some thoughts can be total fiction (wife went to a high school prom with gay neighbor and they are not romantically interested in each other, but still the psychotic husband is suspicious of their relationship);

◆ Exaggeration or Maximization: patients can see a seemingly innocent event but elevate it out of context and give it their own personal spin (neighbor swatted mosquito on wife's arm which psychotic husband sees as a romantic touching);

◆ Temporality: thoughts can show up for a brief period and then go away for long periods of time or the thoughts can be persistent (psychotic working husband only worries about his stay-at-home wife being with the gay neighbor if the neighbor stays home for a sick day—the husband will try to track her every move, calling her frequently on the phone, and may leave work early to come home and try to "catch them together");

◆ Complexity: Disordered thoughts can be the only symptom or can be accompanied by a mixture of other psychiatric symptoms (psychotic husband is sure that neighbor is just pretending to be gay so that he can sleep with the wife, and often the wife has a "three-way" with the gay couple next door);

♦ Duration: the disordered thoughts can appear for a few minutes once or twice a day or may last for most of the day, but usually will disappear during night sleep;

♦ Volition: thought disorders are not under voluntary control and are not intended to take advantage of others (in other words psychotic husband is not fibbing or telling premeditated manipulative lies—he really believes that their gay neighbor had sex with his wife). Husband has nothing to gain from these disordered thoughts.

♦ Beneficence: apart from being out of voluntary control, the disordered thoughts usually serve no benefit to the patient and usually place him in hazardous predicaments when he decides to act upon the wrong thoughts. This can result in violence, suicide, or homicide and will bring the patient into direct conflict with society and its laws (patient attacks neighbor in his front yard, or vandalizes neighbor's car, or patient insists on selling their house and moving away from neighbor).

These thoughts are clearly outside the normal realm for most people, but we need to remember that "normal" refers to what the majority do or sense—what if the majority were wrong?!

Everybody in the whole population has differences of opinion on a variety of topics, but at some point, some differences of opinion must be regarded as different enough to qualify as a thought disorder; hence, abnormal. Truly these differences of thought may be only a difference of quantity, quality, or magnitude; however, when these extremely different thoughts become a severe burden on the patient's functional levels then the difference approaches a level indicating the need for intervention either by police or by psychiatrists.

In psychiatry, the real litmus test for psychiatric disorder is whether a patient's behavior is seriously affecting one or more functional areas of the patient's life. These areas include: interpersonal, occupational, social, legal, marital, financial, and so on. If there is no interference to any of a person's life functions, then the behavior may not need psychiatric treatment—and, in fact this person can not even be ordered to have involuntary psychiatric care until his behavior warrants intervention. Examples of need for intervention would be: interpersonal (spousal abuse), occupational (loss of job for assaulting coworkers, professional probation for possible sexual harassment), social (threatening to attack neighbors or burn down their house), legal (misdemeanor, felony charges), financial (bankruptcy or illicit schemes), and so on. One or more areas of the patient's functioning can be affected. In the best-case scenario, the patient suffers only from psychiatric dysfunction (line four), but if this is not treated promptly the other areas of his life may be altered also:

1-Majority opinion⇆↔⇆ minority opinion ⇇↔⇉ difference of opinion⇨ differing thoughts→confusion
2-Normal functional level.........average functional level........job"stress"....conflict......blaming....suspicion
3-citizen.....................................scofflaw....................dissident...firebrand...renegade ...felon
4-Not psychotic---fixed idea?----schizoid?----psychotic
5-Honest person...little white lie.............Sociopathic liar.......Impulsive liar.....Compulsive liar

---

Diagram IV-1-b   Psychotic Symptom Spectrum*

> *1-First line = personal function   2-Second line = occupational function*
> *3-Third line = socio-political function   4-Fourth line = psychiatric function*
> *5-Fifth line = manipulative function*

This diagram is to show that human behaviors are on a gradual spectrum, and that at some point a person will cross a line into marginally acceptable behavior and then into taboo behaviors. When this seems to have happened, then some designated agency needs to decide when the person is too far over the line: this duty usually falls onto the police and legal system, but psychiatry is sometimes involved, too. Concerning the five lines above, the act of crossing even one line can often attract the attention of the authorities. Psychotics are typically capable of crossing more than just one line.

This is just one way for psychiatry to look at the spectrum of wellness versus illness and should not be construed to have any political import.** This is one way that I visualize the process holistically. Psychiatrists—unlike all other doctors—can become involved in the interaction and integration of social, medical, legal, physical, and mental factors.

Abnormal thoughts can be permanent or temporary and usually cannot be changed by outsiders. Thought Disorders are conditions in which the patient's thoughts are jumbled, unrealistic, unreasonable, and illogical.

Figure IV-1-c: Psychoses

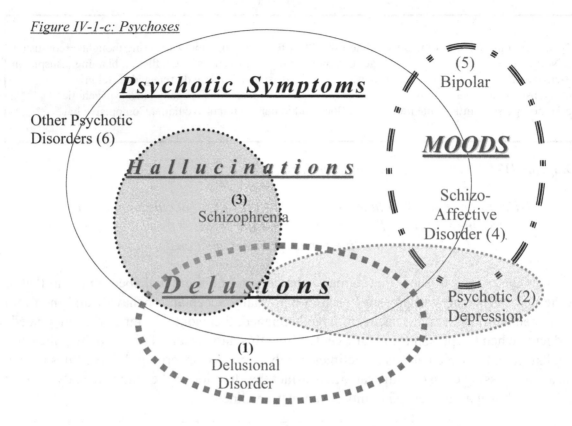

Thought disorders can be classified on the basis of the quantity and severity of disordered thoughts. Having only one disordered thought is a minor problem. Having four kinds of thought disorders is more severe. We can see in *diagram IV-1-c*:

The FOUR Main SYMPTOMS are All UNDERLINED:

MOODS refers to major mood symptoms: these symptoms will occur in major mood disorders such as Psychotic Depression (2), Bipolar (5), Schizoaffective (4) (and any mild depression symptoms due to major thought disorders

HALLUCINATIONS are psychotic symptoms; hallucinations are an essential part of schizophrenia (3) and Other Psychotic Disorders (6)

DELUSIONS are psychotic symptoms and often occur in Delusional Disorder (1), Schizophrenia (3), and Other Psychotic Disorders (6)

PSYCHOTIC SYMPTOMS refers to all the other psychotic symptoms that can occur in any psychotic disorder (6), especially in Schizophrenia (3)

1—Delusional disorder is usually just **one psychotic symptom** (or one major psychotic symptom plus maybe a couple very minor psychotic symptoms without much depression: otherwise the patients are functioning fairly well in all other areas of their lives;

2—Psychotic **depression** might have one or two delusions, but mainly has an element of staggering depression.

3—Schizophrenia has a **number of major psychotic symptoms**—especially hallucinations and delusions—and perhaps some slight temporary depression also: if the schizophrenia comes under control with medications, then the patient faces up to all the things that he did while psychotic and may or may not have shame, guilt, or remorse which can bring on secondary depression symptoms; the modern antipsychotics usually help balance out any of this kind of depressive feeling; Schizophrenia also includes in its gray oval unlisted non-medical problems such as un-employability, housing problems, family rejection, and minimal social/societal safety net;

4—Schizoaffective is a condition in which a person has a **thought disorder plus a mood disorder**.

5—Bipolar disorder includes serious moods disorders that may present with occasional psychotic symptoms;

6—Other psychotic disorders include a whole collection of psychotic symptoms that are a central focus in psychotic disorders: the more of these symptoms, the worse things are; psychotic disorders include hallucinations and delusions (as well as illusions and other symptoms: not listed);

Classification of thought disorders

We just went through the symptoms of thought disorders: illusions, hallucinations, and delusions. (Other symptoms not discussed in this book may come into play when making a diagnosis, but we can dispense with them here.) We can spin out several diagnoses by combining these symptoms based on quantity of symptoms, quality of symptoms, and the presence of non-psychotic symptoms. The following list shows the possible ways that the symptoms can be arranged into differing diagnoses.

These are the diagnostic categories of Thought Disorders:

I—   One isolated Psychotic symptom;

II—   Psychosis;

III— Other Psychosis;

IV— Schizophrenia (there are several types of schizophrenia—not covered here);

V— Delusional Disorders;

VI— Psychotic Depression;

VII-- Psychosis caused by a medical illness. Psychosis due to Dementias (Alzheimer's)

VIII— Psychosis caused by drugs.

IX— Schizo-obsessive

X— Medical Illness worsened by having a psychotic disorder: a person can have a primary medical illness, which is somehow worsened by the psychosis; or, he can have a medical illness caused by the psychosis directly (poor self-care resulting in diabetes) or caused by the psychosis indirectly (due to the anti-psychotic medications side effects that can cause tremors, pancreas disease, liver disease, kidney disease, rashes, and many others).

XI— Illusions or hallucinations alone without real thought disorder.

XII Schizo-affective (see Chapter IV-4)

XIII Schizophreniform Disorder (this is like "early schizophrenia"—not covered here)

XIV Schizotypal and Schizoid (not covered here)

In general, thought disorders have disordered thinking plus some other psychotic symptoms and sometimes include non-psychotic symptoms added onto the psychotic symptoms.

This following diagram shows the general relationship between these diagnostic categories of Thought Disorders.

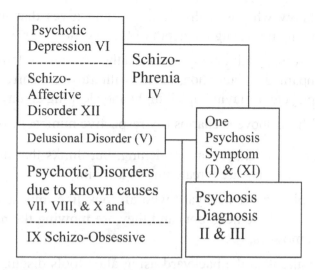

Figure IV-1-d   Family of Psychotic diseases (the Roman numerals refer to the classes listed above) This figure shows the interrelations between the twelve kinds of psychoses I-XII

Thought disorders include all the types of Psychotic Disorders, Schizophrenia and Schizoaffective Disorders, as well as Delusional Disorder Diagnosis. These are all the Psychoses.

I.)-Brad may have just **one psychotic symptom** that may or may not affect his functionality in any way. Most people are probably not aware of this symptom—or if they know of it, they just think that it is one of his personality quirks. This may not need treatment unless it interferes in his life.

Psychosis as a single symptom can also occur in some disorders such as "psychotic depression" in which a person has many depressed symptoms and only one psychotic symptom. In this case, depression is the main disorder.

II.)-**Psychosis** is a condition in which Brad is out of touch with reality. Psychosis can be a whole diagnosis unto itself. This occurs when he has a mixture of unreal symptoms that are not bad enough to be schizophrenia (which is the worst psychotic disorder). A person with Psychosis Diagnosis usually suffers from delusions, and/or illusions, and/or hallucinations. Psychosis Diagnosis includes disordered thinking and unreal sensations.

The diagnosis of psychosis refers to symptoms in which Brad does not perceive reality in the same way that most people do:

1   he may know what is really going on but give it an unrealistic interpretation;

2   he may not understand what is really going on but interprets it realistically and correctly;

3   he may not know what is really going on and gives that interpretation a false interpretation thus furthering the depth of the psychosis; or,

4   he may develop other additional symptoms if the psychosis is left untreated: psychosis can be accompanied by agitation, social withdrawal, bizarre personal habits and reversed sleep cycle of staying up all night and sleeping all day, and so on

Examples of each of these above scenarios (by respective number) would be:

1—he knows that the neighbors are gardening, but thinks that the lawnmower noise contains evil voices that are threatening to kill him;

2—he sees CIA spies in the backyard who all look like imposters or doppelgangers (duplicate copies of the neighbor) and they are mowing the neighbors' lawn with ordinary lawn mowers;

3—he sees space aliens in the backyard using alien tools disguised as ordinary lawn mowers in order to send him terrifying threats; or,

4—Seeing and hearing spies in the backyard, also hearing other voices, having intense anxiety over all this, and believing that "They" are blowing poisons into his house.

Psychosis can rarely occur without a thought disorder (see XI below).

III.)-**Other Psychosis** may have causes that are known or unknown. Known causes such as psychosis due to street drugs, psychosis due to brain tumors, and so on.

IV.)-**Schizophrenia** is the severest form of Thought disorder and is a catastrophic diagnosis. Patients can have delusions, illusions, and hallucinations along with other psychiatric symptoms. Schizophrenics are prone to all sorts of medical problems because they do not take care of their health. Schizophrenia really has biochemical underpinnings—like diabetes. Schizophrenia—like any other medical illness—will get worse and worse if it is not treated promptly.

Unfortunately, prompt treatment is usually not likely because patients do not believe that there is a problem; even if they did acknowledge a problem, they still would not accede to seeing a psychiatrist. Furthermore, the family is usually not able to coax schizophrenic family members into treatment; like most of the young adult patients who are brought in for treatment: they will refuse to take the pills (schizophrenics might think that the pills are poison or just have weird side effects). Even if they do take the pills, the majority will quit the pills after a while and have a relapse (schizophrenics are not good at keeping schedules). Moreover, schizophrenics have a much higher rate of medical illnesses, which get worse also with each psychiatric relapse (probably because it is hard to focus one's health while very psychotic).

If patients are diagnosed early and take the medicines as prescribed, they will have the best outcome—but this also rarely happens because the antipsychotic pills have a lot of harsh side effects (apparently a severe illness requires severe medicines to control it) which results in patient claims that the pills are poison (not too far off the truth). A schizophrenic patient may be a wandering transient and often loses his pills and belongings or may lose pills but not be able to get refills until the month has gone by—and even then, he might simply forget to order or pick up the refills. Often he forgets to take the pills as prescribed. Other people may take his pills (some of these major tranquilizers have street value) and he has such tight finances that he is forced to sell some of his pills on the street to get enough money.

Schizophrenia is the harshest of all the psychiatric illnesses and is the hardest to treat. Patients have to work harder in order to have any good recovery. Their disease robs them of motivation, planning, and follow-through—these are some of the other symptoms of schizophrenia. See diagrams IV-1-e and IV-1-f.

The average life span of a schizophrenic is about half that of non-psychiatric patients (average life expectancy of around forty years or less). Causes of premature death are numerous: exposure to the elements, accidental or intentional suicide, poor self care, uncontrolled medical illness, increased prevalence of medical illness, poor nutrition, and other causes.

Different patients may have different onset symptoms, but the end-point will be about the same.

Figure IV-1-e   Schizophrenia

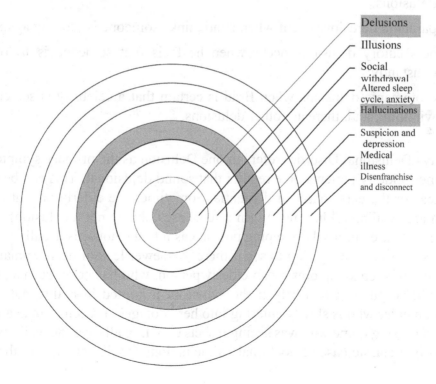

Delusions
Illusions
Social withdrawal
Altered sleep cycle, anxiety
Hallucinations
Suspicion and depression
Medical illness
Disenfranchise and disconnect

diagram IV-1-e shows the core symptoms of psychotic symptoms, starting with illusions, delusions, hallucinations, which result in poor sleep and reversed sleep cycle. The innermost circle is delusional disorder and add this to illusions, and we obtain psychosis, which when added to the next four circles represents paranoid psychosis progressing to paranoid schizophrenia. Then a patient starts avoiding contact with other people. As time goes on, the disease spreads to the outer circles. Prolonged thought disorder is accompanied by medical illnesses, especially "metabolic syndrome" (which is the combination of cardiovascular disease, diabetes, high blood pressure, and high cholesterol).

V.)-**Delusional Disorders** are much simpler. The definition of a delusion is "fixed false belief". Or more completely, the definition of delusion is a "fixed false belief that cannot be changed by logic". A delusional patient cannot be argued out of his delusion by using logic or rational explanations. Assume that Brad suffers from only one delusion. Some of the most common delusions are:

a—jealous delusions occur when one spouse is certain that the other spouse is promiscuous and is always having secret extramarital affairs. Men are more likely to have this delusion, but there are some women with jealous delusions;

b—paranoid delusions occur when Brad thinks someone is plotting against him;

c—persecutory delusions occur when he feels that someone is following him constantly;

d—erotomanic delusions when Brad is certain that a celebrity is secretly in love with him; and, there are other delusions.

Nowadays Delusional Disorder refers to one Delusion as the primary symptom.

Sometimes, elderly patients give reports that sound delusional. This can be caused by "mini-strokes" or the early onset of dementia. Sometimes the elderly patient claims that the children are stealing all her money (in a few cases, this is *not* a delusion). The belief that the neighbors are purposely pumping poison gas into the house is usually not credible, but it might still bear investigating to see if there is a sewer leak or dead animal under the house. Reports of such symptoms by an elderly person, who has never seen a psychiatrist before, should be pursued to verify if the symptom is rooted in reality but incorrectly reported by an elder who is slowly entering into her "dotage". I recently read a case about a woman in a nursing home who was seeing insects crawling all over the walls every night. This is usually a classic case of nocturnal hallucinations (of dementia), but the reporting psychiatrist had a sense that she was not delusional. As it turned out, there really were ants swarming in the early evening!

VI.)-In a **psychotic depression**, an older person named Fred might hear voices, but it is typically a voice which just calls out a single word (often his own name), and the voice does not give orders or give running commentary. The voice is often recognizable as that of a family member or friend saying "Fred...Fred...?" In psychotic depression, he may have disordered thoughts that are obviously part of the depression, such as:

1—self-esteem so low that he thinks "I am nothing—I have no value" (nihilism);

2—self-perception so bad that he thinks he stinks all the time (dysosmia, anosmia);

3—delusions of poverty ("My money is all gone");

4—physiology so bad that he thinks that all his bodily organs have died inside him;

5—Substitution of his nice caring wife with some heartless, insensitive **imposter** who just looks like her and Fred may even leave home to try to find his "real" wife.

VII.)-Psychosis due to Medical Illnesses

Sometimes a real medical disease can make people act psychotic: brain cancer, epilepsy, thyroid disease, viral infection of the brain. Other diseases can attack the brain. Patients with dementias, such as Alzheimer's dementia, can become psychotic—see chapter on dementias.

VIII.)-**Psychosis caused by drugs**. Prescription drugs, herbs, and street drugs are common causes of temporary psychosis: cocaine, Parkinsonism medicines, LSD, excess Vitamin A, Prednisone, Digoxin, Jimsonweed abuse (in Ohio), and many others. Sometimes chemicals or weed killers.

IX.)-**Schizo-Obsessive**: a patient who has severe obsessions with some mild psychosis-like symptoms. These symptoms are so deeply rooted that they can only be controlled by using anti-psychotic drugs (plus anti-obsessive medicines).

X.)-**Psychosis aggravated by medical problems**. Any medical diagnosis which is un-diagnosed or out of control can aggravate a psychosis. Extreme changes in sugar levels in the blood can affect a schizophrenic diabetic's thinking process because the brain might not have enough sugar to function well. Patients with severe thought disorders and with severe mood disorders have a much higher rate of sickness and death than the general population. This is especially true of neurological conditions (Parkinsonism) and metabolic syndrome (the combination of diabetes, cholesterol, obesity, high blood pressure, and heart disease). The medical problems do not apparently cause psychosis, but the presence of a psychotic disorder greatly increases the chances that the patient will have severe medical problems and have poor control over them.

XI.)-**Psychosis** can very rarely occur **without disordered thinking**—i.e., without a thought disorder. Norbert had a brain tumor (pituitary gland) twelve years ago, which left him with partial blindness, illusions, and hallucinations. He continues to maintain reality contact and knows that the illusions and hallucinations are not real. He knows that his symptoms are due to the brain surgery. Norbert has no real thought disorder. Many of these rare cases would usually be found in (VIII) in the above paragraph where a prescription medication or real medical problem causes illusions or hallucinations, and the patients are not psychotic, but have symptoms, and understand that the illusions and hallucinations are caused by their medical medications. These are cases of psychotic symptom without psychosis. Other possibilities would be: visual illusions alone, auditory illusions alone, visual hallucinations alone, or auditory hallucinations alone, without attempts to interpret any of them. Delusions are disordered thoughts and are psychotic by definition; hence, they do not fit in this category. If drugs or tumors or other medical problems make patients delusional, then the *patient is psychotic by definition.*

XII.)— There are some patients who seem to have certain elements of schizophrenia and of manic-depression. These are called **Schizo-Affective** because they have mood (affective) symptoms and thought disorders (schizo–). See Chapter IV-4. Schizoaffective disorder is its own main diagnosis and has symptoms of thought disorders and of mod disorders. It may also have medical illnesses like those seen in schizophrenia, especially "metabolic syndrome.

Here is diagram IV-2-f showing the relationships between various psychotic symptoms and behaviors, social problems, as well as medical and addictive illnesses. Note also the importance of medical illness in these patient populations: they are much more prone to diabetes, cholesterol, and high blood pressure.

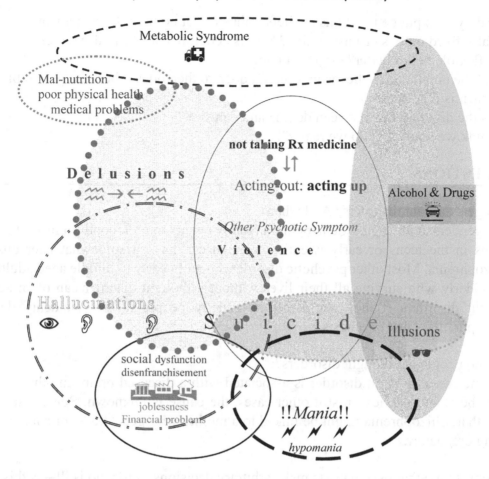

Metabolic Syndrome

Mal-nutrition
poor physical health
medical problems

not taking Rx medicine

⇅

Acting out: **acting up**

Alcohol & Drugs

D e l u s i o n s

Other Psychotic Symptom

V i o l e n c e

Hallucinations

S u i c i d e Illusions

social dysfunction
disenfranchisement

joblessness
Financial problems

!!*Mania*!!

hypomania

Fig IV-1-f Venn diagram of Psychotic Disorders
(*Metabolic Syndrome includes Diabetes, Obesity, High Cholesterol, High Blood Pressure)
(**other psychotic symptoms: impaired judgment, lack of insight, refusal to take medicine, denial [of reality]...)
*(*** Hallucinations can be auditory or visual)*

▶▶ ISSUES

Is it possible that psychotic patients are actually perceiving their own reality just as we are, too?

Who sets up the designations of these classifications?

Who sets the boundaries for Reality? What is reality?

Who is really in a lofty position to judge what is or is not normal?

Try to assume that a patient's fixed false beliefs serve a purpose or feed a need.

Is it our duty to expunge fixed false beliefs if they are of no harm to the patient?
Are unfalse fixed beliefs or false unfixed beliefs better than a fixed false belief?
Is a true flexible belief better? Or preferable?
If 60% of the population believes in a certain dogma, then does it become preferable?
If 80%, then is it normal?
Where is the dividing line between dogma and delusion?
We all think we know, but do we really?!

▶▶ QUESTIONS

Q: Who gets thought disorders? And when?

A: Both genders at any age.[3] Schizophrenia rarely occurs in childhood. In men, it usually begins in the teens or early twenties. Women can have a somewhat later onset of schizophrenia. Most other psychotic disorders occur in early to middle aged adulthood. The elderly who survive all their lives without a thought disorder can often acquire thought disorders if they get dementia. Elderly people do not suddenly develop schizophrenia—just psychosis.

Q: Why do people get thought disorders?

A: In some cases, thought disorder is associated with a diseased brain. In other cases, it might be from genetics. In still other cases, the cause is unknown. Some researchers think that schizophrenia might be linked to a mother who gets "flu"—or some virus—during pregnancy.

Q: It seems to me that psychiatrists make arbitrary decisions as to who is ill—is this so?!

A: That might be partly true, but not really. Non-psychotic patients know that they are ill and come in for appointments because hey have adequate contact with reality. People with thought disorders almost never refer themselves for treatment because they believe in the inherent truth of their thoughts. Why would you refer yourself to a psychiatrist for believing in something that you know to be "true"? In thought disorder cases, patients are brought in by some third party (or authority figure). This is our first clue that patient is quite ill. The next clue is dysfunction in life skills.

*Weighty issues: Sometimes I think that everybody is crazy but "thee" and me—
and sometimes I wonder about "thee"! (old saying)*

---

*I devised this system

**However, this kind of thinking did make former communist governments consider political dissidents as insane. The regime(s) then mandated that State psychiatrists working under the regime must diagnose political dissidents as insane (psychotic). And the psychiatrist was ordered to inject the dissidents with long-acting antipsychotics (which would certainly have calmed down the dissidents and put them into a complacent or even vegetative state).

3-reference 3, section 14.7

Chapter IV-2

Introduction to Mood Disorders

The main mood disorders are depression, manic depression, and bipolar. Manic depression is the original bipolar disorder and it is now called Bipolar I; the other forms of bipolar disorder are called Bipolar II. One could argue that there are only two main mood disorders, those being depression and bipolar. In truth, there is probably only one mood disorder, which probably has a broad spectrum of symptoms, ranging from suicidal depression to extremely abnormal joyousness. All forms of mood disorders are quite common in the United States.

Depression is the best known of the Mood Disorders. It has many forms and affects many people—depression will be discussed more in the next chapter.

Bipolar Disorder has received a lot of attention lately, mainly due to the modern trend of diagnosing bipolar disorder in significantly larger and larger fractions of psychiatric patients. This seems to be directly related to the fact that all the major drug companies are marketing new and costly drugs for the treatment of bipolar disorder. At the current rate, bipolar may soon become the most common of all psychiatric diagnoses—or at least until all the new bipolar drugs become available as generic drugs at which time, we might be able to go back to the previous system of diagnosis, provided that a new suite of costly drugs are not developed and aggressively marketed for some other psychiatric condition, which will then become the "diagnosis *du jour*".

Another reason that bipolar disorder is more commonly diagnosed is that *all mood disorders* are being more commonly diagnosed than in the past. In Medicine, the word "prevalence" refers to the percentage of people who have a disorder in one year (or in some other time period, such as in a lifetime). Here are a few quotes (▶) from experts regarding how common mood disorders are in the United States.

▶ Kaplan and Sadock[3] quote lifetime prevalence of 6% for all mood disorders and in their book they also reference:

▶ the Epidemiologic Catchment Study [3 pp.1021-22] which quotes a lifetime prevalence of mood disorders for women as 15% and as 6% for men (this means that 15 out of 100 women will have some form of depression at least once in their lifetimes; and men, 6 / 100).

Hagop Akiskal is a renowned mood disorders expert whose observations help us understand why we think more Americans are depressed now than in the past:

▶ *"Current conceptualization of mood disorders in the United States embraces a wide spectrum of disorders, including many conditions previously diagnosed as schizophrenia, personality disorder, or neurosis."* [3 p.1067] (in other words, if we expand the definition of "depression", then more people will have that diagnosis.)

As far as bipolar disorder: various estimates place the prevalence of bipolar disorder as a sizable percentage of all mood disorders. In the Archives of General Psychiatry, Merikangas quotes:

▶ *"…4.4% of Americans have had a form of bipolar disorder at some point in their lifetime…"*
[76]

However, the authors are estimating that about half of this 4.4% would be considered "sub-threshold cases" (so mild that the patients have not even come to any medical attention). Here is what the NIMH (National Institute of Mental Health) estimates:

▶ *"About 1% of the population age 18 or older in any given year have bipolar disorder."*
Source: excerpt from Bipolar Disorder: NIMH (NIH Publ. No. 01-3679)

Signs and Symptoms of Mood Disorders

Patients who have depressed or manic feelings, may not feel abnormal, thus their feelings are not technically symptoms from the patients' viewpoint. When the patients begin to perceive their feelings as abnormal, then these feelings technically become symptoms. Long before this time, however, these behaviors can be observed by most observers, and these behaviors are technically "signs" (in general medicine), but in psychiatry these behaviors are nevertheless called "symptoms". The behaviors/signs and symptoms of mood disorders in their spectral nature appear in the next four diagrams.

Primordially, mood disorders are characterized by moodiness and mood changes. The generally accepted descriptions of mood changes or "mood swings" include those of ups-and-downs of mood, which we generally call depression and mania where it is assumed that depression is a "low" mood and mania is a "high" mood. Other characteristics of mood disorders are obvious alterations in emotions, weight, appetite, spontaneity, sleep, pleasure-seeking, and activity levels. Mania is characterized by hyperactivity, rapid thinking and speaking, and lack of need for sleep. There is a whole spectrum of possible signs and symptoms for the diagnosing of Mood Disorders.

I believe that one of the key points of practical diagnosis for depression is that there be a *significant change (for the worse) in a person's previous baseline behavior*. I feel that this is the cornerstone of diagnosis because it allows for comparing past normal baseline behavior to the new onset of current maladaptive patterns that would be considered abnormal for that person.

There are variable intermediate stages in the Mood disorders such as mild depression or mild mania. Mild mania is also called "hypomania" (a "low-flying" manic, something "beneath" full-blown mania). In the same vein, depression can be moderate, severe, or profound. Severe mania is rarely seen outside hospitals. Very severe depression can lead up to the point of having such negative thoughts as to cause delusional thinking. Such a negative delusional depression can cause the patient to think that the world and himself have become nothing ("nihilism").This then would be a very bad case of psychotic depression (see chapter on mixed mood and thought disorders).

Manic depression is the original bipolar disorder and it is now called Bipolar I; the other forms of bipolar disorder have various names, one of which is Bipolar II. There is probably only one mood disorder, which probably has a broad spectrum of symptoms: different people have a different range in the spectrum. I have shown this in the chart below. For example, a person with mild depression has a range of symptoms from unhappy to happy, whereas a person with full-blown manic-depression (Bipolar I) can run the gamut from suicidal depression to elation, exaltation, and mania. (Exaltation is between elation and mania but not shown in the diagram.)

Suicidal ☒	Melancholic ☹☹	Depressed ☹	Miserable ☺☺	Unhappy ☺	☯ base Line	happy ☺	joyous ☺☺	elated ¡↗!	manic 💣

Diagram IV-2-a the range of symptoms in mood disorders (how we see them)

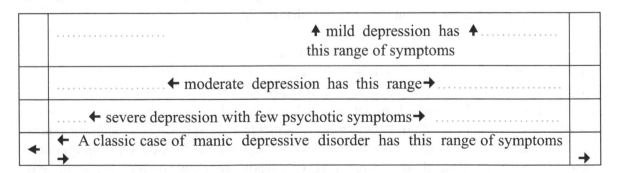

Diagram IV-2-a shows how observers will see a person with mood-disordered behaviors

[the correct jargon would be "dysphoric" (instead of miserable), "dysthymic" (instead of unhappy), "euthymic" (instead of happy), "euphoric" (instead of joyous), and "exaltated" would fit between elated and manic.)]

One fact is obvious: for increasingly severe depressions, the incursions into happiness become less and less attainable with the greater the degree of the depression. Manic-depressives may experience the whole range of emotions, but not always. Some classic manic-depressives never become very depressed, they mainly stay to the right in the "happy" half of the spectrum.

Table IV-2-b This is how doctors would analyze the signs of behavior shown in diagram IV-2-a:
OBSERVABLE SIGNS OF MOOD DISORDER

MOOD SIGNS	DEPRESSIVE	NORMAL	MANIC
Rate of change of mood	unresponsive	Normal	rapid rate of change of moods
Mood	Cranky or flat	Pleasant	overjoyed, elated
Disposition	Grousy		Cheerful
Attitude	Negative	Normal	Positive
Activity level	Slowed	Normal	Hyperactive
Rate of Speech	slow or mute		Rapid
Psychosis(if present)	(Internally focused)		(Internally stimulated)
abnormal speech	Talking to self		Talking to everyone
Weight loss due to	No appetite		Running all over; No time to eat
any weight gain	"Nervous nibbling"		
overall functioning	Doing nothing		Going nowhere fast
Suicide	Intentional (from despair)		Accidental (from carelessness)

A cardinal point of mood disorders is that they are characterized by moodiness and mood changes. Even people who typically have recurrent depressions are capable of having mini-manic episodes, which they really enjoy, but these episodes are rare—all too rare for chronically depressed people who might feel genuinely well only during these brief episodes.

Otherwise, they are "stabilized" on their antidepressants. And chronically depressed people can well understand the joy of other people in a manic episode. Unfortunately, for manics, the mania is usually followed by severe and lengthy depressions.

The symptoms are also relative, depending upon the patient's interpretation. If mild euphoria (hypomania) results in a shopping spree, then a patient might or might not be able to describe the euphoria of the shopping spree, but in most cases, she feels so good while euphoric, that she adopts this as her perceived baseline and does not report this as abnormal. It becomes "normal" to her. People do not come to see a doctor when they feel great—only when they no longer feel good. After the hypomania wears off, then she will feel bad, in comparison to the hypomania. Any mood state below euphoria is not recognized as baseline because it is not pleasurable enough. In cases of mania, a manic patient who is coming down from his manic high may complains of feeling depressed if his mood falls anywhere below euphoria—in reality, his mood might be normal, but he craves the excitement of mania. Of course, he knows that he will continue to descend from normal mood into depression, but he figures that he will worry about that when it happens. The hypomanic woman and manic man adopt the euphoric state as their desired baseline. Anything at or below the normal feeling-state that normal people would consider a normal mood, is perceived by manics and hypomanics as abnormal and depressed. Part of this explanation may be that they know that the descent into n ormal mood will quickly be followed by a full-out depression, and they are dreading this. Thus, when they sink down into a deep manic-depressive depression, they feel even more depressed than a very depressed person with major depression (who has never had mania as a point of comparison).

Suicidal ☒	Melancholic ☹☹	Depressed ☹	Miserable ☺☺ dysphoric	Unhappy ☺ dysthymic	☯ base Line	happy ☺	over-joyed ☺☺ euphoric	elated ¡⚡!	manic 💣☀ exalted

Diagram IV-2-c   Range of symptoms in mood disordered patients (how THEY feel)

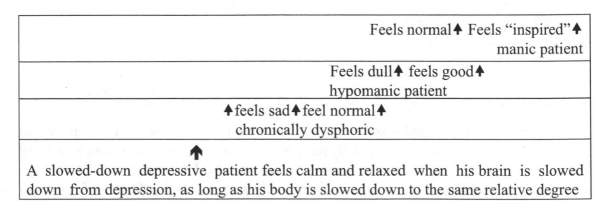

Feels normal♠ Feels "inspired"♠   manic patient
Feels dull♠ feels good♠   hypomanic patient
♠feels sad♠feel normal♠   chronically dysphoric
♠   A slowed-down depressive patient feels calm and relaxed when his brain is slowed down from depression, as long as his body is slowed down to the same relative degree

Figure IV-2A-3   This is how the patients see themselves. This is how they feel. A person with mood disorder "sees" by using his moods as lenses. These are their symptoms, their subjective feeling-states. We observe these as signs as in figure IV-1-a. Mood-disordered patients shift their frame of reference for feeling-states; their feeling-states then become relative. **Manic** *patients adopt "overjoyed" as their "normal" feel-good state, so that "happiness" might feel too slowed-down, like depression. A euphoric manic patient drops down to low-grade hypomania, and then to normal baseline and this feels like a relative depression to him. Relative to feeling manic and euphoric, normal mood feels like a letdown. A* **hypomanic** *patient likes to feel "happiness", and "base-line" feels rather low and uninspiring. The* **chronically dysphoric** *patient rises up to barely baseline and feels relatively better and less depressed. A patient with a* **slowed-down depression** *feels calm and relaxed because his brain and body are moving at the same speed relative to each other, although he is completely unaware that he appears slowed down to outside observers. It is possible that his brain needs this time to rest. Since the brain controls the body, when the brain slows from depression, then the body slows equally (hopefully). If the slowing is not in equal proportion, then he will feel that his brain and body are moving at different speeds, and that becomes symptomatic. It's all relative!*

There are similar happenings on the flip side of the coin. Let's examine a new patient, Edgar, who has low energy levels and sleeps too much. Some slowed-down depressed patients like Edgar feel relaxed and calm and enjoy sleeping and resting. Family members may complain, however, that Edgar is in bed or in his room alone all the time. Edgar is not a good observer of his behaviors. The major mood disorder may slow down everything in his body, including his brain, so that he feels that his body and mind are going at the same speed relative to each other. Outside observers can see that his body and brain activity have both slowed. What they may not realize is that his body has slowed down because his brain (that controls his body) has slowed down from depression. Often the family complains that their young depressed nephew is "lazy" or that their grandfather "probably has Alzheimer's". Despite the family's interpretation, this highlights why background information from the family is very helpful in cases of major psychiatric illness. This is another reason why these are called "Major" psychiatric illnesses.

There are also mood-disordered states during which depressed patients may gain weight and sleep a lot. There are also agitated and irritable states that can occur both in mania and in depression. If depression is accompanied by irritability or agitation then it is an irritable depression. Irritability usually occurs in mild or moderate depression. Agitation and irritation can occur with any kind of manic phase; irritability is more of a symptom whereas agitation is usually an objective sign.

Table IV-2-d SYMPTOMS OF MOOD DISORDER *(this is what patients feel inside their minds)*
Compare to Table IV-2-a and Diagram IV-2-c

	Depressive symptom	Stable	Manic symptom
Mood	Miserable (dysphoric)	Normal	overjoyous—elated
Thoughts	Slowed down	Normal	Racing thoughts
Ideas	Suicidal?	Normal	Unfocused ideas
Delusions	Depressive delusions	--------	Grand plans
Hallucinations	Limited to hearing a word called out (rare)	--------	Visual hallucinations (rarely auditory)
Illusions	Rare (possibly caused by antidepressant medicine)	--------	Visual/auditory

Patients with severe mood disorders can become so depressed that they begin to show evidence of some thought disorders such as false beliefs about themselves or about other people. Depressives may have thoughts such as: "I am nothing and have no value". They may have odd body beliefs "my brain is like oatmeal", false beliefs that he has no money left, that his spouse is having affairs, or that his spouse has been replaced with somebody else, and so on. These beliefs can also form the basis for a suicide attempt in mood-disordered patients.

Patients with severe mood disorders can also become so manic that they begin to show evidence of some thought disorders such as: "I am the messenger of God", "I am the head of General Motors", "My father is Barack Obama". They may imagine themselves to have vast holdings and wealth, to have access to celebrities, and other ideas. They can become so reckless that they may engage in dangerous activites (speeding on the freeway), overexerting themselves (dancing all night and running around all day), or drinking heavily to try to calm the mania. This recklessness can result in their own deaths, technically an accidental suicide.

Patients with major mood disorders may additionally develop minor thought disorders (Chapter IV-1). Some thought disorder drugs might make depressives more depressed. Antidepressant medicines may make manics and thought disordered patients even more manic and psychotic.

Mania and depression can result in accidental or intentional suicide. Severely depressed patients may feel deeply depressed, but not even have the energy to formulate or carry out a suicide plan until they have a little more energy—this is one of the dangers of early treatment of severe depression with anti-depressants: the patient is still suicidally depressed but acquires the minimal activity level to carry out a suicide attempt. Severely depressed patients need to be seen once or twice a week after starting anti-depressants and until they rise up out of this paradoxical emotional "trough". Manic patients do not usually intend to die. They become so hyperactive that they become very careless and feel invincible—like a superhuman. Manic suicide is often accidental. Nonetheless, suicide is a constant and high risk in the mood disorders.

There are many fine medications available for treatment of mood disorders. See Section V.

Essay on Depression

Depression is the best known of the Mood Disorders. Depression is a major cause of lost days of work. The World Health Organization estimates that depression is one of the leading disorders in the world and accounts for a great deal of absenteeism. It is certainly a commonly diagnosed disorder in the United States, where it does account for a lot of absenteeism. Since Americans tend to be diligent in tracking prevalence of diseases, we know how widespread it is. We also know that it may co-occur with other conditions such as alcoholism, chronic pain, HIV/AIDS, and other chronic medical and neurological disorders (multiple sclerosis, for example). We are fortunate to have many treatment choices that are affordable. We are also lucky to have access to temporary (or permanent) disability payments for these conditions. Depression seems to be increasing—or are we just diagnosing and reporting it more frequently? Is it worsened by the (partly self-imposed) stress of our modern fast-paced lifestyles? Or by all the chemical contaminants and pollutants in our environment?

Most people think of depression and imagine a state of sadness. Depression can be more than a state of sadness. It can be irritability, not sadness. Depression can be less than sadness, too, such as a lack of motivation and ambition and a loss of focus and drive. Depression can present as serious changes in appetite (weight loss) and altered sleep patterns (going to bed too early in the evening). This is my definitionof depression:

Depression is an alteration in or deviation from normal/baseline behavior resulting in non-beneficial changes in internal feeling states and in diminished ability to cope with the rest of the world.

And as a corollary, this means that the person's *functional level, effectiveness, and efficiency result in a frank dysfunction usually obvious to other people (but not always) and usually semi-obvious to the depressed person (but not always).*

Signs and symptoms of depression

As mentioned above, the signs and symptoms have a rather wide range. Depressed people have changes in their body weight: they are likely to lose or gain weight or, in some cases, keep the same weight. Depressed people have changes in their baseline activity levels: often they are much more slowed down, but occasionally can be abnormally activated or agitated. Depressed people experience a change in their normal sleeping pattern. Typically they go to bed quite early in the evening to avoid interacting with people and also because their brains are drained by all the hubbub of daily activities. They also have trouble sleeping and might be up in the middle of the night. When they get up in the morning, they feel really tired. And a really good clue to depression is their spending the whole weekend in bed. They almost universally lose interest in pleasurable activities, such as hobbies, pastimes, exercise, food, sex, and so on. Much of the diagnosis of depression relies on how these new behaviors (symptoms) differ from their baseline behavior. And, yes, they may be sad, weeping, withdrawn, socially isolated, and gloomy. Sometimes they say that they wish they were dead but are not actively suicidal. The symptoms that you will *definitely not find in depression* are: happiness, satisfaction, contentment, and enjoyment of life.

If your family member has these symptoms, then prompt consultation with a medical professional is wise.

Some special characteristics of some of the types of depressions

The characteristics of depression can be classified according to:

- severity,
- time duration,
- possible causes—if any,
- precipitants (acts or facts which may tend to bring it on),
- severity of any medical illness, number of medical illnesses,
- total number of medications being taken,
- stress factors,
- substance problems (alcohol, street drugs, pain-killers, sleeping pills, and others),
- family problems/death of spouse,
- previous depressions.
- family members with depression,
- living situation and housing issues,
- and so on.

The severity of depression is usually based on the number, frequency, and intensity of symptoms and might be classified as mild, moderate, severe, or profound (very severe).

The length of time that depression has remained untreated can be a factor in recovery time. Like any other chronic disorder, the longer if festers, the harder it will be to treat.

Causes may be closed head injury, constant pain, or other major medical diseases. Other possible causes are drastic changes in lifestyle, income, family resources, severe trauma, chemicals of all kinds, and so on. In many cases, there may be no apparent cause.

There may be external and internal sources that set off a depressive reaction, as well as worsening physical health. The mixture of all these characteristics acts upon the patient's nervous system. Internal sources may occur if a person is genetically predisposed to depression.

Older people might have medical problems that are accompanied by depression such as chronic fatigue, lupus, thyroid disease, Multiple Sclerosis, etc. If the nervous system had been healthy, then the impact of all this might be lessened.

A few psychiatric medications can lead to depressive symptoms: major tranquilizers.

Stressors can be positive or negative. Most people think only of the negative stressors: divorce, bankruptcy, family death. Positive events can cause stress, too, such as being elected to a high office or winning the lottery. The key is that all major stressors lead to major changes in lifestyle or life circumstances. Adapting to change is fraught with stress.

Chemicals can cause depression such as alcohol and street drugs. Also, some prescription drugs are notorious too: Reglan, Clonidine, Digoxin, Tagamet, and others. And in some cases, it is quite difficult to predict the overall outcome.

Bereavement can be followed by depression, especially in elderly widows and widowers—they begin to feel intense loneliness, which can aggravate a depression.

Some people with a first depression will improve then have a second episode of depression later in life. About two thirds of first time depressions might get depressed again.

Depression in the family can contribute to personal history of depression: either by nature (genetics) or by nurture (childhood). Patients might inherit "depression genes". If not, then just growing up in a household with a chronically depressed parent can predispose to depression, also.

Loss of residence, loss of social supports can bring on unhappiness.

Commonest types of depression

There are many types and subtypes of depression but five of the most common are slowed-down depression, agitated depression, depressive personality, and a couple types of "minor" depression.

In **slowed-down**" depression (we call this "retarded depression"), a person appears slowed down both physically and mentally. His ability to process his inner feeling state is also slower, so he may interpret his depression as a relaxing and calmative state. In other cases he may be slowed down and not even realize it since everything in his body is also slowed down—his mind, feelings, body and so on. Externally, he appears to be moving in slow motion; his internal workings are all on the same slow schedule, so everything may seem status quo to the slowed down depressed patient. Friends and family should keep in mind that his thinking also has slowed down.

In **agitated** depressions, he appears sped up, over-reactive, irritable, and overly sensitive. The patient is usually aware of his new state, but may not equate it to a depressive state, since most people assume that depression is a sad and slowed down state. He usually views it as too much stress overwhelming him—"I can't cram twenty six hours into a twenty four hour day!" he may exclaim in frustration.

The third common category is "**depressive personality**", which we sometimes call "**dysthymia**". Some people seem to be born with a mildly depressive personality state or acquire it in childhood. Others may acquire it as a teenager or very young adult. Dysthymia often becomes a mild lifelong "minor depression". It is "minor" in the sense that it responds well to small dabs of medicine, but having it for a whole lifetime belies the term "minor". These common depressions make up a fair amount of routine psychiatric treatment. People with depressive personality are also prone to get separate episodes of anxiety and major depression added onto their baseline depressive personality.

There are a couple kinds of "**minor depression**", one of which we call mild depression ("Depression NOS"). Another type of minor depression can pop up for a few months as a result of something unpleasant in our environment: this we call "depressed adjustment disorder".

Besides these general states of depression, there are a host of other depressions depending upon the patient's background and baseline. Here are a few of the other common ones:

Psychiatrists working in **geriatrics** will see a number of elderly people who are having the first depression of their lives starting late in life. This depression is due to various factors involved in getting older. This is aging-associated depression. **Elderly depression** can be related to physical, biochemical, emotional, and socio-financial trauma and stresses. The physical aspect of elderly depression is due to the fact that the brain itself is getting old and depleted ("losing its charge"). Biochemical aspects are due to hormonal changes in the body: low levels of male hormones, weak responses to thyroid hormone, low levels of female hormones, and other similar problems.   Some elderly depression is related to "*cosas de la vida*" (Spanish for "things of life"). People reach a certain age in life and look back, realizing that many of their dreams never materialized and their hopes for the future look bleak. They see that the end is near and much has never been accomplished. Expectations and aspirations were never fulfilled. This can lead to regret and remorse: people begin to dwell on "shoulda-coulda-woulda": "I should have finished college..., I could have gone to live in Paris..., I would have married her if only..." and so on. One of the worst and "unfixable" causes of elderly depression is due to loss of a spouse, which can result in prolonged bereavement and a halving of financial resources. Besides all these problems, elderly depression commonly occurs in **dementias** (such as Alzheimer's Dementia) where it is a part of the dementia itself (see Chapter VI-6).

Psychiatrist working with **teenagers** will see a different set of social and family problems causing depressive reactions—including cases of multiple childhood abuses, which can deprive a teenager of life coping skills, and leave a teenager feeling truly stigmatized and unprepared for adulthood. Starting life in a dysfunctional family can be a big handicap. These teens are also prone to drug abuse and experimentation with alternate lifestyles.

Psychiatrists working in **drug and alcohol** rehab centers see a lot of depression secondary to drug addiction and alcoholism. The current vogue is to assign these patients an artificial diagnosis of some sort of "bipolar" disorder, although the addicts and alcoholics are not truly bipolar. There are about four different types of depression subtypes here:

Firstly, in some cases the depression might have occurred first before the addiction. In these cases, the patients might be self-medicating the depression or trying to escape from some depressing situation. Even so, in some of these cases, it is usually a "which-came-first-chicken-or-egg" issue. These people may have been born with a depressive personality or may have started off primarily with a teenage depression that quickly devolved into drug and alcohol abuse.

Secondly, some drug addicts get depressed during the addiction when the drug wreaks havoc on the brain. The brain's natural responses may be temporarily disabled (alcohol) or permanently destroyed (ecstasy, "crystal meth"). All of which can result in temporary depression or permanent depressive symptoms: these people are seriously drug-addicted.

Thirdly, some patients have no true psychiatric illness but fall in love with their drug of choice. When they realize that the drug is killing them, then they do quit using the drug. Without the drug, they then go into a prolonged mourning period (grieving the loss of the drug effects). This can occur with any alcohol or drug addiction, but may be most evident in amphetamine addicts. This prolonged mourning is often diagnosed as a depression, but it can be treatable by prescribing a non-addicting anti-depressant for a variable time period.

Finally, some addictive patients really have no prior psychiatric illness, no dysfunctional family, and have only a primary addiction. They just love the chemical effects of their favorite drug or beverage. After they get clean and sober, they will need no psychiatric medications and rely mainly on Twelve Step programs, church, and various kinds of psychotherapies. This is typical of the high-school football stars, cheerleaders, high-powered executives, high achievers and high functioning people, etc. Some of these people may have one or two on-again off-again depressive symptoms, or brief episodes of minor depression, but do not [need to] see a psychiatrist. They have a minor depression that is brief and can be successfully treated with non-pharmacologic methods, like talk therapy and group therapy (Twelve Steps). They are perhaps quite lucky. Unfortunately, they are a smaller fraction of people in drug and alcohol recovery.

With the exception of the final type above, some of these addicted patients feel entitled to a psychiatric diagnosis that will provide an entrée into permanent disability (SSD). In the first and third scenarios above, it is quite permissible to prescribe as much anti-depressant therapy to get recovering people back on their feet and back into the work force. Failure of these patients to return to work is a failure to implement comprehensive treatment, in my opinion. As long as these patients hold onto the fantasy of being on permanent SSD payments for the rest of their lives, they will—knowingly or unwittingly—sabotage their own treatment. This SSD fantasy needs to be dealt with in therapy. In the second scenario above, if alcoholics and drug addicts have indeed caused permanent brain damage then this should be confirmed by a neurologist. This issue is often more socio-financial rather than medical-psychiatric. Providing permanent disability (based on a rather hasty diagnosis of "bipolar") so early in recovery sends young alcoholics and drug addicts the message that their mood disorder is responsible and that they are not, which tenet is at odds with the teachings of Twelve Steps programs. These treatment issues are addressed in greater depth in the chapters on treatment of alcoholism and drug addiction.

Other less common types of depression

Winter depression occurs in the winter [in northern climates] and takes on the characteristics of animal hibernation behaviors: mental dullness, physical slowness, overeating, gaining weight, tiredness, sleepiness, and withdrawal—and responds very favorable to two weeks in a warm, sunny climate! (The Latin word "hibernation" means "wintering") If you cannot take a winter vacation, then it can be treated with bright light therapy.

Post-partum depression is the clinical depression that women get after baby-birth. "Baby Blues" can be normal at this time, but a deeper, stronger depression usually needs to be treated. Treatment of postpartum depression with prescription drugs will preclude any possibility of nursing the baby with breast milk: the drugs can be passed to the baby.

There are **other depressions** that are not so deep as severe major depression. Such depressions can be caused by a medicine, a medical condition, or even by a depressive adjustment disorder. Depression can be caused by a number of common medicines such as Tagamet (in older men), Reglan, Inderal, Prednisone, Clonidine, and others. Certain disease states can by definition cause a depression in the sense that the disease depresses the body's reactivity: thyroid disease is a good example of this. Other medical conditions could include physical brain diseases (strokes, dementias, multiple sclerosis). Some people are put into a new situation, which depresses them temporarily, but they mostly recover quickly and go on with their lives. Most of these situational depressive conditions lead to a reversible depression, which goes away if the situation can be adjusted, negated, or corrected.

There are also other disorders with some similar underpinnings to those of depression , and these disorders can have partial to full response with certain antidepressants (see chapter VI-5 on chronic pain).

Depression diagnosis

In the United States, we make a diagnosis based on the psychiatric handbook, DSM-IV TR. This is the standard reference book used for making psychiatric diagnoses in this country. DSM-IV-TR recognizes several kinds of depressions some of which might even occur at the same time and in the same patient. This patient could suffer from two—or three—different types of depression all at the same time. A person with "depressive personality" (dysthymia) could have onset of a major depression, and then go on to develop a depression due to a medication like Reglan, resulting in a possible total of three types of depression. Despite being a standardized diagnosis, there can be slight variability regarding which patients might be diagnosed with which kind of depression and by which psychiatrists. Despite best efforts to be objective, the depression diagnosis can have minimal variability among psychiatrists, thus revealing that there is still a certain subjective element present in this diagnosis; however, that variability is not too great. Fortunately, the treatment will probably be the same, despite slight nuances or variances in diagnoses. The DSM-IV-TR lays down the guidelines and common idiom by which North American psychiatrists diagnose depression.

Many decades ago, depression diagnoses tended to be descriptive, using such qualifiers as: reactive, melancholic, neurotic, catatonic, and alcoholic depressions. In some ways, these were more informative as to the patient's symptoms since the descriptive diagnosis seemed to suggest something about the presumed cause of the depression: for example, reactive depression is perhaps a sad reaction to some identifiable stress. These diagnoses lacked standardization and were difficult to interrelate or corroborate. This system also did not provide a clear-cut set of rules for diagnosis that could be subjected to repeat statistical analysis, as the DSM-IV-TR does. Although every doctor thought he was talking about the same type of depression, it actually turned out not always to be the case. Psychiatrists also wanted to try to be more "scientific" and obtain statistically reproducible results. Thus, the first DSM was born out of this endeavor to modernize and standardize psychiatric diagnostic practices. The DSM-I has now morphed over four generations into the DSM-IV-TR soon to be replaced by the DSM-V, which promises to go off on a different tack.

The formalized methods for making the various diagnoses of the various kinds of depressions are all listed in this reference book, the DSM-IV-TR. However, a certain amount of art and experience is required to make a valid and reproducible diagnosis. Currently, there are several types of depression. These are like the ones I have listed above. There are even listings for depression that cannot fit into any of these classes. These paradigms pretty well cover the gamut of all the depressions commonly diagnosed in America. The

DSM-IV-TR brings all the former descriptive depressions into the fold under one or more of these above categories.

More about Minor and Major Depression Diagnoses

Minor depression can be temporary or permanent. If it is temporary, it will usually improve without too much trouble. Some people have a depressive personality style that usually starts before or at adolescence. Since it is/becomes a personality style, it is usually permanent. This can be treated fairly well with low dose of antidepressants or may not need medication but periodically. Minor depression patients are not so likely to have "mood reactivity". Their reactions to good news often or bad news may be somewhat indifferent or they might react pleasantly to good news and, sullenly to bad news but in either case, these feelings are short-lived. These patients have always been somewhat glum, low-key, or un-reactive. The good news is that they will always be about the same year after year (unless they get a second kind of depression superimposed upon the minor depression). The bad news is that this condition is often forever. They can benefit from antidepressants that make them more alert, responsive, and reactive. Some of them may not need or want treatment: they may be in a position or relationship where they are functional, and the minor depression is manageable and is not an overarching concern. They may feel comfortable un-medicated, since this is their psychological "default" state (the only one that they have ever known). They have tried several medicines any of which gave them odd sensations or undesirable side effects. Ongoing psychotherapy can be quite effective but it would need to be weekly—and hence—costly. In the past, this type of depression was sometimes called "neurotic depression". The overall forecast is that these patients are stable in the sense that the symptoms are always the same and they are not so depressed that they will kill themselves.

Major depressions are deeper and more intense than minor depressions. Major depression requires more symptoms for diagnosis. It can be mild, moderate, or severe: the more symptoms, the more severe. Typical symptoms are sadness, tearfulness, moodiness, altered sleep, and changes in appetite and weight. Major Depression is usually a period or phase in a person's life that is not permanent. It will usually go away if untreated (we know this from medical records in the times before drugs were invented). It can come back later, too. Patients sometimes are unaware that the course of major depression will last for many months or years. Nowadays patients can feel relatively better and functional during the time that the major depression runs its natural course. The main treatment now is medication. . Fortunately, there are many antidepressants and other treatments available nowadays.

In the past centuries, very depressed patients would often stay in a state in an institute for many months or years until the major depression improved. Nowadays we use medicine to achieve symptom relief more quickly. Pharmacologic treatment is much more effective and faster. Treatment usually requires high doses of one—or more—major anti-depressants.

Truly severe cases may even call for some type of "shock" treatment. Continuing treatment while major depression is running its course is like keeping a caged monster in the basement: it will make its presence felt and known, but medication can keep it in a subdued state in the hopes that it will eventually perish or disappear. It may get loose and misbehave, but it can be restrained and re-contained, as long as the patient maintains regular treatment. Drug treatment of major depression *does NOT cure* the major depression—medications merely make the patient more comfortable while the major depression is running its course; when the depression goes away, then the medicines can hopefully be tapered off. Do not play around with the pills or dosing schedule and keep regular appointments, which are whenever the doctor tells you to come back: different doctors have different treatment approaches.

In milder cases of major depression, the depression may go away after a certain period of time not to return. Moderate cases are variable. Severe major depression can turn into a "psychotic depression" and this condition requires a lot of medication, possibly even shock treatments. Sometimes major depression gets a lot better, but leaves a person slightly altered for life and also leaves her vulnerable to another episode of depression later on. Treatment of all the kinds of depressions can be a whole subspecialty within psychiatric practice.

Treatment of mood disorders is an important subspecialty of modern psychiatry. Follow your doctor's advice! Take care and be well!

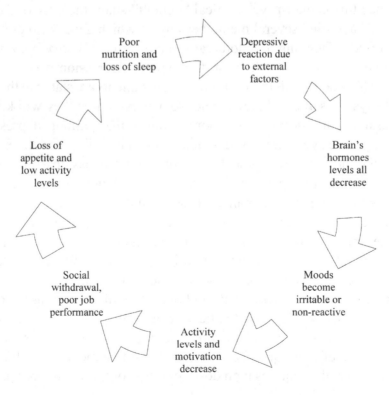

Fig IV-3   The vicious cycle and entrapment of depression until it is treated
    External factors worsen internal factors, which in turn worsen external relationships, which disrupt intimate and familiar relations.

Summary on the burden of depression

Depression is one of the world's leading causes for disability, sick days, and even death (by wasting away or by suicide). A large number of depressed people are not working. In the affluent nations, the patient is usually able to receive some financial support during his time off; in other countries where idleness means hunger, the financial consequences of depression can be harsher. Some people have lingering smoldering untreated mild depressions that result in backaches, headaches/migraines, irritable bowel symptoms, asthmatic anxiety, etc. These people are taking off a couple sick days here and there, which is an inadequate treatment plan. Other depressed workers who do not have these bodily symptoms, will have irritable depression or slowed depression. Their feelings interfere with their ability to work productively. Men tend to self-treat irritable depression with alcohol. The combination of alcohol and untreated depression in men results in disinhibition: men become likely to act out their emotions instead of having them. This can cause angry outbursts and decreased sex-drive, which then makes them even angrier, so that they drink even more, and so on. Depressed women will become quite moody—or moodier; they will often gain weight, oversleep, and withdraw sexually.

Depression can result in death directly or indirectly. The most obvious cause of depression-death is suicide. There are also many indirect causes: accidents due to inattentiveness, self-treating with alcoholism, forgetting to renew health insurance, loss of job and hence loss of medical insurance, starving on the streets (in poor nations), etc. Some depressed people will deliberately refuse to seek treatment for depression thus resulting in a kind of passive suicidal behavior by refusing to do something that might extend the quality and duration of their lives. The impact of depression on the labor pool of able-bodied adults accounts for countless billions of lost revenue dollars worldwide.

▶▶ QUESTIONS

Q: So, what really causes depression?

A: That is not entirely clear, and the answer is probably quite complicated. There are probably a number of factors that determine depression. There also seem to be many types of depressions given that its symptoms can differ from person to person. Some of these factors may be genetic or environmental or as yet unknown.

Q: How many types of depression can be diagnosed?

A: As far as formalized standardized psychiatric terminology, there would be about a dozen and a half. These are based on severity of symptoms and statistics in the DSM-IV-TR, the standard American manual used by psychiatrists to diagnose depression. This is an attempt to diagnose depression objectively rather than subjectively.

Q: Is that all?

A: Probably not. The actual number must be greater. If we ignore the DSM-IV-TR and resort to descriptive diagnosis (which is how depression used to be diagnosed), then the number of diagnoses would be greater, but there would be more subjective personal interpretation of the symptoms and less objective analysis. We believe that depression is biochemically mediated since antidepressants will help the patient to feel better: sometimes she/he will feel a lot better and sometimes, not—with a large range of individual response rates in between. The response rates to antidepressant medications can range from about 20% to 80-95%. And we do not yet know precisely why there is so much variability. Probably because we do not know the exact cause(s) and mechanisms that fuel depression.

Q: What is the likelihood of total recovery after major depression?

A: Outcome is variable; do not be surprised if the patient never completely recovers and possibly needs ongoing antidepressant prescriptions indefinitely. A general rule of thumb might be that one sixth will achieve only a minimal or partial recovery, about a third will have only one episode and no repeat episodes and about a half will continue to need medications indefinitely or might recover but will go on to have a repeat episode(s) later.

Q: What is the likelihood of total recovery after an episode of mild depression?

A: Better.

Q: Which gender is prone to depression?

A: Depression diagnosis seems to be slightly more common in women. In the past, women were estimated to account for 55% of the cases and men, 45% of cases. However, as society has moved forward into modern times shedding some of its previous chauvinism, more and more men are feeling less stigmatized about discussing feelings and emotions. They are now coming in for treatment—or being brought in by family members—instead of self-treating at home with alcohol and upsetting their families with their acting out of the depressive symptoms (anger, irritability, social isolation and withdrawal). Perhaps this is one more of the after-effects of the "sexual liberation" of the 1960's and 1970's. Nowadays men seem to account for almost half of the new depression diagnoses.

Q: How does depression differ in men and in women?

A: Men suffer similar symptoms as do women. Men, however, seem to be more stoic or resigned to the inevitability of the whole process. Because of this practical stoicism, men usually wait longer to come in for appointments than do women. Men are likelier to wait longer before going to see any kind of doctor (except for traumatic or sports-injury-related doctor appointments). In fact, the number of men who self-refer early in depression is still probably rather low; but, if we sum up all the men who self-refer early, self-refer later (when the depression is worse) plus all the men who are brought in grudgingly by family members, the number should be about 50%, same as women. Occasionally, my daily schedule might show a preponderance of men on the list. Not surprisingly, women are more likely to come in early and usually have self-referred themselves, presumably because women are more accustomed to having expressed emotions and perhaps more astute at analyzing the nature and intensity of the emotions, thus being able to recognize early on when something is amiss with their emotions.

Q: At which age does depression begin?

A: First onset can be in childhood or in old age or anytime in between. This sound like a non-specific answer! Depression seems to depend on many factors, but age is not necessarily one of them. Perhaps the better question would be 'what are the circumstances surrounding first onset depression?'

Q: How will I know when the Depression has run its course?

A: Initially you probably will not. It is possible that you will start to feel much better and are beginning to be aware of two feelings: the return to stable mood plus effects of the medication itself. Perhaps, one day you may just start to "forget" to take your antidepressant. Or, your body may start to "reject" the anti-depressant. The answer to this question will require feedback from the psychiatrist, from your body, and from your mind.

Chapter IV-4

Mood Disorders
Bipolar Disorder

Bipolar disorder has become a very popular diagnosis recently. It is frequently referenced on talk shows and in other popular venues where people seem to be quite glib about divulging that they have received this diagnosis. In further listening to their discourse, almost all of them present the explanation that their "bipolar" makes them do bad things, the subtext being that they feel that they cannot take ownership of their inappropriate behaviors, which has usually involved unpleasant interactions within the context of a dysfunctional family. The take-home message often seems to be that "bipolar" causes drug abuse, promiscuity, and antisocial behaviors as well as creating family dysfunction. There is rarely any mention of making amends, showing remorse, taking charge of their lives, or taking ownership of their part of the problem. So what is this new disorder that has seemingly taken the nation by storm? Where was it lurking all these many years?

Do not be alarmed by the specter of a new epidemic! Nothing has changed. America has not changed. The only change that has taken place is that bipolar experts have decided to expand the definition of bipolar from seriously ill manic-depressives to include all manic-depressives plus many people from the following categories: alcoholics, drug addicts, sociopaths, severe personality disorders, and many teenagers who have behavioral disturbances—never mind that adolescence is a time when most teenagers act out a lot anyway. In the *Archives of General Psychiatry,* K. R. Merikangas suggests that almost one person in twenty is bipolar: this includes about half who are considered "sub-threshold cases" (meaning: cases so mild that these patients have not come to any medical attention):

"…4.4% of Americans have had a form of bipolar disorder at some point in their lifetime…" [76]

This is what the National Institute of Mental Health reports:

"About 1% of the population age 18 or older in any given year have bipolar disorder." Source: excerpt from Bipolar Disorder: NIMH (NIH Publ. No. 01-3679). The curious aspect of both these quotes is that classic manic-depression is known to be a permanent disease, like diabetes. These above two quotes suggest that bipolar is temporary and not permanent. These numbers seem very high!

As far as origins of bipolar disorder, Manic-depressive illness is the original bipolar disorder and had been the only true bipolar disorder until recently. Manic Depressive illness can be extremely serious. All of these new additions to bipolar disorder have been documented mainly by statistics and some clinical research. Statistical studies have "revealed" that Manic Depression is merely the gravest from of Bipolar Disorder and that there are many millions of Americans who have milder or moderate forms. Some clinical research (almost always handsomely funded by the drug companies) has shown that many of the new bipolar drugs in low doses can help soften the otherwise excruciating withdrawal symptoms in alcoholics and drug addicts, withdrawal that is always accompanied by drug cravings, insomnia, and agitation. This finding was interpreted to mean that alcoholics and drug addicts must have some sort of bipolar disorder. Forging ahead, similarly funded studies went on to downplay the chemical dependence aspect of these patients and to focus on the mood instability (of early withdrawal) where it was once again shown that bipolar drugs are very helpful. Keep in mind that a lot of these clinical studies may only last for several weeks, coinciding with the early and middle withdrawal periods of alcohol dependence and drug addiction. The bipolar drugs are also excellent for calming down unruly teenagers from dysfunctional families. Hence, all those teenagers must be bipolar also —fortunately, the drug companies all have many new and seriously expensive drugs available to treat all these millions of newly diagnosed bipolar diagnoses, as well as the untold other millions who are walking around without an inkling that they suffer from any such disorder.

In other estimations, the percentage of the population with bipolar diagnosis has soared from way under 1% of the population to perhaps as much as 20-50% of the population— these really high numbers seem to be found in studies paid for by the big pharmaceutical houses. At any rate, this is an increase, which seems to be directly linked to all the new (costly) bipolar drugs coming onto the market. The exact numbers and percentages depend upon who is conducting the studies.

Bipolar disorder is a relatively new term in psychiatry. The name itself refers to the potential cycling of a patient from high points ("up 'poles' ") to low points ("down 'poles' "). This disorder is characterized by mood swings and emotional instability. The use of the term "poles" brings to mind the possibility that we are discussing electrical—or even electro-chemical—phenomena which does seem to be a possible mechanism in severe cases. The nerve [cell] membranes can become unstable, and perhaps this leads to the "polarization" of moods. The nerve cells are subject to electro-chemical forces, somewhat like a car battery. If these electro-chemical forces become altered, they might lead to nerve instability. Treatments that are biochemical or electrical seem to be helpful for damping out the swings between the poles.

As a corollary, please note that the use of electro-convulsive treatment (ECT, also known as electro-convulsive treatment, "shock treatments") is beneficial and seems to help to "re-align" this "polar" defect (although it also releases dopamine, the pleasure hormone). ECT is helpful only in true manic-depression, not the other bipolar disorders—once again highlighting the difference between classical manic-depression (true bipolars) and all of the "new" bipolar patients. The putative mechanism of this treatment is that an electric current comes from one electrical pole on the scalp through the front of the brain and into another pole positioned on the other side of the scalp. Supposedly, this would re-stabilize or re-align the electro-chemical deficiency. This can be a very helpful treatment in severe cases. Some patients will clinically be in need of a once-monthly shock treatment to maintain stability and equanimity. This would describe severe cases of bipolar disorder. Manic Depression was the traditional term for bipolar disorder of such severity.

Signs and Symptoms

The mood symptoms of manic-depression/bipolar disorder are variable: from outright mania to severe depression. The goal of treatment is to move patients from the "minus" section of the chart up as close to baseline as possible. Patients who are too far to the right need treatment to bring them "down" to a state of mild euphoria-euthymia.

psychotic catatonic	-4- melancholic	-3- depressed	-2 - dysphoric	-1- dysthymic	0 BaseLine	+1+ euphoric	+2+ ecstatic	+3+ elated	+4+ exalted
suicidal	psychotic	depression	dysphoria	dysthymia	euthymia	hypomania	mania	mania	mania

Table IV-4-a Full Range Bipolar Symptoms

Mania—exaltation/elation/ecstasy are mood symptoms of Mania. Mania has other symptoms besides mood symptoms: hyperactivity, rapid thinking and speaking, and reduced sleep. "Hypomania" is mild Mania (something "beneath" full-out mania).

Exaltation is an exaggerated state of ecstasy. (++++)

Elation is exaggerated ecstasy (+++)

Ecstasy is a state of exaggerated euphoria and sense of well-being. (++)

Hypomania—euphoria is a mood symptom of Hypomania. Hypomania has other symptoms beside mood symptoms.

Euphoria describes gleefulness and happiness. (+)

Euthymia refers to having a normal stable mood state: not overly happy, not sad. (0). The use of mild medicines in dysthymia should produce approximately a state of euthymia.

Baseline should ideally be mild euthymia. (± 0 ±)

Dysthymia is a constant mild low-grade depression, which is not severely disabling, (-) but over the space of many years, dysthymia can take its toll, too. Untreated dysthymia can prevent a person from realizing his true potential; perhaps he will only be 70% functional. (See chapter on Depression.)

Dysphoria is the opposite of euphoria: feeling miserable, anguished, cranky. (- -)

Depression can be so bad (- - -) that patients think about suicide—suicide is a very common cause of death in bipolar disorder.

Melancholia is a deep slowed-down depression approaching psychotic levels (- - - -). A person might be so slowed down as to be almost frozen without moving (catatonic).

Depression can be mild, moderate, severe, or profound. Very severe depression can lead up to the point of having such negativity (nihilism) as to cause delusional thinking. This then would be a very bad case of psychotic depression (see chapter on mixed mood and thought disorders).

flowchart IV-4-b Here is a whole spectrum of classic manic-depression symptoms (severe bipolar):

suicidality ⇆ melancholia ⇆ depression ⇆ baseline ⇆ hypomania ⇆ mania ⇆ ecstasy ⇆ elation ⇆ exaltation

In some cases, the mania can last so long that the patient will also become psychotic. This is manic psychosis (basically the same as psychotic mania—see chapter on mixed mood and thought disorders). Some people can spend so much time in exaltation that they literally almost die of physical exhaustion (and weight loss). One of the most extreme cases of prolonged exaltation that I ever saw was in a State Hospital: he spent months awake with little or no sleep; not only that, he stayed in front of the nurses station constantly dancing and singing, and telling jokes continuously, non-stop, for about twenty hours a day, every day. He received massive amounts of bipolar medicines. ECT would have stopped those behaviors. After a few months he was transferred to a long-term State Hospital. That was a case of real exaltation in mania.

One likely cause of thought disorder in mania is because the person is up all night and becomes sleep-deprived—which can make anybody feel disturbed and psychotic. Any mixture of symptoms is then possible:

- psychotic symptoms such as: hallucinations, delusions, illusions, poor judgment;
- mania, hypomania, hyper-sexuality, constant talking, light or deep sleep, weight changes, and so on. The number of differences and degrees in signs and in symptoms is almost limitless and as varied as are people.

IV-4-c   Here are Mild-Moderate Bipolar Symptoms:

---

depression⇆dysphoria⇆dysthymia⇆baseline⇆euthymia⇆ mild euphoria⇆hypomania

---

One of the key points of practical diagnosis is that there should be a significant change from previous baseline behavior. This is the cornerstone of diagnosis because it allows for comparing past normal baseline behavior to the new onset of current maladaptive patterns that seem abnormal for.

Mood disorders are best understood when we look at all of these signs and symptoms in a continuous spectrum: in other words there is no concrete wall separating mania and hypomania but rather they all blend together so that some patients might have severe mania or moderate mania or mild mania or mild hypomania or significant hypomania. Likewise, mild, moderate, or severe depressions are possible. There is a whole spectrum of mood disorders and, of course, the severe symptoms imply a severe and medically significant illness for these truly are medical conditions. Mood disorders seem to be biochemically based and probably genetically influenced. The biochemical basis is demonstrated when patients improve while taking mood-specific drugs.

There is a lot of research concerning the genetic basis of manic-depressive illness and much excitement surrounding genetic studies within families where this disease has savaged so many family members. Studies with Amish families in Ohio (where a certain amount of genetic inbreeding occurs) only serve to highlight the genetic transmission.

Mild euphoria---------is-----------happy "up" mood ↗↗
Euthymia   is   normal mood →→
Dysthymia--------------is--------persistently sad mood ↘↘
Dysphoria........is.... anguish and crankiness . . ↯ . ⚡

IV-4-d Euphoria-Dysphoria

Characteristics of Bipolar Disorder

Manic Depression is the original bipolar diagnosis. Some psychiatrists nowadays diagnose bipolar in patients who are subject to "mini-mood" changes, "tantrums", or persistent dysphoria (miserable feeling). In classic Manic Depression, a patient swings from extreme highs to extreme lows. The extreme highs (mania) typically last for weeks or months, and the typical lows (depression) often, longer than the mania. During the high (manic) period, patients will be continuously in very high motion, excited, agitated and running constantly with very little sleep or need of sleep. These periods often culminate in some sort of intervention by the police or other authorities because of the extreme behavior. These episodes may include extreme promiscuity, embezzling, setting up dummy corporations, intense spending sprees—even running down the street naked screaming at 3AM. After the police take a manic person to the psychiatric emergency room, he will be given major tranquilizers and the mania will usually continue for a few days characterized by dancing and singing constantly in the hallways, trying to "help" the nurses, intruding in all the other patients' rooms and so on. Medication usually controls this behavior. He usually calms down and eventually goes home and remains stabilized for many months or years. Then come the depressions that are usually marked by extreme lethargy and possible suicidal thoughts. During this phase, he may need to be re-admitted to the hospital because he becomes suicidal or cannot take care of himself. This is the usual conceptual framework and starting point for diagnosing manic-depressive (bipolar I) disorder.

List of Bipolar and Related Diagnoses (see diagram below)

These are the various types of Bipolar Disorder:
- Bipolar I (classic manic-depression)
- Bipolar II
- Recurrent Unipolar Depression
- Cyclothymia

- Rapid-cycling Bipolar
- Other Bipolar Conditions (Bipolar Not Otherwise Specified, "Atypical" Bipolar, Mood Disorder Not Otherwise Specified)

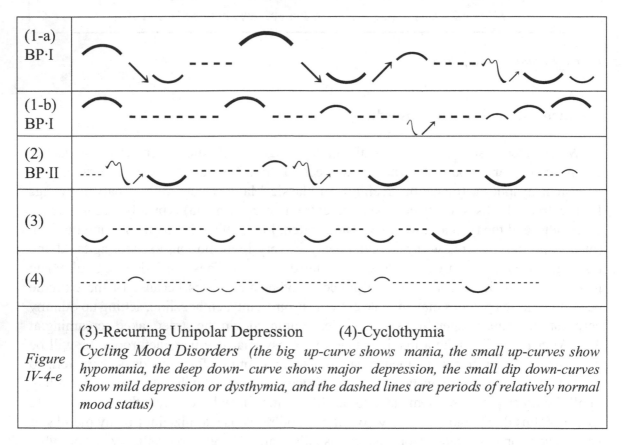

(1-a) BP·I	
(1-b) BP·I	
(2) BP·II	
(3)	
(4)	
Figure IV-4-e	(3)-Recurring Unipolar Depression (4)-Cyclothymia *Cycling Mood Disorders (the big up-curve shows mania, the small up-curves show hypomania, the deep down- curve shows major depression, the small dip down-curves show mild depression or dysthymia, and the dashed lines are periods of relatively normal mood status)*

(1-a)-Bipolar I—manias and deep depressions

(1-b) Bipolar I—manias, hypomanias, and mild depressions (or no depressions)(some Bipolar I patients rarely get depressed)

(2)-Bipolar II—hypomania and moderately deep depressions

(3)-Recurring unipolar depressions: moderate depressive episodes for months or years occurring every few to several years

(4)-Cyclothymia—mild depressions alternate with mildly elevated moods; euthymia is persistent normal mood; in Dysthymia the patients mainly have persistent depression

Figure IV-4-e *(cont.)*	*Rare Bipolar Conditions*
	(5)-Rapid Cycling Bipolar (6)-Other Bipolar Condition(s)
(5)	⌒ ⌒ ⌒ ⌒ ⌒ ⌣ ⌣ ⌣ ⌣
(6)	⌣...⌒...?......⌣............⌣......⌒...?..............⌣......

(5)-Rapid-Cycling Bipolar is like BP-I but these patients might have several cycles in just one year. (shown below).

(6-) Other Bipolar conditions (shown below)

In diagram IV-4-e, we can see:

1)-In patients with BP-I, there may be severe manic depression that goes through high amplitude cycles.

2)-Some patients have recurring depression with cyclically recurring hypomania, which is a much milder form of mania and does not usually involve police intervention: this is typical Bipolar II disorder. Hypomania is not nearly as intense as real mania. During hypomanic cycles, the patient will report feeling really happy and productive and mildly euphoric with some decreased sleep. The hypomania cycles can last for days or weeks (or longer) and then be followed by depressions. The depressions are usually major depressions.

3)-Researchers began to note that there are other types of bipolar or cycling mood disorders: one of the most commonly seen is recurring [unipolar] depressions without any manic episodes (see diagram IV-3-a). This occurs when a person has a deep prolonged depression, receives antidepressant medications and then recovers, and then has another bad (or even worse) depression and goes through the whole cycle again every few years. This relationship between recurring unipolar and bipolar disorder is further highlighted by the fact that anti-manic drugs in low doses can be somewhat helpful sometimes in the control of recurring unipolar depressions.

4)-Cyclothymia is a cycle of mild hypomania recurring with cyclic episodes of mild depression. This is even less severe than bipolar I & II disorders. Cyclothymia is like a very low-grade manic-depressive and is not usually a disability.

5)-Another type of bipolar condition is rapid-cycling Bipolar, which is like having Bipolar I manias and major depressions occurring rapidly several times a year or more. This is a real treatment challenge. It is like the first example (1) above but occurs rapidly.

6)-There are other milder and vaguer Bipolar diagnoses which are usually a temporary working diagnosis or a "stand-in" diagnoses based only on the patient's account of his past behaviors without any other evidence of such a bipolar condition. These diagnoses include: Bipolar NOS, Atypical Bipolar, Mood Disorder NOS. (not all are pictured)

Feelings of mania, hypomania, and depression are called "symptoms" when only the patients can perceive them whereas they are properly "signs" when everybody else can peg them and recognize their presence. However, in psychiatric practice, we often refer to signs as "symptoms".

⇨ *Bipolar Mania disorder is MORE LIKELY when:*

1   Patient thinks her symptoms are just a normal part of everyday happiness, but not at all problematic;

2   He likes himself the way he is and thinks that he is highly productive;

3   He is not even aware of his signs of mania at all, but everybody else is;

4   He is brought in by the police;

5   He runs screaming naked down the street in the wee hours of the morning;

⇨*Bipolar Mania disorder is NOT*:

1   making a weak suicide gesture such as taking six pills and putting a cigarette burn on one forearm;

2   feeling racy for the first month on antidepressants then calming down later.

3   having a temper tantrum whenever you feel that you and your whims are not being catered to (this is immaturity not bipolarity);

4   being happy when receiving good news and unhappy when receiving bad news (this is normal for everybody);

5   having several episodes of "moodiness" per day (unless you are an ultra-ultra-rapid-cycling bipolar which is extremely uncommon);

6   being the only person who is aware of your real mood (symptoms of moodiness without any observable signs of moodiness);

7   disliking to do unpleasant things (disliking visits from your mother-in law is not being "bipolar");

Treatments
Usual treatments for Bipolar I Disorder
The treatments available for Bipolar I Disorder include

- Anti-manic mood stabilizer: Lithium (Chapter V-10)

- Anti-manic mood stabilizers: Depakote, Tegretol, (Trileptal) which are also anti-epilepsy drugs (see Chapter V-12 on AED's)

- One anti-depressant: Lamictal which is also an anti-epilepsy drug (Chapter V-12)

- Anti-agitation drugs: Second Generation Antipsychotics (SGA) Chapter V-4)

- Anti-agitation drugs: First Generation Antipsychotics (FGA) (Chapter V-4)

- Other Antidepressants besides Lamictal

Anti-manic mood stabilizers.

The best known of these is *Lithium*. It was the original FDA-approved anti-manic treatment in the USA. It has only been available for about four decades. It is highly effective in Bipolar I, and less so in Bipolar II. Lithium can sometimes be used in other cyclic mood disorders, but usually at much lower dosages. Lithium is "natural" in the sense that it is a mineral salt (LiCl), extremely similar to table salt (NaCl). Despite being so "natural", anyone taking lithium needs to respect the fact that it is an inorganic chemical and is poisonous in higher doses. Too high a dose is lethal. Unfortunately, a poisonous dose is only about twice that of the usual treatment dose.

For this reason, lithium blood levels are regularly monitored. (see chapter V-10)

We discovered during the latter part of the twentieth century that some of the epilepsy drugs, particularly Depakote and Tegretol are helpful in bipolar disorder and serve very well as *anti-manic mood stabilizers*. They work as well as Lithium, but are less toxic in the sense that the lethal dose is much higher than the usual treatment dose. Thus, Depakote and Tegretol are less dangerous. Depakote and Tegretol have different mechanisms of action than those of Lithium. For this reason these epilepsy drugs can be used with low-dose Lithium in hard-to-treat cases. When we use these epilepsy drugs for treating a psychiatric condition, we think of them as anti-manic drugs. Depakote and Tegretol seem more effective than the others, such as Trileptal.

Trileptal is related to Tegretol, and has some usefulness in cyclothymia. (see Chapter V-12)

Anti-depressant epilepsy drug Lamictal

The anti-epilepsy drug, Lamictal, is a unique anti-depressant for bipolar disorder—unlike the usual anti-depressants, it will not launch a bipolar patient into a manic episode. Hence, Lamictal is often preferrible to the other anti-depressants in Manic-Depression.

Anti-agitation drugs

The anti-agitation drugs are all anti-psychotic drugs originally used for schizophrenia (and other psychotic conditions). These medications are all listed in the third row below. The older ones are called FGA's (First Generation Antipsychotics) and the newer ones are called SGA's (Second Generation Antipsychotics). Not only do they help schizophrenia, but they also work well for any state of agitation, such as drug withdrawal, alcohol withdrawal, extreme anxiety, agitation of dementia, other psychotic disorders, bipolar agitation, and so on. Most of them are now approved for use in both schizophrenia and bipolar conditions. (some of them may work better for mania than schizophrenia, or vice versa, and some of them work equally well in both conditions) And the new ones, the FGA's, are all very expensive.

- Anti-Mania drugs: Depakote>Lithium>Tegretol
- Anti-depression drug: Lamictal
- Anti-Agitation drugs:

  –Zyprexa, Seroquel, Risperdal, Invega, Geodon, Abilify (newer drugs: SGA's)
  –Thorazine, Haldol, Prolixin, and others (older drugs: FGA'

That is how we use the bipolar medications in bipolar patients.

Other Antidepressants (besides Lamictal)

The use of traditional antidepressants in classic Manic-Depressive Disorder (Bipolar) needs to be decided on an individual basis. The psychiatrist and the patient should reach a mutual decision after the patient has been given the pertinent pro's and con's of such treatment: the pro's are that the patient might feel happier, the "con" is that he might become suicidal or launch into a highly driven manic state. In these cases, I usually prefer to prescribe a tiny amount of Wellbutrin and only for several weeks. Anti-depression medicines could cause mania in these patients.

There are some data that suggest that anti-depressants may not be very helpful or effective in Bipolar I patients and should not be prescribed. Nonetheless, some Bipolar I patients do receive prescriptions for mild or non-stimulating anti-depression medicines—but, prescribing of antidepressants is typically much more widespread in Bipolar II patients than in Bipolar I patients. Indeed, some Bipolar II patients may be taking only antidepressant(s). Lamictal is great for bipolar patients who are prone to recurrent stultifying depressions. It is not very effective for the "low-flying" manic-depressives who do not get regular depressions; it may not help Bipolar I patients who are just having a temporary setback that makes them feel depressed. In this case, I use tiny doses of Wellbutrin for a few weeks.

Usual treatments for Bipolar II

These treatments can include low doses of the above-mentioned Bipolar I medications plus anti-depressants, and other medications as indicated. As I noted before, a number of people diagnosed as Bipolar II may just be taking one low dose medication, such as Paxil, although most are taking something more diagnosis-specific, such as low dose Zyprexa. In Bipolar II, there is a trend to treat the specific symptoms and not the "label" (of Bipolar II).

Treatments for Other Bipolar Conditions

These treatments are specific to the symptoms and not to the "label" of Bipolar. Most of these so-called Bipolar conditions are very "soft" (perhaps a default diagnosis or only a temporary working diagnosis). Some of these bipolar diagnoses have been made by well-intentioned psychiatrists for some unstated purpose, such as attempting to get the patient on permanent disability. Sometimes we make this diagnosis in order to justify using tiny amounts of Lamictal, Lithium, or FGA's. Sometimes this is a "stand-in" diagnosis based only on the patient's account of his past behaviors suggestive of an ill-defined mild cycling mood disorder. These cases are all usually mild.

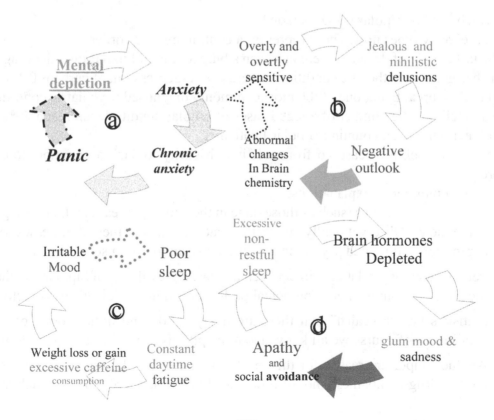

Diagram IV-3-f (ABOVE) shows the complexity of our inner feeling states: the psychic gristmills

a Chronic anxiety can eventually deplete the brain of its neurotransmitters.

b If all these cycles keep grinding away, they can ultimately deplete the brain of dopamine, resulting to a psychotic depression.

c Basis of depression is depletion of the neurotransmitters ("brain hormones").

d Depression can end up as an irritable agitated or an apathetic withdrawn condition.

▶Bipolar disorder can be mild, moderate, or severe. Bipolar can have its usual presentation of ups and downs or unusual presentations ("atypical" or "otherwise"). Most cases diagnosed nowadays are mild or secondary to some other primary condition (like alcoholism or Personality style).

▶Like any other major psychiatric disorder, it should be diagnosed and treated by mental health professionals.

▶ QUESTIONS

Q: So which kind of bipolar is that person?

A: there are many types now. These represent a continuum of disorders.

Over the last couple of decades, there has been a burgeoning of bipolar disorder diagnoses. This has gone from the rare condition, severe manic-depression, of perhaps 0.1% of the population, up to being one of the most commonly diagnosed psychiatric conditions—in some clinics the number of alleged cases of bipolar condition can reach 30% [3] for bipolar II—not even counting Bipolar I patients!

Q:! How could such a disease go from relative obscurity to such a common household word?

A: There are a number of explanations:

1—Some genetic studies (such as those done in the Amish) reveal that there is a genetic component. Observationally, it seems that significant mental illnesses (manic depression and related psychotic conditions) seem to run in some families;

2—Perhaps there is a relationship between increased prevalence of bipolar and the ever increasing amounts of environmental pollution and high societal stress factors;

3—Statistics has "revealed" that there are many subtle and minor forms of bipolar condition—of course we all know about the pitfalls of relying on statistics alone;

4—Another important reason for this mushrooming of bipolar diagnosis comes from the big drug companies who all now have bipolar-approved drugs which are still under patent protection (read: extremely costly medicines). The drugs had cost billions of dollars to develop and bring to market, so the drug companies want to recoup their losses and make profits. Large research centers receive financial backing from the pharmaceutical manufacturers who have hopes of expanding the potential patient pool of people who might need prescriptions for these very expensive drugs. Finally, those research centers will receive significant financial support to study how to expand these diagnostic criteria (how to justify giving more costly medicines to many more people);

5—As a result, the requirements for obtaining a bipolar diagnosis ("inclusion criteria" for diagnosis) have been vastly expanded to include all types of moodiness, irritability, depression, recurring tantrums, and self-reported "manic" episodes. This can include alcoholics, drug-addicts, and some malingerers—plus all the real bipolar patients. That is how the diagnosis has increased to the point of being one of the commonest diagnoses in the USA today.

Q: If ECT (Electro-convulsive treatment: "electro-shock") helps severe classic cases of Bipolar Manic-depression, then would it help mild cases of Bipolar II?

A: Apparently, not, as experience has shown. Electro-shock does not help bipolar II patients or all the other patients usually included in Bipolar II (alcoholics, drug-addicted patients, severe personality disorders, malingerers, etc.). In fact, Bipolar II treatment is often quite different from that for Bipolar I Manic Depression. I see new (to me) patients formerly diagnosed as Bipolar II whose only medication is a single antidepressant like Paxil. Prescribing a single antidepressant to a classic Manic-Depressive would send him immediately into an intense prolonged Mania. This is why I like to specify that bipolar type I is classic Manic-Depression (while remembering that Bipolar II most definitely is *not*). Seemingly, Bipolar II is not true classic Bipolar Manic Depression.

Q: Is it possible that Bipolar II can be so significantly different from Bipolar I?

A: It certainly seems so.

3-reference 3: p.1143, under "Bipolar II", second column

Mixed Mood and Thought Disorders and more on Mania
(continued from chapter IV-3) Also see diagrams IV-1-e-&-f.

Mood Disorders	Mixed Mood and Thought Disorders	Thought Disorders
Major Depression Bipolar Disorder Manic Depression	Psychotic Depression Schizoaffective disorder Manic Psychosis (Psychotic Mania)	Psychosis Schizophrenia

Diagram IV-5-a   Mixed Mood and Thought Disorders represent an intermediate diagnosis

Mood Disorders can occur with equally significant Thought Disorders at the same time and in the same patient. Some people might have a fairly equal mix of thought disorder and mood disorder, as might be found in schizoaffective disorder. In a number of cases, the person might have mainly mood symptoms with a few thought symptoms (psychotic depression or psychotic mania), or mainly thought disorders with some mood instability (manic psychosis). This means that the patient has two serious disorders at the same time. These are incapacitating major mental illnesses. These disorders are the province of psychiatrists and may require long-term treatment and specialized treatments. The specific disorders are named according to what percentage is mood disordered and what percentage is thought disordered. The main conditions include psychotic depression, schizoaffective disorder, and psychotic mania/manic psychosis.

The disordered thought symptoms (psychotic symptoms) are the same as those discussed in the chapter on Thought Disorders. The mood symptoms are the same as discussed in the chapters on Depressions and Bipolar.Here is a more compartmentalized way of looking at these as if they were three separate groups of conditions (which they are not because they all tend to merge into each other at some point, depending on the predominance of the symptoms).

Figure IV-5-b   Simplified grouping of three Major Conditions

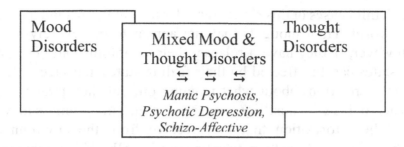

In this chapter we look at the three main mixed mood and thought disorders which are:

- Psychotic Mania (practically the same as Manic Psychosis)
- Schizoaffective Disorder
- Psychotic Depression

We can start out with the signs and symptoms (disease markers) and then describe the conditions.

Signs and Symptoms

In Psychiatry (as in general Medicine)—remember from chapter III-2 (and *diagram III-2-a*) that symptoms are perceived by the patient. Signs are perceived by observers (family, friends, doctors). A patient might not mention his symptoms for two reasons: his memory might be impaired due to having a mood disorder, or his thought disorder tells him that he has no disease.

SYMPTOMS

Thought disorder symptoms (see chapter IV-1)

Mood disorder symptoms (see Chapters IV-2, IV-2A, and IV-3)

Borderline Syndrome (these patients can have bipolar II symptoms and very rare minor psychotic episodes) This is a special condition that is discussed next in Chapter IV-6)

Mixed thought and mood disorder symptoms: special interplay between the mood and thought symptoms (this Chapter)

Symptoms in Schizoaffective Disorder

Patients with mild cases of this mixed disorder may have specialized ways in which they sense the world. Their thoughts may not appear to be severely disordered, just mildly so. (However, if they have a relapse, their symptoms can become moderate). Their thought states can be affected by their feeling states and vice versa. Often they will have misinterpretations about what is going on, but they treat it as a curiosity. They do not react to this with hostility or aggression, usually—unless they are drinking and drugging. The information that they receive from the environment becomes personalized, but does not drive them to acting out, usually. This might not be the same way that most people would interpret the information. There may be misinterpretations of words, body cues, gesture, and suggestions coming from other people. Once again, these are not usually perceived as threatening to these patients, more like a piece of information to file away. There are as many kinds of disordered thoughts as there are patients.

Schizoaffective patients sometimes do not appear very impaired, just somewhat preoccupied with their internal world. Their most apparent impairments may be related to how well they are functioning in general. Mood symptoms and thought symptoms can be mild or moderate. Sometimes the underlying moods and thoughts are partially controlled with low doses of one or two medications. Sometimes they might be taking a third medicine as needed. However, some of these patients have significant alcohol and drug abuse problems, money permitting. As a matter of fact, sometimes drug abuse seems more of a problem than any schizoaffective disorder.

Some of them are not above selling some of their pills; this applies only to the drugs that might have some street value: Seroquel is especially well liked, but so are Zyprexa, Prozac, and all ADHD drugs.

At times, these patients can lapse into episodes of intensified moods or thoughts, but these rarely last long and hopefully do not require hospitalization. Sometimes twenty-three hours of rest and medication in the psychiatric emergency room suffice.

More severe cases of schizoaffective disorder show overlaps between some schizophrenic symptoms and some hypomanic symptoms. They will need more medicine and may occasionally go to the hospital for a week or so, but usually restabilize (return to their baseline) within a few days.

Symptoms in Psychotic Depression

People with psychotic depression have a very deep depression. The psychotic aspect pertains to delusions. Classic examples of such delusions are: "all my money is gone", "I have no value", "the insides of my body are all rotten", "I am really dead now", "this is not my real spouse—my real spouse has been replaced by an imposter", "the food is poison—she is trying to kill me", and so on. "My children are plotting to get hold of all my money." (After interviewing the family, some delusions may turn out to have a basis in reality)

Otherwise, these people have little in common with other psychotic patients. They do not have other psychotic illness. They do not act schizophrenic. They do not stay up all night talking to themselves and then sleeping all day. They are not actively hallucinating and hearing voices all day and night. They do not typically have illusions, either.

What they have in common with psychotic illnesses are the delusions and social withdrawal. They are socially withdrawn but this occurs usually because they are so slowed by the depression that they have no energy for socializing. However, some of the social withdrawal may be due to the delusions, also. Examples of such delusional thoughts are: "I smell bad", "they don't like me", "they are trying to make me do things", "they are trying to control my mind"…

The depression becomes so intense that delusions appear.

They may not have so much in common with other depressions, because a lot of these psychotic depressions are harder to treat and may never come back to their baseline. Other than that, they receive aggressive treatment as for an aggravated depression.

Symptoms in Manic Psychosis

This may occur in psychotic patients who are predisposed to have secondary mood episodes. A person who is extremely paranoid (has extreme paranoid psychosis) may not sleep much because he is afraid that "they" are constantly "after me". He loses sleep trying to find a safe place, watching out the window for "them" and so on. If this loss of sleep goes on, he may also become manic. This mania can further fuel the psychosis, and the result can be disastrous. Sleep loss can cause mania or psychosis, depending upon the person's make-up. (medical interns can become manic after staying up all night in the hospital—if this loss of sleep went on for quite a while, they could then become psychotic—this applies not only to medical interns, but to anyone)

Symptoms in Psychotic Mania

There are two possible causes. Firstly, some manics develop psychotic symptoms as part of their usual manic spree. Secondly, when mania is prolonged and severe, people lose a lot of sleep. This refers to mania that has raged so long that the manic has become extremely sleep-deprived and starts to hallucinate because of lack of sleep.

Diagram IV-5-c   Schematic Look at Mixed Mood and Thought Disorders

Angry	agitated irritable impulsive	hallucination
MANIA *Bipolar* MOOD Disorder *MAJOR* *Depression*	Psychotic Mania↔Manic Psychosis ↔Schizoaffective Disorder↔ ↔Psychotic Depression↔	*Psychosis* *Schizophrenia* THOUGHT Disorder *Delusional* *Disorder*
Sad	Slow lethargic brooding	delusions

(The top horizontal represents speeded up behavior and the lower horizontal represents sluggishness whereas the left vertical is for moodiness and the right vertical is for erratic irrationality; psychotic mania is mostly irritable; manics worsen further and become quite psychotic. Schizoaffective is equally centered on all four parameters of moods, thoughts, and activity levels and tends not to be overtly dramatic, but can have a wide range of mood and thought symptoms. Psychotic depression is mainly depression with a few psychotic symptoms.)

From the positioning in the table, we can see that psychotic mania is an agitated state between mania and psychosis. Schizoaffective disorder is almost an equal blend of all disorders and their symptoms. Psychotic depression is located midway between major depression and delusional disorders.

Diagnosis

The mixed mood-thought disorders can be diagnosed using symptoms of psychosis combined with symptoms of major mood disorders (Bipolar and Major Depression symptoms and signs). However, the mixed mood and thought disorder is still just one diagnosis: schizoaffective, manic psychosis, or psychotic depression. Making these diagnoses is actually complicated, and much has been written and discussed about this topic in textbooks of psychiatry. I am going to limit myself by showing how different degrees of each of the symptom-groups can be arranged—this is shown in table IV-5-d

Table IV-5-d table of Possible Outcomes for Psychiatric Diagnoses in Thought Disorders and Mood Disorders based on combinations of degrees of Symptoms—the resultingMixed Diagnosis obtains from mixing mood symptoms plus thought symptoms and these are shown in gray

↓MOOD symptoms↓

MOOD symptoms➜ ➜ THOUGHT symptoms↓↓	Mild Mood Symptoms	Moderate Mood symptoms	Severe Mood Symptoms
Mild thought Symptoms	Schizoaffective	Schizoaffective *	Psychotic Depression
Moderate thought symptoms	Schizoaffective	Schizoaffective	Psychotic mania
Severe thought Symptoms	Post-psychotic Depression	Manic psychosis	Psychotic mania

*(Bipolar and Borderline Syndrome could slot in here also)

Table IV-5-d shows a way of arranging and thinking about the possible combinations of Mixed Mood and Thought Disorders and how the three diagnoses can be generated.

For especially interested readers, there is an amplified version of this table at the end of the chapter; that table shows all the possible diagnostic combinations for all mood and thought disorders and their combinations.(Table IV-5-D)

This chart provides another look at these intermediate disorders. Schizoaffective disorder is considered to have subtypes, although these are harder to diagnose than Schizoaffective Disorder itself. The current DSM-IV-TR lists bipolar and depressive subtypes; in the previous DSM, there was a schizophrenic subtype. Psychotic Depression is also a somewhat "loose" diagnosis and currently has no exact equivalent in the DSM-IV-TR.

Mood Disorders	Mixed Mood and Thought Disorders	Thought Disorde
Major Depression	Psychotic Depression	Delusional Disord
Bipolar II Disorder Bipolar I Disorder	Schizoaffective Disorder (schizophrenic subtype)→ ←(depressive schizoaffective) ←(bipolar schizoaffective)	Schizophrenia
Mania	Manic Psychosis/Psychotic Mania	Psychosis
	(post- psychotic depression)	

Chart IV-5-e   Mixed Mood and Thought Disorders represent an intermediate diagnosis between psychosis and mood disorders.We can see that there are actually sub-types of schizoaffective disorder, the schizophrenic, bipolar, ,and the depressive subtypes. There is also a depression that occurs after a psychotic episode. This post-psychotic depression usually does not last a long time and may need minimal treatment.

Diagnosis of Related Conditions

Later in the book, you will read about "dual diagnosis". The term dual diagnosis refers to somebody who has one major psychiatric disorder plus chemical dependence. Chemical dependence means addiction to any or all of these chemicals: alcohol, prescription pills, street drugs, and/or other chemicals). Having mixed mood and thought disorder alone counts as just one major psychiatric diagnosis and does not qualify the patient for a "Dual diagnosis" status—unless he is also an alcoholic-addict. Then he would have a dual diagnosis. A person with schizoaffective disorder and alcoholism has a dual diagnosis.

Borderline Syndrome (BPD) is another serious condition, which can present with mixed mood-thought symptoms as part of its greater pathology. The mood aspect of BPD is sometimes coded as Bipolar II. BPD has significant mood swings and periods of brief psychotic behaviors, sometimes referred to as "micro-psychotic" episodes. BPD patients also make frequent suicide gestures. See chapter on Borderline Personality, IV-6.

In any of these disorders discussed in this chapter, the diagnosis will not change much from year to year—for example, the mood disorder will not disappear suddenly, leaving only the thought disorder or vice versa. If left untreated, the patient will get much worse.

Treatment

Mixed Mood and Thought Disorders are sometimes harder to treat because there are two conditions which simultaneously need treatment. So, the patient might end up on two different pills, one depression pill and one psychosis pill. Oftentimes, the antidepressant will be ordered in low doses, and the anti-psychotic will be offered in low dose. Sometimes, only one pill is necessary, Zyprexa for example. The second generation antipsychotics are approved for bipolar and schizophrenia, so they are ideal choices (Abilify, Geodon, Invega, Iloperidone, Risperdal, Seroquel, Zyprexa). Sometimes, an antimanic drug will be used with either an antidepressant or an antipsychotic—or all three together, such as Depakote, Paxil, plus low-dose Risperdal. Seroquel is also popular in combination with other medications. Treating these mixed disorders sometimes requires adjusting and trying a series of doses of medications, and it is often based on patient preference and patient response. A starting dose of Zyprexa might have Paxil added on later, and the patient may feel great but is gaining a lot of weight. If so, other combinations might be tried, perhaps Abilify or Invega with an antidepressant.

There is no one drug that is approved specifically for treatment of "schizoaffective disorder", "psychotic depression", "post-psychotic depression", or manic psychosis. However, combined use of one antipsychotic and/or one anti-manic drug (or anti-depressant) makes so much sense, that there is no rush for any drug company to get approval specifically for one of these intermediate diagnoses. Especially in cases such as post-psychotic depression and schizoaffective where these diagnoses are considered to be more descriptive than scientific.

In reality, Schizophrenia and Psychosis are sometimes harder to treat than mixed disorders. This appears to be due to the fact that these psychotic disorders run very deep and require such high doses of medicine, that the medicine side effects limit the dosage, so that dosages and pills need to be tinkered with.

Some patients might be able to get by with just one of these newer drugs to treat both conditions. Examples are: Risperdal, Zyprexa, Seroquel, Abilify, Geodon, Invega. However, if you require more than one, do not be discouraged! Work with your psychiatrist. Sometimes patients may indeed need two or more medications, but the advantage is that sometimes they can both be used in lowered doses—this is called "pharmacologic potentiation". Consider this: Risperdal 3 mg works well, but you start to tremble and feel nervous inside as well as a little depressed. The Risperdal dose could be lowered to 2 mg and a small amount of Celexa added. You might feel even better with the combination of low doses of two medications rather than moderate dose of just one medication.

The best treatment results may come from one all-purpose medicine or from a combination of lower doses of two or more medicines. The best treatment may require several or many doctor visits to arrive at a point of feeling about 85% better.

Pharmacology is the primary treatment for mixed disorders. Talk therapy is not. The patient, however, might have therapy issues that are unrelated to the primary diagnosis, in which case some therapy sessions might be very helpful. The timing of the talk therapy needs to be adjusted to the phase of pharmacologic treatment. When a person is just starting on new medicines is probably not a good time to start talk therapy, although he could benefit from seeing the therapist for "supportive therapy". Supportive therapy is usually a briefer session to check up on the patient's daily activities and social functioning—not to delve deeply into family dysfunction issues. The one time when supportive therapy is important when beginning pharmacology treatment is when the patient might be homeless, jobless, or have other serious problems like this.

After a mixed disorder patient is stabilized, then she can start working on any secondary problems that she might have: childhood abuse, trouble with boyfriend, and so on.

A person with primary mixed disorder could also have a second psychiatric diagnosis like panic attacks. In reality, a person with a primary disorder of mixed mood and thought disorder could also have all the following problems and disorders: alcoholism, family dysfunction, and panic attacks. These larger collections of problems are often seen nowadays, and each problem needs to be addressed one by one—no wonder these are called major psychiatric disorders! They can require many months or years of therapy.

Complications

Any stress factor can aggravate mixed mood-thought disorders. Any stressor that aggravates mania, depression, or psychosis can aggravate the whole condition. Below is a diagram of what can aggravate the patient before he ever sees a psychiatrist. These same stressors can aggravate the patient after being stabilized on medication. Since these conditions are doubly complex, it is at least twice as easy to set them off again. The patient's therapeutic goal is to stay in the center of the diagram and not allow these encircling factors to put him off balance.

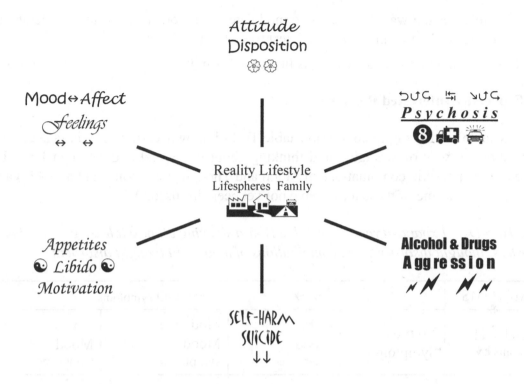

Diagram IV-5-f   Life Stresses that need balancing

In this diagram we can see the relationships between thought, mood, and reality states.

In the center is reality and on the spokes are the ways we act (psychotic or manic) and react (moody and suspicious). Mood and feelings are often unwitting reactions of our internal world in response to the outside world. Disposition and attitude as well as appetites and libido can depend on moods or thoughts. Physical violence of the psychotic person is directed outward toward others while suicide and self-harm are evidence of physical violence directed inward to themselves. The loftiest goal for anybody is to master the art of not responding negatively to disturbing external and internal cues from the environment. This is terminology for *diagram IV-4-d*.

- Attitude—is the way we respond to novel situations which can be positive, neutral, or negative: this is like the handling characteristics of a car, how blithely it cruises over potholes, how well it corners;

- Disposition—is the face (mask?) that we present to the world: this is like the appearance of the engine bay of a car, its styling features, its ergonomic layout, and a list of all its standard and optional equipment;

- Affect—is the way that we try to modulate our moods (this is like acceleration in physics or like taking a car to the test track for an all-out run)
- Mood—is an emotional state (this is like speed in physics or like a car's gear ratios)_

For Especially Interested Readers

This table is the amplified version table IV-F-d shown earlier in this chapter. This tables shows a way of arranging and thinking about the Mood and Thought Disorders. These are the possible combinations of Mood and Thought Symptoms and all their varied combinations. (Some of these terms have not yet been discussed.)

Table IV-5-D   Expanded version of Table IV-5-d showing all possible diagnoses of mood disorders, thought disorders, and combinations of mood and thought disorders

SYMPTOMS	➜ ➜		MOOD symptoms	
THOUGHT symptoms♦♦	No mood Symptom	Mild Mood Symptoms	Moderate Mood symptoms	Severe Mood Symptoms
No thought Symptom	No diagnosis Ø	Minor Depressions — Cyclothymia	Major Depression	Melancholia
Mild thought Symptoms	Schizoid Schizotypal	Mild Schizoaffective	Bipolar II Borderline syndrome	Psychotic Depression
Moderate thought symptoms	Delusional . Disorder . and Paranoia	Moderate Schizoaffective	Schizoaffective	Bipolar I (Manic Depression)
Severe thought Symptoms	Schizophrenia and Psychosis	Post-psychotic Depression	Manic psychosis	Psychotic mania

Borderline Syndrome
(Also known as Borderline Personality Disorder, BPD)

(Pertinent background information is in Chapters IV-1-2-3-4-5 on Thought Disorders, Depression, Bipolar, Suicide, Mixed Mood and Thought Disorders; and in Chapter VI-7 on Impulsivity.)

Borderline Syndrome is a devastating psychiatric illness originally conceptualized several decades ago by Drs. Stern, Knight, and Masterson. Over three decades ago the diagnosis was championed by Otto Kernberg who chose to call it the Borderline Personality Disorder: hence, the abbreviation "BPD". He chose this term for two reasons. First, BPD shares characteristics with other major mental illnesses but in each case, the other major mental illness contributes only some peripheral symptoms. The diagnosis of BPD skirted around on the boundaries—or borders—of depression, psychosis, personality style, high anxiety, (and the later recognition of substance abuse). And secondly, prominent symptoms were those of a disarrayed, undeveloped ("primitive"), or sub-mature personality style. There were prominent traits from the so-called cluster "A" personality disorders: histrionic, narcissistic, and antisocial personalities.

Nowadays we recognize the following markers for BPD:

- Impulsivity
- Dysphoria
- Thought Disorder (trouble separating reality from fantasy)
- Alcoholism and abuse of street drugs and prescription drugs
- Intense neediness and inability to tolerate loneliness
- Self-abuse and minor attention-seeking non-lethal suicide gestures
- Anxiety symptoms (due to loneliness or alcoholism and drugs)
- Disturbing memories of abuses (real or imagined) with possible traumatic stress.
- Inability to bond with other people in the usual manner.
- Emotional embellishment or outright exaggeration of real events in the past

Some mental health professionals find the name of this diagnosis to be a poor description of the real mental condition; they would prefer to diagnose it as bipolar condition, but this term falls even further a-field by implying that it is all about some mood disorder. The advantage of using the original name for the disorder is that we all know exactly what it means. The word Borderline immediately conjures up a set of symptoms that all mental health professionals would understand immediately: an impulsive, volatile, over-reactive [female] in age range from twenty to fifty years old, with stormy relationships, mistrust, neediness, chronic unhappiness, and at odds with just about everyone and everything.

Emma

The reader is probably familiar with depression, anxiety, panic, and people who publicly talk to themselves (who are not wearing telecommunication devices). But the reader has probably never heard of BPD, so I need to give some sort of a psychosocial introduction to this catastrophic condition. Patients with BPD are usually women. Their case histories are usually long and complex and involve many tumultuous psychosocial experiences. There are several types of typical cases.

Let's take for example a thirty year old woman named Emma. She is the middle sister of three and always felt that her mother favored the eldest sister by delegating maternal powers to that sister. Emma always felt that her father favored the youngest sister, perhaps even sexually favoring that sister. Emma had always wanted a third parent to favor her; she got this in a very roundabout way from her mother's youngest half-brother with whom she had been sexually provocative for years. He resisted her coquetteries during these years and up until sometime around Emma's fifteenth birthday (her later recollections were imprecise) at which time he was about twenty-two. They had a few sexual liaisons until he joined the Army. Emma's later recollection was that her uncle had forced himself upon her when she was a girl. She later came to believe that this relationship had caused her to be "bipolar". This belief was reinforced by her fourth female therapist who later confided to Emma a complete understanding of Emma's situation from a "first-person" viewpoint.

Emma's mother was emotionally unstable and divorced Emma's father when Emma was fourteen. Her father drank rather heavily but was not a full-blow alcoholic. Emma earned an MBA degree and was successful in the business world as long as she did not have to deal with handsome young men or other competitive women. Emma found a lot to dislike about her coworkers and wrote up several of her subordinates. One very nice young man who was engaged lost his job because Emma threatened to file a (false and malicious) sexual harassment case against him. After almost three years there, she quit in a huff due to her misinterpretation of some comments made about her. The comments were not completely groundless, and it was true that no one in the office liked her. They were all glad when she quit in a huff and stormed out of the office at 10AM on one Monday. Her reputation for being an aggressive busninesswoman quickly landed her another middle management job where the management was not completely aware of her difficult interpersonal style.

During her mid and late twenties, she had several brief and stormy relationships with all kinds of men, and she seemed to career between these laiasons with a dizzying frequency. Some alcohol abuse was involved also. During this time, she had decided that she was depressed and went to see a female therapist whom Emma adored for the first two months. Later she suddenly turned against the therapist who forgot to answer an after-hours phone call from Emma regarding Emma's disgust with men. Emma took six aspirin pills on a full stomach and then called the suicide hotline. Then she saw a second therapist who diagnosed Emma with BPD and set boundaries with Emma, after which Emma summarily fired her. Additionally, Emma refused to pay for any of the therapy appointments and if the therapist did try to collect, Emma let her know that she would report the therapist to the California State Licensing Board for attempted lesbianisms upon her person. The $400 bill was forgiven. Then Emma decided that she should see a male therapist who could give her advice about her problems with men. That ended badly too with Emma leaving a long man-hating tirade at his answering service and accusing him of touching her inappropriately. And to prove it, Emma, a non-smoker, burned both her arms with cigarettes and then went to the ER at 4AM on a Saturday, telling the female nurses that her male therapist had made her do it by "his lack of therapeutic affection" for her. She also claimed that he had bugged her phone and had hired detectives to follow her. After several more professional debacles, her job instability became habitual and she ended up working as a clerk in an automotive chain. She hated the job, but she loved the good mental health benefits and being surrounded by men. She seduced the owner's great nephew but survived the flack and got a sympathy vote for overdosing on an asthma inhaler. And so it went with Emma's life.

This case would be recognizable to any mental health professional as a typical example of BPD. Some cases may be worse; some, better. Much of the time there is some sort of child abuse and the girls come from families where the mother and the father (if he is even present) are lightyears removed from being Ozzie and Harriet. Male borderlines are severely damaged also, but are sometimes diagnosed as antisocial or narcissistic personalities—or both.

Complex Group of Symptoms

Look at diagram IV-6-a. BPD is at the center where all three circles intersect. This is how the original concept of BPD was envisioned. We now know that the condition is more complex and has elements of other conditions:

Periods of impulsive alcoholism and drug abuse are common as is the impulsive abuse and misuse of prescription pills (taking more pills than indicated): this is one reason that psychiatrists need to dole out only small amounts of non-fatal psychiatric pills in these cases. The pills are taken in an attempt to provide fast relief to the constant swirl of emotions.

There are indeed some cases where the alcohol and drug abuse is more of a problem than the Borderline Syndrome—although not necessarily.

Impulsivity of all kinds is common. This includes impulsive low-grade self-injury, including [usually] low-risk suicide gestures such as self-inflicted cigarette burns and superficial scratches on the wrists and arm; impulsive abuse and misuse of prescription medicines (not taking the pills as prescribed), impulsively bad decisions, and impulsively entangled romantic relationships and impulsive-motivated behaviors in the attempt to salvage these doomed-to-fail relationships. The pills are taken impulsively in response to a sudden stress factor.

The thought disorder symptoms can be fleeting, minor, and mild. These have been referred to as "micro-psychotic" episodes, which is quite accurate.

The mood disorder symptoms basically show up as a long-standing dysphoria (opposite of euphoria), which means feeling miserable. The mood disorder symptoms rarely take on the elements of true manic-depression, although patients like Emma tend to report it as such. Emma's symptoms feel manic to her, but there are really few to no classic signs of mania. Emma is exquisitely aware of her internal feelings, which seem much worse to her than what anybody can observe. Or there are mild manic depression symptoms which are very fleeting (perhaps a day or two). The basic symptoms are dysphoria and a painful sense of recurrent loneliness, aimlessness, self-loathing, social rejection, and abandonment despair.

Interpersonal problems and intense neediness lead to unsatisfying personal relationships and romantic disappointment. This also includes becoming angry with the therapist at least once during therapy.

Transient panic anxiety symptoms may be present but not a significant part of the syndrome and more likely than not are due to side effects of antidepressants (or some other stimulant drugs); anxiety can also be due to mild withdrawal from tranquilizers.

The personality style is a mix of histrionic, narcissistic, and antisocial.

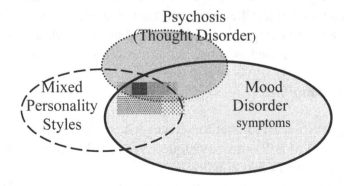

Figure IV-6-a   Venn diagram of Dr. Otto Kernberg's original conception of Borderline Disorder—the shaded area where the three rings overlap is the original core of the

symptoms that made a Borderline diagnosis. Nowadays there are more disease processes recognized—as shown below in figure IV-6-b.

BPD is well depicted by Glenn Close in the movie with Michael Douglas, "Fatal Attraction". (See the second Venn diagram with seven circles.)

All of these symptoms interact with each other. Impulsivity can occur in personal relationships, self-injury, drug abuse, casual sex with strangers, or overindulging in prescription pills to try to get psychic relief (which may or may not help the symptoms). Alcoholism and drug use affect personal safety and judgment about relationships, neediness, and flares of thought disorder when intoxicated and flares of mood disorder when hung over the next day. These symptoms all seem to cluster together and present as one reasonably consistent diagnosis.

Family issues and Upbringing

BPD patients may commonly have BPD mothers. Most—if not all—BPD patients report memories of sexual abuse as children (as boys or girls); or, if not reported, then these memories are frequently recovered or rediscovered during therapy (much has already been written about this controversial aspect of therapy). BPD patients like Emma are very suggestible and can conjure up negative feelings that are distorted into fabricated negative memories. Emma experiences her whole world based on emotion—if her mother always hated Emma's father, then Emma can identify with her mother and turn this negative emotion into a negative memory of something which happened—or surely must have happened in order to give her such negative feelings. The past issues of sexual abuse might be the salient symptom for which male BPD patients will seek treatment. A commoner reason for Emma seems to be centered on romantic letdowns and all past and present interpersonal traumas and disappointments.

Diagnosis

The diagnosis is based on the symptoms and behaviors already mentioned.

The use of the words "Borderline" and "Personality" have been roundly criticized in the past few years. There is a growing trend among psychiatrists to make two diagnoses. We often diagnose it as both BPD and as one of the Mood disorders. It is now common to use these two diagnoses together as compatible and complementary diagnoses, BPD & BP-II (Bipolar II). As we learn more about this illness, the name of the diagnosis may change again or be further revised.

BPD is oftenest diagnosed in women who seem to account for at least 90% of the cases. In recent years, pro-feminist therapists have raged against this system of diagnosis calling it demeaning to women. Diagnosis should come with complete clinical detachment. In psychiatry—as in other medical conditions—certain disorders may be much more common in one gender, but is this really "demeaning"? Therapists need to retain a certain amount of clinical distance and not allow the boundaries between the client and the therapist to get blurred due to "transferring" feelings back and forth between each other and treating each other like some good or bad relationship from the past. Some of these therapists may have had more than a casual personal experience with BPD. This can be an advantage in therapy—after all, who better to understand? The disadvantage is that these therapists might be more prone to have blurred boundaries with their clients. The advantage of this disadvantage is that some of these therapists might have their own therapists or mentors available for discussing these therapists' own issues. Yes, BPD is a very complicated diagnosis! We need to maintain clinical objectivity, otherwise patients may not get better at all.

BPD has no recognized sub-types—BPD diagnosis is all or nothing.

Treatment Issues

The definitive treatment is talk therapy with a psychotherapist. Certain therapists may end up with a large collection of BPD clients. This is highly commendable since a number of therapists and psychiatrists tend to shy away from BPD patients and clients: treatment of BPD moves very slowly and takes many years and can never be cured—only treated. BPD patients require much attention and time. Many other patients can get better quickly and move on while the BPD patients are still engaged in long-term therapy. BPD patients may not show any improvement for years, need urgent office visits and weekly/biweekly therapy sessions, make many after-hours urgent phone-calls, require several brief hospital stays, and do not really respond to any of the psychiatric drugs. In reality, a mental health professional can devote as much attention to one BPD patients as required to treat many depressed or anxious patients. Of course, these "BPD specialists" need to have a much smaller caseload than a general therapist or psychiatrist.

There is no recognized "biologic" treatment for BPD. There is no FDA-approved drug for BPD. Prescription medicines for BPD are for the symptoms rather than for the diagnosis. Most medicines have temporary use: anti-anxiety pills for the current anxiety symptoms; anti-depressant medicines for the current round of depression; small amounts of low-dose antipsychotic medicine for any "micro-psychotic" episode. On certain occasions, the psychiatrist—in consultation with the therapist—may need to admit the BPD patient to a psychiatric hospital for three or four days while the patient is feeling very impulsive and disconnected. These mini-hospitalizations work very well for mini-manic or micro-psychotic episodes. In cases where Emma wants to go to the hospital in order to keep herself safe from herself, then she knows that she must make some communication with mental health authorities using the word "suicide" anywhere within the communication.

The primary treatment for BPD is not pills, but continuous therapy sessions with the therapist: hundreds if not thousands of therapy sessions along with countless phone calls. Primary or general mental health professionals may experience a high risk of "burnout" if their caseload contains large numbers of BPD patients. Since the primary treatment is therapy and not pills, the prescribing doctor has a relatively small peripheral role in treating this devastating condition and his role is for periodic medication adjustments or mini-hospitalizations.

▶Concluding remarks

Borderline Syndrome is serious and devastating because it:
- interferes with enjoyment of life,
- effectively isolates Emma from society,
- negatively impacts occupational relationships, jobs, and earning potential,
- splits and aggrieves families,
- causes erratic, volatile, and unstable romantic involvements,
- involves mood (mini-mania) and thought (micro-psychotic) disturbances,
- places the patient at high risk for self-injury episodes some of which may be lethal (completed suicide).

This diagnosis also exposes patients to a lot of non-specific medication treatment, costs the patient a lot of money (for therapist and doctor visits), results in her working below her technical skill levels, and is often accompanied by drug/alcohol abuse and misuse.

This last diagram IV-6-b shows all the tumult present in this disorder. The conglomeration of these problems are all diagnostic of BPD.

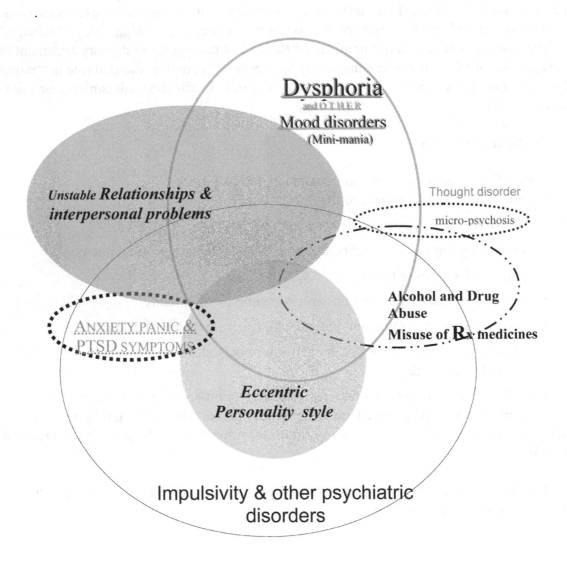

Venn Diagram IV-6-b   Contemporary visualization of Borderline Personality
"eccentric" in the true sense of the word

Essay on Suicide

In this chapter we are going to cover different aspects of committing suicide. These topics are the acts and agents, stages, degrees, volitional controls, risk factors, methods and means, and some special cases of suicidality.

This is a basic chart of the information in this chapter:

STAGES leading up to suicide	**Stage One—psychiatric condition** **Stage Two—persistent depression** **Stage Three—suicidality** (suicidality has six degrees of motivation)
Degrees of suicidality	*Describes the six degrees of motivation to plan and carry out suicide* *(passive death wish, suicidal ideation, intention, gesture, attempt...commission)*
ACTS of suicidality	Are carried out by the Agent or Agency of suicidality, these being the actions of some person that results in suicide— the agent can be the patient or somebody else, who is the "proxy"
Control	Volitional Control: whether pre-meditated, spontaneous, or impulsive

Ted, Ned, Sandi, and Courtney

In this chapter, we meet these four examples of patients.

- Ted is a young many who was jilted by his girlfriend. Ted has a history of acting before thinking. He is impulsive by nature. He lacks any apparent psychiatric history apart from mild to moderate ADHD for which he is currently taking non-addicting medicine. Despite ADHD medications, he barely squeaked through high school and has no ambitious future plans. He is also a compulsive worrier.

- Ned, on the other hand, is a coldly practical man who is given to thinking about life in terms of collars and cents. He is a wealthy man with cancer. He is in constant pain and does not wish to go on. He has a large life insurance policy naming his wife and children as beneficiaries. He does not have access to doctor-assisted suicide.

- Sandi has been born into a wealthy but dysfunctional family. She and her brother are reared mainly by servants or paid care-givers who take them to all sorts of activities such as ballet, soccer, and so on. The parents have their own lives. Sandi is born with a depressive personality (dysthymia), and after puberty, she has started to have episodes of recurrent major depression superimposed upon her depressive personality.

- Courtney is a "party girl". She goes out to discotheques as often as possible, she drinks as much as possible, and loves to use cocaine, ecstasy, and any other drug that is available. She has had a large number of lovers and has had sex at times during blackouts.

Basic terminology and stages of suicidality

(complete terminology follows further in this chapter)

- **–Suicide** means killing oneself. A committed suicide has already happened and the person has died from the suicide attempt. I saw a patient once who told me that she had committed suicide two years before seeing me. Clearly, one cannot commit suicide and still be alive two years later. A suicide means that a person has killed himself.

- **–Suicidality** refers to all aspects of suicidal behavior. I use "suicidality" to refer to all aspects of suicidal behaviors, including thinking about, planning, and acting out a suicide—think of it as:

  SUICIDAL + activITY = SUICIDALITY.

- **–Suicide-planner** is the person who is planning the suicide. He is not yet a patient unless he has already seen a doctor.

- –The **suicide actor** is the person who acts in order to commit suicide. The suicide actor can be the suicide-planner himself or another person. If it is another person, I call that other person a proxy or an agent.

- **–Suicide by proxy**: proxy in this case is an actor whom the suicide-planner is going to enlist to help with the suicide, in case the suicide-planner is apprehensive about carrying out the whole act by himself or feels that he will lose his gumption—or for some other reason; this someone could be a **voluntary proxy**, as when Ned pays a hit man to carry out the full act on Ned; an **involuntary proxy** would be if Ned has left a legal document stating that if he is in a persistent coma, that Ned legally orders his brother to "pull the plug. A Proxy is formally planned in advance unlike suicide by agent which occurs in the heat of the moment.

- ▪ **–Suicide by agent**: this occurs if a suicidal man waves a gun at the SWAT team (agents): the SWAT "agents" will likely shoot the man—whether this is voluntary or involuntary, pre-planned, impulsive, or spontaneeous is moot. This is unplanned, at least on the part of the agents (SWAT team).

- ▪ **Parasuicide** occurs when a person chooses not to do something that is life-preserving. For example, a dialysis patient decides that life on dialysis is just not worth living and refuses to go for any more dialysis treatments, knowing full well that this will cause a lethal outcome. Parasuicide might be less obvious, such as AIDS patients or cancer chemotherapy patients who decide to quit their treatments.

- ▪ **Omission (Act of Omission)** Omission is "a failure to act"; (Parasuicide)

- ▪ **Commission (Act of Commission)** Commission is "something done voluntarily by a person…an expression of will or purpose…a deed or performance…" (Suicide Attempt)

(These definitions of "omission" and "commission" come from *Black's Law Dictionary*)

These terms are further explained below.

The Brain and Suicide

There are a few common themes that accompany suicidality: the most life-threatening theme is coming from the brain.

Some suicidal people have "busy brains" and some have "tired" brains. People like Ted who have busy brains are constantly thinking and obsessing, usually about all the negative aspects of their lives. There is a notable absence of thinking about all the positive aspects of their lives. People like Ted obsess about all sorts of things that are out of their control. Ted is in double danger because he is also prone to impulsive acts. Friends and family are always criticizing Ted's compulsiveness and impulsiveness. Ted habitually seeks instantaneous relief. Ted's impulsivity will eventually be overcome by a moment of utterly hopelessness superimposed upon his baseline impulsivity during which he might drive at a 100 mph and crash his truck into a tree.

The second theme is that some people like Sandi have very tired brains. Their tired brains are tired of causing their tired bodies to stand up every day and move about on top of the Earth's surface. They just want to lie down and vegetate and be left alone. Friends and families are always trying to engage Sandi in activities for which she has no energy or desire. She is obviously suffering from one or more forms of depression. Sandi will eventually become so tired of everybody nagging her, that she will suddenly on an impulse "self-treat" her constant state of utter hopelessness by taking an overdose. Most overdoses are not lethal, and of those, quite a few are not intended to be lethal by the overdoser.

All that Sandi and Ted really want is just to turn off their brains for forty-eight hours. Clearly, they both have overreacted.

Three Stages

Now I am going to present the three **stages** and six *degrees* of suicidality. I have chosen this terminology because it shows that there are three major stages into which a person can fall.

STAGES		
ONE		**Psychiatric and medical illnesses**
TWO		**Persistent depressive symptoms**
THREE	↓	<u>**Suicidality**</u> *(Degrees of motivation (for suicidality)*
	1st 2nd 3rd 4th 5th 6th	*Passive death wish—feeling utter hopelessness* *Ideation— researching possible methods* *Intention—selecting one method and planning it* *Gesture—doing a trial run (to see how much is too much)* *Attempt—completing the plan that is supposed to be lethal* *Commission—resulting in death*
GRIEF		Grief and frustration felt by family, friends, caregivers

The Stages can be non-lethal

Many people might fall into Stages One or Two, and never have suicidal thoughts. A minority of those people, however, may move into Stage Three. Predicting which people might move into Stage Three, however is difficult. Some guidelines suggest that risk factors are based on gender, age, race, ethnicity, psychiatric diagnosis, chronic medical conditions, alcoholism-drug addiction, and family history. Once in Stage Three, the goal is to identify these people and get them out of that stage. Unfortunately, that is not always easy, unless the patient refers himself or unless friends, family, or employers bring him to a psychiatrist. The sad truth is that anyone can kill himself at any time without telling anyone. This chapter is about trying to deal with all these possible scenarios.

The Stages can be lethal

Once a person has entered Stage Three, then he begins a descent into the six degrees of suicidality. There is still time to act, but the situation is dire. The first four degrees can be intervened. The fifth degree is too late if Ted or Ned have chosen violent means. Sandi chooses to overdose, and might survive the fifth degree on her first overdose attempt. However, each time a person like Sandi tries to overdose, she increases her risk of reaching the sixth degree. People who have always remained in Stages One or Two do not have the memory or knowledge of the feeling-state of Stage Three, and thus can not seek it out on that basis. Perhaps they will stumble upon it if they start drinking heavily or have a massive assault of new stresses in their lives. If a person has ever been in Stage Three, then he knows it well, and can find his way back again in the future if he lets down his guard or if he should choose to do so. Stage Three is the most dangerous of the three stages.

The underlying foundations for suicide start with **Stage One**, which involves having a persistent psychiatric condition with or without a chronic medical condition. Most persistent psychiatric conditions can result in depression due to brain 'burn-out" from the ravages of the psychiatric illness. Examples are schizophrenia and depression.

Having a chronic medical condition, in addition to the persistent psychiatric illness, merely worsens the outcome. Since the brain is a physical organ, any medical disease that affects the physical body could affect the physical organ of the brain itself. Good examples of such chronic medical conditions are: multiple sclerosis, HIV-AIDS, chronic pain, cancer, and so on. In one sense, these chronic conditions are not really the first stage toward suicide since most people with depression and schizophrenia do not kill themselves, but in another sense, they are the first stage because a significant fraction of schizophrenics and depressives actually may do something that later results in their own deaths. It is very rare for a person in perfectly good health to skip all these lower stages and go directly to suicide. Therefore, it is reasonable to say that depression or schizophrenia would be a *sine qua non* for suicidality (*there is no suicide without a serious psychiatric disorder, typically depression or schizophrenia*).

As far as **Stage Two**, most suicides pass through a stage of persistent depression. Depression is a regularly anticipated stage in suicidal behavior, except for some manic or psychotic behaviors. Some people who are manic or psychotic may do life-threatening acts as a direct result of being psychotic without being clinically depressed at that moment or without any suicidal intention. Apart from this, Stage Two is typically present in suicides.

Stage Three is the stage of suicidality, which is a very dangerous stage. Better seek help if you are entering this stage.

The aftermath of Stage Three is grief for the survivors.

the Six Degrees of Suicide

These Six Degrees all belong within **Stage Three**. There are various *degrees* of motivation for suicidality. The first degree is "passive death wish" followed by suicidal ideation, intention, suicide gesture, suicide attempt, and finally committed suicide is the sixth and final degree.

"Passive death wish", the first degree, is a symptom of utter hopelessness, typically a symptom of depression. Since this first degree is a depressive symptom, it obviously has been built upon the foundation of persistent depression. Symptoms of passive death wish are expressed when a person like Sandi makes statements such as: "I wish I were dead", "I would be better off if I were dead", "Oh, why was I ever born?!", "today seems like a good day to die, but I don't really want to kill myself", and so on. Passive death wish means that Sandi is questioning the value of her life, but has no specific plans to do anything.

The *second degree is suicidal ideation*, which means researching possible methods that could be used. Women usually prefer a non-violent method, such as overdosing. Men prefer methods that are more violent (hence usually lethal): guns, hanging, and accidents. Overdoses are more survivable than gunshots to the head or hanging.

Third degree is intention, which means that Sandi is making plans that might eventuate in her own death. Her plan is overdose, so she has the intention to go on-line to read about overdosing. She might then decide to order a large bottle of nerve pills (without prescription). If she has the pills sent to her post office box, then she is more serious about suicide than if she had the pills sent to her parents home where she still lives. The chances are high that someone in the home would question a large bag that rattles a lot, originating from a foreign pharmacy. After obtaining the pills, she hides them until one day she feels very sad. Ted, on the other hand, has no intention, but wonders what would happen if he crashed his truck against a tree while traveling at 100 mph. He decides to buy a gun for "self-protection".

The *fourth degree is gesture*. Sandi takes the minimal dose of pills reported to be lethal, which she thinks might not be fatal but will help her sleep for a couple days, thereby allowing her tired brain to rest. She takes the pills alone in her bedroom at her parents' house on a Sunday afternoon, knowing that her brother will come home after playing tennis and that others will be coming into the house around that time, too. Ted might be angry and drive his truck toward the tree but at the last moment apply the brakes, resulting in damage to the truck and deployment of the airbags, with some resulting but survivable injuries to himself. Many of the people who make a gesture with pills are really trying to turn off their brains for about forty-eight hours. Part of the driving factor is brain rest. Other "gesturers" like Ted (or Sandi) are crying out for help: "Help me! Something is wrong with me! Something is wrong in my life!"

The *fifth degree is attempt*. Sandi has learned of the fatal dosage by reading further on the Internet. She drives alone up to her family's deserted mountain cabin. She then proceeds to take the presumed lethal dose, and she does sleep for forty-eight hours, but survives the attempt, thanks to certain unforeseen-by-her physiological and pharmacologic factors. Ted's fiancée jilts him and he becomes impulsively angry with himself, and does attempt suicide by driving his truck into a tree. He might survive this accident, but he will likely have major injuries.

Sixth degree of commission is an act of angry defiance, hopelessness, vengeful impulsivity, and self-loathing. There is often a sense of anger directed toward the survivors. This sixth degree can often be seen as an indictment of the people in the victim's life. It is by extension an indictment of that society in which they all live.

Grief

The person who has committed suicide might intend to inflict guilt and frustration on certain of the survivors. She—or he—fails to realize the full extent of this action. The effects spread out like ripples on a pond. The persons closest to the victim are most deeply affected. These are usually family members, spouses, and friends. They are left to wonder why and what. Why did Ted do that? Why did Sandi do that? What could we have said or done differently? We should have taken her to the emergency room the first time that she cut her wrist. We should have called a psychiatrist. We should not have bought him a new car. And so on…

Then the first ripples affect secondary persons: the friends of the friends of the victim are shocked, the colleagues and family of the victim's treating psychologist may be affected, depressed teenagers who live in that neighborhood may feel the need to act out their own depressive thoughts, and so on. Then the third ripples spread even further: the local community, members of the school board, readers of the local newspaper, and others.

Quick Statistics

—"Up to 10% of schizophrenics die by suicide."

—45% of all suicides had a primary diagnosis of depression"[3]—in another study, 30% of all suicides had depression; and, in another study 64% of all suicides had depression;

—Bipolar rates of suicide range 9-60% in various studies, averaging 18.9% .[3]

—Suicide is the fifth leading cause of years of potential life lost before age 65, regardless of race and gender [ref.77 p.66]

—Suicide is the third leading cause of death in men, ages 25-44 [ref.77p.67]

—Suicide is in the top three causes of death in teenage boys and young men under 25 (the other two top causes are accidents and homicide); a number of these teen suicides are due to mood disorders and schizophrenia[78]

Risk

In one study these were the highest risk factors:[25] being male was the highest risk, followed by being of Native American ethnicity. This study also showed that higher federal aid for mental health and higher density of psychiatrists resulted in fewer suicides.

Other studies have shown that in the general population at large, white males are most at-risk. Currently, teenagers and young adults have the highest suicide risks, which place suicide as the third leading cause of death for these groups.

Risk factors commonly recognized and quoted by mental health professionals are:

- very young adults and very elderly adults, men more so than women
- alcoholism and drug-addiction
- loneliness, isolation, sadness
- financial or legal problems
- poverty (no access to mental health care)
- personal psychiatric history
- family psychiatric history
- dysfunctional, distant, or non-existent family (members)

Acts, Actors, Agents, and Agency

The **actor** of suicide is the person whose actions cause the completed suicide. This is usually the **suicide-planner**, but could be someone else, whom I call the "**proxy**". A proxy has been actively recruited and enlisted in advance by the suicide-planner to be the actor. The proxy is a formalized actor. I use proxy to mean someone who takes on this responsibility voluntarily. I use the word **agent** for an actor who is enlisted involuntarily by the suicide-planner.

I am borrowing the concepts of "omission" and "commission" from the Law (*Black's Law Dictionary*): Omission is "a failure to act"; commission is "something done voluntarily by a person…an expression of will or purpose…a deed or performance…"

When Sandi takes an overdose, she is the suicide-planner and the actor.

When Ted crashes his truck into the tree, he is the actor. The act could have been so impulsive that he had only spent half a second planning it. Or, he could have been thinking about this act for a long time. If he does not survive, then we will never know.

When Ned hires a hit man to kill himself (so his wife can get the life insurance payment), he is the suicide-planner. The hit man is the **proxy**.

If a suicidal man waves a gun at the SWAT team, then they will probably shoot him; in this case, the SWAT team is the **agent**. If the man dies, then we might never know which of three possibilities of suicide had occurred. Had he planned his death in advance, had he been impulsive, or was he so intoxicated that it happened spontantously without his having any idea what was happening?

If he had planned it in advance, then he was the suicide-planner: this is active suicide by agents. He had intended this outcome.

If he had been impulsive in the heat of the moment, then the man turns out to be an impulsive actor in the suicide.

If he had been stabilized previously on Depakote and in men's anger management groups, then we can make a case for Parasuicide—he was neglectful of continuing a possibly life-preserving prior treatment that had probably been beneficial.

If he were so intoxicated that he had had no idea what he was doing, it cold have been spontaneous; if he were an alcoholic who had had black-outs in the past, then he should have not drunk—this is a commissional act.

If he was so psychotic that he thought that he was defending his family from aliens, then he had "diminished mental capacity". If he were a schizophrenic who had had bad experiences before when he quit taking his anti-psychotic medicine, then he should have taken his medicines.

Technically speaking (by my definition) this is Parasuicide because his neglectfulness of taking life-preserving treatment (Risperdal, for example) directly contributed to his death.

In all of these outcomes, the SWAT team plays the role of agent.

---

for Especially Interested Readers
These topics are covered in much greater detail at the very end of this chapter

---

Volitional Controls basic to Suicidality and Parasuicidality

Unplanned suicidal acts can occur in persons who are extremely psychotic and have no contact with reality. They have no idea of what they are doing or how dangerous it might be. They are usually hallucinating and delusional, too. Voices may tell them that Satan is pursuing them. "Jump! Jump now to save your self from the Devil!" yell the voices. Or the voices may urge the patient to wave a toy gun at the invading space aliens (who really turn out to be the SWAT team). The issue is whether the voices have been the product of a subconscious internal impulse to commit suicide or whether it is just an episode of random voices with bad advice. Another unplanned act could be that of a truly accidental overdose in patients with impaired memories, such as in Alzheimer's Dementia. Patients forget that they have taken a lot of medication and end up taking more. In some cases, this forgetfulness may be outside the patient's control.

Partially preplanned suicidal/parasuicidal acts are those that are caused by our studied carelessness—usually while we feel intensely dysphoric (miserable) and ambivalent (indecisive) about continuing to live but also ambivalent about sudden death. These are states in which we do not feel like going on with life, but are reluctant to do something extremely finalizing. In such cases, we make an impulsive decision to push the "envelope" in the hopes that the better and more appropriate outcome will obtain—whatever that might be. Examples might be "accidental" overdoses which occur in people who are misusing their pills, street drugs, or alcohol while in a mentally "diminished capacity". This person knows that this studied forgetfulness is dangerous but simply does not care. Usually patients survive these micro-psychotic episodes (psychotic because they really are out of contact with reality while they are in this altered ambivalent mental state). Medications and chemicals are usually involved. People usually survive. A second possible and foreseeable outcome is a fatality. These ambivalently dysphoric patients, who do not care if they live or die, almost always forget the third possible outcome: surviving but with permanent invalidism such as partial paralysis, minor stroke, and so on. This third outcome can be more common than usually thought. Other examples would include any risky behavior such as unprotected promiscuous compulsive sexual encounters especially where the patient knowingly participates in high-risk sex. Careless and rash behaviors can occur in people with a severe rapidly progressive fatal illness. There are many other examples too numerous to list here.

Preplanned suicidality can be impulsive or carefully planned out over a long period of time. But the act itself is often impulsive. Pre-planned suicide can be based on a sudden impulsive decision that is couched on layers of long-standing unbearable psychiatric misery. Surprisingly, depression is only one factor in suicidality. Most suicidal people do not awaken one day and decide to take their own lives. The person has probably been quite distressed for a long time. There are exceptional cases in which patients receive a diagnosis of a rapidly progressing fatal condition and spend only a short time contemplating suicide. (I remember at the beginning of the AIDS epidemic reading in the

NY Times that a gay couple newly diagnosed with AIDS both jumped off a skyscraper together.) In general, suicidal behavior is based in long-standing primary depressions or in long-standing psychiatric illnesses that have a secondary depression due to the primary psychiatric problem.

Primary depressions include all kinds of depressive illnesses and mood disorders.

Secondary depressions can be due to long-standing medical and psychiatric problems: a lot of people become very depleted and depressed after dealing with grinding primary persistent psychiatric problems, such as: panic-anxiety disorders; compulsive alcoholism and drug-addiction; impulse disorders; during the depression that occurs after a major psychotic episode; and, chronic states of abuses and low self-esteem associated with long-standing stresses (e.g., PTSD—post-traumatic stress disorder). After dealing emotionally with these problems for a long time, the patients may feel emotionally exhausted as well as feeling hapless, helpless, and hopeless. This results in a secondary depression that feels insurmountable. This is the state that can lead up to an actualized suicide.

General Progression toward Suicidality

Firstly, a person like Sandi, is feeling depressed all the time. The depression can become unbearable, especially if she has been to many psychiatrists and taken many medications without relief. She may begin to express a passive death wish ("I wish I were dead"). She can still be helped at this point and various healthful treatments should be tried: exercise, spirituality, self-help, psychotherapy, and antidepressant drugs, and avoidance of alcohol and street drugs.

If she feels no better, then she may start to have suicidal ideation where she is mulling over the possible methods that could be used in a suicide attempt. At this point, she might begin with "herald" signs and symptoms such as giving away treasured belongings to "deserving" friends and family. This can be a red flag—especially, in the elderly. The issue becomes whether they are just giving away cherished items to be certain that the intended heirs receive the items or whether they are disbursing everything of value because they have decided to commit suicide immediately thereafter. If feeling no better, Sandi may have suicidal intentions. Gesturing begins when she starts "experimenting" with suicidal behavior to see which is most tolerable or likely to be successful. Usually this gesture is a "cry for help" and this is the last chance for the rest of the world to try to intervene to save her. Women, however, are especially likely to make repeat gestures in trying to see which method might be acceptable or trying to find out who might really miss them the most. Or in the hopes that somebody will notice the cry for help. Unfortunately, some suicide gestures will—unexpectedly or accidentally—result in a completed suicide. Suicide attempts ensue.

Completed suicide is a condemnation of life by censuring modern society, which seems finally to have failed this person. There is an unfortunate number of young adult and teen suicides in this country each year—far more than there should be. Where has modern American society failed these youths? The constant messages blaring out from the television reminds us that we have to be smart, wealthy, accomplished, successful celebrity "wanna-be's". Both genders feel compelled to achieve, in the vain attempt to capture this mis-labeled "American dream" life and to possess "top-shelf" brand-name merchandise. The number one pastime of America becomes—not baseball—but consumerism. Those who fall short and who feel that they are in the bottom percentiles seem to have such impaired self-esteem that they may be driven to suicide. What a paradoxical indictment of our modern want-it-all-have-it-all society. These people are confused about the priorities necessary for "life, liberty, and the pursuit of happiness".

Methods

Suicide Methods Preplanned: Males tend to use violent and lethal means such as hanging and guns. As a result, males are likelier to succeed in the first suicide attempt than women who have an apparent preference for intentional overdoses, and wrist cutting. Both genders can use any means available, including car-crashes, electrocution, etc.

Suicidal Methods Partially Premeditated: Highly promiscuous unprotected sex while sober; accidental overdoes.

Parasuicidal Methods: Having highly promiscuous and compulsive unprotected sex while chronically intoxicated.

Figure IV-7-b   Suicide culmination by diagnosis, stages, and degrees: notice that each layer builds upon the lower one. We can see that the actual number of completed suicides is small compared to people with depressive symptoms, and even smaller than the number of all the people who have persistent psychiatric conditions.

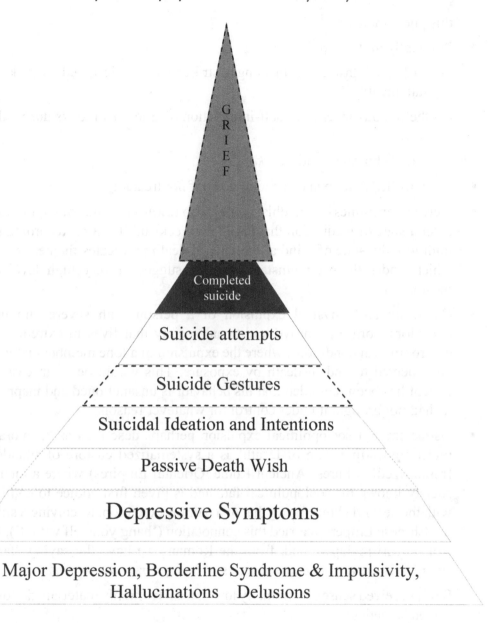

Highly Unusual Circumstances of Death

These are, technically speaking, parasuicides or suicides, which would be expected and intended to end in death. These include psychic suicide, uncontrolled anorexia, politically motivated self-immolation/prolonged fasting, terminal meditative states and so on.

- Psychic suicide is the ability to will oneself to die: there are no statistical data on this phenomenon;

- Politically motivated:

  a—prolonged fasting as in hunger strikes can be designed to make a political statement;

  b—the famous incendiary self-immolation of Buddhist monks during the Vietnam war;

  c—suicide bombers and *kamikaze*;

- uncontrolled Anorexia can end in death if not treated;

- there are examples of Buddhist monks who toward the ends of their lives decided to enter a state of meditation that lasted for weeks until death. According to Buddhist tradition, the state of mind at the time of death predicates the next re-incarnation, which under these circumstances might suggest a very high level of next re-incarnation.

- Ostracism and physical expulsion of a person with severe and uncontrolled behaviors from a primitive traditional society that lives in extreme and adverse environmental conditions, where the expulsion of a lone member on his own would be expected to end in death by exposure. This would occur in cases where the patient has been reminded that his behavior is unsanctioned and inappropriate, but he had not brought it under control for whatever reason.

- Ostracism and sociopolitical expulsion perhaps described as "Honorable suicide under Impending Pain of Death" is a systematized custom of suicide in certain [militarized] cultures (Ancient Rome, Oriental Empires) where a member of that society knows his sociopolitical fate and is given first choice to end his own life with the second choice being that of a painful execution. Receiving a silk cord from the Chinese Emperor carried this connotation ('hang yourself with it'); the practice of hara-kiri in Japan; and, from the Romans we have the saying "falling on his sword". These are the extreme cases of being *persona non grata*.

- Self-perceived sense of terminally low-esteem (in highly materialistic consumerism-driven societies).

Legal Repercussions

A person like Sandi who is suicidal can be psychiatrically hospitalized against her will for a few days or weeks. This is done in order to save her life and to give her the best chance to recover. Sometimes hospitalization can be beneficial. It gives her time to reflect on what she had tried to do, and it likely that she will recant and decide that that had been a very poor decision. Perhaps Sandi had not been taking her anti-depressants properly at home—maybe just taking them "as needed". All of the effective anti-depressants must be taken on a daily basis, regardless of how Sandi feels on that one day. After a certain time, she will begin to feel better. In cases of family dysfunction or relationship problems, hospitalization provides a safe neutral environment where situations with other people can be explored and remedied somewhat. While in the hospital, she will probably sleep better, and restorative sleep can have positive benefits. Very importantly, the nursing staff has the opportunity to see how Sandi is responding to her treatments; if changes need to be made, then this can happen while still in the hospital. Specifically, medications can be adjusted and critical relationship issues can be explored.

Table IV-7-c   Suicide by Gender and Age

	Suicide	Suicide	Passive suicide	Passive	Parasuicide
	Active	By proxy		by proxy	
Male Teens	Hanging Jumping asphyxia	Recklessness Gangs, hustling/sex			Alcohol, drugs, huffing, gangs, sexual asphyxia
Female Teens	Overdose, slit wrists	Promiscuity (STD)*,drugs			Drugs, diet pills, bulimia
Men	Car crash, Gunshot, Hanging, political, self-immolation	By police, In war, self-sacrifice,	*Forego Therapy, (refusing chemotherapy, Dialysis, etc.)	War	Self-stabbing reckless driving, Alcohol O.D. (overdose with or without pills)
Women	Overdose, slit wrists		Severe diets		Sleeping pills Wrist slashing
Elder Men	Gun knife alcoholism	Jaywalking	*Forego Therapy	DNR Status	Grief, Alcohol Omit ADL's**
Elder Women	Overdose	Suicide pact	*forego therapy	DNR status	High anxiety, poverty,loneliness

*STD=Sexually Transmitted Diseases [exposure through reckless behaviors] such as AIDS, Hepatitis C. Cervical cancer risks, Syphilis, Herpes, etc

**ADL's=Activities of Daily Living plus IADL's, instrumental activities of daily living (bathing, cooking, eating, shopping, etc.)

This table gives a run-down on common suicide methods by age and gender.

SUICIDE
ATTEMPT

More gestures cause
physical impairment

Suicide gestures
Overdoses physical injuries
Self-inflicted trauma

Suicidal Ideation
preoccupation with death, self-loathing,
repeated threats of self- injury, dysphoria

Passive Death Wish
Social withdrawal, "Learned Helplessness"
Taking anti-depressants haphazardly, major depression

Depression, Bipolar, severe panic-anxiety, PTSD,
Alcoholism, Drug Abuse, HIV, Hallucinations,
Delusions, Impulse Disorder, Borderline Syndrome

Childhood abuses of all kinds, Learning Disability, Physical
and Mental Handicaps, Chronic Pain, Panic attacks
Anxiety, Drugs & Alcohol, Dementia, Delusions

Figure IV-7-d This is the expanded pyramid shown already in figure IV-6-b

The foundation of the Pyramid consists of: predisposing factors such as chronic untreated emotional illness, extensive family (hence genetic) predisposition, severe stressors, major medical illnesses treated with large doses of many medical medications, post-traumatic issues, traumatic childhood events.

The second level of the pyramid lists common contributing factors, which can lead up to worsening symptoms and behaviors. Any of these factors can aggravate symptoms; the more of the factors which are present, then the greater the possible amount of decline. The chronic anxiety contribution is often minimized since it is not considered to be as major as Psychosis and Manic Depression. However, it also makes an important contribution, statistically speaking. Besides Double Depression, we should add that treatment-resistant depression is a large risk at all seven levels of the pyramid (treatment-resistant depression is a depression that is usually not improved with the routine use of the typical medications—but might be helped by shock treatments). Many severe diagnoses are here: HIV, Borderline Disorder.

The third level lists the psychiatric illnesses that raise the risk of suicide. We should note that if the factors on the base of the pyramid have not been diagnosed and treated, then these undiagnosed and untreated disorders will get worse and lead to the fourth level.

In the fourth level of the Pyramid, the patient is moving beyond medical intervention and going up to a place where there is still time for psychiatric treatment, but time seems to be running out. This level will lead to the next level if untreated. As the patient goes up and up the pyramid, the chances of diagnosis and treatment are lessening.

The fifth level of the pyramid is where the patient is entering a danger zone and is on the verge of having a psychiatric emergency. At this stage, patients may begin to give away precious objects to friends and family. These are the objects that they had intended to pass on after death according to the terms of their Will. This is always a bad sign.

The sixth level of Pyramid is a psychiatric emergency and extreme interventional measures must be taken to prevent an active suicide by commission.

We can observe that many people have predisposing factors and treatable illnesses and that only a small fraction of these people rise up to successive levels, with very few reaching the top (hopefully).

Treatment

Why is all this so important? Why classify the types of suicidal behaviors? The answer is: because this helps us to decide on the treatment approach.

Cases of ACTIVE SUICIDE account for most suicidal patients seen by psychiatrists. In cases of active suicide, the suicide-planner such as Sandi is the actor who plans the suicide.

Sometimes the actor must go through a series of acts: Sandi goes on-line to look at overdosing, she must find the name of a pill, order it from a foreign pharmacy, pick it up at her post office box, find out when no one will be at the family cabin, drive to the cabin, then take the overdose;

The usual response to patients like Sandi is to get them into intensive treatment: talk therapy, medication therapy, and possibly hospitalizing them. The treatment is the same as for whichever psychiatric condition is causing this, but the usual cause is depression.

Impulsive people like Ted usually cannot be intervened because there is often no warning sign

He makes only one act of deciding that this is the day to crash his truck. Impulsive people do not usually volunteer to go to psychiatric treatment unless they are forced by their family or a judge.

Usually, they will not take medications on a regular basis, because they do not believe that medication will help, because they do not believe that they are ill, and because they resent authority figures. The best treatment chance for Ted is to be court-ordered to men's groups where he might hear just one statement that impresses him enough that he will recall it in the heat of the moment when his impulsivity begins to flare.

ACTIVE SUICIDE by PROXY: The suicide planner is the actor who must determine a plan, then find somebody to carry it out in the manner determined. In the case of Ned, he needs to be very cautious in finding someone who knows someone who knows someone who knows a hit man. Then he must contact that person, obtain enough cash without attracting attention, and make the payment. Ned claims to be doing this for his family, but if that is so, then doesn't his family deserve to know before-hand? Active suicide by proxy is not a part of regular psychiatric caseload. I mention it only to acknowledge that it could happen.

PASSIVE SUICIDE (PARASUICIDE): The suicide-planner (actor) decides not to do some life-saving act. Ned decides to forego chemotherapy. Caregivers and family will most likely be quite aware of this decision. In the case of passive suicide where Ned decides that he does not want chemotherapy, his doctors and family will certainly be aware of this. Patients like Ned will usually be sent to see a psychiatrist. If Ned is of sound mind, and knows what his diagnosis is, knows what the proper treatment is, and knows of the outcome with and without treatment, then all that the psychiatrist can do, is to document

Ted's opinions. Contrary to popular belief, we can not intervene in this case to force him to take chemotherapy.

Special Section for Especially Interested Readers

I use **agency** to include three possibilities: active agency, passive agency, or an intermediate agency of parasuicide.

Agency of Suicidality (which actions by which person result in the desired suicide?)

    I—Active Suicide (Comissional suicide)—is deliberately intentional

        A—Suicide by Oneself: see Risk Factors

        B—Suicide by Proxy—the suicide victim has a prearranged agreement with some person whose actions or lack of actions will result in the desired suicide

        C—Suicide by Agency—the suicide victim does some act that will cause someone else to react, and that reaction will kill the patient, resulting in the desired suicide

    II—Passive Suicide (Omissional suicide)—is partially intentional because Ned refuses to take life-saving measures such as chemotherapy

      Ned partially intends to die, just not right away; he feels that death is better than a life of pain

        A—Passive suicide by oneself

        B—Passive suicide by an agent or proxy

    III—Intermediate agency: Parasuicide (non-Commissional) Neglectfulness resulting in self-harm)—is not immediately intentional. I call this "non-commissional" because Courtney is neglectful of a reasonable amount of self-care. She is not actively suicidal by any means. She is not immediately omitting to do something that would keep her alive, either. She chooses to live "on the edge" despite the fact that she knows this lifestyle is dangerous. There are numerous other high-risk (parasuicidal) behaviors besides over-indulgence. All that I require is that the person be conscious of his really dangerous and careless behavior: "Oh, yeah, I thought people could die from that—but not me…" Courtney does not purposely and deliberately intend to die.

Agency in Detail

This section is for those especially interested in all the detail.

Active suicide is the intentional outcome of an *act of commission* (it is something that a person purposely does to himself with the intent of murdering himself). Suicide occurs when a person does something to end his life: hanging himself, shooting himself, taking a fatal overdose of drugs. This is an act of commission that ends in personal death (committing suicide). There are many ways to kill ourselves willfully.

These are some of the reasons and mechanics driving suicidal behavior. It can be a "cry for help": Sandi is using nonverbal communication to express her feelings, saying "I don't like myself or my life—so please help me!" a suicide gesture could be a "dry run" to investigate how much effort is required to cause a completed suicide. Sometimes patients repeat these efforts with ever-increasing determination and willfulness while ramping up the intensity. Very weak gestures may be an attempt to manipulate the legal system in some way, such as to get into a psychiatric hospital for "respite stay" (this is common in people who are in regular jail and want to get into a less horrible environment inside a mental hospital or previous psychiatric patients who are temporarily homeless). These people will take several pills but state to the ER staff that it was a "handful" (which I guess is technically correct depending upon the size of the hand). They might also make some superficial scratches on the wrists with a plastic knife, or some other activity that they know is not a serious attempt.

A failed suicide occurs if Sandi survived what she had considered to be a likely lethal act. In these cases, the effort was not great enough, or her body was stronger than she knew.

A suicide gesture can be a "transparent" attempt to manipulate lovers, spouses, or family members. In this case, it often gets the desired results, e.g. attention, concessions, and sympathy.

Suicide attempts can be mild, moderate, severe, severe and self-aborted, or (profound) seriously severe:

Most patients who make mild suicide gestures will later acknowledge that they did not really think it was a lethal attempt ("without lethal intent"); and, certainly no medical staff would have considered it serious. Moderate suicide attempts could cause slight brain damage: sitting in the garage with the car running for a few minutes. These are the "dry runs" where patients are toying with death but not quite ready to leave us yet. Severe suicide attempts can be accompanied by permanent damage to the body: strokes, dementia, or paralysis. Recovery from these medical problems is very unlikely. Severe and aborted suicide attempts are usually moderate or severe attempts where the patient had lethal intent but shortly afterwards has decided to recant his intentions and ends up calling 9-1-1 (or a family member) for help. Seriously severe attempts are really botched suicides in which the patient has done something to himself that would almost always be fatal, but which the patient has miraculously survived. Such examples are the patients who shoot themselves in the head and survive. They can recover and go about their business (with or without rehabilitation) without too much neuropsychiatric impairment (this is quite rare but it has happened).

The usual outcome of a botched suicide is invalidism of some sort. I have seen two cases of self-inflicted gunshot wounds that went through one side of the head, through the brain, and out the other side. In both cases, the patients had been so impaired prior to the suicide attempt, that their ability to form an intent is debatable—but they survived. One was quite functional and one went on to be fairly functional.

The greatest hazard in suicide gestures and attempts is that the patients are experimenting with something which they do not understand and for which medical science cannot predict the individual outcome in any case. Many times these extreme acts leave the patient alive but worse off physically and mentally. Some may then lack the ability to get hold again of the means to kill themselves—or, they may lose interest in doing any further damage. The greatest tragedy is that people should feel driven or compelled to do any of these behaviors in the first place.

"Suicide by Proxy" occurs when a person has willfully caused some "actor" to end the person's life prematurely according to a plan hatched by the person himself but requiring action by another person, who may be acting voluntarily (as a proxy) or involuntarily (as an agent—in other words, the patient coerces or inveigles somebody to kill him when and where and how he wants). The actor acts voluntarily if the person had planned the suicide by proxy and had given instructions beforehand, and the proxy had agreed to participate in the plan. Perhaps, the patient has a fatal illness (like Ned) with a large life insurance policy. Perhaps the person is abjectly depressed and does not wish to drag on any further "my family will be better off without me and they need the life insurance payout". In very rare cases, one spouse may commit this prearranged act on the terminally ill spouse, as part of a suicide pact. The agent acts involuntary when the agent was not aware of the person's plan to commit suicide: an oft-viewed example of involuntary suicide by proxy is when cornered perpetrators purposely brandish a gun at the SWAT team. These perpetrators appear to be choosing between a long prison sentence or immediate death by execution.

Passive suicide is the intentional outcome of an act of omission (in other words a person can bring on his death by failing to do something to keep himself alive). Passive suicide is only partially intentional. Passive suicide is a lack of action (or a non-action) which a person understands will eventually result in his own death. This could include decisions not to take cancer chemotherapy. A classic example would be a renal failure patient refusing kidney dialysis. These are "acts of omission": the person is refusing to do something that will keep him alive or is doing something that is basically guaranteed to hasten his demise. If he survives longer than expected, he might sometimes feel ambivalence. He does not deliberately intend to die immediately, because he thinks that he can go on for a while. Remember that chemotherapy and dialysis are harsh treatments. These are cases where the treatment is probably about as bad as the disease.

"Passive suicide by Proxy" could include a situation where the patient has given advanced instructions to caregivers to stop giving the patient a life-saving treatment—or to withhold life-giving treatments. For example: a patient who knows that he will lapse into a prolonged and lethal coma may give instructions to staff and family not to put him on artificial life support. Patients can order these kinds of requests by writing a "Living Will" or other documents or by requesting to be given the status of DNR ("Do Not Resuscitate" [in case of heart attack]). Other possible examples might be operative in cases where gang members decide they want to try to leave a ruthless gang knowing full well what will be the likely consequences.

Parasuicide occurs when a person intentionally engages in hazardous activities without any wish to die. These are mainly foolhardy reckless activities. Unlike passive suicide, they do not believe that omitting or committing certain acts will harm them. They feel omnipotential (that they can defy death). These persons harm themselves without clear lethal intent but are nonetheless hurting themselves. This might usually be an outward sign that correlates to symptoms of poor self-esteem, high levels or impulsivity, or internalized rage. Typical examples would be: elderly people who are first-time bungee-jumpers or parachutists, handling live rattlesnakes while on a fancied divine mission, or leading an incredibly dissipated lifestyle that is way beyond just living in the "fast lane".

Table IV-7-a   Acts, Actors, and Agents of Suicidality: ways in which a person can contribute to his own death—the five columns show the categories of causing harm to oneself; the first row gives a general definition; the second row gives a specific example; and, the third row shows the actual method used. The "actor" is the suicide-planner. The act is completed suicide. The "agent" or "proxy" is someone other than the suicide-planner; the agent or proxy helps the suicide-planner to complete the suicide.

(R_x = "treatment")(OD= overdose)(POA=power of attorney)(DUI= driving drunk)

Active Suicide	Active suicide By proxy or agent	Passive Suicide	Passive Suicide By proxy or agent	Parasuicide
ACTOR Acting on Oneself; This is <u>commission</u>	Causing another person to act on Oneself so as to result In one's death <u>Agent or Proxy</u>	Refusing to do an act on one-self that is known to be lifesaving <u>Omission</u>	Ned signs legal papers to force another person to deny a life-saving treatment for Ted so that Ted is put at high risk of death. (guardian ad *litem*, living will, conservator)	Negligent, reckless, or wanton acts on oneself that are commonly known to be harmful to the body—done once or habitually
Ted shoots himself In the head	Ted waves an un-loaded gun at the SWAT team; Ned has cancer and hires a hit man to kill him so that his family might collect his life insurance	Intending to die, Ned refuses dialysis or chemotherapy, which are life- saving treatments (Rx)	Ned writes a living will ordering his family to "pull the plug"; then he writes a final letter stating that if he fails his suicide attempt, he does not want any life-saving intervention(Rx)	Extreme pro-miscuity with many high risk partners, dangerous li-aisons (sexual asphyxia fe-tish), "huff-ing", playing "chicken" with trains, daredevilism
Ted's gun ⤴ Ted ‡	Ted's ┈▶ SWAT gun team guns ⚡ 🚓 Ted ‡	$[R_x]$ →ı ∅ Ted did not receive treatment Ted ‡	*POA →ı ‡ $[R_x]$ ‡ (*Power of Attorney, guardian or conservator, did not authorize Ned's Rx) Ned ‡	"Too many parties, too many pals", high-risk sex ↓↑Courtney↓↑ DUI—drug OD

Bottom Line:

<u>Don't Do It !!</u>

If you have "tired brain" or "busy brain", then go see a doctor.
If you have unbearable depression, then seek medical attention.

3-reference 3 pp. 1744-47   5-reference 5: pp. 24-27, 385;   17-reference 17

Chapter IV-8

Essay on Anxiety Disorders

Anxiety Disorders are conditions in which the symptom of anxiety is the most prominent symptom. Most of these disorders have familiar names such as Panic (Disorder), Anxiety, and PTSD (Post-Traumatic Stress Disorder). Other names that may be familiar include: Phobias, Obsessive-Compulsive Disorder, and Stress. For the purpose of this book, I have labeled the Anxiety Disorders as follows:

- **Anxiety**
- **Generalized Anxiety Disorder**
- **Panic Disorder**
- **Phobia**
- **Short-term Stress Anxiety**
- **Long-term Stress Anxiety**
- **Reactive Stress Anxiety**

In ordinary speech, we sometimes use the term "panic attack" as if it were different from the term "anxiety attack". Currently, psychiatrists use the term "panic attack" to refer to both anxiety attacks and panic attacks. Panic attacks are a symptom. They are the main symptom of Panic Disorder. Panic attacks of Panic Disorder can occur at any time without warning, often unassociated with any apparent stress factor (this is an "uncued" panic attack: it has no cue). Anxiety Disorder refers to a constant state of fretfulness. PTSD is a complicated anxiety disorder. "

Phobia" is Greek for "fear". Some people have a phobia of certain situations, such as driving across freeway bridges (in L.A.) or being in large open spaces. When these people are exposed to the feared situation, then they have a panic attack (a "cued" panic attack: the bridge is a cue). These panic attacks can be prevented by avoiding the situation (cue) that causes the phobia. Invariably, the phobic patients, who come to see a psychiatrist, have a phobia that interferes with their jobs or family life. If a person who lives in the desert (Palm Springs) is afraid of great heights, then he might not come in for a visit—as long as he is not planning to go skiing.

Obsessive-Compulsive patients feel the need to go through certain repetitive behaviors ("rituals"). If they cannot do this habitual "ritual", then they feel anxiously distressed. Stress Disorders can be due to anxiety-provoking situations and/or can cause anxiety symptoms. Examples are short-term stress, long-term stress (PTSD), and anxious adjustment.

"Uncued panic attacks" means that there is no cue to cause the attack. "Cued panic attacks" refers to the fact that some stress factor has probably caused the panic attack. The cues can be external (in the environment) or internal (drugs, foods, or adrenaline rush).

Cued Panic Attacks	*Uncued Panic Attacks*	*Constant Anxiety*	*Off-and-on anxiety*	*High Stress*	*Anxiety-Panic caused by*
Phobias	Panic Disorder	Generalized Anxiety	Obsessive-Compulsive	Stress Disorder	
Agoraphobia Social Phobia				Anxious Adjustment	Street drugs* Medications Foods*
				PTSD	Medical or Neurological Diseases*
Table IV-8: The Anxiety Disorders				Diagnoses are in gray highlight;	
Symptoms are in the first row;			* known causes are in the sixth column		

Sometimes a person could have two anxiety disorders at the same time; this is not unlike situations in which a person could have two depressive disorders at the same time. Some people can have panic attacks with a phobia. This means that the person has uncued panic attacks ("Panic Disorder") plus cued panic attacks (panic attacks when exposed to the feared situation). People with phobias and panic attacks are also exquisitely sensitive to many drugs as well as stimulating foods with excess sugar, caffeine, or chocolate. The list of drugs could be very long, but would certainly include all drugs that might be stimulating, such as antidepressants started at normal adult doses.

I define "anxiety" as a state of mind in which the person feels hyper-aware and distressed all the time and cannot relax or slow down. The person may be up and down all night, pacing. He might wring his hands and feel indecisive. These feelings are usually about the same every hour of every day of every week. Sometimes this state will be so bad that the person might also have the additional symptom of panic attacks.

Some people with panic attacks feel so distressed, that they think about suicide so as to escape the horrible feelings.

Panic attacks can occur in any other psychiatric condition: manic-depression, bipolar, depression, psychotic disorders, and schizophrenia.

Anxiety disorders have effective treatments. Some of the medicines in the Valium family are helpful but are also addicting. Military-related PTSD is the most difficult to treat successfully.

Henry, Gerri, Roberto

Henry is thirty-five year old married truck-driver with two children. He makes deliveries all over southern California from the L.A.-based warehouse. His job has been going well for several years until one evening when he was watching Ice-Road Truckers on the Discovery channel. He became disturbed by the show and did not sleep well. The next day when he was driving in the fast lane of the freeway, he had sudden chest pain and had to be taken to the nearest emergency room, where it was assumed that he was having a heart attack. It was not cardiac, but an apparent panic attack. He was given fifteen tablets of Xanax and an appointment to see his primary doctor in four days. He continued to have unexpected panic attacks whenever driving on the freeway—perhaps once a day or once a week or once every two weeks. The Xanax was continued and was helpful. A few months later, the family decided to go camping and Henry had a couple panic attacks on vacation and his wife did much of the driving. He is having freeway-phobia. He will become dependent on Xanax unless he starts to get mental health treatments.

Gerri is twenty-three years old and has always been anxious. She tends to worry about everything and these feelings are worsening. It is now impacting her first major job in customer relations. She becomes distracted with customers, feels keyed up all the time at work, is irritable, and feels very tired in the afternoons when her customer skills worsen significantly. She has generalized anxiety disorder (GAD).

Roberto was driving to UCLA in rush hour traffic on the freeway when he was in an accident. He was not seriously injured, but the person in the other car was. That night he started to have bad dreams about the accident. He would awaken in the wee hours sweating and with his heart pounding. He had great anxiety and fear of driving on the freeways, so he took major boulevards to travel around the city. In the daytime, he would have sudden anxiety-producing thoughts of and recall of the accident. He also had stressful chats with insurance company representatives. His sleep continued to be fragmented and he often awoke feeling restless and anxious with profuse perspiration. He started to have nightmares about the accident. He goes on to develop mild PTSD.

Anxiety can be a sign, a symptom, or a diagnosable disorder.

Signs of anxiety are visible and noticeable to other people, including to the doctor. Typical signs of anxiety can be fretfulness, restlessness, constant worrying, and wringing of the hands. There are slight differences in the way the two genders perceive this anxiety event. Men often think that they are having a heart attack of some sort. Women are less likely to suspect that they are having a heart attack; nonetheless, they do suspect that some horrible medical event might be happening. They are more likely than men to think that they are having high anxiety or an anxiety attack. Another definite sign is sweaty palms, which I can feel when they shake hands. Sometimes they perspire in the office. They might have trembling hands, hand-wringing, restlessness, or dilated pupils. These are all observable to the doctor. These are some of the signs of anxiety.

Symptoms of anxiety are usually apparent to the patient and perhaps less obvious to other people. These symptoms can be fear of impending doom, fear of dying, racing thoughts, light-headedness, heart throbs, lump in the throat, numb lips, and so on.

Diagnosis of anxiety is based on:

- the history of how this all happened to the patient,
- the signs,
- the symptoms,
- the list of current medications (if any),
- past medical history (any heart condition?),
- past psychiatric history (did this ever happen to you before?),
- family medical history (did your father and uncles have heart attacks early in life, etc?),
- family psychiatric history (does this run in the family?),
- food allergies or reactions (triple chocolate mousse, espresso-grind coffee, cigueratoxin, etc.?)

If the diagnosis is anxiety, then it could be coded as Generalized Anxiety, or as a more specific anxiety disorder diagnosis.

So anxiety might qualify simultaneously as sign, symptom, and diagnosis.

Anxiety Disorder ("Generalized Anxiety Disorder")

Anxiety Disorder is now called GAD (Generalized Anxiety Disorder). The course of generalized anxiety disorder is variable: sometimes it will stay the same for a long time, sometimes it will gradually worsen, and other times it may improve and go away. The severity and the intensity are hard to predict. Most certainly, GAD will get worse if the person has extra stress in his life. It will get better if the person can adequately cope with the stresses.

In the past, there were various confusing terms such as free-floating anxiety, anxiety-tension state, anxiety neurosis, cardiac neurosis, performance anxiety, and so on. These have all been reclassified as one of the official anxiety disorders listed at the beginning of this chapter.

There are some non-pharmacological measures which a person like Gerri can take in order to lessen the burden of anxiety disorders and decrease the stress of anxiety: lose weight, do half an hour of cardiac exercise everyday, get enough sleep, decrease caffeine consumption to the equivalent of one cup of coffee per day (or one cola per day), and learn to manage stressors: commute less, buy less, owe less, need less. Rearrange your mind and your life will follow. In the meantime, here is the story on the different courses that Gerri's anxiety can follow:

- –The first scenario is that anxiety might be a long-lasting condition that may just stay the same more or less.

- –In a second scenario, sometimes anxiety may slowly get better over several months or a couple years and then go away.

- –However, a third possibility is that it may also come back again and be worse than the first time, which will require more vigorous treatment, perhaps with more medications and in higher doses.

- –And in the fourth scenario, anxiety may not go away at all and then slowly evolve into anxiety plus occasional panic attacks which is, of course, a worsening of the anxiety. In this fourth scenario, Gerri has two diagnosable disorders, Panic and Anxiety. The Anxiety Disorder and Panic Attacks can get worse if she needs to take certain medicines for medical or neurological illness.

Generalized Anxiety is usually a long-standing and taxing daily grind of anxiety that often persists until it is medicated. . However, Geri can become drained from the whole process. She will then begin to feel more and more depleted. This can result in a secondary depression caused by persistent GAD.

Anxiety can be mild, moderate, or severe. It can be disabling in a few cases; however, modern medicines can be effective, thus eliminating any need to be on long-term permanent disability.

Panic disorder

Panic Disorder is characterized by panic attacks that appear with quite dramatic symptoms. Many people think that the panic attack is a heart attack, and reasonably so because panic attacks occur with pounding heart, rapid heart beat, chest pain, sense of death, sweating, nausea, dizziness, and numbness of lips and fingers. However, other symptoms may occur, such as feelings of sudden insanity with various psychiatric and non-cardiac symptoms as well as trembling hands, enlargement of the pupils (in the eye), and racing thoughts. Most people in their twenties who have panic attacks are not likely to be having heart attacks—yet. Given all the stress in modern society, however, this is a possible diagnosis, and the emergency room staff will take it very seriously by doing a heart wave test (EKG) and specific blood tests. In the past, panic attacks could even occur with fainting spells (swoons). At those times, some boudoirs had a special piece of furniture called a fainting couch.

Panic attacks can start at any age under any circumstance. Most panic patients are in their twenties and thirties. If first-time panic symptoms start in an elderly person, then this should prompt a search for a serious medical disorder or medication reaction. If there is no such diagnosis, then the attacks might be psychiatric. The list of possible medical causes is very long, so I shall just note a few common medical problems (thyroid or neurological disorders) and medications (antidepressants, asthma treatments, neurological medications for Parkinson's or restless legs).

Phobia

Phobia is the Greek word for "fear". Psychiatrists use "phobia" to refer to a specific fear that will cause panic attacks. Such fears may be: fear of heights, fear of going out in large public spaces, fear of mingling in social situations, and so on. There are many types of these specific fears, hence many types of phobias. In the past, when psychiatrists had less medicine to learn and more time to study Greek and Latin, each different phobia was classified by using its full Greek name. Arachnophobia was fear of spiders, agoraphobia was fear of open spaces, acrophobia was fear of heights, and so on. Nowadays we use the English words such as "Spider Phobia" for fear of spiders. We still recognize Agoraphobia as a specific phobia and continue to use this Greek term as a modern diagnosis. This is literally a fear of going to the "agora", a public market place (large open space) in ancient Greece. Nowadays, it pertains to large open spaces such as malls, fields, and parking lots. Social Phobia also is a special phobia with its own diagnostic code. All other phobias are just diagnosed as a phobia: Spider Phobia, Fear of Heights (phobia), airplane phobia, and so on. Social phobia is a fear of social events, of meeting new people and speaking up in those events.

Some people are afraid of snakes or spiders, but if their fears are not really causing any psychiatric symptoms, then treatment is not necessary. Most Americans are probably afraid of something, but that does not make us officially "phobic".

Short-Term Stress Anxiety ("acute stress disorder")

This is diagnosed when a person such as Roberto has been exposed to some stressful event that would make anybody anxious (bad accident on the freeway). It should be a life-threatening stress that makes Roberto fearful or horrified (he could have died; the other motorist was seriously injured). The stressful event causes anxiety symptoms and other psychiatric symptoms. Some of these symptoms may represent Roberto's trying to get out of his body or out of reality. Roberto begins to have morbid recollections of the stress that intrude into his thoughts daytime and nighttime (he hears the crashing sound, he hears the sound of glass shattering and people screaming). He begins to avoid activities that are closely related to the stress factor (He quits driving on the freeway, and may not want to drive anywhere in any car).

In some cases the short-term stress-related anxiety continues to haunt the person for a longer time, and then it becomes long-term stress anxiety. Milder forms of acute stress disorder should improve and go away with proper treatment. Moderate or severe forms may progress to PTSD

In general, the stress of being in a war zone every day should result in far greater traumatic stress than that of being in a car crash once on the freeway.

Long-Term Stress Anxiety (post-traumatic stress disorder, PTSD)

This is what might develop next if moderately severe Short-Term Stress Anxiety does not improve. This state includes civilian PTSD and military-related PTSD. I am going to discuss mainly civilian PTSD. Military PTSD is ideally handled by the VA Hospital system (Veterans' Administration). A novel article on PTSD appeared in Scientific American April 2009: *"The Post-Traumatic Stress Trap"* by David Dobbs (pp.64-69).

Civilian PTSD occurs when a person is exposed to some event (tornado, earthquake, floods, tsunami) or series of events (inner city riots) that could disturb anybody. In these cases, a person starts to think about these events all the time and begins brooding about the symptoms. He will continue to receive stress cues from his normal surroundings even when the shocking event has passed. A seemingly innocent cue can happen in his everyday life to set off a flood of stressful memories again—a cue, which would not normally upset an unstressed person (a person without PTSD). The bad memories haunt his nightmares with dream-anxiety symptoms that can be moderate or severe, including even nightmares about the event from which he awakens terrified in the middle of the night, perhaps acting out his original responses to the shocking event. In the daytime, he may be thinking about trivia and receiving no innocent cues from the environment and then have a sudden unprovoked "flashback" which is a time of reliving the shock of the stressful event. Or there might be an environmental cue to trigger the flashback. Among civilians, PTSD can also occur after horrific traffic accidents, bank hostage situations, and so on. We are led to believe that PTSD is a regular occupational risk in the armed forces.

Reactive Stress Anxiety ("anxious adjustment disorder")

This can happen to anybody. These are sudden situations that trigger anxious feelings. This can happen when suddenly confronted with adultery and/or divorce, bankruptcy, lawsuit, being fired with no apparent warning, a minor car accident, airplane mishap, etc. Most of these pass within a few days; some may linger on and morph into another anxiety disorder.

Other conditions associated with Anxiety

Anxiety can also be caused by medical medications (asthma drugs, Parkinson drugs, Prednisone, and diet pills), street drugs (amphetamines and steroids), or medical illnesses (overactive thyroid, adrenal disease, and some neurological conditions).

Performance Anxiety is the situation in which a person is called upon to give major speeches, play in orchestras, or be scrutinized while performing before other people.

Some anxious people report having anxiety about the possibility of having anxiety attacks.

Biochemistry and Treatment of Panic-Anxiety

(See Chapter V-9 for the complete treatment guide)

As far as biochemistry of panic/anxiety, there are a couple observations which ring true, regarding adrenaline and lactic acid specifically. First off, panic attacks are believed to be related to surges of adrenaline since the same type of reaction is involved in the so-called "fight or flight" reactions. This is a primitive reaction seen in most animals and humans. Whenever a person or an animal is in grave danger, his body will release a surge of adrenaline to make him feel peppy so that he can quickly and efficiently deal with the danger. The reaction consists of exciting the heart to pump more blood in order to heighten the senses in preparation for taking evasive action. This must work well, otherwise we would not still be here. The adrenaline can be blocked by certain blood pressure pills called "beta-blockers". These same pills can be helpful in panic attacks and performance anxiety. These pills can prevent panic attacks, lessen the impact of the panic attack, or render us non-reactive to the panic attack while it is happening.

The second observation is that panic attacks are related to increased levels of lactic acid in the body.

Anxiety is sometimes difficult to control. There are a number of good treatments available, most of which are not addicting. Antidepressants in low doses often have demonstrable anti-anxiety effect. When used in this way, the antidepressants must be started in tiny doses, not in the regular adult starting doses for treating major depression. Some common examples would be Zoloft 12 ½ mg, Paxil 5 mg, Lexapro 2 ½ mg, Doxepin 10 mg, Elavil 10 mg. Buspar is a failed anti-depressant that works well for generalized anxiety in low doses of 10-60 mg a day, but not for panic attacks..

The fact that anti-depressants can help anxiety lends further weight to the received wisdom that "anxiety and depression are just different sides of the same coin".

The worst scenario in the treatment of panic-anxiety occurs if the symptoms can be controlled only by addicting drugs, such as Xanax. Then habituation or addiction could become a bigger problem than the anxiety. Researchers are still trying to devise novel drugs to control panic and anxiety symptoms.

Beta-blocker drugs are helpful for performance anxiety (Inderal or atenolol).

Also see Chapter V-9 for complete treatment of anxiety disorders.

Outlook

As a single diagnosis, anxiety is not considered a risk for suicide. However, bipolar patients with uncontrollable and constant panic-anxiety are at a higher risk of suicide—of course, bipolar patients have a very high suicide rate regardless of secondary conditions. For those patients who can control their symptoms only with addicting drugs (Xanax, for example), habituation or addiction can become a bigger problem than the anxiety itself.

▶Although it may feel like a heart attack, anxiety is not fatal. Numerous treatments are available.

▶▶ QUESTIONS
___

Q: How is Anxiety different from an anxiety attack?

A: "Anxiety attack" is a commonly used term, but it is no longer a special diagnosis. Our official diagnoses now list Anxiety Disorder and Panic Disorder. Modern diagnosis uses only the term "panic attack" and not "anxiety attack". Some people still use this term, "anxiety attack" to reference an attack that is mainly psychological anxiety (i.e., anxiety symptoms) with less physical anxiety (i.e. signs of anxiety). In common parlance, panic attack is intended to mean the psychological anxiety of an "anxiety attack" plus the physical symptoms, such as perspiration and heart throbbing. (Review the difference between sign and symptom in Chapter I-4, "Introduction to Medicine in General"). I understand if Gerri says she had an anxiety attack when she feels restless and "all wound-up" but does not think that she is having a heart attack.

Section V
DRUG TREATMENTS and PHARMACOLOGY

Superscript numbers refer to references and citations at the back of the book

Chapter V-1

Introduction to Psychiatric Medications

This table gives the reader an overview of the most important chapters in this section. Many of these drugs are interrelated in various ways, mainly on the bases of their structure and function.

Chapter	Topic
V-1	General introduction to psychiatric medications and their date of debut
V-4	Anti-psychotics: (Dopamine and serotonin mentioned)
V-5	Introduction to Antidepressants:
V-6	Stimulating Antidepressants (Psychostimulants)
V-7	Older (Sedating) Antidepressants
V-8	Newer Antidepressants
V-9	Full Alphabetical List of Antidepressants
V-11	Anti-anxiety drugs: GABA

It is often difficult to separate them out in a simplified overview, and this fact has required me to make arbitrary choices. For example, I have tried to avoid using the vast array of chemical names and pharmacologic identifiers. Some of the names have been simplified as shown below:

When I write this name…	…this is the proper medical name or term
Serotonin drug Norepinephrine drug Mixed serotonin & norepinephrine drug	SSRI SNRI SSNRI

Psychiatric drugs exert their effect over behavior by causing temporary changes in brain chemistry (or brain electro-chemistry). Scientists believe that this effect is due to the drug's effects on certain biochemicals inside our brain. This is currently the popular theory.

There are a number of these "certain biochemicals", but we currently hold that the most important ones are serotonin (5-HT), GABA, dopamine (DA), and norepinephrine (NE). Under rare circumstances, the biochemicals related to these psychiatric drugs might cause permanent brain changes but these are usually in the form of unwanted side effects—not desirable therapeutic effects.

Adrenaline is the internal hormone that prepares us for "fight-or-flight". When we are in a tight situation, we get an "adrenaline surge". In general, we refer to the bodily hormone "adrenaline" as "adrenaline" but refer to injectable factory-made adrenaline as "epinephrine".* "Adrenaline" is the Latin name for the hormone, whereas "Epinephrine" is the Greek word. Adrenaline and Epinephrine are exactly the same biochemical.

> *Adrenaline = Epinephrine: these two words refer to the same biochemical*
> *I am using "**Adrenaline**" in this book*

Adrenaline has a counterpart called nor-adrenaline.
Epinephrine has a counterpart called nor-epinephrine.

Noradrenaline = Norepinephrine (same biochemical) *I am using "**Norepinephrine**"in this book* abbreviation **(NE)**	*NE is a major topic In psychiatry*

Norepinephrine and Noradrenaline are also the same biochemical. Norepinephrine is an important brain biochemical. I am using "adrenaline" and "nor-epinephrine" in this book.*

Adrenaline	=	~~Epinephrine~~
~~Nor-adrenaline (NA)~~	=	**Nor-epinephrine (NE)**

The original stimulant antidepressants (amphetamines) have adrenaline-like effects, which means that they act like adrenaline on the body and like norepinephrine on the brain. They can release norepinephrine and other biochemicals in the brain. *Psychiatrists may often use noradrenaline (NA)interchangeably with norepinephrine (NE).*

This chapter gives a general time line of the discovery and uses of important psychiatric drugs. I have made an attempt to link the decade of discovery to the drug's use and relationship to other drugs, with the emphasis on the time line, since the other details will appear in following chapters. There is also a secondary emphasis on the drug's general mechanism of biochemical activity. This emphasis is due to the fact that once a new drug suddenly appeared with a novel mechanism of action, there was usually a stampede by the drug companies to find other drugs with similar biochemical activity. So the time of discovery usually results in an era when a certain similar family of drugs is in vogue. And drugs in a similar family almost always have similar biochemical effects. Being in a similar family, usually denotes that the drugs are all structurally the same, but not always, as is the case with the serotonin drugs. Thus, the drugs will later be presented with their mechanism of action in their own specific chapters.

The first general group mentioned in this chapter are the **adrenaline-like stimulating** anti-depressant drugs. These drugs affect two important brain chemicals, **norepinephrine (NE)** and also **dopamine (DA)**. These stimulating antidepressants are covered specifically in their own Chapter V-6, "Stimulating Antidepressants-Psychostimulants". These adrenaline-like drugs are contemporaries of the barbiturates, which were the first sleeping pills, and barbiturates were also the first anti-anxiety drugs. Barbiturates are dangerous in overdose and especially so, if mixed with alcohol. Barbiturates exert their effects through a brain chemical called **GABA.** Drugs that act on **GABA** have anti-anxiety properties and are covered in Chapter V-11. Drugs in the Valium family are now the best known of the GABA drugs and are commonly callled "minor" tranquilizers. (The "major" tranquilizers are the antipsychotic drugs, a large and important class of medicnes. They control agitation and psychosis. They also affect dopamine, but this effect is not over-emphasized here. See Chapter V-4.) The serotonin antidepressants are mentioned briefly in this chapter, but appear in Chapter V-8. These serotonin drugs are not only useful in depression, but in anxiety disorders. Finally, other less important drugs are referenced.

Order of appearance in this chapter: Adrenaline-like drugs: stimulants	Note on the names of brain biochemicals
GABA-acting drugs: "minor" tranquilizers	1)-I am using "chemical" to refer to something from outside our body and "biochemical" (or "brain hormone") to refer to a natural substance made inside our body
"Major" tranquilizers	
Serotonin drugs: depression and anxiety	2)-the most important "biochemicals" are serotonin, GABA, norepinephrine, and dopamine
Other drugs	

The practical history of the use of mood and mind altering drugs goes far back into prehistory—how far, we do not know. There are inferences that Europeans have been using Valeriana for thousands of years. Anthropologists believe that shamans used powerful drugs for ritual purposes. All over the world, these practices are found: absinthe (wormwood), belladonna, and numerous herbs in Europe; peyote, jimsonweed, tobacco, and mescaline in the New World; khatt, hemp, poppies in the Old World, countless herbs in China; "ordeal beans" in Africa, and so on. (Alcohol too has a long history: ancient Sumerians loved to make beer, five to six thousand years ago.) And now salvinorin extracts from *Salvia divinorum* are becoming a focus of research.

History of Modern Pharmaceuticals

The modern history of psychiatric medications began in Japan well over a century ago when a scientist named Nagai isolated ephedrine from the *Ma Huang* plant. Ephedrine is a natural stimulant with effects somewhere between those of caffeine and amphetamine, more or less. Very soon thereafter in Germany, the first amphetamine was made from ephedrine by a simple process. Later they learned to turn amphetamine into methamphetamine, also a powerful stimulant (homemade methamphetamine is the notorious "crystal meth").

Also, right around this time, adrenaline was identified in Poland. Chemists were able to determine the chemical make-up of adrenaline. They wanted to make an antidepressant or "pep pill" that would produce results like adrenaline because they thought that this would make people (workers, soldiers) livelier, more active, and activated. Adrenaline and its sibling compound **norepinephrine** cannot be absorbed by mouth. So, the search was on to find a modified adrenaline stimulant drug that could be absorbed by mouth and could retain this stimulant activity.

At the beginning of the twentieth century in Germany, Emil Fischer and Joseph von Mering made the first tranquilizer, a barbiturate. They combined urea (from urine) and malonic acid (from apples). It was promptly brought to market in 1904 by Bayer and marketed under the trade name of Veronal. (Fischer had traveled to Verona, Italy, which he considered to be a delightfully calming city and travel experience; thus, the name Veronal). The barbiturates exert their effects by changing levels of **GABA** in the brain.

The next phase took place in Germany also but took a very dark and sinister fork in the road around the 1930's. The Axis powers (Germany and Japan) started to give amphetamines (methamphetamine) to their soldiers to make them more alert and active. Hitler also was apparently taking large daily doses of these drugs. Amphetamines taken at high doses for a long time can cause mania and psychosis. There are anecdotal reports that Japan—after World War II—continued to avail themselves of amphetamines and had ten times the prescription rate of amphetamines as in the USA. Americans also liked to use amphetamines such as: Benzedrine, Dexamyl, and Desoxyn. Desoxyn is pharmaceutical-grade methamphetamine, known on the street as "crystal meth".

Amphetamines act on the brain where they cause the rapid release of brain biochemicals such as **dopamine** resulting hopefully in a state of euphoria. This euphoria is an indirect effect of the drug. The drug causes the release of stored dopamine. Eventually the dopamine will all be released and depleted, and the drug-user will experience an agitated depression due to direct activity of amphetamine on the brain, which may eventually lead to a state commonly referred to as "crashing" which doctors call dysphoria (the opposite of euphoria).

Undeterred by all this, scientists continued to research compounds with chemical properties similar to those of **adrenaline**, ephedrine, and amphetamines. They learned to manufacture pseudo-ephedrine from ephedrine. Pseudo-ephedrine can be used to make methamphetamine, the highly addicting and damaging drug ("crystal meth").

Next Parnate was manufactured. It is an adrenaline-like stimulant antidepressant, but was given the special family name of MAOI Antidepressant. There are other MAOI antidepressants, but they are not so closely related to adrenaline. Their names are Nardil, Selegiline, Emsam, and Marplan. (Still others are available in Europe). Please note that St. John's Wort has mild MAOI activity as part of its antidepressant activity.

The mid-twentieth century became a time of frenzy in its own way. Some of the most dangerous stimulants and sedatives debuted in this time. Dangerous stimulants such as Eskatrol and other amphetamine derivatives. Cylert and Ritalin followed. And a host of "diet pills", the most notorious of which turned out to be "Fen-Phen" (now off the market). A lot of dangerous sedatives appeared at this time. These drugs were very dangerous in overdose, and fatal overdose could occur from mixing a one month supply with alcohol. They have mostly faded into history with names such as Doriden, Noludar, Placidyl, Equanil, Miltown, et al.

Fortunately, the sedative Valium was synthesized around this time and became vastly preferred by doctors —and most patients. Valium is much safer in overdose, even when mixed with alcohol. There are now many drugs in the Valium family. Apart from the fact that they are habit-forming, they are reasonably good. Their main activity is due to acting on the brain hormone that relaxes us, called **GABA** (see more about GABA below).

Another old anti-anxiety drug, Vistaril, is still popular. It is also called Atarax. It is almost never dangerous in overdose and is not habit-forming.

As far as "major tranquilizers", Reserpine is a drug that comes from the *rauwolfia* plant of India. The Hindus have used it for countless centuries to treat psychotic behaviors, but reserpine can also cause suicidal depression in addition to controlling psychosis. It was the only natural anti-psychotic available. It was also the only anti-psychotic available until Thorazine was invented in mid-twentieth century.

Around 1950, a whole new class of mind-altering drugs was discovered. The first drug in this class was manufactured by the French Navy as an accessory anesthesia drug. Its name is Thorazine. It is a major tranquilizer. Soon Thorazine showed that it had remarkable powers to calm down psychosis and schizophrenia. This was the beginning of a whole new class of psychiatric drugs never imagined before—they all had a tricyclic chemical nucleus (so technically, Thorazine is the first tricyclic anti-psychotic, but psychiatrists do not refer to it as tricyclic). Tricyclic means that the drug has three aromatic carbon rings (with side chains attached). These Thorazine-like drugs could make very psychotic people slow down and calm down. Schizophrenics could collect their thoughts and focus. Thorazine was followed by other major tranquilizers in the same class but with slightly different properties. Some of these new drugs similar families to Thorazine were: the Mellaril family, Navane family, Prolixin family, and Loxitane. A new class of drugs was next discovered, of which Haldol is the best known (in the USA). Then came a different drug, Moban. Orap was also produced. All these drugs became known as major tranquilizers. Most of them are chemically related except for Moban, Haldol, and Orap. Other equally good major tranquilizers (unlike Thorazine) were never brought to the USA (sulpiride, for example).

These became known as the "First Generation Antipsychotic drugs (FGA). They all have a tendency to make patients feel mentally dull, and all of them might cause Parkinsonism (uncontrollable shaking and stiffness). Apart from these side effects, some of them have additional effects on other organs in the body (heart and liver, particularly). Nonetheless, all of them are lumped together and referred to as the class of major tranquilizers, which are also called neuroleptics, thymoleptics, or FGA's. Each of these four terms has a slightly different nuance to psychiatrists. These drugs all have a huge advantage over reserpine.

As a result of the introduction of Thorazine, many new spin-off drugs were being created and tested. One of these very early drugs was Imipramine. Imipramine differed from Thorazine by only a few small chemical changes, but had no major anti-psychotic properties. Schizophrenics who volunteered to try it, however, did report feeling happier. Imipramine was brought to market as an antidepressant. This was the first so-called "tricyclic" antidepressant. Many other tricyclic antidepressant drugs were made and sold, and then researchers found other new antidepressants that were not related to adrenaline or to Imipramine.

By the 1980's, the search for new antipsychotics had resulted in Clozaril. This began a new era in anti-psychotic treatment. After Clozaril, new and unique anti-psychotics came to market. These are: Risperdal, Zyprexa, Zydis, Seroquel, Geodon, Abilify, and Invega. And now comes Fanapt (Iloperidone). These were given the name of SGA's (Second Generation Antipsychotics). Although they do not produce an unpleasant sense of sedation, they also turn out to have significant side effects. Some of them are associated with diabetes, obesity, and high cholesterol. One of them has a possible cardiac side effect, and three of them could cause a minor form of Parkinsonism (like the FGA's). They typically cause a relatively pleasant sense of relaxation or sedation.

The FGA's and SGA's are mainly differentiated on their **dopamine** activities. This is the original basis for separating the SGA's from the FGA's. This dopamine activity relates to their propensity to cause Parkinsonism.

Back to antidepressant research: Further work on the chemistry of adrenaline-like drugs finally produced non-addicting Prozac. Prozac—like Parnate—has an obvious chemical resemblance to adrenaline and **norepinephrine** (as do some asthma and sinus drugs). Parnate and Prozac are not habit-forming and are not classified as addicting drugs.

Prozac is of very major importance because it was the first of a new kind of antidepressant. Even though Prozac has an adrenaline-like structure and can stimulate some people, by and large, its antidepressant activity focuses on **serotonin**, another important brain hormone, which we have not mentioned until now. Researchers were delighted with Prozac and the search was on for more serotonin-active antidepressants. These were eventually discovered, and curiously, none of them share a common chemical structure with any other serotonin drug. These serotonin drugs are totally unrelated to each other chemically. They are now famous and include: Prozac, Zoloft, Paxil, Luvox, Celexa, and Lexapro. They are not addicting (like stimulant antidepressants) and are not lethal in overdose (unlike all the previous classes of antidepressants, such as tricyclics and MAOI drugs).

Later research has now created new antidepressants with a **mix of norepinephrine and serotonin** qualities: Effexor, Cymbalta, and Pristiq. Otherwise, these are quite similar to the serotonin-drugs such as Prozac and Paxil.

Trazodone was a novel antidepressant that appeared just before Prozac. It is still a popular medication and it spun off other similar medications such as Serzone and Buspar (and gespirone in Europe).

Other Medications

Before barbiturates were invented, bromides were used as sedatives. These were not really manufactured, but are earth salts. Barbiturates were the first manufactured sedatives.

Brain Biochemicals

Our current understanding of the effects of psychiatric drugs on the brain is referred to as the "neurotransmitter theory". Neurotransmitter is our technical word for brain biochemicals. The theory is very complicated, but these are the basic foundations of the theory: Norepinephrine drugs make people feel active. Dopamine drugs create a sense of pleasure. Serotonin drugs help people to concentrate and feel composed. Drugs that raise brain levels of GABA possess anti-anxiety properties and help people feel very relaxed and calm. Obviously, drugs that act on any of the four main brain biochemicals are of immediate interest to psychiatry.

Symptoms of depression, anxiety, and psychotic states do improve when most patients begin taking diagnosis-appropriate medicines. On the other hand, some patients have paradoxical reactions to common drugs whereby their target symptoms actually get worse. This suggests that this "neurotransmitter theory" of the "brain biochemicals" might need more explanation. It may even need serious revision, although what I have presented here is the state of current knowledge about these neurotransmitters' mechanism of action.

Researchers still do not know if psychiatric drugs act directly on the "brain biochemicals" (neurotransmitters, "brain hormones") or on some other brain system that results in alterations of the "brain hormones". There are brain chemicals called BDNF (Brain-derived neurotrophic factors) that affect the size and numbers of brain cells. Changes in BDNF may correlate to mental illness. Changes in the brain due to BDNF may account for the observed abnormalities of "brain hormones". This remains an active field of research.

Other biochemicals of much interest are glutamate (glutamic acid) and aspartate (aspartic acid). These are both amino acids which are the building blocks of proteins. Glutamate and aspartate are found in great abundance in our bodies and are most certainly "natural". Glutamate is becoming a very important focus of research in the neurotransmitter theory.

These are the four main "brain biochemicals" which are targets for the current understanding of brain function and brain response to psychiatric drugs:

	DOPAMINE (DA)	SEROTONIN (5-HT)*	NOREPINEPHRINE (NE)		GABA
	Pleasure and reward Sense of well-being Euphoria Attention Anti-depressant	Concentration Focus Inspiration Anti-anxiety Attentiveness Anti-depressant	Activation Motivation Energy Anti-apathy Anti-depressant		Relaxation Serenity Inhibition
Cocaine Amphetamine LSD	++++++ +++++	+ + +++++++	+ +		Valium++++ barbiturates+++

*V-1-a (see V-5-a)   three important neurotransmitters (cocaine stimulates all three brain hormones, amphetamine stimulates dopamine, and LSD causes so much serotonin stimulation as to result in psychotic symptoms). Norepinephrine (NE) is the same as noradrenaline. GABA is a counterweight to excess anxiety from any cause (stress, DA, NE); its activity of inhibition means decreasing apprehensiveness. *The full name of serotonin is 5-hydroxy-tryptamine.*

For especially interested readers,

this is a list of other biochemicals that act on the brain and serve as important messengers in the nervous system[ref.5-p.19] .

1- Acetylcholine, (Butyl-choline, too?)—possibly deficient in Alzheimer's Disease;

2- Tyramine, phenylethylamine—both closely related to adrenaline;

3- Melatonin—a hormone from the pineal gland regulates sleep (day-night cycles);

4- "Real" hormones: growth hormone, thyroid hormone, vasopressin—promote physical well-being and some effect on mental well-being;

5- "male and female" hormones (steroid hormones) testosterone, androgens, estrogens—provide motivation, drive, desire, and libido;

6- Amino acids: glycine, glutamate, aspartate—all help to maintain normal nerve functioning;

7- our natural internal narcotics: various enkephalins and endorphins—these make us feel good: the source of a long-distance runner's "high"—they are peptides (like very short proteins);

10- intestinal hormones acting on the nervous system: secretin, gastrin, motilin, CCK, VIP;

11- natural "cannabinoid": anandamide, a fatty acid (cannabinoid=marijuana family);

12- other hormones: bradykinin, carnosine, neuropeptides, bombesin, galanin, oxerin, neurotensin, delta sleep factor;

13- other substances: substance P and neurokinins;

14- nicotine stimulation (mediated by our natural Acetylcholine, #1 above), and others.

---

* explanation about norepinephrine for especially interested readers

Clarification of often Confusing Terminology:

Adrenaline = epinephrine
I am using "**Adrenaline**" preferentially
because the readers are probably already aware of "adrenaline rush"

▶Adrenaline is the same biochemical hormone as Epinephrine. Adrenaline is preferred in England. You will probably hear American doctors use epinephrine and adrenaline interchangeably, to refer to the same exact biochemical. The reason that Americans started to prefer epinephrine is because a trademarked version of epinephrine was sold in America as Adrenalin® (without the final "-e"). Even more curious, American doctors often use adrenaline to refer to the natural hormone and epinephrine to refer to the injectable drug (an injection of "epi"). It's not confusing to us, but the reader needs to be able to sort this out.   Adrenaline is usually not of immediate interest to psychiatrists.

▶Adrenaline (epinephrine) can be "stripped down" to produce Nor-adrenaline (noradrenaline) that is the same as Nor-epinephrine (norepinephrine).

▶Noradrenaline = Norepinephrine
I am using "**Norepinephrine**" preferentially
Because it is very important in psychiatry: we write it as NE
Psychiatrists often use norepinephrine NE interchangeably with noradrenalin NA

▶**Phenyl-ethyl-amine** (Ph-Et-NH$_2$ *or* φ·Et·NH2) *is the correct name for the chemical family that includes adrenaline, norepinephrine, dopamine, amphetamines, Prozac, Parnate, et al.*
▶*The pharmacologically correct adjective for norepinephrine is not "norepinephrinic"—it is "noradrenergic", which I am not going to use in this book. I will write "norepinephrine-like". Likewise, "adrenergic" is the only adjective in use for both adrenaline and epinephrine (I am using "adrenaline-like"). Sorry, but Medicine has a huge vocabulary of words and word usage.*

Chapter V-2

"Mechanics" of Prescribing Psychiatric Medications

This chapter involves understanding the goals of treatment, the origins of medications, and the basic techniques of consuming the prescribed medicines.

The doctor who prescribes psychiatric medications is responsible for all the effects caused by the drugs. He needs to understand that medicines are chemicals. He needs to understand what kind of chemical it is: whether it comes from animals, plants, minerals, or some other source. What class of chemical is it? Is it a mild acid, alkali, protein, or salt? Is it dangerous in overdose? How can such an overdose be treated? Can the drug cause permanent damage? What are the most common side effects in most people? Which drugs can be taken with it and which other drugs must be avoided?

The use of prescription medications for any medical purpose should require any doctor to understand all of the following guidelines:

1) understanding the chemistry of the drug;

2) understanding the origins of the medication (how it is derived or created);

3) absorption of the drug into the body and brain;

4) duration of its effects (how long will it stay in the body and brain);

5) toxicity to the body—if it is a dangerous chemical;

6) reactions of the body to the drug;

7) expected benefits, relief, and side effects of the drug;

8) degradation of the drug: whether it is torn apart into active or inactive daughter chemicals (or none at all);

9) its reaction with other drugs in your body; and,

10) its route of elimination from the body—how the body gets rid of it.

This is the usual gamut of medication information.

Medications can come from many sources, some sources being quite unusual or rare.

These are some of the possible sources of medications:

- mineral and elemental (lithium, bromide, calcium, potassium, magnesium, bicarbonate, iron);

- animal origin (thyroid extract, omega fish oils, porcine insulin, vaccines grown in chicken or duck embryos)

- inspiration from animal origins (steroids, Prozac (adrenaline-like), amiodarone (formed from four thyroid molecules), epocrit;

- plant origin (digitalis, rauwolfia, reserpine, cocaine, opium, belladonna);

- found naturally in plants but synthesized in the laboratory because the amount of medication needed is far more than that which can be easily isolated from the plant itself (galantamine from crocus bulbs, vincristine from periwinkles);

- inspiration by the plant world (benzodiazepines based on Valeriana extract), Sudafed (similar to natural ephedrine), opium derivatives which do not exist in nature and are not addicting such as dextromethorphan;

- mimics of natural substances but are not known to occur in nature: valproate as a mild organic acid, gabapentin based upon a hexose sugar, EDTA (four vinegar molecules);

- combinations of simple known natural substances joined together to form a novel chemical substance (barbiturates);

- totally synthetic products with no known natural basis (Paxil);

- "monstrosities" and exotic structures (nonachlazine, Ludiomil, Trazodone);

In the case of psychiatric drugs, there will be all of these variables plus the sundry effects that the drug will have on the central nervous system.

New Technologies

New technologies are bringing hopefully better prescription drugs to market. There are three new areas of technological advances. These can concern the activity of the drug, the purity of the drug, or its "delivery system". "Delivery system" refers to new types of slow-release pills and injections.

Active forms of the drug and its by-products

In order for the drug to help us, it needs to be in its "active form". In the active form, it can act on our brain to produce the desire effect. Some drugs are swallowed in an inactive form (Vyvanse). The body needs to turn this into an active form so that it can help us. Other drugs are active when swallowed. Some drugs are turned into two or more active forms in our bodies, and each active form is a slightly different chemical, like non-twin siblings. In this case, an active drug is processed in the liver which turns the drug into a few by-products by rearranging or tearing apart the original drug. These by-products can have therapeutic effects, or they may cause annoying side effects. (The biochemical name for these by-products is "metabolite".) These are the possible effects of these by-products:

1 the processed by-products may have no activity and no side-effects;

2 the by-products may have activity like the parent drug and no additional side effects;

3 some of these byproducts can intensify the action similar of the parent drug—with minimal or variable side effects; and,

4 some may cause new side effects with or without any beneficial effects.

In all these cases above, some of the side effects might be related to dose. If the main drug is helpful but you get some delayed side effects (possibly from the by-products), then you might be able to lower the dose of the parent drug and find this drug tolerable. A few examples of number three (#3) above are: Ludiomil (Maprotiline) turns into Oxaprotaline, Valium into nor-Valium, Vistaril (Hydroxyzine) into Zyrtec (cetirazine), Soma into meprobamate, and so on.

New Techniques to make "Purified" Active Forms of Medications
These are the left-sided form ("Levo-form"), or right-sided form ("Dextro-form"):

Drugs have left-sided forms and right-sided forms both present in 50/50 combinations. They form randomly as mirror images of each other when they are produced in chemical reactions. Often one form is the active form (often the left-sided form), and the other form is inactive. This inactive form can be responsible for many of the drug's unpleasant side effects. In an attempt to reduce side effects, chemical engineering of these forms involves separating the drug into its two mirror images, left-sided and right-sided. Then only one mirror-image form of the medicine, the active form, is packaged into the pill. In these cases below, only the therapeutic mirror-image is packaged into the pill and the other mirror image with annoying side effects is discarded.

- **Lexapro** is the active form of Celexa;
- **Pristiq** is the active form of Effexor,

- Provigil has its own new active form, **Nuvigil**.

- Vistaril/Atarax is an old sedative and antihistamine; in our body, Vistaril is turned into its active form of Zyrtec, and from this, they have made the left-sided Zyrtec, which is Xyzal

The technological advances in being able to produce these new mirror image forms of drugs will hopefully result in fewer side effects while maximizing pharmaceutical benefit. This technology is expected to reduce adverse drug reactions (ADR's).

Here is the full example of what is going on with these drugs as technology marches forward: Vistaril is an old sedative used by psychiatrists. It causes side effects of dulled drowsiness and hunger. Hunger is not usually a desired side effect (except in anorexia). Sedation is a good side effect because that is its desired effect. Vistaril is also an antihistamine used by dermatologists and family doctors for allergic reactions and allergies. Zyrtec is a refined by-product of Vistaril, having less sedation, less mental dulling, and less hunger. Xyzal is the mirror image of Zyrtec and Xyzal is thus a third generation drug, actually a "granddaughter" of Vistaril. Xyzal is said to be highly effective for allergies without causing any undesirable side effects. These "spin-off" next generational drugs are becoming more popular. I mention this one example in order to help you understand the basic process. Expect to see a lot more of these mirror-image by-products coming to market.

Parent drug	→	active form for allergy	→	Levo-form
Vistaril/Atarax (hydroxyzine) 1-Sedative and 2-Antihistamine (allergy pill)	→ →	Zyrtec (cetirazine) allergy pill	→ →	Xyzal (levo-cetirazine) improved allergy pill

Blood levels of Psychiatric Drugs

Some medications have readily available drug levels and some do not.

Some of these drugs have mandatory blood levels: *Lithium* blood levels must be checked often because the toxic blood level is about twice as high—or less than—as the beneficial blood level. The beneficial blood level is about 0.5-1.5 (different labs have slightly different standards) whereas a toxic level could be anything over 2.0.

Some psychiatric drugs have blood levels that are readily available and provide guidance for adjusting the number of pills needed. *Pamelor* is such a drug. This also applies to *Tegretol, Depakote, Klonopin.* Tegretol and Depakote levels should be checked with some regularity. Klonopin blood levels are available, but I usually do not order these, unless I plan to taper someone off Klonopin. Some alcoholics are sent to me while they are taking high-dose Klonopin, and I feel the need to lower the Klonopin dose before the person has a bad reaction from mixing alcohol with that drug. I can monitor progress with a blood level.

Some drugs have blood levels that are available, but the blood levels do not necessarily give clear guidance on how many pills to give the patient. Examples are *Elavil and Doxepin.* The purpose of these blood levels is for special circumstances, usually to allow us to infer if the patient is a slow or rapid user of the drug (see Chapter II-4). For example, a patient named David who was a quarterback now has injuries resulting in constant pain. He is forty years old but still exercises in a swimming pool. Two years ago, his sports medicine doctor sent him to psychiatry for control of chronic pain. David is feeling about 80% better on very high dose Doxepin, 375 mg a day. He does have dry mouth and some weight gain, but is not overwhelmed with a lot of annoying Doxepin side effects. Most psychiatrists would view this as a probable and reasonable dose for such a person. However, I would worry about the heart in patients who are large, less active, formerly athletic, and taking high dose Doxepin. So, I order a heart wave test (EKG) which the cardiologist reads as "probably within normal limits". I also order a Doxepin blood level, which shows the blood levels are in the middle range of normal. (actually the test has two results, one for Doxepin and one for nor-Doxepin). So, I can confidently tell David that all is going well medically, and he can continue on the same dosage.

Some blood levels of drugs are available but are costly and are of questionable value, because sometimes the drug level interpretations can be ambiguous. These kinds of blood levels are done only under quite unusual circumstances. I would include herein the blood levels for *Trazodone, Haldol, and Prolixin.*

New "Delivery Systems"

Some medications are now available in time-released forms, which are like small "drug-spheres" (spherules) of medicine: Effexor-XR pills and Risperdal-Consta injection. After such a drug enters the body, it is slowly released over an extended period of time in the hopes of keeping the drug levels stable for longer periods of time.

Some drugs are available as "pro-drug" which means that the pill contains an inactive form of the drug which has to be swallowed. After it is swallowed, our bodies will convert it into the active form of the drug: the amphetamine Vyvanse is an example.

Some drugs are available in forms where the whole pill is layered like an onion. One by one, each layer is slowly dissolved away allowing gentle absorption and prolonging the drug's action: Wellbutrin-XL, Ambien-CR, and Invega.

Some drugs are available in "depot injections": the drug is "dissolved" in an oily substance which is injected into a muscle (the "depot") where the drug is slowly released over weeks. The oil is very thick and enters the body (from the muscle) over a typical period of weeks.

Dissolving tablets are a convenient way to take doses while on the go: this offers the advantage of a portable pill that dissolves in the mouth and is absorbed in the mouth. There is no need to take the pill with water: examples are Zyprexa-Zydis, Risperdal M-tab, Klonopin wafers, Fazaclo (Clozaril), Abilify Disc-melt, and Remeron Sol tab. Dissolving pills are also useful for people who cannot swallow or who must not swallow pills before a medical procedure.

"Pharmaco-economics"

In other words, saving money at the pharmacy. Some medications are priced about the same, no matter which size of pill has been prescribed. This is the case with generic Zoloft, for example where the 25 mg, 50 mg, and 100 mg tablets all cost about the same. If you are prescribed 50 mg a day (per month), then you can save money by buying 100 mg tablets and taking only half a pill. This will allow a one-month supply to last for two months. This might be very important for people who have limited pharmacy insurance benefits. Another possible way to save money would involve procuring liquid medicines (see below under "customized dosing").

"Customized" Dosing

There are ways to customize dosing of medications. The main way is by using liquid medications. This allows dosing that is as personalized as the person's ability to measure liquids. This is especially practicable for the very elderly who need comparatively tiny doses as compared to healthy young adults. For example, if an extremely elderly and petite lady has tried Lexapro 2½ mg and found that too weak, and has tried 5 mg and found that too strong, then she could be given 3¾ mg of Lexapro. If she responds well to that, then that dosage could be continued. This is how to achieve fine-tuned dosing:

- Lexapro is available as a peppermint flavored liquid. The bottle comes with a measuring device for teaspoons.
- The concentration of Lexapro in the bottle is: 5mg/5mL = 5 mg/tsp.

- In order to obtain a dose of 3¾ mg, you will need to administer ¾ tsp.(3¾ mg = ¾ tsp)

- The desired amount is therefore ¾ teaspoon which might be easy for you to measure—if so then give that amount;

- If you have trouble measuring out ¾ teaspoon, then you can do this: obtain a measuring cup (Pyrex measuring cup, for example) and put 3 tsps. of Lexapro liquid into 1 cup of water (or orange juice). Then give your elderly patient ¼ cup of that water to drink. That ¼ cup will not be too much for her to drink (hopefully) and it will contain 3¾ mg of medicine. (3 tsp = 15mg; 15 mg/cup is a concentration of 3¾ mg per ¼ cup).

- Refrigerate the measuring cup and use it up over the next three days.

- Each bottle contains 240 mL of Lexapro

- HMO insurance often will not cover the cost of liquid medicine (unless the patient is perhaps in a nursing home), so this can be a financial strain on the family. However, remember that your patient will only consume ¾ tsp per day. At that rate, one prescription bottle of Lexapro liquid will last for 64 days (slightly more than two months).

This system can permit fine-tuned dosing and may result in a "positive pharmaco-economic effects" (money saved). The pharmacist can help you with these kinds of calculations.

Chapter V-3

"Indications" for Psychiatric Medications

THIS IS VERY IMPORTANT INFORMATION!!
Skip the drug information if you like, but be sure
to read this chapter!!

At the end of this chapter are useful tables. Table V-3-c lists some common off-label uses of some common psychiatric medications. Table V-3-d presents branded names of drugs alphabetically corresponding to their generic names. Table V-3-e presents a list of drugs arranged alphabetically by their generic names corresponding to their branded names.

This chapter covers the very important topic of how a drug becomes available for use in our country. Most people complain about the price of medications in this country—as well they should. We are an extremely profitable market. We pay a lot and thus are entitled to expect a lot. The cost of bringing a new drug to market in the USA is astronomically high, both for Americans and for drug companies doing business here. Sometimes, Americans end up subsidizing more than their share of these costs.

The drug company usually applies to the FDA to obtain the legal right to sell that drug here. The FDA regulates the sales of all drugs and medical products and devices. Once a drug company has received approval to sell its new drug here, the drug is legal—it has its foot in the door, so to speak. Doctors can choose to use that drug for any medical condition whether that use is FDA approved or not. Firstly, you can read the brief summary on FDA approval. If you want more information on this subject, then you can read about the detailed approval process. Otherwise, you can skip ahead to the list of Facts.

Summary on FDA Approval:

- If a drug company wants to sell a drug in the USA, then the company must obtain approval from the FDA.

- The FDA will require that the drug company submit extensive medical research to show that the drug is both safe* and effective.

- If the FDA likes the medical research, then the FDA will approve that drug for sale in the USA.

- Once the drug is legal in the USA, doctors can prescribe it for any purpose.

Detailed Story on FDA Approval (optional)

The FDA is the branch of the federal government that oversees the safety of drugs available in our country. If a drug company wants to sell a drug in the USA, then the drug company must go through a legal regulatory process to obtain permission from the FDA to do so. The drug company must state the purpose of the drug and give the FDA proof that the drug is safe and effective for a certain diagnosis. The purpose for prescribing the drug is called its "indication". Practically speaking, "indication" is diagnosis is purpose. Prozac is indicated for treatment of a diagnosis of depression. Prozac's purpose is for treating depression. So, the purpose, indication, and diagnosis for prescribing the drug are all the same basically. After a drug company submits reams of information and research on its new drug, the FDA will review all these data. If the FDA finds the proof and evidence credible, then the FDA will approve that drug for treating that diagnosis in the United States. Then the FDA will list the indication for Prozac. That is its labeled indication and defines its therapeutic purpose. In other words, Prozac was approved for the purpose of treating the diagnosis of depression in the USA. That indication is "on its label". Any doctor who decides to prescribe it for a purpose that is not indicated (not FDA-approved), is prescribing the drug "off-label". Indications for drugs are obviously very important because they specify the diagnosis needing treatment, and carry a certain amount of *gravitas* in a court of law.

There is more to this story, however. Some drugs might have a different indication in Europe from their American (FDA-improved) indication. Sometimes all prescribing doctors—including the FDA—know from word-of-mouth and years of medical experience (in the USA or worldwide) that the drug is very helpful for more than one indication, but the drug company usually brings the drug to market in the USA for just one indication. The reason for this strategy is cost. Each indication can cost up to a billion dollars for each separate round of the FDA-approval process. Law states that the FDA can grant an indication if and only if the drug company presents hard evidence that the drug is effective (and safe*).

Thus, an indication names the diagnosis that a drug is intended to treat. If a doctor decides to prescribe a drug for some other diagnosis (as used in Europe), then he should have a good reason. Prudent doctors document this situation in writing in the patient's medical record. On the other hand, if a "respected minority" of doctors use this drug off-label, then precise documentation might not be as important. Sometimes, American doctors may end up prescribing the drug preferentially for its European indication rather than its American one.

Some drugs might have more than one indication. Here is an example for Paxil. Paxil is an antidepressant in Europe. When it came to this country, its stated purpose was to treat major depression. The diagnosis under consideration was major depression. The FDA approved it for the indication of treating major depression. It was sold here and did well as a treatment for major depression. Psychiatrists started to use it for other kinds of depression, such as minor depression. Psychiatrists began to notice that it seemed to help anxiety occurring in some cases of "anxious depression". Researchers had also reached a similar impression from studying Paxil chemically. Its sponsoring drug company learned that it was helpful in a number of anxiety disorders. Then the drug company applied for approval to use Paxil for the indication of specific anxiety disorders. Eventually, Paxil earned FDA approval for treatment of five anxiety disorders. Including the original indication for major depression, Paxil now has six indications! That is a large number! But wait—we began to hear from some men that Paxil caused delayed ejaculation, which they perceived as a big problem and annoying side effect. Doctors started to use it as treatment for premature ejaculation. It worked well and it still works well. It has no indication for premature ejaculation, but doctors know of this side effect, which can be turned into a beneficial side effect for some patients. Internists, psychiatrists, and other specialists prescribe Paxil for premature ejaculation—Paxil is probably the most commonly prescribed drug for this treatment.

There is no drug currently FDA-approved for this kind of sexual dysfunction. So, in this situation, Paxil is being prescribed "off-label". "Off-label" means the drug is not being prescribed for its FDA-approved purpose. Prescriptions for some drugs are mainly off-label!

Apart from safety* and effectiveness when used in a certain diagnosis, cost is another issue when trying to obtain FDA-approval. The drug company adopts a strategy in regards to pricing. Usually, the drug company applies for a standard indication. For example, if a drug is used as an antidepressant in Europe, then the drug company will usually apply for FDA approval to sell the drug as an antidepressant in our country also. However, an alternate strategy is to market the drug for a secondary use or in a niche market. Luvox is an antidepressant in Europe. It works the same—as an antidepressant—in America, also. However, it also has powerful anti-obsessive properties. There are many similar antidepressants on the market in the USA (too much competition) but only one other drug indicated for obsessions (Anafranil). And Anafranil is very different chemically from Luvox. So Luvox entered a niche market where there was really very little competition. This strategy allowed for the sale of Luvox for OCD (Obsessive-Compulsive Disorder) as well as allowing psychiatrists to prescribe it "off-label" as an antidepressant, its original purpose in Europe.

Facts

FACT ONE: an ***Indication*** is the FDA-*approved use* of a prescription medication. This indication appears "on the label" of the new drug. This means that the FDA has approved the drug for this specific (labeled) use and *in this specific diagnosis*. This does not mean that the drug is not useful for other purposes—this means that the drug company has already spent one billion dollars to get the drug "indicated" for one medical use in one diagnosis. The drug company may later decide to spend another fortune to do a second set of clinical trials to get the drug officially approved for a second medical use (a second indication). And quite frankly, the drug will have the same biochemical effect on patients, regardless of what does or does not appear in print. Psychiatrists—and any doctors—may choose to use a drug for a second diagnosis based on anecdotal reports that we read in psychiatry journals, learn at medical conferences, and hear from colleagues. Prescribing a drug for this second diagnosis is called "**off-label prescribing**" and is not illegal. Many doctors prescribe many drugs for secondary uses, or uses that patients might not find listed in the PDR (Physicians' Desk Reference). A surprising number of drugs are used "off-label". In the case of some drugs (Neurontin, for example), the off-label uses account for much of the drug sales. *See figure V-3-a and Table V-3-b.*

Diagram V-3-a: How FDA-approved Drugs acquire Off-Label Uses

(1)–Neurontin is originally approved for certain types of epilepsy—this is the original FDA-approved neurology-indication

(2)–Then neurologists expand its use to other kinds of neurological conditions (diabetic nerve pain).

(3)–Then psychiatrists learn to use it for anxiety

(4)–Then psychiatrists expand its use further outside of this scope for all sorts of chronic pain disorders (with secondary psychiatric symptoms).

Diagram V-3-a: (1) FDA indication for Neurontin is only for Epilepsy (central gray area) (2)Expanded neurology use in regular font;
(3) and (4) *off-label Psychiatry uses in talics*

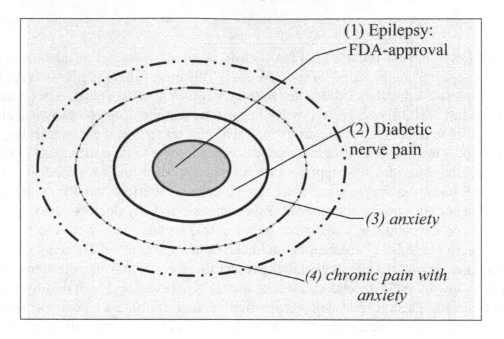

(1) Epilepsy: FDA-approval

(2) Diabetic nerve pain

(3) anxiety

(4) chronic pain with anxiety

I am spending a lot of time on FACT ONE because it is one of the biggest sources of patient confusion about psychiatrists' prescribing patterns and practices. Patients will check the PDR or other source and discover that a psychiatrist prescribed an epilepsy drug when the patient knows in fact that he has pain not epilepsy. This awareness is followed by a frantic phone call to the psychiatrist. However, modern patients often check the Internet where all sorts of off-label uses abound. Next, please note this tabulation V-3-b that refers to the flow chart and target diagram V-3-a:

V-3-b (table) FDA-indications and off-label use   How Neurontin came to be more popular for off-label uses than for certain types of epilepsy

Drug Neurontin	**FDA-indicated for neurology use in certain epilepsies**	new neurology use for diabetic nerve pain	Psychiatrists use it for Anxiety	Psychiatrists use it for Chronic Pain Disorders with psychiatric symptoms
Use	epilepsy	nerve pain	anxiety	chronic pain-anxiety
FDA Approval	original first approval **YES**	No, but neurologists use it anyway	No	no
Comment	ends up **not** being a major epilepsy treatment	however, it helps other neurology conditions	of little use in Bipolar	Other specialists start to use It for chronic pains (without psychiatric symptoms)

EXAMPLE OF THE RATIONALE (How doctors find new uses for old drugs):

Usually, when a new drug like Neurontin appears, only neurologists will use it and only for its special epilepsy condition. As time goes on, neurologists may learn to use it for other kinds of epilepsy. Then neurologists may begin to use it for diabetic nerve pain. Then a few prominent psychiatrists may try it for stabilizing nerve membranes in psychiatric condition. The prime goal was to try it for bipolar disorder, but it did not work. A few prominent psychiatrists might have noted its calming effects and later prescribed it for anxiety. After its good effects on diabetic nerve pain, then Neurontin was tried on other types of chronic pains. This is Neurontin's story:

- Neurontin is discovered to stabilize nerve membranes in lab rats.
- Drugs that stabilize nerve membranes can help epilepsy.
- Drug company tests it in rats with epilepsy.
- Drug company tests Neurontin in humans with epilepsy. Positive results.
- Drug company applies for and receives FDA approval to use Neurontin in certain kinds of (human) epilepsy. Neurontin is now an approved epilepsy drug.
- Psychiatric conditions sometimes benefit from any drugs that might stabilize nerve membranes.
- Psychiatrists try Neurontin "off-label" for Bipolar, but results are very disappointing: it does not seem to stabilize "mood swings". However, it is tranquilizing.
- Psychiatrists start to use it off-label as a tranquilizer in special conditions (liver failure, and so on).
- Neurologists start to use it off-label for diabetic nerve pain.
- Psychiatrists start to use it off-label for all chronic pains with anxiety components.
- Neurontin used off-label helps relieve suffering in millions of Americans
- FDA [unfairly] punishes Pfizer Pharmaceuticals with enormous fines (because of… off-label uses)—this is a long story.

The Neurontin itself is just a chemical. Like all chemicals, it has hundreds or thousands of effects on the human body. Neurontin just happens to stabilize the nerve membrane. Neurontin does not know anything about the FDA or FDA-approval, and probably would not care anyway what the FDA said about it. It still works chemically just the same. Maybe you were hired into your job because of one certain skill that you possess. After working there for a while, your supervisors see that you are even more skilled at other tasks. Should this mean that you are not to be approved to perform other tasks at which you excel?

In summary, psychiatrists are now using Neurontin "off-label" for two separate diagnoses.

FACT TWO: Nowadays the drug companies spend upwards to a ***billion dollars*** in order to bring a drug to market for just one indication. In many cases, a drug has more than one therapeutic effect, but the drug company picks the one disease that will be helped the most. They choose the indication most likely approvable. They also pick the indications and diagnoses likeliest to generate as much profit as possible.

So at this point, the readers exclaim: "So what?!—the drug companies have too much money already!" Well, I have no specific response to that but will remind you of the following. Between the constant barrage of frivolous lawsuits, outlandish jury verdicts, and lack of revenues, it is sometimes a wonder that any drug can be brought to market in the USA. If the costs of doing business here continue to go up, the drug companies might be obligated to retreat from the American market. So then how would you get the latest diabetes drug on sale in Europe but not FDA-approved here? I suppose you might say that you will just order it from Europe…I have no response to that, either.

As a counterpoint, I will also point out that these same drugs are a lot cheaper when sold in other countries. Many of them are also available without prescription in some countries.

FACT THREE: Once the drug has been FDA-approved for one indication, then the drug can be sold legally in the USA—under any condition, as long as is prescribed by a licensed physician.

FACT FOUR: All drugs are just synthetic chemicals. All synthetic chemicals are poisonous. .

"Synthetic" here means "not occurring naturally" or "found in nature but in only tiny trace amounts" which necessitates synthetic production of the drug (Galantamine for example). What is the difference between Neurontin for anxiety and Neurontin for epilepsy? As far as I can see, there is no difference. We all know that drugs have many side effects. That is because poisons have many side effects. Truly, there is no difference between therapeutic effects and side effects, except as our senses and bodies make it so.

FACT FIVE: Synthetic chemicals have many effects on the body, which humans have divided into "good" effects and "bad" effects (therapeutic effects vs. side effects). When some of the effects make us feel better then these are called the good effects; and, when some of the effects make us feel bad then we call them side effects. The drug is just a chemical made in a chemical factory—there is nothing "good" or "bad" about it, but that labeling it so, makes it so.

How can that possibly be? Patients have many bodily experiences from prescription drugs:

    1—in many cases there is improvement in the disease and the patient feels good;

    2—in some cases the disease improves but the patient has minor side effects;

    3—in a few cases the disease improves, but the patient has unbearable side effects;

    4—in a few cases the drug does nothing at all;

5—in rare cases the only action of the drug is to produce a lot of side effects, and,

6—in rare cases, the drug makes the disease itself worse.

7—worst-case scenario is that of a lethal outcome: hopefully never.

This goes to show that the drug has many activities in many circumstances in different people. An otherwise innocuous drug can be felt as toxic in people who might be taking many other drugs already. Also, see how our genetics affects our ability to process drugs (Chapter II-4).

FACT SIX: When the drug is inside our bodies and working well, it can be causing dozens or hundreds of effects which most of us do not even feel. Ideally, we should feel only the intended good effects. People who are more sensitive will become aware of these dozens or hundreds of effects inside their bodies. Most people experience mainly the intended side effects. (see Chapter V-19).

COROLLARY TO FACTS ABOVE: Some drugs under certain circumstances can also be beneficial for certain conditions for which they are not indicated. This discovery usually occurs after the drug has been on the market for a while. An example is Effexor which came to market for the indication of depression (to treat patients with a diagnosis of depression). After some time on the market patients reported that it helped anxieties too. Many antidepressants in very low doses have anti-anxiety properties, so this was not a shocking discovery. Then later doctors observed that it helps chronic pain. A few other antidepressants were already known to help chronic pain, also. So, Effexor was an antidepressant that also helped anxiety and chronic nerve pains, and doctors began to prescribe it for these conditions, also. In these cases, the patient can feel better despite the fact that the drug was prescribed for some disease other than the FDA-approved indication. Once again, this is called *off-label prescribing* and is done by doctors all the time. The good news is that patients get better and feel better but the bad news is that the drug is used "off-label". This is not illegal—as long as your doctor is prescribing it. It is not unethical either. Although it can be a complaint in a lawsuit, it is unlikely to hold up in court especially if all the other doctors are doing it too as "usual and customary" prescribing practice. Or if the "respected minority" of doctors are following this practice. Anybody who holds a medical license can—in theory and in practice—prescribe any FDA-approved drug for any reason, whether for its indicated diagnosis or for some other diagnosis. The main point is to make patients feel better. Doctors—and patients, especially!—would not be happy if everything had to be to the letter of the FDA regulations. The drug itself has not read the FDA approved indications, so it does not know that it can only help FDA-indicated diseases—it is perfectly willing to try to work well in all practical circumstances.

In some cases the drug may work so well for other indications that the drug company will actually pay another half billion dollars or so to do the clinical trials for a second indication—this is the case with antidepressants (finding uses in anxiety disorders) and with the SGA (second-generation anti-psychotics' finding uses in bipolar disorder).

I will sometimes hear that a patient refuses to take the prescribed medication because it has been prescribed off-label. I regularly discuss this with patients while writing out the prescription. This issue can be discussed depending on the circumstances: does a patient demand a cheap generic drug? Is this the best drug for this condition? Are there alternative treatments? Sometimes the pharmacy will panic the patient. Some patients will call from home complaining that the pharmacy references Depakote as epilepsy treatment, and the patient does not have epilepsy. Depakote has carried an FDA indication for Bipolar (and migraine) treatment for a long time. This is what happens at the pharmacy without my knowing it. Some patients call me in a somewhat accusatory manner. On this basis, some patients even refuse to fill the prescription.

Some patients read all the possible side effects and refuse to take the medication—see Chapter V-19.

In my experience, *the main cause for the development of most side effects occurs very shortly after patients read the hundreds of possible side effects that might occur.*

SECOND COROLLARY—In some cases, where the patients feel better while taking a drug "off-label" they begin to believe that the original indication for the drug is now their true diagnosis. Example: Lithium helps cluster headaches but is not FDA-approved for cluster headaches; if headache patients improve on Lithium, then some of them will come to believe that they are manic-depressive (the FDA-approved indication for lithium). Yet they are not manic-depressive! The beneficial results of off-label use of a drug for a non-FDA indicated diagnosis, does not drive the diagnosis.

▶ Chapter Summary and take-home points:
- Drug companies usually choose the best indication that was the primary focus of research on that drug, but sometimes may be forced to bring the drug to market for a secondary indication that had not been the focus of research. Reglan is a failed antipsychotic brought to market as a digestive drug. Buspar is a failed antidepressant brought to market as an anti-anxiety drug. They both work fairly well for their new second-choice indications; however, their side effects are referable to their now-scrubbed first-choice indications (Reglan like other anti-psychotics can cause Parkinsonism; Buspar like other antidepressants can cause "buzziness" in high doses).
- Sometimes, the number of prescriptions for off-label use far exceeds the originally indicated uses (psychiatrists constantly use the antidepressant trazodone primarily as a sleeping pill nowadays. We use Neurontin as treatment for chronic pain and anxiety-tension states).
- All prescription drugs are chemicals.

- All chemicals are poisons.
- All drugs, therefore, are poison taken in small amounts.
- All chemicals cause many biochemical changes inside our bodies.

---

* some drugs are not "safe" but necessary as a last-resort treatment: Clozaril for schizophrenia, for example. Try to think of Clozaril as "chemotherapy" and the picture comes into focus.

There are now three tables following to end out this chapter. The first table shows off-label uses in the USA. However, this is arbitrary: Luvox, for example, is an antidepressant in Europe. There was more advantage to bringing Luvox to market in the USA as a treatment for obsessive-compulsive disorder.

Table V-3-c **Examples of common off-label uses:**

DRUG NAME	INDICATION	OFF-LABEL USES (USA)
Lithium	Mania	Cluster headaches
Elavil	Depression	Chronic pain, sleeping pill
Cogentin	Parkinson's disease	Antipsychotic "antidote"
Luvox	Obsessive-Compulsive	Depression
Seroquel	Schizophrenia & Bipolar	Sleeping pill in agitated disorders and restless legs
Urecholine	Urination problems	Antidepressant "antidote"
Periactin	Antihistamine	Weight gain
Zyprexa	Schizophrenia, Bipolar	Dementia and agitated depressions
Paxil	Depression, anxiety, Panic	Premature ejaculation
Melatonin	Jet lag	Sleeping pill
Trazodone	Depression	Insomnia
Clonidine	Blood pressure	Opium withdrawal
Inderal, Atenolol	Blood pressure	Performance anxiety
Zantac	Ulcer symptoms	Antidepressant-related stomach aches
Doxepin	Depression	insomnia
Droperidol	Anesthesia	High blood pressure psychosis due to PCP
Strattera	ADHD, ADD	Depression
Provigil	Narcolepsy, excessive daytime sleepiness	depression
Neurontin(gabapentin)	Epilepsy Nerve pain	Chronic anxiety, insomnia, chronic pain, Migraines
Triavil	[psychotic] depression	Chronic pain

Tables V-3-d and V-3-e

The following is a chart of the branded names of the drugs cross-referenced to their generic names. Its companion chart is presented afterwards. These lists of charted drug names provide an easy way to find the generic name of a branded drug or the branded name of a generic drug. This is the only purpose of these tables.

Table V-3-d: Alphabetical listing by branded name (these same drugs appear alphabetized by generic names in the next Table V-2-e)

1	Abilify	Aripiprazole
2	Ambien	Zolpidem
3	Anafranil	Clomipramine
4	Antabuse	Disulfiram
5	Asendin	Amoxapine
6	Ativan	LORAZEPAM
7	Buspar	Buspirone
8	Campral	Acamprosate
9	Celexa	Citalopram
10	Chantix	varenicline
11	Clozaril	clozapine
12	Compazine	prochlorperazine
13	Depakene	valproic acid
14	Depakote	valproate
15	Desyrel	TRAZODONE
16	Dexamyl	dexedrine
17	Elavil	AMITRIPTYLINE
16	Equanil	meprobamate
19	Eskalith	Lithium
20	Geodon	ziprasodone
21	Halcion	triazolam
22	Haldol	haloperidol
23	Inapsine	Droperidol
24	Invega	paliperidone

25	Klonopin	clonazepam
26	Lamictal	lamotrigine
27	Lexapro	escitalopram
28	Lithium	Lithium, Li_2CO_3 / citrate
29	Lithobid	Lithium carbonate/citrate
30	Loxitane	Loxapine
31	Ludiomil	Maprotiline
32	Luvox	Fluvoxamine
33	Lyrica	Pregabalin
34	Mellaril	Thioridazine
35	Miltown	Meprobamate
36	Navane	Thiothixene
37	Norpramine	DESIPRAMINE
38	Pamelor	Nortriptyline
39	Paxil	Paroxetine
40	Pexeva	Paroxetine
41	Placidyl	Ethcholorvynol
42	Prolixin	Fluphenazine
43	Provigil	Modafanil
44	Prozac	Fluoxetine
45	Restoril	Temazepam
46	Revia	Naltrexone
47	Ritalin	Methylphenidate
48	Seconal	Secobarbital
49	Serax	Oxazepam
50	Serentil	Mesoridazine
51	Seroquel	Quetiapine
52	Serzone	Nefazodone
53	Sinequan	DOXEPIN
54	Stelazine	Trifluoperazine
55	Surmontil	Trimipramine

56	Symbyax	Zyprexa plus Prozac
57	Tegretol	Carbamazepine
58	Thorazine	Chlorpromazine
59	Tofranil	Imipramine
60	Tranxene	Clorazepate
61	Triavil, Etrafon	Elavil plus Trilafon
62	Trilafon	Perphenazine
63	Trileptal	Oxacarbazepine
64	Valium	DIAZEPAM
65	Vivactil	Protriptyline
66	Wellbutrin	Bupropion
67	Xanax	Alprazolam
68	Zyprexa	Olanzapine

Generic names which have come into very common use are CAPITALIZED.

Table V-3-e   Alphabetical listing by generic name (these drugs are also alphabetized by their branded names in the preceding Table V-3-d)

1	Abilify	aripiprazole
8	Campral	acamprosate
67	Xanax	alprazolam
17	Elavil	AMITRIPTYLINE
5	Asendin	Amoxepine
66	Wellbutrin	bupropion
7	Buspar	buspirone
57	Tegretol	carbamazepine
58	Thorazine	chlorpromazine
9	Celexa	citalopram
3	Anafranil	clomipramine
25	Klonopin	clonazepam
60	Tranxene	clorazepate

11	Clozaril	clozapine
37	Norpramine	DESIPRAMINE
69	Pristiq	desvenlafaxine
16	Dexamyl	dexedrine
64	Valium	DIAZEPAM
4	Antabuse	disulfiram
53	Sinequan	DOXEPIN
23	Inapsine	droperidol
61	Triavil, Etrafon	Elavil plus Trilafon
27	Lexapro	escitalopram
41	Placidyl	ethcholorvynol
44	Prozac	fluoxetine
42	Prolixin	fluphenazine
32	Luvox	fluvoxamine
22	Haldol	haloperidol
59	Tofranil	imipramine
26	Lamictal	lamotrigine
19	Eskalith	Lithium
28	Lithium	lithium,Li2CO3,Li-citrate
29	Lithobid	lithium,Li2CO3,Li-citrate
6	Ativan	LORAZEPAM
30	Loxitane	Loxapine
31	Ludiomil	maprotiline
16	Equanil	meprobamate
35	Miltown	meprobamate
50	Serentil	mesoridazine
47	Ritalin	methylphenidate
43	Provigil	modafanil
46	Revia	naltrexone
52	Serzone	nefazodone
38	Pamelor	nortriptyline

68	Zyprexa	olanzapine
63	Trileptal	oxacarbazepine
49	Serax	oxazepam
24	Invega	paliperidone
39	Paxil	paroxetine
40	Pexeva	paroxetine
62	Trilafon	perphenazine
33	Lyrica	pregabalin
12	Compazine	prochlorperazine
65	Vivactil	Protriptyline
51	Seroquel	quetiapine
48	Seconal	secobarbital
45	Restoril	temazepam
34	Mellaril	thioridazine
36	Navane	thiothixene
15	Desyrel	TRAZODONE
21	Halcion	Triazolam
54	Stelazine	trifluoperazine
55	Surmontil	trimipramine
14	Depakote	valproate
13	Depakene	Valproic acid
20	Geodon	ziprasodone
2	Ambien	Zolpidem
56	Symbyax	Zyprexa plus Prozac
10	Chantix	Varenicline

Anti-Psychotic Medicines
(Technical information on the drugs is in this chapter)
(practical anecdotal information is listed in Chapter V-9)

Antipsychotic medicines are also referred to as Major Tranquilizers. These drugs have major effects on major psychiatric disorders and have major side effects, too. They are truly major in every sense of the word. We use them to control the most severe of psychiatric illnesses (psychosis). In large doses, they can control many types of psychotic symptoms such as mania, hallucinations, delusions, illusions, and other psychotic manifestations (see chapter IV-1 on Thought Disorders). Some patients need very high doses of anti-psychotics in order to control psychotic symptoms. In very small doses, they may be useful as "helper-drugs" to control high anxiety, delirium, agitated dementia, chronic pain, agitated depression, Tourette's Syndrome, drug withdrawal, and other agitated states. In low doses, they mainly help to control excitability and have minimal anti-psychotic effect. None of these drugs are addicting, and they are not controlled substances. The anti-psychotics have had two waves of evolution, the so-called "first generation anti-psychotics" (FGA) and the "second generation" anti-psychotics (SGA).

First Generation Anti-psychotics with psychiatric use (FGA'S)

Some of the First Generation Anti-psychotics have been around for half a century, and their names are fairly well known: Thorazine and Haldol are both well known. There are other drugs in this class which are still on the market and some which are no longer on the market. Some of the other first-generation anti-psychotics were less popular, or had less advertising budget, or other issues (side-effects, tolerability, availability, effectiveness, safety issues) and are no longer on the market (in the U.S.), having gone the way of Hudson, Packard and Studebaker. There are other very good FGA's (butyrophenones and Sulpiride), which were never marketed here, having come to the party too late, so to speak, but have always been available overseas. Some of these drugs were not marketed here due to the high costs of getting FDA approval. Nowadays, if one truly needs any of these medicines, they could be ordered from Canada or Europe via Internet.

The major side effect of these drugs is the possibility that long-term use can cause movement disorder (known as secondary Parkinsonism which has the special name of

Tardive Dyskinesia). This is a most unpleasant and sometimes permanent side effect. Patients with movement disorder certainly look uncomfortable; however, most patients do not report feeling uncomfortable. There are also other possible side effects which are numerous but not as much of a deal-killer as is the Parkinsonism.

Those FGA's which have survived and are still on the market are the following: Stelazine, Trilafon, Haldol, Prolixin, Thorazine, Navane, Loxitane, and Mellaril. Stelazine is the least sedating and Thorazine, the most sedating. Navane and Mellaril are calmative. Haldol and Prolixin are available as long-lasting injections. Trilafon is well rounded as far as effects and side effects.

Mellaril has recently received negative publicity about cardiac side effects; however, it has always had cardiac effects. I have always monitored the cardiovascular status of my Mellaril patients and have not had any problems. Mellaril is likeliest to lower blood pressure. Most men refuse to take Mellaril since it usually causes impotence. It is quite sedating and less likely to cause Parkinsonsim. It can also very rarely cause visual changes that need to be seen by an eye doctor (ophthalmologist). Mellaril may also have rare side effects that I have never seen (rash or bone marrow suppression). Mellaril has helped millions of patients over the last four decades, and can be reasonably safe when used and monitored correctly. It is available in its "purified form" called *Serentil*, which gradually lost its market share, so it is not locally available.

Serentil is FDA-approved and can be ordered from Canada. It is less sedating and, in general, has fewer side effects. Correctly speaking, it is really the active form of Mellaril.

Thorazine is notorious and rightfully so. It is extremely sedating and very powerful. It can be used in very high doses at which time all the possible unpleasant side effects may appear: mental dulling, constipation, urine retention, blurred vision, dry mouth, and dizziness or light-headedness. Do not give by injection. Thorazine Spansules® once daily in the evening were helpful for some people (to decrease the side effects).

Stelazine is the opposite of Thorazine: not sedating, fewer side effects, but likely to cause twitchiness.

Trilafon is a good all-around drug with moderate effects and side effects. Available injectible.

Navane is sedating but not overly so.

Prolixin is sedating but not overly so.

Loxitane is mildly to moderately sedating and theoretically has mild antidepressant effects. It is very closely related chemically to the antidepressant Asendin.

Taractan is in the same subfamily as Navane and just as effective, but somewhat less sedating with somewhat milder side effects. It is FDA approved and can be ordered from Canada.

Others –Tindal, and others are FDA approved but no longer sold here: order from Canada.

Haldol is another notorious FGA drug and is not chemically related to the others listed above. It is less sedating, can cause Parkinsonism, and is still popular. It is available in pills, liquids, and three kinds of injection.

Droperidol is in the same family as Haldol. I have used it in the ER for extreme agitation for which it produces a pleasant sense of sedation. It can lower blood pressure significantly, thus extremely agitated young men are the prime recipients. It is available here only as an injection and is used with anesthesia in the operating room. It is available as a pill in Europe. The other two members of the Haldol family (*Benperidol* and *Spiroperidol*) are also sold as pills in Europe.

These FGA's can typically cause varying degrees of mental dulling, constipation, urine retention, blurred vision, dry mouth, and dizziness or light-headedness. Rarer side effects are breast enlargement, and milk letdown (in women). They can cause tender nipples or even breast swelling in men.

The worst long-term side effect is Parkinsonism. This can happen to 10-20% of patients and may appear anytime during continuous treatment. This could appear within six months of starting the drug (extremely rare) or at anytime over the next fifty years of taking the medication. If the Parkinsonism starts up with one FGA drug, then it should probably be stopped and changed to another medication.

The most life-threatening effect is called NMS which is a medical emergency and requires hospital admission—often to the ICU (intensive care unit). The early symptoms are stiffness, fever, confusion, high blood pressure, high pulse rate, and rapid breathing. NMS is extraordinarily rare but sometimes fatal. The patient should be told never to take that drug again.

Most FGA's are available in liquid form. Some are available in a short-acting injection: Haldol, Prolixin, Trilafon. Haldol is available in a once-monthly injection and Prolixin is available in two forms: a weekly and a biweekly injection.

Some First Generation Anti-psychotics lack significant psychiatric use. This would include drugs used to control nausea (such as Compazine), to control allergic reactions (such as Phenergan) or to control trembling (Parsidol/Parsitan). Compazine has adequate anti-psychotic properties, but I have used it only once for this purpose. I do not know of any cases of Parkinsonism caused by Phenergan. Parsidol can be temporarily helpful for trembling (Prakinsonism). Several others in this category are available overseas. These drugs are usually used only on a short-term basis.

Second Generation Anti-psychotics (SGA's)

Clozaril

In an attempt to find safer antipsychotic drugs, these new waves of drugs were developed. The first was Clozaril which is still in use but is very toxic—and sometimes lethal (more often than one would like) – and only used as a drug of last resort for the most desperate cases, but in those cases it may provide tremendous relief from the misery of severe and persistent psychotic illness. Clozaril is called a "dirty" drug: this refers to the fact that even when it is providing excellent control over psychosis it still has a large number of unpleasant or "messy" side effects. The prescribing of Clozaril is such a time-consuming, medically intensive, and elaborate endeavor, that large institutions will try to set up a separate "Clozaril Clinic" usually requiring the dedicated services of one psychiatrist, one nurse, and one pharmacist who will all be working in tandem to monitor this drug. This drug has many interactions with other drugs and requires an intensive amount of monitoring.

Zyprexa

Starting with the Clozaril basic chemical structure, an attempt was launched to seek a newer but similar drug hopefully without so much toxicity. This was Zyprexa. Its basic molecular structure was inspired by Clozaril and by Valium. Zyprexa causes little movement disorder (unlike the FGA's). Zyprexa has received a lot of publicity in the media recently due to the fact that it seems to be associated with weight gain, high cholesterol, high blood pressure, and diabetes. This combination of medical problems is collectively referred to as "Metabolic Syndrome", and it is—in some ways—worse than movement disorder because these metabolic side-effects can occur within the first months or year(s) of treatment whereas the movement disorder(s) may not appear for years or decades—or never. So, in this case, the side effects of some of the second-generation drugs (SGA's) may be worse since they occur early in the treatment (usually when the patient is still young).

I have no vested interest in any of these drugs, but in defense of Zyprexa, I must add that my elderly patients usually do not experience diabetes or high cholesterol while taking Zyprexa (and I do not ordinarily prescribe Zyprexa to the elderly who already do have diabetes or high cholesterol). However, diabetes and elevated cholesterol are a regular feature in many of the younger patients. Younger patients are often taking relatively higher doses. It seems as if elderly people who have eaten healthy food for all of their lives and not been exposed to junk food and fast food in childhood, seem relatively spared from this effect. And Zyprexa is worthy of being defended because it has helped so many people with so many conditions ranging from high anxiety, mania, psychosis, and mild Valium withdrawal, to dementia. If I were stranded on a desert island practicing psychiatry and could bring only one drug, then Zyprexa would probably be my choice.

As far as the younger generation of junk food and fast food consumers are concerned, many of their peer group are overweight and in the process of developing high cholesterol and weight gain without ever being exposed to Zyprexa. On the other hand, a Zyprexa patient's triglyceride levels can rise as early as the first month of treatment, so Zyprexa certainly seems to have some possible involvement in Metabolic Syndrome. Curiously, many of my patients who are experiencing these side effects do opt to continue on Zyprexa anyway despite the given risks. They make this choice because they feel so much better emotionally and mentally. Other patients will routinely opt to switch to another SGA medication—or rarely, to one FGA. My (few) Zyprexa patients who exercise a lot and eat a Mediterranean-type diet do not gain weight—or not much weight. Still, one has to wonder about Zyprexa's overall complicity in this affair. Nonetheless, doctors do need to inform patients about the benefits and possible perils of Zyprexa and other SGA's.

Zyprexa has been noted to cause trembling and Parkinsonism, but this has been exceedingly rare in my experience.

Other drugs in this SGA class include Risperdal, Invega, Seroquel, Abilify, Iloperidone, and Geodon. Abilify and Geodon seems to have the fewest side effects but also may be less potent overall. Zyprexa and Seroquel seem to produce a pleasant state of relaxation. Some of these other SGA drugs may also be associated with some risk of developing metabolic syndrome (weight gain, blood pressure, diabetes, and elevated cholesterol and triglycerides), but it is often less of an issue than with Zyprexa. All of these second-generation anti-psychotics have their own advantages and disadvantages and must be prescribed by someone who is very familiar with them (psychiatrists).

Risperdal

Risperdal has been on the market so long that it has become available in generic form. It can cause Parkinsonism. It is a very effective antipsychotic. Most people can only tolerate a certain amount before they start to feel trembly. It is less likely to cause metabolic syndrome (diabetes). It is available in a long-lasting injection (2 weeks) and a dissolving tablet ("M-tab").

Seroquel

Seroquel is the most sedating of all the SGA's. This effect can be very pronounced within the first couple weeks or months of treatment. This sedation seems to be partly due to its potent antihistaminc effects to which patients gradually adjust and become less sedated with time. This antihistaminic effect also causes a ravenous appetite and carbohydrate craving, so patients are likely to gain weight. But there is often less time to eat since patients may spend much time sedated or asleep. Because of this sedation, many patients take a large dose in the evening or at bedtime. As a result of other effects, Seroquel can cause lowered blood pressure which might cause dizziness when standing up. Seroquel is second likeliest to cause metabolic syndrome (diabetes), but not nearly so much as Zyprexa. Sometimes Seroquel is used in tiny doses as an off-label sleeping pill. Seroquel requires a lot of monitoring and up-adjusting of its dosage.

Abilify

Abilify is a mild medicine with few side effects. It is fairly effective as an antipsychotic and can be a helpful accessory drug for serious mood disorders. It requires little monitoring. It is available in regular pills and dissolving pills.

Geodon

When Geodon first came on the market, there was much concern that it might cause abnormal rhythms of the heart, but this seems to be rare in clinical practice. Nevertheless, these patients should be followed closely for any possible cardiovascular problems. In very low doses, Geodon is stimulating (possibly because of serotonin-like effects), but this is not a problem at higher doses. It may be as—or more—useful in severe mood disorders than in psychoses. It is available as a short-acting injection which patients find very pleasant.

Invega

Invega is a "purified" form of Risperdal and seems to have slightly fewer side effects. It can produce effective antipsychotic activity and be tolerated at relatively higher doses than its parent compound, Risperdal. The pills cannot be split.

Special Preparations

Zyprexa and Geodon are available in short-acting injections. Risperdal is available in a 2 week long-acting injection. Dissolving tablets are available for Zyprexa-Zydis, Fazaclo (Clozaril) and Abilify Disc-Melt. Risperdal is available in a liquid form (any of the dissolving tablets could be dissolved in water and thereby become a liquid form also).

Apart from their primary purpose as antipsychotic drugs, SGA's can be used in low doses for high anxiety. Some have mild antidepressant properties in their own right, and some can boost antidepressant effects of the primary antidepressant.

Other similar drugs

- Moban (Molindone) is another of the old anti-psychotics, which is not related to any other prescription medication. It will cause **weight loss** in some people. It is believed to be reasonably safe without causing Parkinson's movement disorders or Metabolic Syndrome (diabetes).

- Orap (Pimozide) is another antipsychotic not related to the others. It can cause the heart to beat irregularly but has much less chance of causing other side effects. It is classified as an "orphan drug" in the USA and is used for Tourette's disorder (involuntary tics).

- Reglan(metoclopramide) was developed as an antipsychotic drug for the treatment of schizophrenia. But, in the high doses needed to control schizophrenia it caused too much parkinsonism. Since Reglan—like most anti-psychotics—had anti-nausea properties, the dose was lowered, and it was brought to market as an anti-nausea pill destined to be used in the severe cases of nausea or stomach dysfunction, such as diabetic stomach (gastroparesis) where it works quite adequately. However, true to its origins it can still cause parkinsonism and a "wooden" depression (patient looks stiff and zombie-like). "This drug is useful, but the patients need to be aware of these possible neuro-psychiatric side effects.

- Promethazine is an ingredient in cough medicines. It has apparently never been associated with long-term toxic side effects. It is usually taken in very small doses for short periods of time. Its chemical properties suggest that it will probably never cause Parkinson's movement disorders of diabetes.

▶Psychosis is a major disease that is treated with "major" tranquilizers which, can have "major" side effects that generally fall into two main possibilities: (1) Parkinson's movement disorder or (2) diabetes with high cholesterol.

Chapter V-5

Introduction to the Antidepressants

This chapter covers biochemical activity in relation to each family of antidepressants (chemical structure).

There are hundreds of antidepressants on the market here and abroad, and they are not always easy to classify because of overlaps and other reasons. The two common ways to classify them is either by their **chemical structure** or by their **biochemical activity**. One would think that similarity of chemical structure endows them with similar antidepressant properties, and in general it does. But they can also be classified by their biochemical activity in our body, in which case they may be from very different chemical families. Some readers might want to know about other similar drugs with similar chemical structure; this would be in case the reader were seeking out a new drug to try for himself, but a drug similar to one that he likes. Other readers might want to find a drug with a certain kind of biochemical activity. finally, some readers might want nothing more than to read one paragraph on a certain antidepressant of interest in order to learn a little about it. These three types of readers all have different purposes and needs.

"Quick Study"

▶For those who want to read only a short paragraph about the drug, go directly to Chapter
V-9, where you will find each drug presented individually accompanied by a short story about that particular drug along with some commentary based on experiences with real patients.

Biochemical Activity

▶ For those of you who want to know about the antidepressant drug's **biochemical activity**, you can read Chapters V-6, V-7, and V-8.

Chapter	Topic
V-6	Stimulating Antidepressants (Psychostimulants)
V-7	Older (Sedating) Antidepressants
V-8	Newer Antidepressants

Chapter V-6 discusses the Psychostimulants, which are the first real antidepressants. These are the amphetamines, Ritalin, and Cylert. Also included is Wellbutrin that is derived from an old diet pill and by rights should be stimulating, although patients may find it calmative after they have been taking it for a month. The MAOI Antidepressants are included in this chapter because they can be stimulating and result in loss of sleep.

Chapter V-7: I have labeled as "Older Sedating Antidepressants", which description some patients might find off-putting. Describing this group of older antidepressants with one word is not easy: they could also be called "classical" antidepressants. They can affect serotonin and norepinephrine but have not received this accolade—but the newer ones have. Older is not always a bad thing. These older drugs have been on the market a long time, and we think we know everything about them, including long-term side effects. The older sedating antidepressants embrace the Tricyclic family, Trazodone family, and Remeron (although Remeron is the "youngest" in this group).

Chapter V-8: The newer antidepressants start in *Chapter V-8* when Prozac appeared in the late 1980's. These newer drugs have prominent effects on serotonin, although the older tricyclics do, too. These new drugs have been touted for their norepinephrine effects, although the older tricyclics do, also. These newer drugs have usurped this distinction for acting on serotonin and norepinephrine and are referenced as serotonin and norepinephrine drugs—and that's just how it is.

The drugs will be presented with their mechanism of biochemical activity in their own specific chapters. The first group mentioned are stimulating anti-depressant drugs. These are covered specifically in their own Chapter V-6, Stimulating Antidepressants. The serotonin antidepressants are dealt with in Chapter V-8. Some of the newer (SGA) antipsychotics also affect dopamine, but this effect is not emphasized in this book. The older sedating antidepressants have a mixed set of actions: adrenaline-like, serotonin-like, and other effects too complicated to appear here. They appear in Chapter V-7. Chapter V-9 discusses each individual antidepressant in its own little "biographical vignette".

Chemical Structure

▶For those of you who want to know how the actions of the drugs are related structurally to each other, then this is your chapter. Their structural activity usually means that drugs with similar structures have similar beneficial effects, but with a slightly different suite of good effects and annoying side effects. Readers with this interest, for example, might already be taking one tricyclic to good effect, but are curious to know if switching drugs can give them a "fine-tuned" effect. This tactic, however, can be somewhat confounding. All the serotonin antidepressants are structurally very different from each other, but their effects are more or less similar—not exactly. Prozac is structurally modeled on norepinephrine, but has no significant norepinephrine activity—it has mainly serotonin activity! Parnate also is structurally modeled on adrenaline and does have some stimulation like adrenaline might, but Parnate belongs to the family of MAOI antidepressants.

The rest of this chapter covers biochemical activity in relation to each family of antidepressants based on their common chemical structure.

Here is another reminder about the terminology (for more details see Chapter V-1 footnotes)

Adrenaline = epinephrine: *I am using "__Adrenaline__" preferentially*	*Noradrenaline = Norepinephrine* *I am using "__Norepinephrine__"* *preferentially* abbreviation **(NE)**

▶**Phenyl-ethyl-amine** (Ph-Et-NH$_2$ *or* φ·Et·NH$_2$ *) is the correct name for the chemical family that includes adrenaline, norepinephrine, dopamine, amphetamines, Prozac, Parnate, ephedrine, "diet pills" et al.*

Here is a quick review of what all this might mean. In the 1950's, doctors and scientists began to understand that brain biochemicals can make us feel good when we have enough or more than enough of these chemicals. If we have too small an amount of the brain chemicals, then this might make us feel depressed. We already knew that drugs like Reserpine could deplete our brain biochemicals and make us feel depressed. Other drugs that seemed to increase the brain chemicals, made us feel happy. These chemicals under discussion were norepinephrine, dopamine, and serotonin. This came to be called the "Amine Hypothesis" of how antidepressant drugs make us feel better. Recently, we have come to understand that other biochemicals besides just amines can make us feel good. So, we include all of those non-Amine chemicals in the expanded theory and call it the "neurotransmitter theory" of antidepressant activity. The tables below show that a number of antidepressants are related structurally to norepinephrine. Most of these drugs were designed specifically by starting with norepinephrine and modifying it until that experimental chemical seemed to make rats "happy". (It's more complicated than that). However, a number of these drugs may also affect serotonin as well as norepinephrine.

The following table shows the effect of each biochemical on our brain.

	DOPAMINE (DA)	SEROTONIN (5-HT)	NOREPINEPHRINE (NE)
	Pleasure and reward Sense of well-being Euphoria Attention Anti-depressant	Concentration Focus Inspiration Anti-anxiety Attentiveness Anti-depressant	Activation Motivation Energy Anti-apathy Anti-depressant
Cocaine Amphetamine LSD	++++++ +++++	+ (+) +++++++	+ (+)

V-5-a (see V-1-a)   three important neurotransmitters (cocaine stimulates all three brain hormones, amphetamine stimulates dopamine, and LSD causes so much serotonin stimulation as to result in psychotic symptoms). The full name of serotonin is 5-hydroxy-tryptaminE (5-HT).

The next tables show the relationship—if any—between an antidepressant drug's family and its biochemical activity.

The amphetamines and some of the MAOI Antidepressants (to a certain extent) all belong to the same drug family (phenyl-ethyl-amine) as adrenaline and norepinephrine. The basic structure of the molecule is PHenyl-EThyl-Amine ("phetamine"); the specific name of amphetamine is α-*methyl*-β-*phenyl*-*ethyl*-*amine* = "Am-Ph-Et-Amine". (also known as β-*phenyl-iso-propyl-amine*). Amphetamines and MAOI's act on all three main systems of DA, NE, and 5-HT.

Remeron has many unique activities. Ludiomil is a potent but non-stimulating NE medication. Provigil has many effects, but we do not know how it causes these effects (this shows that there is something that we do not understand about the "neurotransmitter theory / amine hypothesis". There are scads of MAOI available outside the USA. Serzone is quite similar structurally to Trazodone, but Serzone can cause liver failure.

Table V-5-b	Structure may be based on NE or on some other chemical structure (** see below ***)	Biochemical Activity DA = raising Dopamine activity 5-HT = raising Serotonin activity NE = raising norepinephrine activity
PSYCHOSTIMULANTS		
Amphetamines	NE	DA, NE, 5-HT
Ritalin	(NE)**	like amphetamine

Cylert	Oxazolidine	Stimulant
Wellbutrin	NE*	DA, NE
Provigil, Nuvigil	diphenylmethyl thioketone·amide	unknown (stimulant)
Strattera	NE***	NE
Mazindol (diet pill)	Imidazo-isoindole	NE, DA
TRICYCLICS (Older Drugs)	3 rings	various effects
Elavil, Tofranil, Doxepin, Surmontil, Anafranil	"	5-HT, NE
Asendin	"	NE, DA
Vivactil, Desipramine, Pamelor, Ludiomil	"	NE
Remeron	4 ring-piperazine	NE, 5-HT, others
Trazodone	Triazolo·piperazine	5-HT
(Serzone)	Ditto	5-HT

MAOI Antidepressants		
Parnate	NE	NE, DA, 5-HT
Nardil	NE**	ditto
Selegiline-Emsam	NE**	DA, NE, 5-HT
Marplan	phenyl-hydrazine	ditto

NE = structurally resembling norepinephrine: DA has a similar structure to NE (as explained above: this would properly be "structurally related to Ph-Et-NH$_2$")

NE*= similar to NE but with some modifications

NE**=similar to NE but with a major modification

NE***=there is a NE foundation somewhere in the molecule

NEWER DRUGS		
Prozac	NE***(F$_3$-Ph)-Ph-Pr-NH$_2$	5-HT
Zoloft	Chlorophenyl·naphthalene	
Paxil	phenyl·piperidine	5-HT (NE)
Celexa-Lexapro	Bicyclic·phthalane	5-HT

Luvox	NE**(butyl)-Ph-Et-NH$_2$	5-HT
Effexor-Pristiq	NE** phenyl·ethyl·cyclohexane	5-HT, NE
Cymbalta	Naphthyloxy-propylamine	NE, 5-HT

What we see from these tables is how much we do not know. Remember that our understanding of these drugs is still a theory.

For more details on how these structural relations might relate to biochemical effects, see the respective chapters. Also see Chapter V-9.

Chapter V-6

Stimulating Antidepressants
Diet Pills (see Chapter V-18)
(Technical information on the drugs is in this chapter)
(Practical anecdotal information is in Chapter V-9)

The history of psychiatric antidepressant medications actually dates back to the years 1895-1901 when scientists made extracts of animal adrenal glands. Independent researchers at this time were able to identify adrenaline and then later to determine its chemical make-up. This new chemical isolate received its international name, adrenaline, because they found it in adrenal glands (but Americans also refer to adrenaline as epinephrine). Adrenaline had two interesting properties that were immediately obvious: it could be made in the adrenal glands but was discharged into the bloodstream that delivered it all over the body. The second interesting property was that it causes excitation and stimulation.

This first property of adrenaline was that it could be made in the adrenal gland but could be distributed quickly to the whole body via the bloodstream. Biochemicals with this ability are called "hormones". Here is my general definition for "hormone"

"Hormones" are biologically active chemicals that are produced in one part of the body and have off-site effects (effects nearby or at a remote part of the body). Hormones can travel in the bloodstream or remain by their site of production. (The definitions given in Harrison's and Dorland's are wordier.)

The second interesting property was that adrenaline causes excitation and stimulation. Adrenaline can surge through our bodies and result in the "fight or flight" reaction when we are suddenly excited or stimulated with intense emotions, The "fight or flight" reaction gives us instantaneous abilities to respond to emergencies. When we have this adrenaline surge, we prepare ourselves to react quickly to any life-threatening event. In a natural state, "fight" usually refers to addressing an enemy and "flight" may refer to escaping from a scary situation (disaster) or from a predatory animal (saber-tooth tigers, buffalo stampede). The system must work well enough, because we are still here.

Adrenaline has no specific antidepressant effects. However, adrenaline has a chemical sibling called norepinephrine abbreviated NE (see footnote Chapter V-1). Norepinephrine can be produced very easily from adrenaline. Norepinephrine is an important antidepressant biochemical in the brain. Psychiatrists think of norepinephrine as a neurotransmitter ("brain hormone" or "nerve hormone"). This means that norepinephrine can be released in one part of the brain and have effect in other parts of the brain. Sometimes it might travel over only a microscopically small distance, or maybe a few inches.

Amphetamine is also stimulating like adrenaline and norepinephrine and is very closely related to them chemically. Although amphetamine had been discovered in 1887, it went overlooked for a couple decades. Twenty-some years later, methamphetamine was made from amphetamine and was found to be activating and stimulating. Methamphetamine became very popular as an endurance drug and performance enhancer.

Also in the late 1800's, chemists (Nagai, et al.) had extracted ephedrine from a Chinese plant (the *Ma Huang* herb). They later determined that ephedrine, too, had similar effects upon the body as adrenaline and amphetamines because it too had an adrenaline-like structure and was also in that same exact family of chemical stimulants (properly called the phenyl-ethyl-amines). Ephedrine was modified slightly to produce pseudo-ephedrine. Both ephedrine and pseudo-ephedrine are useful for respiratory and sinus problems and are stimulating in higher doses. Pseudo-ephedrine is well known under the branded name of Sudafed.

All of these kindred drugs taken in excessive doses can raise blood pressure and turn stimulated activity into an unpleasant state of hyperactivity and agitation.

After all these discoveries, pharmaceutical scientists wanted to make an antidepressant or "pep pill" that would produce results like adrenaline and amphetamine but with milder side effects. Adrenaline and its sibling compound norepinephrine cannot be absorbed in the stomach when taken by mouth. Amphetamines cold induce a roller coaster of emotions. Ephedrine and pseudo-ephedrine were useful, also, but not so much in psychiatry. So, the search was on to find new drugs like adrenaline and norepinephrine that could be absorbed by mouth and could provide a pleasant sense of stimulation without other side effects such as "crashing" emotionally. The search fanned out and included new medications as well as new amphetamines and new adrenaline-like drugs, mostly used in cardiovascular and respiratory disorders, though.

Dopamine was incidentally discovered, and it also had cardiovascular and neuro-psychiatric effects. Dopamine is another natural "brain hormone" that is very important for making us feel good. Dopamine is also in the adrenaline-family (phenyl-ethyl-amines). Our brains and bodies make dopamine. It is also related to all these substances listed above and is a useful injection for heart diseases. (And no, its name does not come from the word "dope"—the real name is DOPAmine, DihydrOxy-Phenylethyl-Amine). Dopamine has also become important as a target for pharmaceutical research.

Soon thereafter, L-DOPA was also discovered. It is in the adrenaline-family and also occurs naturally in our brains. L-DOPA is useful for the neurological disorder of the brain called Parkinson's Disease. Psychiatrists are familiar with Parkinsonism because some anti-psychotics can cause this as a side effect.

This ongoing search resulted in the development of Parnate. Parnate is a major antidepressant that—like L-DOPA and dopamine—was fabricated around the middle of the twentieth century. Years later, Prozac was created. Parnate and Prozac are antidepressants with activating antidepressant properties. Parnate is in the adrenaline-family and very similar to adrenaline. Prozac is an antidepressant that is a kind of modified and "fluoridated" adrenaline. Neither one is addicting.

In summary, these are the important members of the adrenaline (phenyl-ethyl-amine) family:
The first three are found naturally in animals, and the fourth is from a plant:

1—adrenaline causes brief bursts of high energy and alertness; it is available medically as an injection

2—noradrenaline results in energy, tenacity, and motivation;

3—dopamine has a central role in [human] movement disorders and aids us in the ability to feel pleasure and alacrity; Dopamine and dobutamine (injections for the heart) (dopamine can be found in plants as well as animals: one plant source of dopamine is Chinese peapods.)

4—ephedrine (from a botanical source, the Chinese Ephedra plant, *Ma Huang*) is useful for asthma and stimulates the brain mildly; it can easily be turned into pseudo-ephedrine, which can then be turned into methamphetamine.

Dosages

Dosages for most of these drugs are standardized. Adults usually have a specified dosage range and children have a similar but smaller dosage range, adjusted for a child's age and weight.

Psychostimulants derived from Norepinephrine

All these drugs listed below are stimulant drugs derived from adrenaline, but with the advantage, that they can be taken by mouth and retain a goodly amount of pharmacologic effect. In many ways, these drugs are superior to adrenaline (which does not last very long and can not be taken as a pill).

These drugs, including amphetamines, all belong to the same drug family as adrenaline and norepinephrine, the so-called phenyl-ethyl-amine family. The basic structure of the molecule is PHenyl-EThyl-Amine ("phetamine"); the specific name of amphetamine is α-*methyl*-β-*phenyl*-*ethyl*-*amine* = "Am-Ph-Et-Amine". These drugs can act on some or all three main systems of anti-depressant brain biochemicals, which are DA, NE, and 5-HT.

Some patients who take these stimulant drugs actually report improved concentration, but these patients also have to deal with the usual side effects of these pills such as agitation, insomnia, emaciation, heart activation, and loss of appetite. It should be noted that loss of appetite results in less food intake hence less growth and fewer vitamins and trace minerals absorbed, too. Since some of these drugs are used for ADHD in children, weight and height effects on growing children should be monitored. Most of these drugs will increase the heart's activity rate and raise blood pressure, effects I find to be of concern.

Under normal circumstances and usual dosing, these stimulating drugs will increase norepinephrine and dopamine levels. Increased norepinephrine will result in increased diligence. Increased dopamine is often equated with a pleasurable sensation. However, if the drugs are given every day, some of these effects may be perverted into annoying side effects. This is likely in cases where the patient has the genetics for addiction. This could be possible in cases where the drugs have released all the brain's natural stores of dopamine and norepinephrine. If the patient is taking the drugs every twenty-four hours, but the brain needs thirty-six hours to replenish its supplies naturally, then there will be no brain biochemicals to release. In this case, the daily drug dose will have direct stimulation on the brain (causing agitation) instead of the indirect effect of releasing a bolus of pleasure "hormones". In the case of the addictive personality, the patient needs to be prescribed a non-addicting ADHD** medicine (Wellbutrin, Strattera, Effexor, Desipramine, possibly Pristiq). In the case of constant direct stimulation, the patient will need to develop a different dosage schedule or switch to the just-listed non-addicting drugs. Taking the addicting drugs on a regular basis is much more problematic than using the non-addicting ones.

In cases of excessive dosage, these psychostimulants can release not only norepinephrine and dopamine, but also serotonin and perhaps other "brain biochemicals". Under these circumstances norepinephrine causes great excitation, dopamine results in over-stimulation, and serotonin can provoke all sorts of hallucinations.

Therapeutic uses of Psychostimulants:

- they may improve concentration and attention (or worsen agitation and result in impulsivity or rash judgment)
- they have antidepressant properties (amphetamines are the first antidepressants)
- they can cause a temporary reduction in body weight (that is regained after quitting the drugs)
- they may open the airways to the lungs and help asthmatics (and the asthmatics may

develop constant anxiety, trembling, and insomnia, requiring psychiatry visits).

- they may be helpful in some neurological conditions such as narcolepsy, Parkinsonism, Excessive Daytime Sleepiness.
- cocaine applied to the skin is a local anesthetic.
- Dopamine (as does the similar drug dobutamine) helps a failing heart.
- Injectable Adrenaline (Epinephrine) is helpful for severe allergic reactions.

Therapeutic Classes of Psychostimulants

These drugs listed below all share a common adrenaline-norepinephrine structure and most of them have similar effects:

- amphetamines (a family of stimulants) including methamphetamine, Dexedrine, benzphetamine, hydroxy-amphetamine, and Ionamin
- MAOI Antidepressants, Parnate and Nardil
- Asthma and respiratory drugs: phenylephrine, ephedrine, albuterol, and pseudo-ephedrine (which can be sedating in low doses for some people, but in higher doses becomes stimulating)
- Various diet pills, including Pondimin, Ionamin, PPA (phenyl·propanol·amine)
- -L-DOPA for Parkinson's disease of the brain (also has an absorption problem in the stomach)
- Other antidepressants that contain a simple adrenaline structure that has been highly modified into a larger structure: Wellbutrin, Strattera, Luvox, Nardil, Selegiline-Emsam, Effexor, Pristiq, Prozac
- Various other "diet" pills (also called "anorexiants", meaning "drugs causing anorexia") that contain a simple adrenaline structure that has been highly modified into a larger structure: Tenuate
- Prozac antidepressant (a fluorinated and modified derivative of norepinephrine)
- Ritalin
- Cylert
- Provigil and Nuvigil
- Schedule I stimulant drugs

Amphetamines

The similarities among adrenaline, norepinephrine, ephedrine, and pseudo-ephedrine, eventually led scientists to fabricate amphetamines. These chemicals are so similar that any one of them could be used as the starting ingredient to make the others. Drug-dealers soon discovered this, too and they found a ready supply of Sudafed available in any pharmacy without a prescription. Sudafed is a basic ingredient for making a cheap source of street-grade amphetamine, called methamphetamine (crystal "meth"). "Cooking" Sudafed tablets (pseudo-ephedrine) results in "crystal meth" (methamphetamine), which is quite addicting. Eventually, a federal law was promulgated to limit the sale of Sudafed.

Amphetamines are addicting because they produce a state of pleasure upon initial usage. They improve concentration and motivation in the short-term. Repetitive tasks are not so intimidating or dreaded. As a matter of fact, one of their side effects is called stereotypy. This is Dorland's definition of stereotypy: *"persistent repetition of senseless acts or words. It may be a persistent maintaining of bodily attitude, of senseless movements, or constant repetition of words...".* People who have dull repetitive jobs might find the jobs more bearable with amphetamines. One would think that stereotypies are an annoying side effect. In the long-term, these drugs can also alter judgment and cause impulsivity, which is a combination for disaster: irrational violence, for example. Amphetamines produce insomnia and disrupt sleep cycles with the result that people become irritable and irrational, resulting in further deterioration of judgment and unacceptable behaviors.

Usage of amphetamines has swung back and forth. Amphetamine was invented and then ignored for a couple decades until the methamphetamine derivative was produced. Methamphetamine proved to be very popular. It is still available in pill form (Desoxyn), but is rarely prescribed. Most amphetamine prescriptions nowadays are for dextro-amphetamine, and not for any of the other types of amphetamines. These drugs became very popular as **performance enhancers** in the early and middle parts of the twentieth century. Then they fell out of favor for a while, but had a resurgence in the drugged out era of the 1960's when amphetamines were popular as party drugs. The government tried to suppress their use, and was moderately successful, but only briefly, as they made a resurgence and assaulted society once again at the end of the twentieth century as a popular remedy for Attention Deficit. The recent prescribing trends of these dangerous drugs has gone from overly cautious to downright promiscuous.

This new use was found when we started to use them for the new diagnosis of "minimal brain dysfunction(MBD)", a diagnosis that was newly applied to overactive boys in the 1960's-1970's. This terminology was soon changed to the more politically correct Attention Deficit Disorder (ADD) and Attention Deficit Hyperactivity Ddisorder (ADHD). These boys were given stimulants, Ritalin or dextro-amphetamine. Cylert was another stimulant available. The non-addictive drug, Desipramine, was also helpful in some cases. The use of stimulants had a paradoxical effect of quieting hyperactive boys. Technically, **performance enhancement**, once again. But, drug effects on children's brains can sometimes appear "paradoxical". Once the boys reach puberty, however, a lot of them start to experience the usual and anticipated adult sensations of excitation and erratic judgment. Many boys nowadays receive the newly modified diagnosis, ADD Hyperactive-Impulsive Type. Not to be left out, girls eventually received their formalized entrée into the world of psychostimulants when they received the diagnosis of ADD Inattentive type. The percentage of children diagnosed as ADD seems to be increasing in direct proportion to the number of new and expensive ADD drugs entering the market place.

I am not a child psychiatrist, but I see adults regarding ADD/ADHD diagnosis under certain conditions. The first condition is when a child with severe ADD grows into an adult who still has severe ADD. The second condition occurs with previously normal adults without any compelling evidence of childhood psychiatric problems who come in claiming to have a first-time onset of ADD in adulthood (when this is really a childhood disorder that children grow out of). The third issue occurs when a young adult with resolving childhood ADD wants to continue taking amphetamine apparently for the rest of his adulthood.

Although I am not a child psychiatrist, I have witnessed this whole history unfold from the days of performance enhancement ,"Mother's Little Helper" of Rolling Stones fame, through the late 1960's party scene, up to the current era of arguably contrived "ADHD" diagnoses. My concern is the onslaught of adults now claiming to have "ADD". ADD was originally considered to abate by early adulthood. Diagnosis of ADD in adults was once so unusual a diagnosis, that it had no diagnosis. Research and clinical experience did reveal that a few cases persist into adulthood. At that time, there appeared a new diagnosis of "Adult residual ADD". These adults are quite rare, but I have had two men who truly fit this category: poor concentration, erratic, impulsive, prone to blurting out, restless, and occupationally-impaired. Eventually, thanks to research funded by the drug companies, we "discovered" that a sizable proportion of men now have ADD. Curiously, they are often diagnosed based on symptoms classically attributed to major depression. They do improve on stimulants. I maintain that this is because stimulants are antidepressants. If these men are depressed, then give them anti-depressants. Muddling through contrived diagnoses and manipulations by the drug companies should not be a way to make diagnoses.

As an example of the drug companies' insidious exploitation, look at these examples:

Here is an ad in *Psychiatric Annals* by Shire Pharmaceuticals: "*adults with ADHD were almost 2 times more likely to be divorced...Diagnose. Address. Assess.*". This is also true of adults with drug abuse. This one fact is hardly the basis for an ADDH (ADHD) diagnosis. (One of these ads features a brideless bridegroom, and the other a woman's driver's license.) Another ad sponsored by www.AdultADHDisReal.com trumpets the fact that "10,000,000 adults in the US have ADHD". Is that not about 5-6% of the entire adult population? The Vyvanse ad refers to problem areas such as memory, focus, organization, discipline, impatience, intrusiveness. These rather vague types of symptoms could apply equally well to major depression, anxiety, or agitated depression. What makes these symptoms so specific to ADHD, apart from wanting it so?

In the past, I have seen ads for adult ADD medications listing three classic symptoms of depression as the criteria. The ads have recently become more likely to list the symptoms of childhood ADHD and apply those to adults. ADD in adults may be far less frequent than ADD in children. The current trends in overdiagnosing it seem to be highly subjective. (The TOVA computerized test is an objective measure of ADHD.) Even the official handbook of the American Psychiatric Association, the DSM-IV-TR, indirectly acknowledges this fact:

> *"**Coding note:** For individuals (especially adolescents and adults) who currently have symptoms that no longer meet full criteria, [the diagnosis of] "in partial remission" should be specified."*

The DSM-IV-TR makes no comments on treatment or treatment-status. This above quote echoes the previous suggestions of the previous editions of this handbook in which the diagnosis of "adult-residual ADDH" symptoms are [statistically] more likely than a full suite of childhood symptoms persisting into adulthood (an unlikelihood). So how do we arrive at ten million adults with ADD in the USA?? The reader can form his own opinions.

We should be asking ourselves the following questions. What is the real cause of this sudden increase in ADD diagnoses in children? Why does the diagnosis increase when societal stress increases, when world pollution increases, when affluence increases, and when family size decreases? I have seen children dragged into my office by parents who want the children to study long and hard so that the children can attend Stanford or Harvard. Is this the dream of the child or of the parent? **Performance enhancement**.

I do not object to adults taking stimulants, except that the DEA (Drug Enforcement Administration) makes it so. The DEA monitors the quantities of amphetamine prescriptions for each doctor. I met a doctor once at a medical luncheon who himself acknowledged taking 2 ½ mg of Dexedrine (dextro-amphetamine) twice a day—he felt productive and happy (no surprise), but complained that the DEA was "harassing" him (no surprise). If people are afraid of losing their jobs, then let them come in and talk about it. If people are feeling depressed or anxious, then let's talk about that, too. If people want a performance-enhancing drug, there are various antidepressants that are better than amphetamines and Ritalin. We can talk about that, too. The one vexing situation is when successful and educated adults show up for a first-time psychiatry visit and claim that they have ADHD and demand branded amphetamines or Ritalin. They usually claim that they read it on-line, in a magazine, or a friend has suggested this diagnosis. Sometimes their therapist "diagnosed" them.

The real situation is that they are usually over-stressed or starting to become depressed—or both. They arrive to their first session with a fixed notion that they know more about this than the doctors and often demand controlled drugs, sometimes by brand name. If they are becoming stressed and depressed, and if they are offered an antidepressant prescription, they often are annoyed or offended. They do not want an antidepressant, they want amphetamines! They are ignorant of the fact that all antidepressants help ADD and that amphetamines are merely one of several antidepressants available for treatment. Amphetamines were the first antidepressants. Some of these new adult patients assume that ADD drugs are completely distinct from anti-depressants and have forgotten that all these drugs are just chemicals with a lot of good effects and bad side effects. Amphetamines have various uses, and amphetamines themselves do not care about which way they are used. (see Chapter V-3). Adult patients in LA see that a new drug is available for ADD and they want it. Most of these drugs are not really new: they are still either dextro-amphetamine or Ritalin. The only things new about them are the drug delivery systems. The first (expensive) advance was to provide a pill that was time-released. Now the newest advance is to provide the stimulant as a "pro-drug" which is then turned into dextro-amphetamine in the body and then time-released (Vyvanse). Technology aside, the child or adult is still awash all day long in amphetamine.

Another challenge to adult psychiatrists is seeing young adults who have been taking ADD drugs for ten or fifteen years since childhood. Most of them assume that they will continue these drugs indefinitely into and through adulthood. I have reasons for not continuing these drugs indefinitely into adulthood. Firstly, stimulant drugs have cardiovascular side effects apart from their potential to cause psychological agitation and irrationality, all of which makes the drugs of questionable benefit to adults. Secondly, teenagers are notorious for selling their amphetamines or giving them to classmates to cram for final exams. This provides opportunities for a lot of pharmacological misadventure. Thirdly, most teenagers go through aging processes, which change their reaction to the stimulants from one of calmness to one of overreaction. Fourthly, most of these young adult patients have few symptoms of ADD apart from some possible over-stimulation referable to the amphetamines and Ritalin. The astute reader may at this point exclaim, "Aha, the teen is stable on his stimulants, and that is why he is not symptomatic!" Nonetheless, I do not maintain adults on amphetamines. I explain to them the reasons why this is. Most of them can be engaged to participate in the change from addicting stimulants to non-addicting medications such as Wellbutrin, Effexor, Prozac, Vivactil, and so on. Once stabilized on these new medications, they report feeling much better than they had during their last year on amphetamines. Perhaps ADD is better visualized as some sort of agitated mood disorder of childhood (that responds to antidepressants).

This above commentary applies to the highly addicting amphetamines, which the DEA calls "schedule II drugs". Some amphetamines (MDMA ecstasy) are considered addicting and dangerous and are classified as "schedule I". These drugs are not available on prescription to anyone. (They are available only for research, provided that one has the proper authorization).

For the sake of completeness, here are other amphetamines: biphetamine, TMA (tri-methoxy-amphetamine), DMA, MDA (methylene-dioxy-amphetamine), STP, PMA (para-methoxy-amphetamine). These following drugs are related to amphetamines: Dinintel, Pondinil, Fenisec, and Captagon (caffeinated amphetamine). Access to all addicting stimulants is under the control of the DEA branch of the federal government (Drug Enforcement Administration).

MAOI Antidepressants Parnate and Nardil

Parnate is very similar to norepinephrine and is capable of stimulating the three major brain biochemicals, norepinephrine, dopamine, and serotonin. Nardil is also structurally similar. Parnate is the more stimulating of the two. Parnate can be a good antidepressant in select patients. Nardil has multiple uses in depression, anxiety disorders and phobias (social phobia, agoraphobia, and panic), and bulimia[3].

Other MAOI Antidepressants and MAOI-active medications

These include Marplan and Selegiline tablets, and Emsam. Other MAOI drugs are available in Europe.

The MAOI Antidepressants are rarely used nowadays because they could have dangerous side effects such as stroke. The risk of stroke is greatly heightened by eating aged cheeses—cheddar cheese especially. Thus, we call this the "cheese reaction". This reaction occurs in the stomach area. So, patients taking MAOI must restrict their diet and avoid consumption of aged, pickled, preserved, or moldy foods (e.g., Bleu cheese). Any food that is the product of bacterial, fungal, or yeast-like activity is probably not safe. (The complete list of MAOI dietary restrictions is somewhat lengthy). Three of the four original MAOI's are still available. Some of the newer MAOI drugs are safer because they have little or no risk of "cheese reaction"; however, they lack corporate sponsorship in this country (read: would not earn enough profit to warrant bringing them to market in the US, and do not qualify for "orphan drug" status). Selegiline is a "newer" MAOI available in the US. It is less likely to cause "cheese reaction" but only at low doses. If taken orally in high doses, it might cause this reaction, too. Fortunately, Selegiline is now available as a skin patch, further reducing the risks of a "cheese reaction" (by bypassing the stomach areas). This patch (Emsam should serve as an ideal depression treatment for select patients.

St. John's Wort has mild MAOI Antidepressant activity. Also, be aware of several non-psychiatric drugs having MAOI effects, which are Eutonyl for blood pressure, Isoniazid for TB, linezolid (Zyvox), and Matulane for cancer).

Respiratory medicines

Experimenting with the Chinese Ephedra plant was more productive, because chemists were able to isolate the active ingredient, ephedrine, which can be absorbed in pill form. Ephedrine was originally used for asthma treatment, but people began to realize that it had mild brain-stimulating properties. Chemists were able to manufacture Ephedrine in laboratories and factories and then later learned to refine Ephedrine thus creating Sudafed (pseudo-ephedrine), which is also helpful for mild respiratory problems (common "cold" and sinus problems). Sudafed is likewise mildly stimulating for some people and sedating, for others, depending on dosage and other factors.

Phenylephrine and phenylpropanolamine (PPA) are two other spin-off drugs useful for sinus problems and the common "cold"; phenylephrine is also mildly stimulating to some people, and PPA is stimulating to most people. Both of these drugs can raise blood pressure. PPA is also used in over-the-counter diet pills.

Diet pills related to norepinephrine (also see Chapter V-18)

Plegiline and Preludin (phendimetrazine, phenmetrazine)

L-DOPA

This is a neurology drug used for Parkinson's disease of the brain. Like its parent drugs, adrenaline and norepinephrine, it is not well absorbed from the stomach; however, manufacturers have devised a system to enhance its absorption. Parkinson's disease of the brain is related to a deficiency of Dopamine (DA) in that part of the brain. L-DOPA can be taken orally and helps the brain to make more Dopamine. Eventually, some Parkinson's patients will develop side effects from the L-DOPA. These are psychotic side effects such as visual hallucinations and agitation. Some of these patients need to see a psychiatrist for the psychosis. This is a delicate balancing act between neurology and psychiatry because some of the necessary psychiatric drugs could make the Parkinson's symptoms worse. Seroquel is a good choice, but it can lower blood pressure and aggravate diabetes. Abilify is free of these problems but may not be strong enough.

Zyprexa and Risperdal have their proponents but could aggravate the Parkinson's. Theoretically, Mellaril might be helpful except for its cardiovascular side effects. Serentil is nominally better than Mellaril.

Other antidepressants and diet pills with highly modified norepinephrine structures
Effexor, Luvox, Wellbutrin, Prozac. (see Chapter V-9)

Prozac

I have listed Prozac separately because it is special in a few ways. It is a moderately modified norepinephrine drug, but has serotonin activity, except in high doses when it might have mild norepinephrine activity in some people. This drug started a new class of drugs, the serotonindrugs (SSRI antidepressants: selective serotonin reuptake inhibitors, is the full name). Prozac is stimulating to people with manic or psychotic tendencies. And when it stimulates those patients, they become more psychotic or manic psychotic. What we learned from this drug has made most psychiatrists cautious about using any of the SSRI antidepressants in manic or psychotic patients. As a matter of fact, there is an ongoing debate among psychiatrists if manic or psychotic patients *ever* need antidepressants

Wellbutrin

Wellbutrin *(bu·propion)* was inspired by the old diet pill Tenuate (di-ethyl-propion); chemically, they are like fraternal twins. Wellbutrin is an effective non-addicting antidepressant that does not cause any sexual side effects. Wellbutrin might cause constipation, especially in the elderly. Wellbutrin should not be prescribed to bulimics or epileptics. Bupropion and psycho-stimulants (amphetamines, e.g.) are the main anti-depressants which act on the Dopamine system in the brain.

Other Psychostimulants

Other psycho-stimulants do not share a common "platform" with epinephrine and have different stimulant effects from those of the diverse norepinephrine family of psychostimulants. They are also chemically distinct from each other. The one common factor they all share is the ability to create a state of arousal and alertness. This alertness results from the fact that they all raise the levels of stimulating brain hormones, presumably dopamine and norepinephrine (possibly serotonin—and others). Provigil falls in this class, along with its"purified" form, Nuvigil.

Other antidepressants

Not available in the USA: Amineptine (stimulating to some people) and Nomifensine (dopamine activity)

Other various Diet Pills

There are a number of diet pills that have antidepressant properties such as Tenuate, Mazindol, Meridia.

In the category of diet pills are various unrelated drugs such as Tenuate, Mazindol (that acts on dopamine DA and on norepinephrine NE), et al. These are rarely prescribed nowadays. A newer diet pill is Meridia (sibutramine, a highly modified phenyl-ethyl-amine). These drugs can be stimulating and may decrease appetite while they are being taken orally; however, stopping the medications will result in appetite returning to its baseline or to its "default" setting with the likelihood of regaining some or even more weight. These drugs have little use as antidepressants.

Ritalin

Ritalin and Cylert are chemically unrelated to any of the above medications and to each other. Ritalin is a schedule II drug like most amphetamines.

Cylert

Ritalin and Cylert are chemically unrelated to any of the above medications and to each other. The DEA considers Cylert to be less addicting than the other psychostimulants (it is a Schedule III drug). Cylert can stress the liver and is not currently available in the USA—whether it will be available again is not known. Cylert is FDA approved. Anyone who needs it, can order it from Canada.

Provigil and Nuvigil

Provigil (Modafinil) is a stimulant used to promote daytime wakefulness in patients with excessive daytime sleepiness. A "purified" version has recently been released: Nuvigil (armodafinil). Provigil is less addictive (it is only schedule IV). It helps to counteract EDS (excessive daytime sleepiness): that is basically its FDA indication. Provigil can cause headaches, "buzziness" and nausea.

Access to all addicting stimulants is under the control of the DEA branch of the federal government (Drug Enforcement Administration).

"Schedule I" drugs

These drugs are not available on prescription since they are considered to be highly addicting and/or dangerous, possibly damaging the body. These are not available to the public: Ecstasy, oral cocaine, and Crystal Methamphetamine. Ecstasy causes permanent damage to some of the brain cells resulting in permanent depression. Cocaine is available as a schedule II prescription drug only when used by ENT (ear-nose-throat) doctors. Crystal

Methamphetamine is one of the most addicting drugs known. It can be snorted, injected, or ingested (eaten), but in any case, it causes physical damage to the body. It dries out the mouth and is the number one cause of tooth loss in young adults. It causes long-term dopamine loss in the brain and permanent brain damage that shows up psychiatrically as permanent depression or psychosis. It shows its handiwork as brain defects that are visible in functional brain scans (PETScans). A more pedestrian version of methamphetamine is available on prescription as Desoxyn.

Toxicity notwithstanding, people still have an irresistible taste for the effects of amphetamines and other "psycho-stimulants", and there is an ever-widening chorus touting them for use in ADHD-ADD, Excessive Daytime Sleepiness, and states of vegetative apathy. In Latin America, one of them (Captagon) is indicated for "climate sensitivity". It seems likely that these drugs will soon experience another renaissance as Americans constantly overfill their 24-hour schedules with 26-hour agenda. Or, perhaps, a new, safer, spin-off Amphetamine-like psycho-stimulant will be created as the next *"drug du jour"*.

Chemical Imbalance?

When people say that they have a "chemical imbalance" they are referring to the fact that current theories suggest that they might not have enough "brain hormones", particularly norepinephrine, dopamine, and serotonin; but, there is no way yet to prove this scientifically—not even by sampling spinal fluid. The only physical proof would be to extract brain tissue and submit it to the laboratory for studies. That sampling technique could cause permanent brain injury to a live person.

I tend to cringe when people tell me that they have been "diagnosed with a chemical imbalance" because:

- We do not know what the mechanics of any such "imbalance" would be—or how they would operate. Supposedly, they are referring to the twentieth century theory about "brain hormones" based on studies in rat brains (and a few human autopsies). This is not conclusive proof that serotonin deficiency causes depression in Man.

- We do not know exactly which neuro-chemicals are involved—there are actually a lot of substances in the brain that may be important; I have only mentioned the few which we think are important for psychiatric drug actions.

- Even if we knew which chemicals were imbalanced, we still would have no way to measure the deficiencies (or excesses) of these imbalanced substances inside the brain with current technology—unless the patient were to have a P.E.T.Scan—which might or might not be definitive.

- This "imbalance" diagnosis also suggests that if we could restore the "balance" then the patient would feel better. There is no way to measure brain hormones before and after treatment in order to show medications have been effective inside the brain. The fact that people do feel better after the medicines does suggest that the medications have had some kind of effect.

- A diagnosis of "chemical imbalance" also suggests that we have a deep understanding about the subject of brain functioning—which we really do not.

These suppositions are not verifiable by current technology. Hence, "chemical imbalance" is an opinion or surmise and not a diagnosis.

Furthermore, some researchers are moving beyond the current biochemical theories into new realms of neurochemistry. Recently, a small cadré of progressive psycho-pharmacologists have been advancing theories that go beyond these known brain hormones: some researchers are suggesting that these alterations in the hormone levels may be markers of a completely different and unknown process, and that any such alterations may simply be incidental to the real cause—which is still totally unknown and unidentified. (It is true that spinal fluid samples of some suicide victims do show apparently altered levels of "brain hormones", but it is possible that low levels are a marker for depression and not a cause or effect of it.)

In defense of current theories, it is quite clear that depression, anxiety, and psychotic states do correct themselves when patients begin taking diagnosis-appropriate medicines. Researchers still do not know if psychiatric drugs act on the "brain hormones" or on some other system that indirectly affects the levels of the hormones. This remains an active field of research. So, if you are told that your diagnosis is "chemical imbalance", then you should ask which "chemicals" are "imbalanced" and request [written] details on this putative diagnosis (then you can send me a copy too!).

Once again, here is the table of the three main brain hormones which are targets for the current understanding of antidepressant function:

Dopamine (DA)	Serotonin 5-HT	Norepinephrine (NE)
Pleasure and Reward	Inspiration	Activation
Sense of well-being	Focus	Motivation
Euphoria	Anti-obsessive	Anti-apathy
Attention	Anti-anxiety	Attentiveness
Anti-depressant	Anti-depressant	Anti-depressant

Table V-6-a   Table of three main "brain hormones" *(neurotransmitters)
NE is the abbreviation for Norepinephrine, same substance as Noradrenaline (NA)

▶There is much to learn about the brain's chemistry. Many other substances in the brain have been targeted for further research, so the next twenty years should be very interesting times for depression research.

*N-O.R.-adrenaline stands for "*N-ohne radikal*-adrenaline (German): demethylated adrenaline

** Truly, we cannot tell if a child has an addictive personality yet, but if most of the family members have drug and alcohol problems, then that should be taken into account.

Chapter V-7

Older Sedating Antidepressants

Tricyclic Family, Trazodone Family, Remeron
(Technical information on the drugs is in this chapter)
(practical anecdotal information is listed in Chapter V-9)

There is no text book of psychiatry that will list these drugs officially under the name of "older" drugs. I have arbitrarily adopted this terminology "older" and "newer" (Chapters V-7 and V-8) in order to avoid introducing complicated pharmacological classifications into this book. Most psychiatrists will understand this terminology, although it is not official. The first members of the "older" drugs, technically speaking, were the amphetamines: these are already covered in Chapter V-6. If confronted with this terminology, psychiatrists would tend to reference Tofranil in the late 1950's as the debut of the older drugs. The era of the older drugs extended up until the late 1980's, when the first of the so-called "newer" drugs, Prozac, appeared on the market. Prozac ushered in a new era of antidepressant treatment. Antidepressant drugs introduced to market since that time (except Remeron) may be considered "newer" antidepressants (Chapter V-8).

These older drugs have been on the market for a long time and we think we know all of the good effects and bad effects of these drugs. There are now millions and millions of people worldwide who have taken these medicines for thirty or forty years. Some people have taken them since youth and have grown old with the drugs and even passed away while on the drugs (deaths not necessarily or apparently related to the drugs). The Tricyclics are the oldest in this group, some going all the way back to mid-twentieth century origins. Trazodone has been on the market for over two decades. Remeron is the youngest in the group, but it is merely the "purified" version of mianserin, a European antidepressant that has decades of longevity, also. Mianserin would fall into the group of older drugs. At this point in time, there are not likely to be any new surprises in this group of medications.

This is the list of sedating older medications covered in this chapter:

- Tricyclics (including Asendin and similar drug Ludiomil)
- Trazodone family

- Other Cyclic drugs (Non-tricyclic, "Heterocyclics") (Remeron, Ludiomil)

- European sources: Mianserin, Amineptine, and others

- Merital (Nomifensine) is not particularly sedating and not quite like any other antidepressant; it might warrant being in its own category.

- Low doses of certain SGA anti-psychotics (Second Generation Antipsychotics)

- Low dose of the FGA anti-psychotics Triavil (Etrafon) and Loxitane / Asendin

General Principles for all of them

Uses and Purposes (Indications)

These drugs are primarily antidepressants, although some of them have a number of off-label uses and have been used off-label for decades without any serious problems (see Chapter V-3 to learn about "Indications").

Commonalities of Function

These medications have varying effects on the body and brain. Most of the effects are believed to act on serotonin, noradrenalin, and dopamine receptors and on less well-known receptor sites (sites involving neurotransmitters—see chapters V-1, V-5, and II-2). No matter the intended function, antidepressant effects typically predominate among all the drugs' effects.

Most of these older sedating antidepressants have anti-anxiety properties at low doses and antidepressant properties at higher doses, a fact that has not been overlooked by researchers and is of constant benefit in psychiatric treatment. Most of them have mixed therapeutic effects and mixed side effects. Most have serotonin activity and some have norepinephrine activity. Asendin has minor dopamine effects, and nomifensine has significant dopamine effects. Their chemical structure imparts a number of mildly sedating effects, which tend to counterbalance any stimulant effects, resulting in a sense of calm alertness. Patients will ideally feel focused. Apart from treating anxiety and depression, these medications also have many other uses in other conditions such as: bedwetting, pain control, itching, sleeping, ADD, and obsessive compulsions.
Sinequan has been used for stomach ulcers.

Commonalities of Side Effects

These drugs have varying degrees of similar side effects. These side effects can be grouped into two large sets of side effects. The first set of side effects peculiar to these drugs includes sedation, appetite and weight gain (except the Trazodone family which is just sedating). The second set of sedating effects may result in dry mouth, constipation, blurred vision, urinary "slowness", and dry sinuses (once again, the Trazodone family has minimal amounts from this set of side effects).

As far as the first set, the factors leading to weight gain can be partly or wholly controlled by diet and exercise. There are four possible mechanisms by which these drugs cause weight gain. Firstly, these drugs tend to stimulate the **appetite center** in the brain and this makes food more desirable. Secondly, the drugs also slow down the digestion process ("**decreased peristalsis**") so that food moves more slowly and thus has a longer time and more opportunity to be absorbed. Thirdly, antidepressants in general and Tricyclics especially, make food taste better as part of the **antidepressant effects**. And finally, if the drugs cause **insulin release** (norepinephrine-like activity), then the patient will also have "carbohydrate craving"; this means that bread products and pastries will become very appealing. Understanding these mechanisms can help patients try to thwart these insidious side effects. If a person can do daily exercise for half an hour, count calories, and avoid fast food-junk food, then there should not be much weight gain. Despite these four mechanisms, weight gain can be minimized.

The second set of side effects is dry mouth, blurred vision, dry sinuses, and urinary slowness. Dry mouth creates a sensation of thirst. If a person drinks a lot of water, that is very helpful. But if the beverage of choice is soda, then your body will need to deal with all the chemicals in the soda. Full-strength soda with sweetener can add undesirable calories. The ideal beverage is water or any drink without "caloric consequences" (a beverage having zero calories). The side effect of dry sinuses is very appealing to people who are prone to allergies and hay fever. Any side effects resulting in dry eyes, blurred vision, or urinary "slowness", can be treated with a side effect pill (yes, that would require taking a second drug in addition to the sedating antidepressant). Some patients welcome the addition of side effect pills, whereas many are content to consume more fluids. I recommend the latter choice, but the available side effect pills are innocuous, if you should so choose.

Although these medicines may improve focus and attention as a beneficial effect, other properties of the drugs can cause the side effect of short-term memory impairment. This side effect ceases once the drug has been stopped. It is not a permanent memory problem. However, this side effect definitely limits the use of these drugs—especially the Tricyclics—in the elderly, who are already prone to short-term memory problems.

A corollary to memory problems is next-morning grogginess. The more sedating the pill and the better sleep that it produces, then the more likely is grogginess in the morning. This can occur with all these sedating antidepressants, although Serzone is least likely to cause this problem, followed by Asendin and Surmontil, which are less likely to cause this.

Sexual side effects are not a common complaint in this group of medicines unlike the newer serotonin drugs, which often do cause sexual side effects. A few of these antidepressant drugs lack annoying sexual side effects such as Serzone and Remeron. Tricyclics have minimal effect on sexual function one way or theother. Trazodone family drugs may even enhance sex slightly.

Specifics of each Antidepressant Family

Tricyclic Antidepressants

The Tricyclic antidepressants are still in use nowadays, but much less so than in the 1960's through the 1980's. In psychiatry they were originally used for major depression. Then we learned to use them in lower doses for minor depression. Then in even lower doses they were observed to help various anxiety disorders. Some may help obsessions in moderately high doses, and some help chronic pain in still higher doses. Many of them have multiple medical uses outside psychiatry (itching, bedwetting, gastric ulcer symptoms). The Tricyclics all share a common molecule made up of three conjoined aromatic carbon rings. Psychiatrists sometimes combine Tricyclics with the newer serotonin drugs. In these cases it is advisable to use a non-serotonin Tricyclic with the newer serotonin drug, because the combination might cause excessive serotonin activation, a medical emergency, otherwise known as "Serotonin Syndrome" (muscle twitching, fever, sweating, confusion). This is a rare condition. I would not suggest that your family doctor mix and match psychiatric drugs, as there are many pitfalls. Here are some suggested standard combinations for mixing newer with older drugs.

Table V-7-a   Commonest Combinations of Antidepressants

Desipramine or Pamelor plus	Prozac, Zoloft, Paxil, Celexa-Lexapro
Ludiomil plus	Prozac, Lexapro
Vivactil plus	Prozac, Effexor
Trazodone plus	Prozac, Zoloft, Paxil, Celexa-Lexapro, Effexor

Luvox has complicated reactions and interactions with other drugs and is not ideal for mixing with older sedating antidepressants. As a matter of fact, Luvox is not ideal for mixing with most prescription medications. Anafranil has too much serotonin activity to mix with other serotonin drugs. I have less experience with combinations involving Surmontil,

Pristiq, Remeron, or Cymbalta. Nonetheless, we do use all sorts of combinations in an attempt to make people feel better. Any effective treatment within reason is possible.

This is a list of the Tricyclics:

Pamelor (Nortriptyline) Pamelor is effective as an antidepressant, its main use. At one time, it was considered an ideal treatment for geriatric depression; however, some of the newer drugs are preferable. This is the only one in this category to have readily available drug levels that are useful for monitoring therapy. (see end of chapter V-2 about drug levels). In a certain sense, Pamelor is the "active ingredient" of Elavil.

Elavil (Amitriptyline) is useful for various conditions at various dosage ranges:
~at low doses it can help anxiety and bedwetting
~at medium doses it can help mild depression and headaches
~at higher doses it can help serious depression and chronic pains, such as backache, diabetic foot pain, chronic nerve pains present in certain neurological disorders. Elavil is also helpful for persistent nerve pains, such as those from Shingles.

When our bodies break down Elavil, one of the by-products is Pamelor, an antidepressant in its own right, but this does not mean that the uses and advantages of Elavil are the same as those for Pamelor. Each medicine has slightly different uses. In theory Pamelor could be helpful for chronic pain, but is rarely used this way. I have had a couple chronic pain patients start on Elavil and then go on to need high doses, which in turn caused side effects. Elavil side effects in these cases was improved by changing to Pamelor, but this may not always be the outcome. Pain control was about as good with Pamelor as with Elavil, and the Elavil side effects abated.

Sinequan (Doxepin) can be useful for allergies, itchy skin, stomach acidity, anxiety, depression, and chronic pain. It also causes low blood pressure, so that elderly patients should be encouraged to switch to another medicine. Doxepin is the most sedating of the sedating antidepressants.

Tofranil (Imipramine) is useful in low doses for bedwetting and panic-anxiety, and at regular doses for depression, and obsessions. It has been used in the past for ADHD, but has fallen out of favor recently. Tofranil and Norpramin might be associated with rare side effects of heart attack in athletic teenage boys. The human body turns Tofranil into an active by-product, Norpramin.

Norpramin (Desipramine) Norpramin is mildly stimulating and has minimal side effects. The only Tricyclic that is more stimulating is Vivactil. It is like the "active ingredient" in

Tofranil. Tofranil and Norpramin might be associated with rare side effects of heart attack in athletic teenage boys.

Vivactil (Protriptyline) Vivactil rarely causes weight gain, but can cause rashes (any drug rash is a reason to stop taking the drug). Vivactil is mildly stimulating. It also has cardiac effects, rendering it inappropriate for elderly patients. Vivactil can be very effective in major depression when combined with Effexor or Prozac. This combination should be monitored by a psychiatrist. Vivactil was used years ago for snoring (sleep apnea).

Anafranil (Clomipramine) This is an antidepressant which is marketed in the USA for the indication of obsessive-compulsive disorder. It has rather significant side effects but is helpful to some people. It has powerful serotonin activity.

Surmontil (Trimipramine) This is not used very much. It is somewhat sedating and does not last very long. It is ideal for prescribing at bedtime for people who like bedtime Doxepin but feel too groggy in the morning from Doxepin. Try Surmontil in these patients.

Asendin (Amoxepine) Asendin is somewhat different from the other Tricyclics, but I have added it here. It is the only one with dopamine activity. It is very closely related to its sibling drug, Loxitane, which turns out to be anti-psychotic and not an antidepressant. Loxitane is unique among the FGA anti-psychotics by having some mild serotonin activity. In other words Asendin and Loxitane both share dopamine and serotonin activity, but Loxitane has more dopamine activity (and less serotonin activity), whereas Asendin has more serotonin activity (and less dopamine activity). In theory, Asendin is ideal for psychotic depression or schizoaffective disorder.

Ludiomil (Maprotiline) Although Ludiomil has a basic tricyclic shape, it is unique in having a different size ring as well as a (fourth) three-dimensional hoop-ring". See below under Cyclic drugs. It is sedating in lower doses and stimulating in higher doses. It is very popular in Europe and Latin America. It never gained popularity in the USA because it arrived too late to the "party".

Weight Gain and Tricyclics

Weight gain is the most bothersome Tricyclic side effect. This is the ranking of these medications and how much weight a woman might gain (men, as usual, might gain less or more). Doxepin is most likely to cause weight gain, and Vivactil is essentially "weight-neutral" (no weight gain). The weights listed are the additional weight above the woman's normal baseline weight.

Some people with agitated depression will drop below baseline. When the depression is treated, they typically regain weight back up to their baseline; and, then gain some more weight while on Tricyclics, more or less in accordance with the following table. For example, a woman who usually weighs 135 lbs. drops down to 120 lbs. with agitated depression. After starting treatment with Tofranil, she regained 15 lbs. to bring her back up to normal baseline, and then gained an extra 17 pounds, putting her at a total weight of 152 lbs while taking Tofranil. She might opine that she gained 32 pounds, but it is technically only 17 lbs.

Table V-7-c *Expected Weight Gain from Tricyclic Antidepressants by Gender*	
♀ Women	♂ Men
<u>Weight Gain in a typical Woman</u> Doxepin—25-50 lbs ↑↑↑ Tofranil, Elavil—15-35 lbs ↑↑ Pamelor, Surmontil, Anafranil—15-20 lbs ↑↑ Asendin—10-15 lbs ↑ Desipramine, Ludiomil—10 lbs ↑ Vivactil—few pounds gained/lost ↕	**Active men** will gain fewer than the minimum pounds for women, **Semi-inactive men**, about the same as for women. **Inactive men** may gain more than the maximum for women

In my experience, weight gain in men mainly depends on their activity levels. Weight gain in women taking Tricyclics is more complex and seems not to be the result of any one factor. Weight gain in women is also more predictable and probable than in men.

Dosage Guidelines

Starting dosages: Start low! Go slowly!

Complicated drugs with complex side effects should be started at lowest dosages and increased slowly in order to minimize early side effects (sedation, nervousness) and to minimize toxic reactions related to fast dosage increases (seizures, for example). Treatment with Tricyclics usually requires more medical supervision—at least twice as much oversight—as with the newer drugs.

Therapeutic Dosages

These drugs have an immensity of possible dosage ranges. Some people will require ten times as much dosage as other people, although the dosage range variation is more like fourfold to fivefold. Since these drugs have many uses at many different dosage ranges, I have included the general guidelines for dosing. These guidelines are given in milligrams of dosage, abbreviated "mg".The dosing guidelines are important since these drugs can become somewhat toxic at higher doses. They are also toxic in overdoses. At the end of this chapter is a table of approximate dosing ranges depending upon the diagnosis. Blood levels are available for a few drugs and serve as treatment guidelines: Pamelor levels are especially useful. (Dosing guidelines had not been necessary for stimulants or for the newer drugs, since the dosage ranges for adults and for children are more standardized. The dosages might vary only depending upon how much one person can tolerate or how much he needs. The newer drugs are not toxic even in really high daily doses)

This is the dosage table showing the range of milligrams dose depending on diagnosis. This table lists only the commonly used medications. This list reflects my practice habits.
Table V-7-c

Dosages in milligrams	Anxiety disorder	Minor Depression	Major Depression	Chronic Pain	Other uses & dosages
Elavil	10-40 mg	50-75mg	100-250 mg	150-275	
Pamelor	10-30 mg	30-50 mg	50-150 mg		geriatric depression 20-30 mg
Tofranil	10-50 mg Panic 10-50 Phobia 100	40-100 mg	100-300 mg		bedwetting 10 mg compulsions 200 ADHD 25-75 mg
Norpramin		40-75 mg	75-100 mg		ADHD 25-50 mg
Vivactil		5-15 mg	30-60 mg		ADHD 10-30 Snoring 10 mg
Doxepin	20-60 mg	50-100 mg	125-300 mg	150-300	IBS 30$^+$ mg*

*IBS = Irritable Bowel Syndrome (nervous acid stomach)

The Tricyclics dry out the nose, digestive system, eyes, and urinary bladder (and prostate). The sedating ones might lower blood pressure in the elderly and could cause dizziness and falling down, especially at night. Most of them usually cause some level of sedation or calmness. They are, however, ideal for depressed patients with diseases of excessive secretions such as hay fever, stomach acidity, bedwetting, and ongoing diarrhea. They are all calmative for agitated patients.

Trazodone family

Trazodone is representative of the next family. It is the best known and most widely used of these drugs. These are the members of this family with their generic names first then (branded names):

- Trazodone (Desyrel)

- Nefazodone (Serzone)

- Buspirone (Buspar)

- Gespirone (not available in USA)

Trazodone

Trazodone is used constantly by psychiatrists as an antidepressant and as a sleeping pill. It has three basic methods of use. It can be used alone as an antidepressant. It can be used alone as a non-addicting sleeping pill. Or it can be a secondary antidepressant when combined with a primary antidepressant (preferably an antidepressant from the class of "newer" antidepressants). Trazodone is FDA-approved for use as an antidepressant. It never went through a formalized vetting process to obtain an indication as a sleeping pill, but sleep-enhancement is now its primary use. I frequently prescribe it alone as a sleeping pill. It works well in about ninety percent of the cases. Patients may complain of some morning grogginess, which they say improves within an hour of awakening. Most choose to continue taking it. Some people only need one pill at bedtime, and some need three to four or even more. Bedtime absorption is improved if the Trazodone is eaten with a light carbohydrate snack, such as a couple unsalted crackers. If it is taken with crackers, then the number of pills can often be reduced, for example from three pills to just two or two and a half.

Another advantage of bedtime use as a sleeping pill is that patients can take Trazodone as needed and whenever they please: once a week or every night. Patients are allowed to increase the dosage slowly if they need to, just as long as they keep me informed of what they are doing, and why. I usually have Trazodone patients come in about every three to four weeks until they reach a period of stabilization when they are taking the same dose every night for months. Then they can continue to take the drug according to plan and need only come in once every three or four months—of course, anyone is welcome to come back sooner. The sooner, the better—before some untreated problem compounds itself.

The second method of use for Trazodone is to use it alone as an antidepressant. As such, it can be given all at bedtime or in two or three divided doses throughout the daytime, especially for agitated or anxious depresssion. Trazodone is a sedating antidepressant, so it is ideally given in daytime divided doses in cases of anxious depression or agitated depression.

The third method of use is to add it on to a primary "newer" antidepressant, such as Prozac or Zoloft. There are two reasons to do this: firstly, some patients do really well on Prozac but find that Prozac disturbs their sleep cycle. Trazodone can normalize their sleep. In other case, people are doing fairly well on Prozac, but need to increase the dosage of Prozac in order to feel less depressed. The further increase in Prozac may make them feel more animated but also more stimulated. Trazodone can be useful in divided daytime doses or as one dose at nighttime. The same can be said of using Zoloft, Lexapro, Paxil, or Effexor as well as Prozac. When used in combination this way, Trazodone can be considered both as a sleeping pill, as well as a secondary antidepressant. Patients who are taking a newer antidepressant such as Prozac might have trouble sleeping, and Trazodone provides excellent relief.

A fourth uncommon use of Trazodone is to use it as if it were Buspar, i.e. using it for anxiety treatment—although some of these cases are closer to a mildly anxious depression. In this case, the trazodone would be taken at least twice daily, perhaps as much as four doses a day, in small doses.

Not everyone likes Trazodone. Some people complain that it causes strange dreams, nausea, or dizziness and stop taking it. These are indeed the three most common side effects and reasons for stopping the medicine.

The only limitations for trazodone use are certain heart conditions and in men. Heart patients who have "ventricular tachyarrhythmia" (a very serious but rare heart condition) must not take Trazodone as it can lead to a life-threatening aggravation of that condition (death). As far as men, Trazodone can—on rare occasions—cause permanent erections that might lead to a urological emergency, the surgical treatment for which could lead to permanent impotence. Men who are still sexually potent reject Trazodone on this basis. Men who are reasonable candidates for Trazodone are those who have long-standing impotence from diseases, such as penile cancer or diabetes. Diabetic men often express a wish for even a faint chance of this side effect (which is not ever likely to happen). None of my patients has complained of this sexual side effect, except for one woman who complained of a clitoral itching sensation.

Original animal research in the 1980's showed that beagles (dogs) on Trazodone developed cataracts, but it turns out that beagles have a genetic predisposition to cataracts, and that has not been a known side effect in people.

The maximum recommended dose for Trazodone (as an antidepressant) is 600 mg. I do not recommend using it at 600 mg bedtime in one dose as a sleeping pill. If this much is needed, there are other choices such as Doxepin, Remeron, high-dose Neurontin, or Seroquel. If using Trazodone at very high doses, I would recommend obtaining a heart wave test (EKG) while on this high dose; a blood level would also be desirable.

Serzone

On the other hand, Serzone is hardly ever prescribed nowadays since it was linked to a few dozen cases of liver failure worldwide. It is still available in generic form in the USA, but its original corporate sponsor has stopped selling the branded product (legal liability). Apart from that, Serzone is/was a very good medication. It had no negative effects on usual sexual functioning of normal men or women. It was calmative but not so sedating as its sibling drugs. A few of my long-time Serzone patients opted to continue taking it despite the extremely rare liver side effect. They are aware of the risks and go to have blood tests every three-four months for monitoring purposes, although experts believe that the liver failure can start so suddenly that quarterly blood tests would not be of much use. This is not certain. I do not start new patients on Serzone except for patients in end-stage kidney failure for whom it seems to work very well.

Buspar

Buspar was created to be an antidepressant like Trazodone but people could not tolerate it at the high doses required to treat depression. So, the dosage was lowered and it was brought to market as a treatment for general anxiety (see beginning of this chapter). It is marginally successful as an antianxiety pill. About thirty percent of patients find it useful. It can be taken as the only pill for anxiety treatment. It is also useful added on to other medications—it can be combined with almost any medication except for the MAOI Antidepressants. When adding Buspar to any antidepressant, one must remember that it is really an antidepressant and any side effects from the combination are referable to this fact. It is an excellent add-on anti-anxiety medication for people who are taking the newer antidepressants, such as Prozac, Lexapro, Effexor, Zoloft. In this way, it functions about the same as Trazodone used as an add-on antianxiety treatment. The advantage is that men can safely get the Trazodone-like benefit but by taking Buspar instead.

When Buspar first appeared, it was hailed as the first effective non-addicting anti-anxiety agent. This is not true because Vistaril and Atarax were the first non-addictive sedative-anxiety medication(s). (Vistaril and Atarax both contain the same active ingredient, hydroxyzine, but have slight chemical differences—one is compounded with hydrochloride, and the other, with pamoic acid). Buspar is not typically mixed with addicting anti-anxiety agents, since the primary purpose of Buspar is treat anxiety on a long-term basis without invoking the risk of addiction. Buspar is not addicting like drugs of the Valium class (or barbiturates or Equanil). In cases of extremely high anxiety (we call this "pan-anxiety"), Buspar could successfully be added to Neurontin or Zyprexa, for example. The advantage here is that the add-on Buspar would allow us to prescribe a very small dose of Zyprexa, which is not really indicated for anxiety, but can be used off-label for treating agitation ("pananxiety").

This is the dosage table for the Trazodone family, showing the typical range of milligrams (mg) dose, depending on symptoms and diagnosis (Serzone is not shown):

	Trazodone as a sleeping pill	Trazodone as Antidepressant (up to 600 mg)	Trazodone for anxiety (mildly anxious depression)	Buspar for anxiety
Typical dosage	50-150 mg at bedtime	50 mg twice a day & 100 mg bedtime	25-50 mg three or four times a day	5-7 ½ mg thrice daily
Maximum range	350-450 mg At bedtime	100 mg twice /day & 200 mg bedtime	— —	15 mg x 4 = 60 mg a day

Other Cyclic drugs include Ludiomil, Remeron, and others. High-dose Ludiomil has more stimulation and less sedation than regular tricyclics. Remeron is sedating and often a good choice for agitated depression and insomnia in [dry] alcoholics. Asendin would warrant a second listing here as well as with the tricyclics.

Ludiomil has been on the market for nearly forty years and is much more popular in Europe and South America than in the USA. At the time of its debut in the USA, Ludiomil acquired an ill-deserved reputation for causing seizures. As long as Ludiomil is started at a low dose and increased slowly, the risk of seizures is tiny. Many of these antidepressants have seizures as a possible side effect. None of my patients has experienced a seizure as a side effect from antidepressants—at least not that they have told me.

Ludiomil has been used for neurotic anxiety in Europe and South America in the manner that American psychiatrists use Elavil or Doxepin. Ludiomil is available in those countries as 10 mg tablets to use one tablet a few times a day. Faced with the same cases, we will sometimes prescribe Elavil 10 mg tablets or Doxepin 10 mg capsules, a few times a day. At intermediate doses, Ludiomil is effective for Dysthymia: 50-100 mg a day. For major depression, Ludiomil can be used at higher doses 150-200 mg.

Asendin has its main listing earlier in this chapter.

Remeron is the active form of the European antidepressant, Mianserin. Remeron is sedating. It has unique pharmacologic properties besides sedation to enhance its effectiveness. It can also be used as an "off-label" non-addictive sleeping pill. It is especially useful as a sleeping aid for insomniac alcoholics in early recovery. The main side effects are weight gain and swollen ankles (women usually). The causes of the weight gain are not quite clear, but probably related to the mechanics of weight gain with the Tricyclics listed above. Analogous to swollen ankles in women, Remeron may also cause them uncomfortably swollen wrists. Doctors may tell patients to lie down and elevate the feet; however, the only way to get rid of the swollen ankles, is to get rid of the Remeron. Possible substitutes would be one of the Tricyclics, perhaps Vivactil (younger patients) or Desipramine (middle-aged). Effexor is also a viable option. Remeron is also very potent when used with Effexor.

Remeron can cause dizziness. Remeron can suppress bone marrow early in treatment. The symptoms of this are infections that get worse, such as a bad sore throat or fevers.

Remeron is available as Remeron-sol tab. This is a dissolving tablet that can be taken on-the-go without water. Sol tabs are also ideal for people who cannot swallow pills for any reason.

European Antidepressants

Amineptine is a three ringed cyclic antidepressant, resembling some of the other three-ringed antidepressants. It is stimulating to some people. Mianserin is a standard old cyclic antidepressant. It is not available in the USA, but its "purified" form is available here as Remeron. Nomifensine is one of the few dopamine active antidepressants. It was prescribed in the USA for about a year before the FDA withdrew it due to a couple cases of blood disease (hemolytic anemia). It is still available but should be used by a psychiatrist who is familiar with its properties. Because of its blood effects, it is another drug of last resort. Vestra (Reboxitene, Edronax) is a norepinephrine acting antidepressant that was going to appear in America about ten years ago, but that still has not happened. It is available in and can be ordered from Europe.

SGA (second-generation antipsychotics)

The SGA medications can fulfill four purposes. Some of the so-called atypical anti-psychotic (SGA's—see chapter V-4) medicines possess very modest antidepressant properties in their own right (very low-dose Geodon, especially). Others can be helpful in very low doses for boosting the antidepressant effect of primary antidepressants, being especially helpful if added to serotonin antidepressants (SSRI's); examples of these would be Risperdal, Zyprexa. A third use of the SGA's is that they can be used in very low doses for very high anxiety. They can help control mania. And of course, their primary purpose is to act as an antipsychotic, which is covered in Chapter V-4.

FGA (first-generation antipsychotic)

Loxitane would theoretically fit into this category due to its slight serotonin activity. It could be added to an antidepressant at a dose of 5-10 mg. (lower doses of 2 ½ mg are possible by using the liquid form of Loxitane)

Depression Treatment Outcomes

In some cases where anti-depressants have provided about 50% relief of depressive symptoms—but not much more—then there are other options. A secondary antidepressant can be added to the primary antidepressant. Sometimes "helper" medications can be added to the primary antidepressant. Examples are: Lithium, thyroid hormone (Cytomel), tiny doses of stimulants or old diet pills (Sanorex), and others. Other examples of "helper" medicines are the FGA and SGA medications listed above. Sometimes these maneuvers of adding extra medicines to the antidepressant will provide a "jump start" and help boost the antidepressant effect of the primary antidepressant. However, the initial effect is sometimes lost after a period of months. We have many treatment choices available nowadays. Unfortunately, the patient might need to try each new treatment strategy for upwards of six weeks to six months before declaring it ineffective. I believe that at least 85% of depression can improve by at least 85%, given enough treatment attention by the doctor and diligent follow through by the patient.

In summary, most Antidepressants act as anti-anxiety drugs at lower doses leading to the unofficial quip that "depression and anxiety are just different sides of the same coin". A better description might be that anxiety disorders and mood disorders may present as if being a collection of symptoms belonging to a broad spectrum of emotional turmoil. Curiously, bipolar mood disorder is often preceded or accompanied by very significant levels of anxiety symptoms, too. It is possible that there is just one spectrum of psychiatric illness, and that different treatments are aimed at small zones of salient symptoms in that spectrum. Trazodone, Serzone, Tricyclic and other Cyclic Antidepressants in low-doses are commonly used for anxiety-panic and in higher doses for depression, obsessions and chronic pain. This is curious because they all belong to different and unrelated chemical families yet remarkably seem to have calmative effects on the body, albeit different kinds of calmative effects. We still have much to learn about psychoactive drugs.

Chapter V-8

Newer Antidepressants

(Technical information on the drugs is in this chapter)
(Practical anecdotal information is listed in Chapter V-9)

There is no textbook of psychiatry that will list these drugs officially under the name of "newer" drugs. I have arbitrarily adopted this terminology "older" and "newer" in order to avoid introducing complicated pharmacological classifications into this book. Most psychiatrists will understand this terminology, although it is not official. The first of these so-called "newer" drugs was Prozac (late 1980's), and all the drugs introduced to market since that time (except Remeron) are "newer" antidepressants.

These medications have varying effects on the body and brain. As mentioned in previous chapters, three brain chemicals seem to be involved in producing antidepressant effects in the brain. Most of these effects are believed to act on the three chemicals, serotonin, norepinephrine, and dopamine—and on less well-known chemicals (see chapters V-1-2 and II-2-3). Antidepressant effects typically predominate among all the drugs' effects, although many of them have anti-anxiety properties at lower doses. The term SSRI refers to a serotonin drug ("selective serotonin reuptake inhibitor"). SNRI refers to a norepinephrine drug ("selective norepinephrine reuptake inhibitor") and SSNRI, is selective for both serotonin and norepinephrine ("selective serotonin and norepinephrine reuptake inhibitor"). This is the list:

- SSRI: Prozac, Zoloft, Paxil, Celexa, Luvox, Lexapro
- SSNRI: Effexor, Cymbalta, Pristiq
- SNRI: (Strattera, an antidepressant that is marketed in USA as an ADD drug—see Chapter V-6)
- European sources: SNRI e.g. Vestra/Reboxitene
- Miscellaneous medications

Uses and Purposes

These drugs tend to have a broad range of uses and the dosage will depend a lot on the diagnosis under treatment. When used for Panic attacks, the dosage ranges are usually quite small. Anxiety usually requires a low-to-moderate dosage. Treatment of major depression is usually from mid-range to high dosage. Treatment of obsessive compulsions is usually in the high dosage ranges.

Most of these drugs have multiple purposes (indications, see Chapter V-3).

Common Side Effects

Despite being so different in chemical structure, they all seem to have similar biochemical effects on our bodies. By virtue of their serotonin activity, they can improve concentration and attention, boost depression, and decrease constant worrying. Rashes may occur. Any skin reaction to a medication is probably an allergic reaction, and the drug should probably be stopped, after talking to your prescriber. During the first week of treatment, the drugs can cause headaches, nausea, sleepiness, jitteriness. These side effects usually subside within a couple weeks. This is why I prefer to start (even) adults on half-doses for the first week. There is no point in feeling depressed *and* having annoying side effects. The symptoms will come under control just as quickly by starting half-doses as full-doses.

Panic patients, especially, are extremely sensitive to these SSRI drugs, so I occasionally start them out on only ⅓ or ¼ dose (Paxil 5 mg, Zoloft 12½ mg). Adding Xanax or Ativan during this difficult time may be wise. Not adding Xanax or Ativan may end up in needless trips to the emergency room for sensations of "heart attack"; but, patients need to understand that Xanax and Ativan are only intended for the first several weeks. Ideally, give a panic patient tiny starting doses of Paxil or Zoloft and during the first three weeks have them take the Xanax or Ativan a few times daily to prevent any breakthrough panic attacks. After the first few weeks, decrease the Xanax or Ativan to "as needed" dosing only and not all day long. Addition of Atenolol may be useful for some patients.

Equally annoying, most of these "newer" antidepressants can cause varying degrees of sexual side effects. The resultant sexual dysfunction can range from mild to very annoying: in men and women. These drugs can cause not only loss of interest in sex but also difficulty in having orgasm. The drugs do not typically interfere with having full erections, but do delay ejaculation significantly. Strattera can cause impotence; besides that, Strattera has one unique sexual side effect in men: a sensation of cremasteric contraction (the uneasy feeling that the testicles are being drawn up into the pelvis). See below for more on this. Also see Chapter VI-9 on "Men's Issues".

SSRI (selective serotonin reuptake inhibitors)

"Serotonin Antidepressants"

- Celexa
- Lexapro
- Luvox
- Paxil, Paxil-CR
- Prozac, Prozac Weekly
- Zoloft
- Available in pills or as a liquid: Celexa, Lexapro, Paxil, Prozac, Zoloft
- Injectable: none available in shot form

The **SSRI**'s are the most famous and popular group of modern antidepressants and are used extensively as the first line drugs for treating depression. SSRI's can be helpful in treating panic-anxiety, too (in lowered doses). Curiously, none of the drugs in this loosely affiliated SSRI category is related to each other chemically, and yet they all seem to have similar effects, which is one more reason why researchers have begun to question current theories about anxiety, depression, antidepressants' mechanism of action, and the exact roles of the known "brain hormones". Prozac, for example, is a kind of modified fluorinated adrenaline and none of the others is even remotely based on adrenaline. They all seem to belong to very different unrelated chemical families.

In modern practice, low doses of Paxil and Zoloft are often used for panic-anxiety; the other SSRI's may also be useful for panic-anxiety on a case-by-case basis. All SSRI antidepressants are useful for treating depression, and the dosage range can be from average to very large dosage. Additionally, they all have anti-obsessive properties but Luvox is strongest in this regard. These drugs are truly "broad-spectrum" psychoactive drugs because they all seem to be effective throughout the spectrum of mild anxiety-depression symptoms.

Certain details about each drug may make it theoretically more useful than any one of the other five. Here are some examples regarding age differences. Prozac is not ideal for treating the elderly because one dose lasts longer than twenty-four hours and thus accumulates in the elderly body. Lexapro ideally does not interact much with other drugs so is often preferred when patients—especially the elderly—are taking a huge number of medically necessary pills. Prozac is the only SSRI that is FDA-approved in children, although Lexapro has recently been approved to treat depression in teenagers (over age twelve).

These drugs are easy to use, often requiring only one dose a day. All are available in liquid form, except Luvox. The SSRI drugs are also safe in overdose,

Celexa has intermediate properties among all the SSRI—it is not too stimulating or too sedating. It lasts for the day. If taken at night, it can cause strange dreams and nausea.

Lexapro is the "purified" form of Celexa. The "better half" of the Celexa is isolated chemically and then it is compressed into a Lexapro tablet. It has fewer side effects and is more effective. When using it for anxiety disorders, the best starting dose is 2½ mg for the first several days and then increase to 5 mg.

Luvox is an antidepressant with prominent anti-obsessive properties. The other powerful anti-obsessive drugs are Anafranil (an older tricyclic) and Nardil (MAOI antidepressant).

Paxil—has multiple uses official and unofficial. Officially, Paxil has FDA approval for treating depression, panic disorder, social anxiety disorder, posttraumatic disorder, obsessive-compulsive disorder, generalized anxiety disorder, and Paxil-CR is approved for "PMS" (Paxil-CR, controlled release form). Paxil is used "off-label" to treat premature ejaculation. Besides having prominent serotonin activity, Paxil has mild anti-histamine properties, which translate into weight gain. Paxil patients should expect to gain weight. Researchers believe that high dose Paxil possesses mild norepinephrine properties in some patients. Common side effects are rash and weight gain. People who quit taking Paxil may experience the so-called "discontinuation syndrome" (see in chapter V-9). Paxil is FDA-approved for treating six disorders!

Prozac is a well known antidepressant. It is useful for major depression, minor depression, borderline syndrome, bulimia, and has some anti-obsessive properties. Some people find it calmative and some find it stimulating. Patients with a history of mania or psychosis can become extremely stimulated on Prozac and might act out homicidal and suicidal urges. It is also available in a large 90 mg capsule that can be taken once a week (Prozac Weekly capsules).

SSNRI (selective serotonin and norepinephrine reuptake inhibitors)
"Serotonin-Norepinephrine Antidepressants"

The next classification includes the **SSNRI**'s such as:
- Effexor, Effexor-XR
- Cymbalta

- Pristiq
- None available as a liquid or injectable
- By virtue of their norepinephrine activity, any of these three can raise blood pressure unacceptably

Their common benefits accrue from helping depression and chronic pain. They are all effective antidepressants, probably because they act on both serotonin and norepinephrine in the brain. Their benefits in chronic pain are made obvious clinically when patients report feeling better.

Their common side effects include jitteriness and high blood pressure.

Effexor was the first of these to appear in the mid 1990's. It debuted as a tablet, Effexor-IR (Immediate Release) and in this form it was famous for causing upset stomach. A few years later, it was repackaged in a different "delivery system" of time-released beads inside a capsule, Effexor-XR. This was better tolerated by patients. Another drawback of the tablets was that they did not last very long and had be taken more often: usually three times a day—possibly four times. A few people did well with twice daily dosing. The controlled release XR form lasted longer and needed to be taken only once or twice a day (for possible reason why, see Chapter II-4).

Effexor is effective at low doses for anxiety and quite effective at higher does for controlling depression, anxious depression, and chronic pain. Effexor can raise blood pressure. It is often constipating. In some patients Effexor may disturb sleep (stimulating antidepressant effect), and in others it seems to promote sleep (anti-anxiety effects). Those who are stimulated, usually take the last dose in the late afternoon, and by bedtime, the stimulation effect has yielded to sedation. Then the person can sleep well through the night. Those who are sedated by Effexor, usually take the last dose at bedtime and sleep well through the night.

Effexor often needs to have its dosage adjusted over the space of several months. Once patients are finally stabilized, they can usually stay on that same dose indefinitely. Younger patients should check their blood pressure once or twice a month and report back if the blood pressure is rising. Elderly should check blood pressure at least once a week. If Effexor results in high blood pressure, the person should see his family doctor.

Effexor can also cause constipation and/or upset stomach. Treatment of constipation is the same as for regular constipation. Upset stomach is often a regular feature with Effexor-IR tablets and I treat it with Zantac 150-600 mg per day, taken with the Effexor tablets. The same technique can be used with Effexor-XR, although upset stomach is not common with the XR.

Pristiq is the "purified" form of Effexor and is used to treat depression. One pill lasts all day. Most adults start with the 50 mg tablet and continue taking that dose. Thus, Pristiq is very easy to dose, unlike Effexor which often needs a lot of dosage adjustments.

Cymbalta is FDA approved for both depression and chronic pain. It works well for both conditions. It can produce a range of stimulation from mild to moderate. It has been associated with blood pressure issues, but less so than with Effexor.

SNRI

"norepinephrine antidepressants"

There are currently no SNRI antidepressants on the market in the USA. Strattera is a SNRI antidepressant, but it is only FDA approved for treating ADD. It could theoretically be used to treat depression, since it is available on prescription.

Reboxitene is an SNRI that can be ordered from Europe. Savella (milnacipran) is now available in the USA.

Treatment by Age Groups

This table shows which of the SSRI antidepressants are approved for which age group and if dosage adjustments are necessary. As always, remember, that the amount of dosage (the number of milligrams) depends mainly on one's genetics—not on one's age. Active teenagers often need dosing in the young adult range; however, their bodies are in a state of flux, so dosage may vary; and, they are not accustomed to being exposed to synthetic chemicals (SSRI), so the dosage might need to be lower on this count. The elderly require less dosage for many reasons, such as having slowed down bodily functions and taking many other pills. Also, remember that very low dosing is possible if the liquid form is prescribed.

Child	Teenager	Adult	Older Adult	Very Elderly
Prozac	Prozac Lexapro	All SSRI	All SSRI	Lexapro, Zoloft preferred (Celexa is OK) (Discourage use of Paxil)
				Avoid Prozac, Luvox
¼ dose	-1-*	-1-*	-1-*	Start with ½ dose for men, ⅓ dose women
	one (1) average adult starting dose			

Table V-8-a: Treatment by age group (SSRI Antidepressants)

Information on the above chart:

- Prozac alone is approved for use in children. Starting dose of 5 mg seems reasonable. (this is ½ of a 10 mg scored tablet or ¼ teaspoon of liquid Prozac)

- Recent alarmist reports suggest that suicides are increasing for anyone under the age of twenty-five, who is taking SSRI antidepressants. The rate of depression is also increasing in that age group, for whatever reasons—whether they are medicated or not. Suicide is one of the commonest causes of death in this age group, regardless of medications. Suicide is a constant risk of any depression, whether it is treated or not. Suicide attempts may occur earlier in treatment when the teen is beginning to feel better; suicide attempts may be due to excessive blood levels (possible in teens) or due to ongoing alcohol and drug abuse (very likely in teens).

- Only Prozac and Lexapro are approved for treating depression in teenagers.

- All SSRI drugs are approved for all adults

- In the elderly, Lexapro and Zoloft are relatively "clean" drugs (fewer side effects) and thus more suited to use in this age group; Celexa is acceptable for use, as it is the parent compound of Lexapro and is available more cheaply as a generic drug; Paxil might worsen memory problems and cause weight gain (Paxil has mild anti-histaminic properties), Prozac accumulates in the elderly body, Luvox has too many interactions with other prescription drugs;

- The number "-1-" refers to one average adult starting dose: Celexa 20 mg, Lexapro 10 mg, Luvox 50 mg, Paxil 20 mg, Prozac 20 mg, Zoloft 50 mg.

- A good rule of thumb in the very elderly is to start men on half-dose or even less, and women on about a one-third dose, more or less.

Dosages

The dosage range for most of these drugs is standardized for adults. There are different dosage ranges for different purposes of the pills. If used as anti-anxiety drugs, the dose will be lower than the doses used to treat major depression and chronic pain. At the end of the chapter is a table of usual dosage ranges for the drug's intended purpose (indication), reflecting the patient's diagnosis. The doses are listed in milligrams, abbreviated as "mg".

Table V-8-b   typical dosage ranges of SSRI, SNRI, SSNRI antidepressants based on diagnosis in everyday treatment (all dosages should be halved in the elderly)

	Depression	Anxiety* Disorder	Other FDA Approval	"off-label" uses
SSRI				
Celexa	20-80 mg			
Lexapro	10-25 mg	GAD 5-10 mg	(panic)	
Luvox	(varies)***		OCD 100-300 mg	antidepressant
Paxil	20-80 mg	P, SA:5-10 mg GAD 10-20 mg PTSD varies	♀ "PMS" 12½-25mg every day / month** or 2 weeks / month	Premature ejac. ♂ 10-25 mg
Prozac	20-80 mg	(Panic)	Bulimia 20-100 mg ♀ "PMS" 20 mg**	
Zoloft	50-200 mg	SA: 25 mg PTSD/OCD: varies	PMS** 25-75 mg Panic: 12½-25(200) mg	♂ Premature ejaculation
SSNRI				
Cymbalta	20-60 mg		Diabetic nerve pain	
Effexor	75-375 mg up to 450	GAD, P, SA		Chronic pain: 150-450 mg
Pristiq	50 mg			
SNRI				
Strattera	(varies)***		ADD	Antidepressant

* Anxiety Disorder abbreviations:

P (panic) SA (Social Phobia/Social Anxiety) GAD (generalized anxiety disorder)	OCD (obsessive-compulsive disorder) PTSD (post-traumatic stress disorder)

**"PMS" is premenstrual syndrome, now called "premenstrual dysphoric disorder" or "late luteal phase dysphoric disorder"; Prozac for "PMS" is sold as "Sarafem®" (pink & lavender capsule)

***Luvox is an antidepressant but is FDA approved only for treatment of OCD in the USA; Strattera is likewise an antidepressant but is FDA approved only for treating ADD in the USA.

Notes on the table above table:

DEPRESSION:

Celexa is recommended as 20-40 mg a day for depression; some patients need 60 or up to 80 mg. The HMO will usually approve this dosage range as long as the psychiatrist provides good evidence. It is not likely that the HMO will extend this same courtesy to non-psychiatrists. The HMO is likelier to approve higher doses of antidepressants available in generic form ($).

Lexapro is the purified "half-form" of Celexa and thus dosage can be half that of Celexa: 10-20 mg. Unlike the parent compound, Celexa, patients rarely require over the allowed maximum dosage of 20 mg.

Paxil dosage in depression is usually 20-60 mg. The HMO will approve 80 mg usually.

Effexor doses as high as 450 mg or more may be required to treat certain depressions.

Pristiq is the purified half of Effexor and thus is needed in lower doses, usually 50 mg a day.

OCD and PTSD usually require higher doses, which can slowly be increased until the patient feels relief

ANXIETY: Treatment of the other anxiety disorders—Panic, GAD (generalized anxiety disorder), SA (social anxiety/social phobia) in most patients requires only tiny doses—moderate or high doses can cause some anxiety symptoms.

CHRONIC PAIN treatment dosage is usually a high dose

BULIMIA treatment is variable, depending upon how much depression—if any—is present with the bulimia (there usually is depression to a certain degree).

SEXUAL DISORDERS

♀ PMS dosage in women is usually rather low dose, and often for only ten to fourteen days per month.

♂ Premature ejaculation in men likewise requires low doses. Usually the man needs to take enough to maintain a low blood level, such as one half-one dose every day or every other day. Then the man can take a bigger dose a couple hours before sexual activity. This is practical information not found in textbooks. If Joe has premature ejaculation almost at the moment of penetration, then he will need to take at least 20 mg Paxil (or 50 mg Zoloft or 50 mg Effexor) every day. A couple hours prior to sex, he can take an extra dose. If Mike has only a mild case and he has endurance of a few minutes, then he can probably get by with 10 mg of Paxil every day or every other day, and take 15 mg about an hour and a half before sex. If Jimmy can last up to eight or ten minutes, but there is pressure on him to have extended stamina, then he could probably take 5 mg Paxil every day or other day and then 10-20 mg about two hours before sex. If any of these men take the "booster" dose an hour or so before sex, he will first feel a surge from the antidepressant effect itself, which enhance his libido. The ejaculation will be delayed because he has maintained a regular blood level. A few hours after taking the booster dose, the man is going to feel a loss of desire whether he has ejaculated or not. The initial enhancement feeling is the antidepressant effect; the delayed ejaculation is a sought-after side effect, and the loss of libido is an unavoidable and undesirable side effect. Timing can be everything, and you may need to fiddle with the dosage on your own. Men who feel that the erection does not last until ejaculation should go to a sex shop and purchase a "cock ring" to maintain erections.

Premature Ejaculation Plus Impotence: ask your doctor about medications such as Viagra, Cialis, Levitra. Or go to a sex shop and purchase a "cock ring". This device is like a semi-snug tourniquet that helps to maintain erections. The rings are available in an assortment of fixed sizes as well as adjustable ones.

▶   In summary, SSRI's and SSNRI's in low-doses are commonly used for anxiety-panic and in higher doses for depression, obsessions and chronic pain. The SSRI's are curious because they all belong to different and unrelated chemical families yet remarkably seem to have similar effects on the body.

Full Alphabetical List of Antidepressants
Arranged also by family / group:

Antidepressants arranged by family

1) The SSRI-SNRI-SSNRI family: this is a large family: the SSRI medications are rather well known by now: Prozac, Zoloft, Paxil, Luvox, Celexa, and Lexapro; the SNRI-SSNRI drugs are Effexor, Cymbalta, and Pristiq. (Edronax-Reboxitene can be ordered from Europe). These antidepressant medications are listed together because they all have similar effects on the brain, but curiously, most of them are completely unrelated to each other chemically (unlike the tricyclics).

   a) Celexa

   b) Cymbalta

   c) Effexor

   d) Lexapro

   e) Luvox

   f) Paxil

   g) Pristiq

   h) Prozac (is chemically similar to amphetamine)

   i) Zoloft

   j) (Edronax from Europe)

2) Wellbutrin; Wellbutrin was developed from the old "diet pill" Tenuate (diethylpropion); apart from that it is an "only child" (of Tenuate); they are distantly related to Amphetamines.

3) Trazodone family includes three other medications: Trazodone has three cousins Buspirone, Gespirone (in "Europe), and Serzone (no longer routinely used in the USA)

   a) Buspirone used in the U.S. as an anti-anxiety medication

b) Trazodone (Desyrel)

c) Gespirone (Europe only)

d) Serzone (no longer routinely used in USA)

4) Tricyclics and Heterocyclics *FAMILY*: *The* tricyclics are like fraternal twins; the Heterocyclics are like half-siblings of the Tricyclics (Asendin, Ludiomil) or step-siblings (Remeron)

a) Anafranil

b) Asendin

c) Elavil

d) Desipramine

e) Doxepin

f) Ludiomil

g) Norpramin

h) Pamelor

i) Remeron (derived from Mianserin)

j) Sinequan (Doxepin)

k) Surmontil

l) Tofranil

m) Triavil / Etrafon

n) Vivactil

o) (also both Mianserin and Amineptine from Europe]

5) Stimulants include Amphetamines, Amphetamine-derived medications, and various other unrelated stimulants. The amphetamines are the oldest family of antidepressants. They are similar to adrenaline. Adrenaline cannot be swallowed in a pill form and can only enter the body as injections. In an attempt to find oral adrenaline, the basic structure of adrenaline was modified slightly to produce a stimulating drug, which indeed could be taken by mouth. This was amphetamine and was invented more than a century ago. All sorts of modified amphetamines have been devised over the last century: some are very similar to amphetamine, some are modified, and some have been modified so much that they cannot be considered a part of the family anymore. Phentermine is an amphetamine sibling. The MAOI Parnate belongs to this Family, too. *Prozac, Parnate, and Selegiline* are antidepressants that are siblings or half-siblings of the amphetamines; *PPA*

and *Phenylephrine* are also in this family. *PPA is phenylpropanolamine* used in diet pills and respiratory disorders. Phenylephrine is a decongestant. Any of these members of the Amphetamine Family can cause seriously high blood pressure. *Ritalin* is not closely related to any other stimulants. *Cylert is* like a second cousin twice removed and is not currently available in USA at this time. *Provigil* is like an identical twin of Nuvigil, except that Provigil was born first as a "breach birth" and *Nuvigil* was born second and "pure"; but, otherwise these two are orphans together and not related to any other stimulating antidepressants. Other "diet pills" used as stimulants are remotely related to amphetamines, like second cousins. Mazindol, however, is very alien from all the other stimulants/diet pills. In the list below, Amphetamine Family medications are marked with a hatch mark # , drugs distantly related to amphetamines (~), and non-Amphetamines are explained or otherwise unmarked:

a) Adderall # (This name reminds us to treat ADD diagnosis; yet "adder" is also a poisonous snake.)

b) Amphetamine #

c) Bupropion (~)

d) Concerta (Ritalin)

e) *DANGEROUS AMPHETAMINES (street drugs) are methamphetamine ("meth"), MDA , and MDMA ("ecstasy")* Ecstasy and [crystal] "meth" are capable of causing temporary or permanent brain damage and should be avoided.

f) Desoxyn # (methamphetamine)

g) Dexedrine/dextroamphetamine #

h) Diethylpropion (~) (Tenuate)

i) Fenfluramine #

j) Fen-Phen (fenfluramine-phentermine) # – # (both) This combination—not surprisingly—caused heart disorders: all the amphetamines can raise pulse and blood pressure, and cause other undesirable cardiac side effects.

k) Focalin (Ritalin)

l) Ionamin #

m) Mazindol (diet pill primarily)

n) Meridia (diet pill primarily)

o) Metadate (Ritalin)

p) Nuvigil—"purified" form of Provigil

q) Parnate (#) has an amphetamine structure but acts like MAOI

r) Phendimetrazine (~)

s) Phenmetrazine (~)

t) Phentermine #

u) Pondimin (fenfluramine) #

v) Provigil—also see Nuvigil

w) Sanorex (Mazindol)

x) Strattera

y) Tenuate (diethylpropion)

z) Vyvanse #

6) MAOI Antidepressants: a *less common FAMILY/GROUP is that* of *MAOI antidepressants*—most of these are somewhat related chemical compounds (called hydrazines) like half-siblings and their names are: *Nardil, Iproniazid, Eutonyl, Marplan, and Parnate (as well as Nialimide and Moclobemide from Europe);* Parnate behaves like an MAOI but it belongs structurally in the amphetamine class—this makes Parnate quite unique. Thus Parnate is not structurally related to the other MAOI medications, but curiously, it has similar effects on the brain as do the other MAOI medications which are:

a) Emsam (is a selegiline skin patch, effective and reasonably safe)

b) Eldepryl (is a selegine pill)

c) Nardil (related to (d) and (e))

d) (Iproniazid and Nialimide) (related to (c) and (e))

e) Marplan

f) Nardil

g) Parnate (related to amphetamine)

h) (Moclobemide is available in Europe)

7) European and Canadian antidepressants (such as mianserin, amineptine, nomifensine, Zelmid, Edronax, Moclobemide, et al.)

The specific drugs are listed here alphabetically, as it is assumed that the reader does not want any further comprehensive lesson in pharmacology or chemistry.

<u>Antidepressants listed alphabetically by name</u> (as well as useful terminology)
(listed by both generic name and branded name)
Including important activity as antidepressants as well as salient facts for patients

---

Adderall—see Stimulant antidepressants

Amoxapine—see Asendin

Amphetamines—see Stimulant antidepressants

Amitriptyline—this is generic Elavil; when this generic form first became available, some patients complained that it did not seem the same as brand-name Elavil; this has not been reported as a problem in later years; see Elavil

Anafranil—is a potent tricyclic antidepressant with pronounced serotonin (5-HT) effects that give it good anti-obsessive properties. Apart from that, its side effects are listed with the other Tricyclic antidepressants below.

Antidepressants in general—can cause dry mouth, nervousness, insomnia. Various antidepressants are used to treat ADDH: Effexor, Imipramine, Strattera, Wellbutrin, and the stimulant antidepressants such as Ritalin, Concerta, Adderall, Vyvanse, et al.

Asendin—is a tricyclic, but is also closely related to an antipsychotic medication, Loxitane. Both have serotonin activity. Asendin has milder side effects than the [other] tricyclics. It is unique among the tricyclics for having both serotonin and dopamine activity—this is probably why it is less sedating. However, it can cause Parkinsonism that is often permanent. Its use should be restricted to psychiatrists only. It is good as an alternative for mixed mood and thought disorders or psychotic depression.

Atomoxatine (antidepressant used for ADDH)—see Strattera

BRAND-NAME DRUGS, BRANDED DRUGS, PATENT MEDICINES, TRADE-NAME MEDICATIONS: these are the original medications which were first marketed by the parent drug company; when the drug company's seventeen year patent expired, then generic versions of the branded drug were allowed to be sold; when very popular branded drugs become generic, there may be two or more generic companies marketing generic versions—if this is the case, some patients may notice a difference between the branded and generic drugs—and may also notice a difference between generic versions made by different generic drug companies; for this reason, it is wise to try to stabilize on particular version and stick with it; unpopular branded drugs may not have any generic alternatives available—or the parent company may simply repackage its own branded drug in a different sized and colored pill and make a virtual monopoly of the branded and the [only] generic version (in this case, the generic will not be cheap); if the parent company continues to make only its branded version and if one generic drug company is the sole provider of the generic version, then the generic version will also not be cheap; In these latter cases, you might ask, 'so what's the big deal about a costly generic?'—the big deal is that your HMO will offer you the generic at a cheaper rate (the same generic co-pay you pay for all your other generic drugs: the costly generic is only costly if you have no health insurance prescription plan);

Bupropion—see Wellbutrin

Buspar (Anti-anxiety medication with mild antidepressant properties) Buspar was originally developed as an antidepressant, but at the higher doses required for antidepressant activity it caused too many side effects in human volunteers. This highlights the fact that early experiments with effects on rats do not always translate to humans. The dosage was lowered and Buspar was brought to market as an anti-anxiety agent. Many antidepressants in very low dose can have anti-anxiety effects, an observation that is of constant benefit to doctors and drug companies. The typical side effects of Buspar are: dizziness, queasiness, headache, nervousness. The biggest side effect is that it does not always provide any significant effect to some people. It is not addicting and needs to be taken on a daily basis for best results, although some people use it on an "as-needed" basis. Its anti-anxiety effects appear after a few days. Buspar will not help Panic attacks at all; it can not be used with MAOI antidepressants because it is an antidepressant, technically speaking; Buspar may be used successfully with other antidepressants such as Effexor or Prozac with the reminder that the patient will technically be taking two antidepressants—not one plus Buspar. Buspar belongs to a group of three other drugs (Desyrel and Serzone are both antidepressants) none of which has any negative effect on sexual function—indeed, some of these might slightly enhance sexual function.

Buspirone—see Buspar

Celexa—this is the fourth medication in the SSRI class. It offers another treatment option for people who do not do well with other SSRI medications. See side effects of SSRI under SSRI's. Celexa is less likely to cause "discontinuation syndrome". Some people require higher doses of Celexa, and the HMO insurance plans are very reluctant to authorize this (extra expense). Fortunately, Celexa is now available in a less expensive generic presentation. And, Celexa is now available in a "purified" version called Lexapro. See Lexapro.

Citalopram—see Celexa

"CLEAN" drug—has very few unpleasant side effects (in the majority of patients): Lexapro and Desyrel (Trazodone) are examples. Serzone was also—until we learned that it has the risk of liver failure. See "dirty drug".

Clomipramine—see Anafranil

Concerta—see Stimulant antidepressants

Cylert—currently off the market in USA; it is FDA approved and can be ordered from Canada; it is not highly addicting, but may cause liver stress—especially in children; Cylert is a stimulating antidepressant and has some use in ADHD.

Cymbalta—is a SSNRI which means that it acts on serotonin and nor-adrenaline which are two of the three actions that confer presumed antidepressant activity. (The third action would be on dopamine which is not affected by Cymbalta.) Cymbalta is also approved for diabetic nerve pain. (see Effexor); it can raise blood pressure and is mildly to moderately stimulating;

Desipramine—see Norpramin

Desoxyn—see Stimulant antidepressants

Desvenlafaxine—see Pristiq/Effexor

Desyrel—is a multi-purpose antidepressant related to Serzone (and Buspar) that is so frequently used, that it is usually called by its generic name, Trazodone; It functions as a calmative antidepressant to be given twice or more per day; it has found its market "niche", however, as a sleeping pill for patients who are mildly Depressed and who have trouble sleeping; even more commonly it us used with the SSRI and SSNRI antidepressants either as a secondary antidepressant or as a sleeping aid; it is very popular with psychiatrists; most people who take it, report good success; a few people stop taking Desyrel because it makes them dizzy or nauseous; it is best absorbed with a very small carbohydrate snack; it should not be used in men who are not impotent since it can cause priapism which becomes a medical emergency that in extremely rare cases can result in permanent impotence: I discuss this with male patients, and nobody wants to take it except for those men are permanently impotent from diabetes or prostate surgery, or who have had a penis removed for penile cancer (one case)—I had one female patient who once reported clitoral discomfort—I have prescribed it to thousands of women without any other such reports; Desyrel *must not* be prescribed in cases of severe heart problems called ventricular arrhythmias; Trazodone blood levels are available, but are almost never necessary; Trazodone does not cause cataracts as once thought (the early research had been done with beagles who are well known to develop cataracts naturally);

Dexedrine—is available in several sizes as well as timed release preparations— see Stimulants

Dextro-amphetamine—see Dexedrine and Stimulant antidepressants

"DIRTY" drugs—have a large number of unpleasant side effects in the majority of patients; examples would be Clozaril; (Nardil, too). See "clean" drugs.

DISCONTINUATION SYNDROME—Some patients experience several days of "flu-like" symptoms after stopping a serotonin drug (SSRI or SSNRI). This is not a true withdrawal and does not equate to addiction. This episode is harmless. If warranted, patients should be given a doctor's note of excuse from work for a few days.

Dopamine—one of the three main brain chemicals ("brain hormones") that are thought to play a role in Depression: it is theorized that a deficiency of one or more of these chemicals might cause Depression; Depressed persons who take an antidepressant that boosts these chemicals will often feel better while taking the antidepressant—and feel worse sometimes if the medication is stopped; the other two brain chemicals are norepinephrine (noradrenalin) and serotonin (there are many chemicals that have recently been identified as being involved in Depression, and research is continuing in this arena); most antidepressants affect of one these three chemicals more robustly than the other two: patients who take two or more antidepressants are deemed to be in need of boosting two or more brain chemicals;

Doxepin—see Sinequan

Duloxetine—see Cymbalta

Effexor—is a SSNRI medication which is active on serotonin at lower doses and active on both serotonin and nor-adrenaline at higher doses; this activity results in decreasing nerve pains and chronic pain; Effexor is also an effective antidepressant; it has a few side effects such as headaches and dizziness, but these usually disappear after the first or second week of treatment; Effexor can cause constipation; Effexor can aggravate high blood pressure or even cause high blood pressure which is sometimes difficult to control with the usual blood pressure pills; Effexor can also cause discontinuation syndrome (see chapter on terminology); Effexor is available in rapid-release tablets and delayed-release capsules; the commonest side effect with the tablets is stomach irritation which can be treated with "Histamine/H_2 blockers" like Zantac (see below); Effexor is now available in a new "purified" version, Pristiq;

Elavil—is one of the older tricyclics; it has been used for many psychiatric, neurological, and medical purposes, including but not limited to: depression, anxiety, insomnia, migraines, and chronic pain; It has all the usual tricyclic antidepressants and is the most commonly prescribed in the USA; It has effects on the nor-adrenaline and serotonin systems; see Tricyclics, Amitriptyline, and Pamelor; Our bodies make Pamelor out of Elavil, but this does not mean that the uses and advantages of Elavil are the same as those for Pamelor. Each medicine has slightly different uses. In theory Pamelor could be helpful for chronic pain, but is rarely used this way. I have had a couple chronic pain patients start on Elavil and then go on to need high doses, which in turn caused side effects. Elavil side effects in these cases might be improved by changing to Pamelor. Pain control was about as good and the Elavil side effects were better.

Eldepryl (is a selegine pill—also see Emsam)—Edepryl is Selegiline which is a MAOI antidepressant. It is useful for Parkinsonism and depression; it is available for use as an oral antidepressant, also. Eldepryl does not require a special diet when given at low doses but at high doses does require a special diet, which is rather complicated. When used as an antidepressant, it is more likely to require a higher dose than that used by neurologists to treat Parkinsonism. If a Depressed patient is taking a higher oral dose, then he will have two choices: either learn to follow the diet; or, use the Emsam patch which is absorbed directly.

Emsam (is a selegiline skin patch, effective and safe—see Eldepryl) If the patch irritates your skin, you can ask your doctor to prescribe a steroid inhaler to pre-treat the skin. The patch can be cut into pieces to make different sized doses, such as 7 ½ mg.

Epinephrine—see Dopamine

Escitalopram—see Lexapro

Etrafon—see Triavil

Eutonyl—an old blood pressure pill that was rarely used as an antidepressant—it belongs to the MAOI Antidepressants

Fenfluramine—see Pondimin

Fluoxetine—see Prozac

Fluvoxamine—see Luvox

GENERIC DRUGS—see branded drugs; see Chapter V-14 on Generic Drugs

Imipramine—see Tofranil

Ionamin—is an amphetamine derivative primarily used as a diet pill. It is effective for weight control, but only while it is being taken continuously. Once the pill is stopped, the person is likely to regain weight unless she has made major modifications to her lifestyle in the meantime: daily aerobics, non-caloric beverages, low fat diet incorporating protein with high biological value, and so on. It has occasionally been used in Depression as a secondary drug. Like all the amphetamines, it can have cardiovascular effects in the long term.

Isocarboxazid—see Marplan

Lexapro—is a SSRI which is the "purified" form of Celexa (also a SSRI).

Ludiomil—is a medication similar to the tricyclics, but having a unique structure and somewhat differing side effects as well as desirable effects. Low-dose Ludiomil is used extensively in Europe and Latin America for anxiety and mild depression. When it was first marketed in the USA, its competitors created the impression that it causes seizures—this risk is minimal but can increase if it is used in very high doses. A few other antidepressants can cause seizures when used [at very high doses]: Anafranil and Wellbutrin, for example. Any possible risk of seizure can be minimized by starting at a low dose and increasing slowly—which is really how most psychoactive medications should be prescribed, anyway. It can be used for anxious depression, dysthymia, or depression. It has a well-rounded spectrum of beneficial effects and side effects. Not overly stimulating or sedating and results in less weight gain. It favors activation of the nor-adrenaline system, and hence, can be used—if necessary—with low dose SSRI's (Lexapro or Prozac) to favor a broader range of antidepressant activity.

Luvox—is another of the SSRI antidepressants. It has good antidepressant effects and is used to treat Depression in Europe. So why isn't it an antidepressant in the USA? It is. Yet apart from its antidepressant effects, it exerts even more anti-obsessive properties than any of the other SSRI's. All of the SSRI's have some degree of anti-obsessive properties, but Luvox has it in abundance. Its parent drug company decided to bring it to market here as a treatment for obsessive-compulsive disorders, with its only competition at that time, having been Nardil (a complicated MAOI drug) and Anafranil which is a tricyclic and not a SSRI; hence, each of these three drugs carved out its own unique place in a "niche" market (for the treatment of obsessions and compulsions). American psychiatrists already knew that Luvox was also a potent antidepressant and did not hesitate to use it in depressions that had been resistant to many other medications, and in these cases it often worked well. The big drawback of Luvox is that it interferes with many other medications. For this reason it is not ideal for elderly patients or anyone who is taking a lot of other medicines.

Maprotiline—see Ludiomil

Marplan—is one of the old MAOI medications and has a very small following. It should be *prescribed only by psychiatrists* who are familiar with its effects and complicated side effects.

Mazindol (an old diet pill)—this has dubious antidepressant effects, but has been used in very rare instances.

Meridia—this is a diet pill with questionable effects on Depression.

Mirtazapine—see Remeron

Modafanil—see Provigil/Nuvigil

Nardil—this is an old MAOI antidepressant. It *should be prescribed only by psychiatrists* who are familiar with its complex suite of side effects and beneficial effects. It is very helpful for selected patients. It is hard to believe now, but Nardil was once a novel antidepressant with a popular following. It debuted at a time when there were only three families of antidepressants: amphetamines, MAOI, and a few Tricyclics. When Nardil was a big "hammer", it was used on many "nails". It has since then been superseded by many new classes of antidepressants, most of which are safer (Prozac). Nardil is still very effective for certain types of depression, panic, obsessions, and "hysteroid dysphoria" . A person taking Nardil needs to follow a very specific and restricted diet, otherwise she may run the risk of having a stroke or other cardiovascular misadventure. When it is prescribed in the usual method, it will not have any effects until between the fifth and sixth weeks of treatment. These patients need to have regular monitoring of their vital signs (blood pressure, pulse, temperature). Side effects can include flushing, dizziness, sexual dysfunction, and insomnia—these will appear after the sixth week of treatment.

Nefazodone—see Serzone

Noradrenaline—see Dopamine.

Norepinephrine—see Dopamine

Norpramin—this is a tricyclic antidepressant with fewer side effects. It is the "purified" form of Tofranil (Imipramine) and has minimal side effects, compared to the other tricyclics. Norpramin is mildly stimulating. The only Tricyclic that is more stimulating is Vivactil. It favors the nor-adrenaline system and can be used with low doses of SSRI's if need be.

Nortriptyline—see Pamelor

Nuvigil (a stimulant with secondary antidepressant properties); this is the "purified" form of Provigil—see Provigil.

Pamelor—this is a Tricyclic and the "purified" form of Elavil; its popularity is waning somewhat. It has effects on nor-adrenaline. Our bodies make Pamelor out of Elavil, but this does not mean that the uses and advantages of Elavil are the same as those for Pamelor. Each medicine has slightly different uses. In theory Pamelor could be helpful for chronic pain, but is rarely used this way. I have had a couple chronic pain patients start on Elavil and then go on to need high doses, which in turn caused side effects. Elavil side effects in these cases might be improved by changing to Pamelor. Pain control was about as good and the Elavil side effects were better. See Elavil,

Parnate –see MAOI, tranylcypromine

Paroxetine—see Paxil

Paxil—is similar to the other SSRI drugs with a few exceptions. Paxil can have histamine-like effects which can cause hunger and, thus, weight gain. At very high doses, it may demonstrate mild stimulation due to a slight norepinephrine-like effect that might appear in some patients. Paxil is probably the likeliest of the SSRI medications to cause "discontinuation syndrome". Paxil is also very effective for premature ejaculation (see SSRI).

Phenelzine—see Nardil

Phentermine—see Ionamin

Pondimin (fenfluramine)—is an amphetamine marketed for weight loss.

Pristiq—is the "purified" form of Effexor—see Effexor.

Protriptyline—see Vivactil

Provigil—a stimulant with secondary antidepressant properties

Prozac—Prozac has a long history dating back to the 1980's. Prozac has a chemical structure based on that of amphetamines, but is not addicting. When it first appeared, it was quickly recognized as a vast advance in the treatment of depression. It was active on the serotonin system. It was activating (in some cases too much so), it was safe in overdose (very important property); as time went on we also learned to mix it with other antidepressants for enhanced depression activity. Most antidepressants should not be prescribed to manic or psychotic patients (patients who might have post-psychotic Depression or Manic Depression). In these cases, any antidepressant might set off a manic or psychotic episode, which can be a very harrowing experience for patients and those in their surroundings. In the mid-to-late 1990's, Prozac received a bad [undeserved] reputation from which it has never fully recovered, in the sense that I still see first-time patients who refuse even to try Prozac. It can be used in Depression, Bulimia, and obsessions. It is approved for use in children and teenagers. See also SSRI's.

Psychostimulants—see Stimulants

Remeron—is a sedating antidepressant which can be given in the evening to promote sleep for the night and antidepressant effects on the following day. It is also quite agreeable for use in recovering alcoholics. Remeron can cause hunger and fluid retention—and hence, weight gain. A number of patients do not like its sedation or other side effects. For those who tolerate it well, it is very helpful. It is available in a special "Sol-tab" table that dissolves on the tongue. The Sol-tab is very effective for patients who can not or will not swallow. It is the active ingredient ("purified version") of Mianserin, an old sedating antidepressant.

Ritalin—see Stimulant antidepressants

Selegiline—see Eldepryl and Emsam

Serotonin—see Dopamine

SEROTONIN SYNDROME—is a serious emergency medical condition that can suddenly arise from having too much serotonin stimulation in the body: it would be associated with many of the usual antidepressants that have any effect on the serotonin system; it can arise most commonly if two such antidepressants are used together; the symptoms are: restlessness, twitching, jerking, sweating, shivering, confusion, fever, visual hallucinations, as well as changes in heart beat and blood pressure; if this happens, the patient needs to be taken to the nearest ER. Migraine pills such as Midrin and the "triptans" could also set off this cascade of events.

Sertraline—see Zoloft

Serzone (no longer routinely used in USA)

SIDE EFFECTS: a few generalizations can be made about side effects (derived from my experience): (1) rashes are likelier with stimulating drugs: Vivactil, Prozac, Paxil, Effexor, (Merital); (2) serotonin drugs can cause serotonin syndrome when drug levels are too high—wheras serotonin drugs can cause discontinuation syndrome symptoms when their blood levels fall toward zero; (3) norepinephrine drugs can raise blood pressure—permanently; (4) dopamine drugs can cause agitation, twitchiness, and repetitive movements; (5) the rates of sexual dysfunction in men taking SSRI/SSNRI drugs is higher than officially listed;

Sinequan—is the branded name for Doxepin. Doxepin is a very popular Tricyclic antidepressant. It is almost as popular as Elavil. (In Europe and Latin America, Ludiomil would typically be used in low doses in the way that Elavil and Sinequan are used here.) Doxepin has effects on Serotonin and nor-adrenaline systems. It also has a lot of anti-histamine effects, which result in sedation, weight gain, deep sleep, and drying effects (ideal for hay fever or sinus sufferers). It also has anti-acid properties and enjoyed a certain vogue in Sweden in the 1970's as a stomach pill for ulcer patients: it has drying and soothing effects on the stomach and helps control constant low-grade burning pain (of stomach ulcers). It also causes low blood pressure. In low dosage, these effects make it ideal for anxious young men, and for patients who want to dry out some part of their organ systems (hay fever, stomach acidity)—but too much drying and slowing can result in constipation, urine retention, blurred vision, and dry mouth. It lasts a long time in the body. It has some interactions with regular medical drugs. It causes excess sedation when used with other sedating medications. For all these reasons, it should usually be avoided in geriatric patients—unless they have been taking it for decades and are already stabilized on it: in these cases, the baseline dose should, however, be further reduced to the lowest possible dose, because it *will* cause these side effects in elderly patients.

In other words, in elderly patients, these will be all the possible problems: (a) fainting spells in the daytime, and even more so in the wee hours while urinating; (b) worsening of prostate symptoms (difficulty in producing a stream of urine); (c) other possible cardiovascular problems (although in low doses it usually should not cause irregular heart beats); (d) constipation; (e) general weight gain which in itself can aggravate arthritis by creating more weight to be dragged around; (f) any weight gain which can aggravate any diabetes or "early" diabetes; (g) abdominal weight gain can aggravate the labor of breathing in emphysema; (h) worsening of glaucoma and cataracts due to Doxepin's proclivity to cause blurred vision—and it should really be avoided altogether in glaucoma patients—if eye patients want to continue taking Doxepin, then I insist on ophthalmology approval. It was used extensively in Dermatology for drying the skin or for decreasing itching. It does not cause a spectacular weight gain in Anorexia. It is available as a liquid also.

SNRI—Vestra (reboxitene, Edronax) and Strattera (Atomoxetine) are two SNRI drugs

SSNRI—Cymbalta, Effexor, Pristiq: these drugs have varying effects on serotonin and nor-adrenaline, depending on: (1)-which drug is taken; (2) the person's genetic ability to use the drug; and (3) the dosage range. For example, Effexor affects serotonin in low and medium doses, but then at higher doses, Effexor affects serotonin and nor-adrenaline. Effexor might cause "discontinuation syndrome" (see under SSRI).

SSRI—this is a heterogeneous group of medications that includes Celexa, Lexapro, Luvox, Paxil, Prozac, and Zoloft. As a group they have a number of similar properties and side effects. ~~Beneficial effects include the large number of psychiatric diagnoses that may be treated with these drugs: anxiety disorders, Depression, and Obsessive-Compulsions: in low doses these medications can help anxiety disorders whereas higher doses are often needed for Depression and Obsessions; in low doses they may control premature ejaculation (e.g. Paxil) ~~ Side effects can include dizziness, nausea, diarrhea, headache, confusion, nervousness, sedation, as well as rash and bruising; Any rash requires stopping the medication immediately; bruising is related to the location of serotonin receptors on the platelets in our blood; the other side effects are typical of the first week of treatment, and patients should be encouraged to continue the SSRI—this is the reason why I usually start patients with a half dose in the first week: less discomfort; ~~One of the more distressing side effects is that of the so-called "discontinuation syndrome". Discontinuation Syndrome represents a group of symptoms that may occur in patients who quit taking a SSRI medication. This occurs in only a fraction of patients. It usually occurs in patients who have adapted well to the drug and like its positive effects but have decided to quit it—for one reason or another. The patients who did not like the SSRI are glad to be rid of it because it either did not help them or caused a lot of annoying physical side effects. The Discontinuation symptoms will appear within a day or two (or longer time interval with long-acting SSRI's such as Prozac) and will last for a few or several days. The symptoms are usually those of "flu", such as aches, headaches, dizziness, as well as racing thoughts or lethargy. This is technically not "withdrawal". "Withdrawal" is a term we use for the possibly life-threatening symptoms and signs that occur when a drug addict or alcoholic experiences if they do not get their regular dose of drug or alcohol; symptoms of withdrawal are vastly more disabling that those of Discontinuation. Discontinuation Syndrome produces no [direct] lethal effects. Symptoms of Discontinuation do not ever approach the severity or lethality of the symptoms of Drug-Alcohol Withdrawal. It is entirely reasonable to give a Discontinuation patient time off from work (a couple or few days). If a second SSRI is being chosen as a replacement for the first annoying SSRI, the switch can often be done expeditiously over a long weekend without too much discomfort (but there may be some for two to five days). The maneuver of this depends upon the half-life of the first SSRI, the patient's reaction, and the psychiatrist's philosophy / experience.

Stimulant Antidepressants—also called Psychostimulants which name should give you a good idea of their effects and potency; in a sense, any antidepressant that causes euphoria could be a psycho-stimulant, but it is generally accepted that this term refers to the amphetamines and several other types of medications, all of which are habit-forming or addictive;

Strattera (a European antidepressant used for ADDH in the USA)

Surmontil—is a Tricyclic antidepressant with short-acting properties; it is like Sinequan but with all the side effects much reduced; it may help onset of sleep; the biggest advantage is not awakening in the morning with such grogginess as with Sinequan; Surmontil may be rather stimulating for some people;

Tofranil—is a Tricyclic antidepressant with all around generalized side effects and with a number of uses: most importantly, it is an effective antidepressant which tends to be sedating in lower doses, but more activating in much higher doses; it can be used in obsessive compulsions and panic-anxiety—it worked fairly well when it was about the only prescription we had for these purposes (when Anafranil was available in Canada but not here); it could be used in ADHD/ ADD but its use in teenage boys has been possibly loosely associated with two or three sudden heart attacks per year in this country; its "purified" form is called Norpramin (Desipramine);

Tranylcypromine—see Parnate

Trazodone—see Desyrel

Triavil—is a fixed combination of Elavil and Perphenazine and seems to work better than taking each drug in two separate pills; it was used in psychotic depressions, involutional melancholy, and depression linked to chronic pain; also marketed as Etrafon;

Tricyclic antidepressants—this broad family of medications includes all those listed above in the section alphabetized by chemical family. They all share certain side effects: mild sedation, dry mouth, blurred vision, constipation, urine retention, dry skin, changes in blood pressure and pulse. Any of these side effects is possible, but most people only have one or two of the side effects most of which improve by using "helpful" drugs listed below in the section on side effect pills. Some may cause a rash, whereas Sinequan can be used to decrease itching (due to its antihistamine properties, not its antidepressant properties); they can be helpful for certain kinds of chronic pain (shingles, back pain, other pains); Vivactil can cause some cardiovascular side effects and should not be used in the elderly; Doxepin can cause low blood pressure and likewise should be avoided in the elderly. (See Chapter V-7)

Trimipramine—see Surmontil

Venlafaxine—see Effexor (and its "purified" version, Pristiq)

Vivactil—is an activating Tricyclic which I use a lot as a second or third tier medication in depressed women; it is especially helpful if these women report extreme stimulation from the SSRI's, (Effexor, or Wellbutrin); It can have cardiac effects and it use should suggest the need to obtain a baseline EKG; it can be used in ADD, it can be used in combination with low-dose Effexor; it is not for use in the elderly;

Vyvanse—see amphetamines: this medication is taken in its "pro-drug" form which means that it can not be artificially altered [easily] in a drug-dealer's laboratory in an attempt to turn it into street-grade amphetamine; it can only be turned into the active drug when ingested by a human. But it is then turned into a stimulant just like any other stimulant drug.

Wellbutrin—can be stimulating to some people due to the fact that it can activate two antidepressant effects (dopamine and adrenaline). ~~Its stimulating side effects are most apparent in the first one to three weeks of treatment (especially in the first week). This is one reason that it is not usually considered a first-line medication for agitated Depression, Psychotic Depression, or in any Depression that could not tolerate stimulation (such as patients who are already over-stimulated from asthma medicines, prednisone, or who have a family history of bipolar depression, and other clinical situations). I do not use it as a first-line or second-line medication in most people who are trying to recover from alcoholism and sedative drug addiction, since these people can be quite sensitive to its stimulating properties and may also be more prone to seizures in general. It can be effective in recovering "speed" addicts (addiction to stimulant drugs); When I start patients on Wellbutrin, the experience is much more tolerable if we start with very very small doses and then increase up to normal adult doses after one to three weeks—this maneuver is also thought to reduce the risk of side effects, especially seizure. None of my Wellbutrin-treated patients has experienced a seizure, perhaps due to this practice of "go low-go slow". ~~In its earliest clinical trials, Wellbutrin raised an index of suspicion that it might aggravate or cause seizures. Therefore, it is not to be used in patients who have Epilepsy or Bulimia, as it might cause seizures. I have never used it in these two types of patients. None of my Wellbutrin-treated patients has experienced seizures, despite the FDA warnings that 2% of all patients might have seizures—even if they had never had epilepsy or bulimia. Most psychiatrists do not report any increase in seizures with Wellbutrin—no more seizures than with any other semi-stimulating antidepressant.~~ Its main short-term side effects are overstimulation; its main long-term side-effects are constipation and dizziness. Since it is derived from the old diet pill, Tenuate, it is rarely associated with weight gain. Wellbutrin and Serzone are the only two antidepressants which are least likely to cause sexual side effects. Wellbutrin can cause cardiovascular side effects with symptoms of dizziness or head buzzing. Rashes are possible. Oftentimes, patients may report that they felt stimulated in the first week of treatment, but then started to feel calmer after three weeks: they like this effect and it seems to parallel what happens when we use antidepressant medication to treat ADDH (All the treatments for ADDH are simply antidepressants of various classes). ~~ Wellbutrin has an added convenience of being available in short-acting pills, intermediate-acting pills, and long-lasting pills. Some people who like Wellbutrin's mild stimulation derive great benefit from it in the daytime, but then complain of insomnia (at bedtime). These people can be given a form of shorter acting Wellbutrin that should wear off by nighttime.

Zoloft—is a SSRI drug with a general well-rounded side effect profile and useful for various kinds of Depression and Anxiety Disorders. See SSRI's; useful in geriatrics.

Weak Antidepressants

These are medications that have mild antidepressant activities of their own and can be used as "boosters" for the primary antidepressants.

a) Abilify—can be used in small to moderate doses for serious mood disorders; it has few side effects;

b) Aripiprazole—see Abilify above

c) Buspar/Buspirone (see above)

d) Lamictal/Lamotrigine—is very effective for bipolar depression. Lamictal should be started in tiny doses and increased slowly to avoid a possible life-threatening skin reaction. For this reason, Lamictal needs to be started preventively since it will have a lag time of a month or two before it becomes beneficial; hence, it cannot be used as an emergency treatment.

e) Lithium—can be helpful for serious depression (agitated, bipolar, recurrent unipolar, or schizoaffective depression). Lithium can be very toxic and dangerous and should be taken only by prescription from a psychiatrist. Its lethal dose is only slightly higher than its therapeutic dose level. It can reach poisonous levels quickly. Fortunately, if it is used only as a secondary drug for depression, it is needed in small enough doses that high blood levels are unlikely. Most Lithium patients gain weight, retain fluid, have mild hand tremors, and occasional diarrhea—even when it is not at a lethal dose. However, patients with these serious depressions may only need low-dose lithium and maybe only for a few months, depending on the case. If the lithium level is too high, there will be much trembling and spasticity. This poisoning is related to the fact that Lithium levels are very dependent on the amount of water and table salt consumed. Hot weather and sweating can affect Lithium levels as can alterations of salt in food and amount of water and fluids consumed. Also over-the-counter pills like ibuprofen or naproxen can cause altered lithium levels. Anyone who takes Lithium needs to have regular monitoring. Even if Lithium patients feel really well for years or decades, they will usually need to face the reality that long-term Lithium use can also lead to thyroid and kidney problems.

f) Olanzapine—see Zyprexa—see Chapter V-4

g) Risperdal/Risperidone—see Chapter V-4

h) Thyroid hormone / Cytomel (T$_3$)—may animate a depressed person who is already taking one or two antidepressants.

i) Trazodone—can be added at bedtime in low doses to help onset of sleep. It can be used with any of the SSRI-NSRI-NSSRI medications—however, Trazodone can interact with these medications in rare cases, causing a serious condition called "Serotonin Syndrome" (see above). Your psychiatrist is aware of this possibility; if your primary doctor is prescribing these medications, he may not be aware of this rare but serious condition. I do not use Trazodone with any other primary antidepressants apart from the SSRI-SNRI-SSNRI medications. I do not encourage family doctors to mix and match psychiatric drugs.

j) Zyprexa—has mild antidepressant effects and can be helpful for psychotic or agitated depressions. It works very well. Younger patients may gain a great deal of weight (25-50 pounds or more). The weight gain may cause diabetes. (see Chapter V-4).

Minerals (Lithium)
Herbs
Prescription-Grade "Natural" Drugs

Chapter Outline
MINERALS: Lithium and Bromide
HERBS: St. John's Wort Valeriana Kava kava
"NATURALS": barbiturates caffeine galantamine guaranà melatonin L-Tryptophan

Some people want to be "natural" and eschew use of synthetic chemicals made in factories. These people feel reassured by resorting to the use of so-called "natural" treatment substances. Unfortunately, these therapies are fraught with their own drawbacks, too. It is true that modern antidepressants are usually purified synthetic (artificial) chemicals. These are definitely poisons consumed in small sub-lethal amounts. Our body (liver) will not acknowledge these as "natural". Ever. However, many of the so-called natural treatments are a mixture of chemicals, also, which can be just as harmful to our bodies.

Minerals such as lithium or bromide can be very dangerous. Lithium occurs naturally as lithium chloride. We can take lithium as this salt, but nowadays it is reprocessed and chemically combined with carbonate or citrate of pharmaceutical grade. Bromides need to be chemically combined with minerals to produce bromide salts. Although lithium and bromide are simple elements, they are both *inorganic* chemicals whereas our bodies are composed mainly of organic chemicals.

As far as herbs, our livers must work very hard when we take herbs. This is because our liver has to process the herb. Herbs are dried plants (plant parts), and dried plants contain most of the same chemicals as a live plant, in other words, hundreds or thousands of plant chemicals coming from a living organism. Our liver needs to assess and address all these botanical chemicals—each chemical needs its own special processing.

There are also natural substances that can be derived from the plant world and isolated down to a single chemical. That single chemical may be the active ingredient with the desirable medicinal value. Examples would include Reserpine, Ephedrine, galantamine, and Digoxin. Although these substances occur in Nature, the process of collecting and isolating the medicinal substance is too expensive, so they are also made in a factory. Perhaps these are the safest—from the "natural" viewpoint—because they do occur in nature and they are one purified chemical compressed into a tablet.

There are a lot of herbs and natural treatments, which are very good. We have co-existed on Earth with these herbs for a long time and have learned to harvest and use them medicinally.

MINERALS

Lithium

(Also see Chapter VI-10)

Lithium and its family members: Sodium and Potassium

Lithium is one member of the six-member alkali earth metal family. The members of this family in order from lightest to heaviest are: Lithium, sodium, potassium, rubidium, cesium, and francium. Lithium is the smallest member of the family. Sodium is the second lightest member. The two natural earth elements just above lithium are the well-known minerals, sodium and potassium. Rubidium has not panned out as a suitable medical therapy, whereas cesium and francium are downright poisonous. Lithium is a naturally occurring salt as are its "chemical siblings", sodium and potassium. They are all three very abundant and common salts. This is the same sodium we know as table salt (sodium chloride), also found in baking soda and Alka-Seltzer® (sodium bicarbonate). This is the same potassium used as potassium chloride (KCl) in salt-substitutes (Morton Lite Salt®, No-Salt®). Likewise, Lithium salt (LiCl) was once used as a salt substitute, but some heart patients used too much of it. Lithium salt and sodium salt are obtained from salt deposits and salt mines.

Since lithium, sodium, and potassium are inorganic chemicals as well as being alkali earth metals, humans can get very ill from consuming too much of any one of them. If we have twice the amount of potassium, sodium, or lithium that are bodies will tolerate, we can get sick and die.

Actually, we cannot even tolerate a doubled amount of sodium in our bodies, so we are least tolerant to excesses of sodium; however, our body (kidney) is more proficient at dealing with abnormal levels of sodium. Lethal doses of lithium and sodium usually involve nervous system malfunction; potassium can cause heart attack or heart failure.

Sodium and potassium are important minerals that are found in every cell of our bodies. (Lithium is not—lithium is not normally even in our bodies.) Our bodies need sodium and potassium salts in order to maintain health and to stay alive. Like all chemicals and minerals, however, we can be poisoned by too much sodium or potassium—and medically compromised by too little (See Chapter VI-10). Therefore, our bodies maintain rather strict controls over the levels of sodium and potassium in our bodies (in health). Any significant imbalances result first in sickness and then in death. For example, if levels of these salts in our bodies increase or decrease by 8-25% (8% sodium-25% potassium), then we can die from heart or nerve problems. If sodium levels drop too low, this will cause permanent brain damage, progressing on to seizures and death. The same is true of patients taking lithium: any significant excess can lead to seizures and death.

These are the percentage tolerances in variation that our bodies will tolerate:

- Sodium 8% variation (up or down)

- Potassium 25% variation (up or down)

- Lithium 50% variation (above maximum dose)

(there is no direct brain or heart damage from too little lithium in our bodies, since it is not normally present at all in our body; the indirect lethal outcome of too little lithium occurs only in the case where a manic depressive quits taking his lithium pills and becomes so manic that he does something reckless that results in his death)

Our kidneys are in charge of keeping sodium balanced. Kidneys also are involved in keeping balanced lithium levels. When the kidneys work well, then our sodium levels will hopefully be normal; likewise, when the kidneys work well in lithium-treated patients, the kidneys will also help maintain reasonable levels of lithium, by balancing sodium levels. Since Lithium is so closely related to sodium, it can move around the body as if it were sodium. The kidneys treat lithium as if it were sodium. In the kidneys, Lithium has the same "security clearance" as does sodium. Anything that lowers the levels of sodium will raise the levels of lithium and vice versa. Lithium levels do not need to increase very much to become toxic: the warning signs of high lithium levels are jittery hands, trembling, and diarrhea (see below).

Sodium and potassium are naturally very prevalent everywhere in our bodies, whereas lithium is not naturally found in our bodies. The only way to get Lithium into our body is to eat Lithium salt.

Lithium belongs to the family of alkali earth metals.

Table V-10 Lithium   Sodium (NaCl) is what we use everyday as table salt.

Chemical	Lithium **Li⁺**	Sodium (natrium) **Na⁺**	Potassium (kalium) **K⁺**
Edible salt Substitute	LiCl (No longer in use)	NaCl Table salt	KCl* Still in use as table salt
Current Medical use	Psychiatry	Internal Medicine e.g. Normal saline Intravenous fluid	Cardiology, Internal Medicine 1-For low potassium levels 2-Salt substitute*

(there are many salt substitutes containing potassium; for example, Morton's Lite contains sodium, potassium, calcium, and magnesium—plus iodide.) Ask your doctor before using!

In table V-10, we see that Li⁺, K⁺, and Na⁺ all have one (+) positive charge. Magnesium and Calcium have two (++) positive charges (Mg⁺⁺, Ca⁺⁺). Calcium and magnesium have no specific use in psychiatry but imbalances of these two metals can present with symptoms that may look like psychiatric symptoms: sluggishness, agitation.

Lithium

Lithium is as old as dirt—that's because lithium *is* dirt! (The Greek word "lithos" means "stone"). Lithium is extremely abundant in the Earth's crust and in rocks. Lithium comes from lithium mines: one of the largest is in North Carolina, another is in Bolivia. There are also natural spring waters that are rich in lithium and have a particular taste. These spring waters were used in the past as a beverage. Since lithium is so old and stable, lithium itself really has no expiration date—or at least the lithium crystal has no known expiration date.

When Lithium is sold as a prescription pill, it comes as lithium carbonate or lithium citrate. Both carbonate and citrate are also natural substances. Carbonate is commonly found in baking soda and stones (e.g. limestone) and in carbonated beverages (soda pop). Citrate (citric acid) is a natural molecule found in citrus fruits, animals, and human bodies. Lithium carbonate is a powder at room temperature and will dissolve in water. Lithium pills are available as tablets, capsules, or slow-release timed tablets. Lithium citrate is available as a liquid (this liquid can be used for patients with swallowing problems or who might require unusually small doses).The carbonate part and the citrate part, however, can degrade with time; hence, the pills themselves have an expiration date, but the Lithium part of the pill is good for eons.

Lithium is used in psychiatry for manic-depressive illness and has been also used off label for the treatment of cluster headaches. The history of therapeutic lithium goes back to ancient Roman times when it was observed that manic patients thrown into a lithium spring or lithium pool sometimes calmed down although one wonders if it was from ingesting the very dilute lithium water or was just from the shock of being involuntarily submerged (technically the forerunner of "hydrotherapy"). Lithium chloride was marketed as a salt substitute (sodium chloride) for heart patients but then they consumed too much and got lithium poisoning which worsened the heart condition. The Australian psychiatrist Cade resurrected the use of lithium in the 1970's and it became a first-line treatment for manic-depressives.

Therapeutics

Lithium is FDA approved for the treatment of manic depression (Bipolar disorder), specifically Bipolar I disorder. It was the first choice treatment for this condition until Depakote took over as first choice in the 1990's and Lithium was relegated to second choice. Lithium mainly controls the mood swings and the mania. It tends to prevent the mood cycling and puts a "governor" on the manic episodes so that they do not spiral out of control. It has less effect on severe bipolar depressions. Many drugs had been tried for treatment of these debilitating emotional troughs. Finally, Lamictal has emerged as the first choice to prevent the recurrences of disabling bipolar depressions. It works very well, but needs to be added slowly to avoid the risk of life-threatening rashes. Lithium may be used with any other bipolar treatment, including Depakote and Lamictal.

The dosage of lithium varies upon how much a person needs to control mania. Mild cases may need only 600 mg a day; typical doses are 900-1200 mg a day; some people need 1500 or even 1800 mg; we had one patient who took 2100-2400 mg a day, but he was a very rapid excreter of lithium and was an unusual case. Men may need more lithium each day (than women) if they are younger, large, very active, or very thirsty.

Lithium is available as tablets, slow-release tablets (Eskalith-CR, Lithobid), capsules or liquid. The usual dosages achievable with pills are: 150, 225, 300, and 450 (milligrams). Odd doses will need liquid. Lithium is available in two preparations, carbonate and citrate. I have not had occasion to use the chloride form.

Lab tests required are blood levels of lithium. For those who have bad veins or squeamishness, lithium levels can also be derived from the saliva in which the salivary level of lithium should be around 1.0-2.0.

The usual side effects of Lithium are the following:

- weight gain from fat (appetite stimulation causes overeating)

- weight gain from fluid build-up and swelling

- acne

- lithium does not directly interact with most other pills.

- diarrhea

- hand tremors

- thirst and metallic taste

- light-headedness

These side effects are annoying to patients who may request a change to another drug.

Besides these side effects, lithium causes internal medical problems. It can cause:

- Sluggish thyroid function (the thyroid gland makes people more active, so if its activities are slowed by lithium, then the thyroid gland could become sluggish and then the patient becomes sluggish, too)

- Early mild kidney failure of very slow and gradual onset—Lithium dosage should be lowered or stopped. This is rarely life threatening.

- Lithium has no effect on the liver, a question I hear often.

- Using Lithium on a long-term basis involves blood testing. These blood tests are used to monitor:

  1—kidney function

  2—thyroid function

  3—lithium levels (contrary to popular belief, normal humans have *zero* detectable levels in their blood: I have had patients come to me from "St. Elsewhere" and tell me that the former psychiatrist prescribed them Lithium because their body levels of Lithium were too low! This is not true. We have no detectable lithium in our bodies unless we swallow lithium.)

Lithium and sodium are freely exchanged in your body. If you are stabilized on a regular dose of lithium, then you will need to maintain a regular level of table salt too by consuming the same amount of sodium daily. Unfortunately, sodium levels can rise and fall based on the food you eat, the amount you perspire and the amount of water that you drink: if sodium and lithium become unbalanced then you can get lithium poisoning which starts out with serious trembling of the hands and body, but if not corrected can cause dire medical consequences.

Danger Signs

These are some warning signs of Lithium levels that are too high:
- Trembling hands followed by jerkiness and spasticity of arms, legs, body
- Serious diarrhea
- Nausea, followed by vomiting
- Confusion
- Irregular heart beat and dizziness

Watch out for foods that are high in sodium such as certain soups, ham, and ethnic foods.

▶Summary of information on Lithium:

- it is a salt
- our normal body level is zero
- it has no effect on the liver
- Lithium poisoning is a medical emergency
- it works well in manic depression (Bipolar I)

Bromide is a natural element and is another natural substance. It is in the chemical family of inorganic halogens that includes fluoride, chloride, and iodide. We put fluoride in our water to prevent dental cavities. Chloride (sodium chloride, table salt) is in the same halogen family. Iodide we put into table salt to prevent goiters. These are the facts on bromide:
- Bromide is a natural tranquilizer. It was sold over the counter, the last formulation that I can remember seeing on pharmacy shelves was Miles Labs Bromide salts marketed as "Nervine®".
- It commonly causes skin rashes.
- It can occur as a single atom joined to a larger molecule, such as brompheniramine, a sedating antihistamine, in which case it is safer and contributes to the sedative effect.

HERBS

There are hundreds—or thousands, if we include Chinese herbals—of herbs and herbal products in use in the Occidental world (European and Euro-American). The best known is probably St. John's Wort, which is one of the most commonly used in Europe and America. *Ma Huang* (known to us as Ephedra, ephedrine) was used in China as a respiratory stimulant; it also provides animation and energy. Guaranà is a Brazilian herb which contains chemicals from the caffeine family, of which about 97% is in the form of caffeine, <1% cocoa (theobromine), and 1-3% theophylline (an older asthma drug). Valeriana is a popular sedative and inspiration for Valium. Other substances that are not frankly antidepressant, but do augment antidepressant activity include: SAM-e, Yohimbine, Ginseng, and Gingkoba. Deficiency of Vitamin D may be linked to mild neuro-psychiatric symptoms also. In fifteenth century Europe, Paracelsus briefly popularized the use of some heavy metals, which are no longer used (due to toxicity).

Important difference in terminology: in Europe and America, the word "herb" refers to a plant product. In China, an herb is any "found object": with origins as a plant, animal, mineral, etc.

Herbal products contain parts of dried plants. And, plants themselves contain many bio-chemical substances of which only one or several are usually the sought-after psycho-active ingredient. For example, St. John's Wort has two large classes of active ingredients (hypericins and hyperfolins) and both classes include one or more active chemicals. Valeriana contains a number of classes of active ingredients, including GABA, a natural brain relaxant. The sought-after psycho-active properties are usually anti-depressant or anti-anxiety properties, but might include stimulant, anti-psychotic, or psychedelic properties. Eating dried herbs is not necessarily as "natural" as one might think since these herbs can actually contain dozens of chemicals, some of which our bodies recognize as poisons. We come genetically equipped with all the machinery necessary to detoxify these plant poisons suggesting a long and intimate relationship between the plant and animal kingdoms— indeed, this might be the only part of the process that is truly "natural". (Chapter II-4) Whether we eat a hundred trace poisons or just one purified synthetic drug-poison, our bodies are forced to rework those chemicals and render them harmless. Hence, depression treatment might often require the patient to consume one or more natural or synthetic chemicals, which is unfortunately not a part of his normal daily intake.

St. John's Wort is still widely used and can be effective for milder cases of depression. However, three caveats apply to the use of St. John's Wort:

- As with all herbs it is a concoction containing dried botanical ingredients and contains many chemicals some of which (the hypericins) are imbued with healing properties while many other chemicals are present but not therapeutic and might even contribute to some toxic side effects. The quality of herbs also depends upon soil, rainfall, sunlight, and the presence of insecticides and herbicides.

- It can cause birth defects when used in pregnancy; for this reason, it is available in

Germany only on prescription (the thalidomide tragedy is not forgotten there).

- It also possesses mild MAOI effects (see later in this chapter under MAOI) which can result in toxicities if mixed with high doses of a number of synthetic drugs and antidepressants. St. John's Wort has become a popular herbal treatment in the United States and is available in a number of strengths and formulations (Bottled herbs sold in pharmacies are regulated by the FDA.)

If Americans intend to use St. John's Wort, then they should study up on it, just as they should with any synthetic pharmaceutical.

Valerian (Valeriana) is also a natural herbal product and a calmative herb. Reportedly, it has been used for thousands of years in Europe. Valeriana is an herb, so it does contain many chemicals that must be detoxified in the liver. It contains several classes of psychoactive drugs, mostly tranquilizers. As direct evidence of its potency, scientists have also isolated GABA, which is the tranquilizing brain hormone. GABA is also probably the link to the habit-forming properties of Valeriana and other habit-forming tranquilizers. Valeriana is the inspiration for the name "Valium". And like the synthetic drugs of the Valium family, it can also become habit-forming. Valerian is available in the USA without a prescription (see Herbs)

Kava Kava is an exotic herb (root) that has natural tranquilizing properties. It is processed heavily in the liver. In the Pacific islands, some people find it seductive, if not habit-forming—those who use it excessively may develop scaly yellow rashes and their palms may turn yellow. It has GABA-activity (see Chapter V-11) It is banned or regulated in some Western countries. It is still available in America.

Prescription-grade "NATURAL" DRUGS

Barbiturates were first manufactured from urea (from horse urine) and malonic acid (apple juice acid). Nowadays they are made in a factory. They were commonly used in the past as tranquilizers and sleeping pills. Barbiturates are dangerous and were a frequent cause of fatal overdose (Dorothy Kilgallen, Marilyn Monroe?, Elvis?, and many other victims…). Nowadays barbiturates are no longer routinely used [in psychiatry], although neurologists still use Phenobarbital for epileptic seizures and Butalbital (Fiorinal, Fioricet) for headaches.

Caffeine Derivatives there are various compounds (e.g. *Vivarin*) containing pure caffeine without the need to consume coffee that might have ingredients causing upset stomach. Other chemicals in the caffeine family are theobromine and theophylline. These are both stimulating, too. Theophylline was popular as an asthma medication. Caffeine is also found in Yerba Maté and Guaranà.

Galantamine is the active ingredient in one of the Alzheimer Treatments, Razadyne (formerly known as Reminyl), and is naturally found in the crocus (bulb); however, the cost of extracting galantamine from flowers is more expensive than fabricating it in a pharmaceutical laboratory—which is its current source.

Guaranà is a South American plant that contains guaranine (caffeine), theobromine, and theophylline (both caffeine derivatives also).

Melatonin is the natural "brain hormone" that starts our sleep cycle every night. As we get older, our pineal gland (in the brain) produces less melatonin, one of the many possible reasons that the elderly have more sleep disorders. The pineal gland is a tiny gland in our brain. The pineal seems to respond to cycles of light and dark. The original purpose of packaging melatonin in pill form was to help people who have bizarre or "unnatural" schedules that interfere with sleep: airplane pilots and crews, shift workers, and people who have advanced phase sleep disorder or delayed phase sleep disorders (see Chapter V-13).

Melatonin was finally purified and released to the public in the mid-1990's. Melatonin can be purchased in pill form in pharmacies in various strengths such as 0.5 mg, 1 mg, 3 mg. Opinions vary as to whether it should be taken every night—the best answer at this point is probably "no". Save it for use as a sleeping pill on an "as-needed" basis. The long-term effects of taking a brain hormone in pill form every night are not well known. Adults can take up to 9 mg each evening.

As a zoological curiosity, the tuatara (animal) still has a parapineal gland (beside and connected to the pineal gland) which seems to respond to light and darkness (this is the tuatara's "third eye"). If the tuatara is the living fossil that it seems to be, it may have much to teach us about sleep cycles.

Reserpine is extracted from the plant *Rauwolfia* and is considered to be a natural antipsychotic. This drug is hardly ever used in the USA anymore since it makes patients feel suicidal.

L-Tryptophan is an amino acid (a natural substance) which is found extensively in our bodies. A bedtime dose of 3-5 grams can induce sleepiness. Natural sources high in this amino acid are turkey, warm milk (the warming releases more of the bound-up Tryptophan) and bananas. This amino acid is the building block for serotonin, one of the antidepressant "brain hormones". Serotonin deficiency has been linked to types of depression.

This is a common mistaken belief by many patients:

> *That herbs and non-prescription drugs lack medical importance*
> *since these drugs are sold without a prescription.*

As a result, they forget to mention all their herbs and vitamins when listing their current medications. It is important that we know all the chemicals that you are putting into your body.

▶Herbals, hormones, and metals are effective for some patients some of the time. However, they fall short in the presence of major diseases such as schizophrenia, mania, panic, and severe depression. In just the last century we have increased our pharmacologic arsenal by a factor of thousands in effectiveness compared to all the previous historical and pre-historical periods.

> *We've come a long way, but we're still not there yet!*

Chapter V-11

GABA and the Treatment of Anxiety
Anti-Anxiety Medications

This is a directory of the anti-anxiety drugs. The first four on the list are in this chapter. The others are discussed in their own chapters as noted:

Anxiety Treatments listed in this Chapter

- Minor tranquilizers with addictive potential: (this Chapter)
- Minor tranquilizer without addictive potential: Buspar (this Chapter)
- Antihistamines with dual action on allergies, agitation, and anxiety:
  Vistaril, Atarax, and Benadryl (this Chapter)
- Blood pressure drugs that block adrenaline outflow: Inderal, Atenolol (this Chapter)

Anxiety Treatments listed in other Chapters

- Major tranquilizers used in "minor" doses (see Chapter V-4)
- Sedating antidepressants (see Chapter V-7): Tricyclics, Remeron, Trazodone
- Serotonin antidepressants (see Chapter V-8): Zoloft, Paxil, Celexa, Lexapro, and Effexor-XR
- Stimulating MAOI antidepressant (see Chapter V-6) Nardil
- sedating anti-epilepsy drugs (see Chapter V-12, AED's)
- calmative herbs: Valeriana, Kava (see Chapter V-10)

Introduction

Back to the theory of how modern psychoactive drugs act on the brain: this was called the "Amine Hypothesis" in the 1950's and is now more recently referred to as the "neurotransmitter theory" (Chapter V-1). This theory refers to "brain hormones", a term that I am using here. The "brain hormones" are more formally referred to as catechol-Amines or neurotransmitters. This theory supposes that when "brain hormone" levels fall too low, we get depressed. If we take antidepressant drugs to raise the levels of these "brain hormones", and if the drugs seem to offset the depression, then depression must be due to low levels of brain hormones.

Then more recently, we discovered more "brain hormones"—a lot more. The brain has a natural marijuana substance, natural narcotic substances (enkephalins and endorphins), GABA, and many more (see list at very end of Chapter V-1).

Then we went on to apply part of this theoretical reasoning to GABA, the natural tranquilizer of the brain. Low levels of GABA might relate to high anxiety: high levels of GABA might correlate to great tranquility. Drugs that normalize brain levels of GABA (the tranquilizing "brain hormone") have been noted to possess anti-anxiety properties. These drugs with anti-anxiety properties may possess capacities that directly or indirectly affect GABA levels. The best-known drugs in this category are all the drugs in the Valium family. Other anti-anxiety drugs and some of the anti-epilepsy drugs have positive effects on GABA, a fact not lost on their corporate sponsors who have even given them GABA-reminiscent names such as gabapentin, gabitril, and pregabilin.

The GABA-active drugs are often habit-forming, and the more powerful the GABA-action, the likelier the drug is to be even more addicting. Examples are drugs in the Valium family, Barbiturates, and others. However, some of them are not addicting. Neurontin is a good example. (also See Chapter V-12 on anti-epilepsy drugs).

Researchers still do not know if anti-anxiety drugs act directly on GABA or on some other brain system that results in alterations of GABA. There are brain chemicals called BDNF (Brain-derived neurotrophic factors) that affect the size and numbers of brain cells. Changes in BDNF may correlate to anxiety disorders. Changes in the brain due to BDNF may account for the observed abnormalities of GABA and "brain hormones". This remains an active field of research. Until then, we shall continue to prescribe GABA-active drugs for anxiety states.

Anti-anxiety medications are used to counteract symptoms of panic and anxiety disorders, such as: restlessness, fretfulness, racing heart, sense of impending doom, trembling hands, poor concentration, and poor sleep. Anti-anxiety drugs can be classified in various ways, perhaps one of the most useful classification systems is based on their addictive potential:

Addictive anti-anxiety drugs—these are usually drugs in the Valium family although other types of addictive agents are available (but no longer commonly used in the USA):

- Valium family drugs
- Xanax subgroup of Valium family drugs
- Addicting sleeping pills—see Chapter V-13

- Other older, dangerous, and addicting drugs: Miltown and barbiturates for example. These anti-anxiety drugs are also called "minor tranquilizers". (The antipsychotic drugs are the major tranquilizers, based on the observation that psychotic agitation is apparently "major" compared to anxiety.)

The definitions of habituation (habit-forming use), abuse, and addiction are given in Chapter I-7, "Introduction to Pharmacology".

Addictive Anti-Anxiety Drugs (Valium family *drugs*)

The addictive anti-anxiety drugs in common use are those from the Valium family, of which Valium is the best known, because it was the first one. The prescription of Valium has slowly decreased over the years. Valium is effective for long-standing anxiety and prolonged seizures. Nonetheless, I once witnessed a paradoxical reaction (seizure) to emergency use of injectable Valium in a young boy. Librium is still used sometimes for anxiety. I prescribe a fair amount of Serax, which is the fully degraded form of Valium. Valium, Librium, and Klonopin are long-acting drugs, whereas Xanax, Serax, and Ativan are short acting. Ativan is usually the universally preferred drug in the whole Valium family, because it is safe in the elderly, causes the fewest side effects, and is most appropriate for emergency situations. Patients with anxiety often receive a small amount of Ativan (or Xanax) in the emergency room. (Patients who are seen in emergency rooms for panic-anxiety typically receive a small amount of addicting medicine because it takes effect quickly. When the person leaves the emergency room, he is typically given only a small number of these pills because: (1) the drugs are addictive and need medical supervision; (2) anybody seen emergently needs to follow up quickly with a doctor; (3) a large dose of these drugs can be harmful if swallowed with huge amounts of alcohol.)

The Valium family has at least twenty drugs, some of which have fallen out of vogue (Centrax, Paxipam, Doral), some of which are good but rarely used (Tranxene, ProSom), some of which should no longer be used (Dalmane) and some of which are quite good but were never brought to the USA (Mogadon, nitrazepam). Restoril is a popular sleeping pill that is in the Valium family.

Addictive Anti-Anxiety Drugs (Xanax subgroup *of the Valium family*)

Other addictive anti-anxiety drugs in common use are those from the Xanax sub-family of the greater Valium family. These are Xanax and some others (Halcion, a sleeping pill, and Versed, used for surgery and medical procedures). Patients with panic attacks often receive Xanax in the emergency room. Xanax is the most addicting non-narcotic on the market in the USA, and Xanax addiction is often very hard to treat. Treatment of Xanax addiction requires a slow reduction of the dose, usually over weeks or months, with the use of secondary medications to control withdrawal symptoms and minimize panic attacks. Klonopin is similar to Xanax; it is long acting but can also be quite addicting. The original use of Klonopin was in Epilepsy. It is also effective—but addicting—for anxiety-panic. Klonopin is the only one that has routine blood levels available (because epilepsy patients need specific blood levels of the drug). Halcion was withdrawn from the market in the U.K. due to its apparent role in causing strange nighttime behaviors (like black-outs or sleep-walking). I had one elderly patient who injured herself at night while taking Halcion from her family doctor (I usually refuse to prescribe Halcion—there are other options such as Lunesta, Sonata, Restoril or Ambien-CR). It is still on the market in the USA. I try to avoid using all the drugs in the Xanax subgroup because they all seem to beget more problems than medications from the "main" group of the Valium family.

Duration of Action→ Purpose↓		Very Long acting	Long acting	Short acting	Very Short acting
Valium family→ ↳	Anxiety	Valium Tranxene	Librium	Serax Ativan	
	Sleep	Dalmane	Restoril	Prosom	
Xanax subgroup	Epilepsy·Panic Anxiety·Sleep		Klonopin	Xanax	Versed* Halcion**

Table V-11-a   Valium family drugs in first two rows   (*anesthesia injection)
Xanax sub-family drugs are in third row   (**banned in UK)

There are other older, dangerous, addictive medications that are hardly ever used (Miltown).

Addiction Risks

These are some of the risk factors and warning signs for addiction, including who is likely to become addicted to these drugs, and how can addiction be minimized or prevented:
- Any patient who comes from an alcoholic family is probably at higher risk, too (due to genetic loading)
- Recovering alcoholics and drug addicts especially should avoid these drugs, because these drugs can cause alcohol craving and lead to a relapse of alcoholism in recovering alcoholics. (I have seen a few recovering alcoholics who could tolerate bedtime Ativan, but this is definitely not advisable practice.)
- The longer the period of exposure to addicting anti-anxiety drugs, the greater the

risk of future dependence or addiction

- Anybody who has taken the medicines for only a couple weeks and already shows withdrawal signs after one missed dose is at risk

- Anybody who feels the need for higher doses than the average patient

- People with addictive traits should avoid these drugs: addictive traits would include any person with a history of unchecked compulsive behaviors such as compulsive gambling, overeating or binge eating, compulsive shopping and overspending and so on...

Other Concerns

The only drug in this class with measurable drug levels is Klonopin: we can check blood levels of this drug to estimate how much the patient is taking and possibly how much benefit the patient is getting; however, all these drugs will show up on pre-employment screening urine drug testing. Some of these tests have a cut-off point below which the urine test will come back negative (acceptable) in cases where the person is just taking a small ordinarily prescribed amount. The urine testing is intended to ferret out people who have a serious addiction to high amounts of these drugs. A positive test for any of these drugs is viewed with much concern by prospective employers.

People who are addicted to the Valium family of drugs are more likely to have other drug addictions. Sometimes patients resort to using these drugs to control drug-induced highs. Any practicing alcoholic who drinks all day on his days off can take a Valium on working days to stop his alcohol withdrawal symptoms until he can get home in the evening and resume drinking. Even worse, Valium addicts are more likely to be slowed down which results in clumsiness and industrial accidents, which in turn leads to Workers Compensation claims.

The government made an excellent decision of refusing to pay for any of these Valium-family drugs if prescribed to patients on SSI or SSD. This is a commendable decision, because the drugs can easily create more problems than they cure. SSI is for the elderly who should not take Valium drugs because they suffer side effects (memory loss and falling down: bone fractures. Anybody younger (on SSD) should avoid these drugs since the drugs cause addiction and depression (unless they are prescribed by a specialist for temporary muscle relaxation or for control of seizures).

Treatment Issues

Some patients with sudden onset panic attacks have been prescribed small doses of Xanax by the family doctor or in the Emergency Room. They will usually come in to the psychiatrist's office feeling some sense of stability. In these cases, we need to make a *bona fide* attempt to introduce a non-addicting drug because this is the wisest decision for the long term. The patient needs to understand and agree to this. The solution here is to continue the Xanax for a few or several weeks while slowly introducing an efficacious but non-addictive agent after which Xanax can be slowly tapered off after a couple months. The patients need to be educated that addictive drugs give instantaneous relief and that is part of the [addictive] appeal. A corollary to this is the fact that patients learn to take extra doses of the addictive drug in an attempt to feel even better, which can eventuate in escalating addiction. This extra dosing (misuse of drug) is rarer with non-addicting drugs.

People who stay on the addicting drugs note that over time the addicting drugs begin to lose effect unless the dose is continuously raised to the point where the patient has all the side effects that come with taking excess medicine. The longer the patient spends on the addictive drugs, the greater the likelihood that the patient will begin to experience daily symptoms of withdrawal, which on the long-term basis creates a fair amount of misery.

Quitting addicting drugs after long-term use causes severe withdrawal symptoms that are uncomfortable, are accompanied by intense craving for the addicting drug, and may cause serious medical reactions such as high blood pressure and seizures.

There are some panic attacks that can be controlled only by Xanax; in these cases, ongoing Xanax can be continued as long as there have been reasonable documented attempts to wean the patient off the Xanax. Hopefully, that patient does not have a lot of risk factors for addiction (see section above). Patients need to understand all the risks of using addicting drugs.

Conversely, short-term results with the non-addicting drugs are somewhat less predictable than with the addictive ones but the elimination of the risk of addiction is worth it. That is why addicting drugs are addicting: they make patients feel really good immediately whereas the non-addicting ones do not take effect immediately but require a long period of adjustment after which the patient will actually feel better in the long run, than on the addictive drug.

Other Treatment Specifics

Valium was the first drug of this class for anxiety and it still works well
Klonopin is useful for seizures, anxiety, and panic
Serax does not stress the liver
Librium this is a standard drug used for alcohol treatment
Dalmane this is an old drug: one pill can be detected in the urine four days later! Not an ideal treatment for sleep disorders, and especially not in the elderly.

These drugs will show up in pre-employment urine tests: the short-acting ones clear from the body sooner than the longer-acting ones. A person who has been taking these daily for months or years will return a positive urine test for *at least* one to three weeks after the last pill is taken.

Non-addictive Anti-Anxiety Medications

(The definition of addiction is given in Chapter I-7, "Introduction to Pharmacology".)

This is a large group of medicines that are not necessarily related to each other chemically or in any other way. This very diverse group of drugs attests to the fact that tranquilization either has multiple mechanisms of action or that most of these drugs have some sort of unknown or poorly understood GABA-like activity, perhaps due to indirect properties of raising levels of obscure "brain hormones" not yet studied. Most of them are not "minor" tranquilizers. You can see that in the group there are sedating antidepressants, non-sedating antidepressants, major tranquilizers, blood pressure pills, antihistamines, herbs, and epilepsy drugs (AED's). This is the full list:

- Minor tranquilizers, Addictive anti-anxiety agents (covered in this chapter—see above)

- Minor tranquilizer, Non-addictive anti-anxiety agent: Vistaril, Atarax, and Buspar. These may be helpful for anxiety but not for panic attacks: fortunately there are other non-addicting medicines which can be quite helpful for panic.

- Minor doses of major tranquilizers (none of which is addicting) may be helpful, especially tiny doses of Zyprexa, Risperdal, or Thorazine. See Chapter V-4.

- Curiously, very small amounts of antidepressants can often have anti-anxiety properties thus spurring a lot of new research into the biochemical relationships between the theories of anxiety and depression. The antidepressants most useful for these purposes are:

  i— Zoloft, Paxil, and others (Celexa/Lexapro), also Effexor: see Chapter V-8

  ii—Tricyclics (Imipramine, Doxepin, and Elavil): see Chapter V-7

  iii—Trazodone: see Chapter V-7

  iv—Nardil, an MAOI antidepressant: see Chapter V-6

  (v)—(Buspar was actually developed as an antidepressant but brought to market as an anti-anxiety medicine)

- Some of the anti-epilepsy medicines may be helpful—especially Neurontin and Gabitril. Less so, Lyrica. (see Chapter V-12 on anti-epilepsy drugs)

- Antihistamines with calmative action include Atarax and Vistaril which are good for both sedation and allergies. Psychiatrists prescribe Benadryl for certain purposes.

In this chapter

- Calmative herbs are Valeriana, Kava-Kava. (these have GABA activity) See Chapter V-10

- Adrenaline blocking drugs are also helpful at times, especially the beta blockers. If used on a daily basis then Tenormin (Atenolol) is best; if used only rarely for "performance anxiety" then Inderal is preferred but Atenolol and Wytensin are quite helpful also. see this chapter

Buspar, Vistaril-Atarax-Benadryl, and Beta-blockers

These are the medications covered in this chapter.

The others have already been covered in the previous chapters.

Buspar

Buspar is a non-addictive medicine specifically indicated for generalized anxiety disorder (GAD). Like most non-addictive medications, the patient must take it daily for a couple weeks before the full effect is felt. Buspar helps some people to feel better. In truth, fewer than half of the people who try it, opt to continue it after a few weeks, citing concerns about side effects such as dizziness or lack of impressive tranquilization. This is not surprising when we remember that Buspar is not a traditional anti-anxiety medication, but rather a failed antidepressant that was brought to market at a lower dose and used for anxiety. On the positive side, Buspar has no negative effects on sexual performance and may even enhance performance slightly (in men), probably due to the fact that it is in a family of drugs that lack negative sexual side effects (Serzone and Trazodone). I have never had a patient develop a rash, gain weight, lose sleep, or become aggressive while taking Buspar. It seems to help recovering alcoholics, suggesting an element of subtle underlying depression in [those] alcoholics. It is ideal for recovering alcoholics and drug-addicts because it is not addicting. It can be mixed with the serotonin antidepressants. It must not be mixed with MAOI antidepressants. There is questionable value of adding it to Wellbutrin or other sedating antidepressants. It may be helpful as an add-on drug in schizophrenia.

Because of its delayed onset of action and weak GABA properties, Buspar is not very effective in Panic attacks.

Vistaril, Atarax, Benadryl

These are all sedatives and antihistamines. At the usual doses they are all sedating, but at higher doses, they may be surprisingly stimulating. They must be avoided in persons with prostate problems, severe glaucoma, urinary retention, or severe stomach ulcers.

Vistaril and Atarax are different compounds but both are a form of Hydroxyzine, which is the active ingredient. In low doses, they are sedating. These are of great use for producing a pleasant sense of sedation or sleepiness without risk of addiction.

Benadryl is an antihistamine that psychiatrists use regularly. It is used for two purposes: for sleep and for counteracting side effects of FGA antipsychotics (first generation antipsychotics). It functions well at bedtime as a non-addicting sleeping pill. At higher doses its mild stimulation can counteract some of the major sedation of the FGA's. The stimulation is produced in relation to functional similarities to atropine-like drugs. (Atropine comes from belladonna and is important for understanding medical pharmacology, but is beyond this book.)

Beta-blockers

These drugs are typically used for blood pressure and heart conditions. Some of them block the outflow of adrenaline that is often a central feature in panic-anxiety states. Inderal can be used on an "as-needed" basis for performance anxiety; it should not be taken everyday as it can cause depression and weird dreams. Atenolol is ideal for everyday use in panic-anxiety conditions. Typical dosage for Inderal is 10-20 mg before the performance. Atenolol can be given at 25 mg a day in healthy young adults. If you are already being treated for high blood pressure or a heart condition, then do not take these drugs (without input from your primary doctor).

Treatment Issues

Short-term results with the non-addicting drugs are somewhat less predictable than with the addictive ones but the elimination of the risk of addiction is worth it. That is why addicting drugs are addicting: they make patients feel really good immediately whereas the non-addicting ones do not take effect immediately but require a long period of adjustment after which the patient will actually feel better in the long run, than on the addictive drug. Patients must learn that the non-addictive drugs must be taken daily. Patients also need to be schooled about the effects of the non-addicting drugs: they will slowly start to exert their therapeutic effects after the first few weeks or even months. That is how long before the treatment would begin to show its maximum anti-anxiety or anti-panic properties. If the patient has a good response to non-addicting drugs, then he can maintain long-term prevention of panic attacks—*unless* he stops the treatment on his own judgment—and then all bets are off. If the patient stops the treatment prematurely, then usually the panic/anxiety may come back and sometimes be much harder to control while in relapse mode. After several weeks on non-addicting medicines, the patient should begin to feel good in a natural sort of way. Medications like Zoloft and Paxil might cause some sexual dysfunction and the other non-addicting drugs might cause elevation of sugar, cholesterol, or liver tests. Most patients and most psychiatrists feel that the benefits of non-addicting drugs outweigh the risk of the non-addicting drugs.

Favorable initial adjustment to non-addicting treatment usually gives long-lasting effects for years, although the patient might become resistant to the full effect after several years, but at least will not experience a daily cycle of withdrawal symptoms. Rather, he will slowly sense that the drug is not having so much effect as before. This may be the patient's body telling him that he no longer needs the drug, or this may be a separate phenomenon of the body slowly becoming resistant to the beneficial effects of the drug.

Other Concerns

There may be some minor withdrawal symptoms caused by quitting non-addicting drugs, but this is not medically catastrophic and the process is called "discontinuation syndrome". It may feel like having the "flu" or headaches. It is not life threatening (like Xanax withdrawal). Quitting addicting drugs causes severe withdrawal symptoms that are truly uncomfortable, are accompanied by intense craving for the addicting drug and may cause serious medical reactions such as high blood pressure and seizures. Hence, the preference of non-addicting drugs over the addicting Valium family drugs. If you take a group of a hundred Xanax patients and compare them to a hundred of Zoloft or Paxil patients you will see that the Zoloft-Paxil patients feel better and more satisfied overall.

In the following table you can see a chapter summary showing the advantages and disadvantages of addicting versus non-addicting tranquilizers. The best outcomes may come from educated patients.

Drug type	Addicting Valium, Xanax	Non-Addicting Antidepressants	Non-Addicting Major tranquilizer	Non-Addicting Buspar, Atarax, et al
% relief	High	Higher	Moderate/high	Fair
Max. effect	immediate	Weeks-months	Days-weeks	Day/Days
Worst effect	Addiction	Rash	Weight gain	Sleepiness
Long-term	Addiction, Memory loss, Falls, accidents	Headache, Impaired sex	Diabetes Cholesterol Tremors	Slowed thoughts Weight gain Dryness
withdrawal	Seizures	"Flu" symptoms	Minimal	Anxiety returns
Overdose	Maybe fatal	Some are safer	Safer	Safe

Table V-11-b   Table of anti-anxiety medications

►In addressing anxiety, it is important to try to differentiate between Panic Attacks, Anxiety, and Agitation, because the treatments are different.

Chapter V-12

Anti-Epilepsy Drugs (AED's)
And GABA

Because some anti-epilepsy drugs are also used in psychiatry, they may be considered neuropsychiatric although they are not normally classified as such. These drugs stabilize the nerve membrane and the nerve itself which results in apparent stabilization of certain unstable neurological and unstable psychiatric disorders. The number of neurological medications is many, but only a few are used routinely in psychiatry: Depakote, Lamictal, and Tegretol are the three main ones used; there is a fair amount of usage of Neurontin also and to a considerably lesser extent: Gabitril, Trileptal, Lyrica and Topamax. (I use the terms anti-epilepsy drug and epilepsy drug interchangeably in this book.)

Depakote is an excellent drug for controlling Bipolar Disorder and is now the most frequently used medication for this indication—even more so than Lithium which has now dropped to second place for Bipolar treatment (lithium is covered in Chapter V-10). Chemically speaking, Depakote is a small organic acid (not unlike acetic acid from vinegar, or butyric acid from butter, or malonic acid from apples). Depakote has an unknown mechanism of action. Presumably, it stabilizes the nerve cells. Neurologists prescribe Depakote for epilepsy and also for migraine headache symptoms. It is available in several forms for oral administration:

- liquid
- capsules/gelcaps
- tablets
- controlled release tablets
- extended release tablets.

It can be somewhat hard on the liver especially in children. Drug levels and liver tests are a regular feature of Depakote therapy. It should be avoided—or used very cautiously—in anybody who has hepatitis or cirrhosis. Blood levels are much more predictable than with lithium. Even if blood levels of Depakote rise significantly, that is not a life-threatening medical event as with Lithium. It also has far fewer annoying side effects, but can typically result in weight gain of 5-12% above baseline.

Lamictal is a good treatment for bipolar depression, especially in manic-depressives with a history of recurrent disabling depression. It is also sometimes useful in patients who have repeated severe depression episodes that cannot be controlled by the usual antidepressants. Lamictal can cause a potentially fatal skin disease if started in too high doses too quickly but otherwise is usually well tolerated. As a result of this skin sensitivity reaction, Lamictal needs to be started at a very low dose and very slowly increased over a span of a few weeks or months. Obviously, Lamictal can not be used for any emergency purposes because it takes so long to reach an effective level. So it usually is started when the patient is relatively stable in anticipation of yet another recurring depression sometime in the future. Routine blood tests are not regularly required. It is used usually as preventive maintenance in patients who are prone to severe recurrent depressions.

Tegretol is an older AED which structurally is very closely related to Elavil (the tricyclic antidepressant, Chapter V-7), but the Tegretol molecule is different enough from Elavil to give it a different biochemical profile and a different set of uses. Tegretol is useful for bipolar disorder.

Unfortunately, Tegretol has several side effects that make it less "user-friendly" than Depakote. Tegretol can make patients very susceptible to infections, usually starting out with sore throat or bronchitis symptoms. This bad side effect occurs because Tegretol suppresses bone marrow. If this dangerous side effect is not detected, then the infections might become serious. This is a regular feature of Tegretol treatment in my patients: most of them have a 50% drop in white blood cells while on Tegretol: from a white cell count of 5-6,000 down to 3-4,000 and sometimes close to 2,000 which is a danger level. That is the bad news. The good news—relatively speaking—is that the white counts settle at a certain reduced level and doggedly stay at that level for the whole duration of Tegretol treatment. Patients who maintain a constant level of uder 3,000 white cells get blood-tested more than those above 3,000. Thus Tegretol might not be a good choice in diabetics who are already so sensitive to infections.

Tegretol can also cause low sodium levels (table salt is half sodium). If sodium levels drop very low this could cause permanent brain damage, but this would be exceedingly rare. Tegretol can affect the liver, but that is quite rare compared to the potential problems posed by the reduced white cells (and sodium).

Besides that, many patients also feel "weird" on Tegretol. Because of these side effects, Tegretol has now been relegated to a third or fourth choice in bipolar treatment. There is a small group of patients who feel really good on Tegretol. Good for them, but they are a small minority.

Trileptal is a newer and slightly modified version of Tegretol and is better tolerated. Trileptal has fewer unpleasant side effects. It is occasionally helpful in mild mood cycling disorders, such as cyclothymia. Not all insurance plans will pay for it. Like Tegretol it can rarely lower sodium levels, but overall Trileptal is more "user-friendly" than Tegretol. It does not require many regular blood tests and does not effectively suppress bone marrow. And its sedating effect is usually more pleasant. Its potency for bipolar treatment, however, is less than that of Tegretol.

Neurontin is used by psychiatrists to control chronic pain, to alleviate anxiety, and to help promote sleep; it makes an excellent sedative for use in patients with severe liver problems since it is not processed in the liver; it is not processed anywhere in the body and leaves the body unchanged in the urine. It has a chemical structure partially similar to that of natural sugars. This drug is safer than Tylenol or aspirin. The dosage does usually need to be increased gradually, but once a patient is stabilized on a certain dose, then he may continue that dose. After stabilization, he may need come in for a visit every few months. Overdose with Neurontin is not a life-threatening problem, but should still be sent to the emergency room.

Gabitril has been shown to be effective in some cases of generalized anxiety disorder, but is not a regular treatment of anxiety. Some patients find it mildly effective.

Topamax is for epilepsy, but psychiatrists use it in very low doses (25-50 mg) to suppress the appetite; this effect is slow and subtle, and the weight loss is slow, but ultimately will allow a patient to lose dozens of pounds over the space of a year or two. (This is "off-label use"—see Chapter V-3.) The patient ought to drink at least eight glasses of water a day to lower the risk of kidney stones; Topamax would not be an ideal medication for patients who already have a prior history of kidney stones or kidney disease. Topamax might cause vitamin B-6 deficiency and so the patient will need to take B-vitamins. The only annoying side-effect is the possibility of feeling slowed down mentally which does happen in many cases; if this happens to you, the only specific treatment is to stop taking Topamax. If this is not a problem and you have no kidney stones, then Topamax may indeed help you lose some weight. (Neurologists use it for epilepsy and migraine headache.)

Lyrica is another AED which is rarely used by psychiatrists. It might be helpful as a last resort in severe anxiety but not likely. It is approved by the FDA for treating fibromyalgia. Psychiatrists who are consulted for chronic pain control could find Lyrica to be a valuable resource (see chapter on chronic pain)

Other neuropsychiatric medications

Psychiatrists use some of the "first-generation" **anti-Parkinsonism medications** to a much greater degree than Neurologists. These would include Cogentin, Artane, Akineton, and Kemadrin. Cogentin is the most commonly used. Artane is mildly stimulating and has been used as a street drug (powdered and sprinkled into cigarettes). Akineton is pleasantly mild with fewer side-effects. Kemadrin is the most potent in this family.

Parsidol/Parsitan is very effective for suppressing abnormal movements due to antipsychotics. Sales of Parsidol dipped so low in the US that it was no longer profitable. (neurologists and psychiatrists mistakenly thought that Parsidol might cause Parkinsonism.) Parsidol can still be ordered as Parsitan from Canada.

Other neurology drugs rarely used by psychiatrists: Mysoline and Requip. Requip can be used for RLS (Restless Legs Syndrome). I do not prescribe Requip. For RLS, I use Neurontin or Seroquel. If these are not effective, then the patient needs to see a neurologist.

▶Drugs originally developed for neurology can be useful in psychiatry (and vice versa: psychiatric drugs such as Elavil and Effexor can be useful in neurology). This serves to highlight the overlap between the two specialties. These drugs improve nerve instability [presumably], which seems to be linked to neuro-psychiatric conditions.

Chapter V-13

Sleep and Sleeping Pills

Chapter Overview:
Sleep Problems can be a Symptom or Disorder
Sleep Problems can be Life-long or Temporary
Sleep Cycle and Healthy Sleep (Sleep Hygiene)
Treatment of Sleep Disorders: four Methods of Sleep Induction

Sleep is a normal part of our daily cycle and is considered important to daily functioning. It is generally believed that a lack of sleep has never been the direct cause of death, but it certainly seems self-evident that some people have died as an indirect lack of sleep, for example falling asleep while driving a car or other inattentiveness.

People who do not sleep well do not feel well. It is for this reason that I almost always take a brief sleep history of my patients not only upon initial evaluation but also at follow-up visits. You might not be surprised to learn that the majority of my new patients do report some abnormality in sleep cycle. That is the bad news. The good news is that almost all of these problems can be resolved by thoughtful use of appropriate medicines or referral to a neurologist or sleep lab.

The first thing that I need to do is to take a sleep history and have the patient share any other important information.

Symptom or Disorder?

Sleeping problems can be merely one symptom (of another disease) or a whole disorder unto itself:

Sleep Problem as Symptom of Other Diseases

As one symptom of another disease, sleep problems can occur with:

- psychiatric illnesses (thought disorders, anxiety disorders, stress disorders, major mood disorders). If the main illness is brought under control, then the person should be able to sleep better. People who have major mania or psychosis cannot sleep because their minds are constantly "revving". There might be agitation or frightening hallucinations. Anti-psychotic and anti-manic drugs should be very helpful in providing good sleep.

- Developmental disorders (Autism, Down's Syndrome and others) require prescribing by a doctor who is knowledgeable about these cases.

- Medical disorders can cause insomnia for many reasons: overactive thyroid hormone can cause agitation; emphysema can cause sleep disruptions; chronic pain patients awaken from pain; some disorders inherently cause sleep problems because they occur at night/during sleep such as restless legs and other movement disorders.

- Use of chemicals (alcohol, caffeine, cocaine, amphetamines, diet pills, and so on). Alcohol can disrupt normal sleep cycles. Valium family drugs decrease REM sleep (not good). Stimulants can release adrenaline-like chemicals and hormones, which lead to insomnia. Some Parkinson's drugs as well as asthma drugs can cause insomnia.

Sleep Disorder as its own Diagnosis

As a whole disorder unto itself: Doctors have a scientific way of classifying sleep disorders that involves four basic categories: not enough sleep or poor quality sleep (the commonest one), excessive sleep (for which snoring may be a symptom), irregular, altered, or disturbed sleep (like jet lag and working the nightshift), and the fourth sleep disorder includes other disorders that occur during sleep cycle (like sleepwalking). These are four recognized kinds of sleep disorders:

- not enough sleep (insomnia): people report problems falling asleep too early, awakening in the wee hours, or awakening too early in the morning—or any combination of these sleep problems. This is the commonest sleep disorder. It may have some aggravating factors which need to be addressed (strange work schedule, anxiety over anything or everything, snoring spouse, worries about family matters, job stress, and so on). Or, it may be an on and off problem for years. Most patients think they just need a "sleeping pill" and then they will be fine. This is the one sleep disorder that has so many possible causes and outcomes. The treatment of insomnia has as many causes and remedies as there are patients.

- Too much sleep (hypersomnia): this occurs when people sleep too many hours every twenty-four hours. I have had middle-aged and older patients who have late-life onset of going to bed in the early evening, sleeping until late morning, then taking an afternoon nap, too! They are not uncomfortable with this and feel rested. However, their families complain and the patients themselves know that this is not normal—not for them or for anybody. They are actually sleeping more than fourteen hours in total. On the other hand, there are other patients who complain of spending too much time in bed, but further discussion reveals that they are often lolling in bed or tossing around and they probably sleep eight-nine hours at night with a two-hour nap. The rest of the time, they are in bed dozing or resting. These patients may complain of "too much sleep", "too much tiredness", or "spending too much time in bed but not having restful sleep". These cases may have an underlying depression that can be treated with fair success.

- Irregular sleep (dyssomnia): permanent alterations in sleep such as having a brain that is on a 22 hour or 26 hour cycle The temporary cause of this can also be occupational for time-zone travelers (airplane crew), factory workers on graveyard shift, or first responders (emergency medical personnel, police, and firefighters).

- Disrupted sleep (parasomnias): sleep-walking, frequent nightmares, recurring sleep hallucinations, or sleep paralysis.

Narcolepsy

This is a neurologic disorder in which people have attacks of suddenly or repeatedly fall asleep during the daytime. Sometimes, their bodies go limp while they are momentarily awake. Sometimes exciting events or environmental stimuli can trigger an attack. The attacks occur on a regular basis and may appear in adulthood. This is not mere drowsiness after a large lunch. This is very dangerous while driving, even while crawling along bumper-to-bumper in LA traffic. (This is how one patient presented: every afternoon while driving home: his diagnosis was confirmed at Huntington Hospital). This problem is usually diagnosed by a Multiple Sleep Latency Test and treated by neurologists. Psychiatrists may treat these patients under certain circumstances, for example, if there is no neurologist in a region or if the psychiatrists run the sleep lab. Stanford University has an active narcolepsy research program using narcoleptic dogs. (narcolepsy is limited to predatory animals and not their prey, for obvious reasons).

Excessive Daytime Sleepiness (EDS)

This is what its name suggests. People who are sleepy all day. Usually this is due to poor nighttime sleep, typically due to sleep apnea and snoring. This is not dramatic like narcolepsy. Provigil and Nuvigil may be very effective.

Life-long problem or Temporary?

For practical purposes we can divide sleep problems into three general kinds which are life-long or temporary symptoms:

Lifelong problems and concerns with sleeping

Chronic lack of sleep negatively affects daily functioning. There may be a few possible subtypes here:

- There may be a permanent problem in the patient's timing center in the brain (the so-called *Zeitgeber*, German for "timekeeper"). His brain may lack the ability to clock the constant cycles of day and night. Or the clock may have the ability but the pineal gland may not give the correct readings. (The pineal gland entrains nightly sleep cycles by releasing melatonin around the same time each night—see chapter V-10) The result is that the patient does not follow normal sleep cycles (he is not "entrained"). He does not experience "restorative sleep" and hence feels miserable every day, thus compounding the original sleep problem by adding the anxiety that he will probably not be able to sleep well the next night, etc. These sleep concerns are often the main reason that the patient is coming in. The patient's first statement will usually be about the sleep problem. These kinds of sleep problems are hard to treat and require vigorous prescribing of medicines that are effective without causing addiction or excess sedation in the daytime. In the following diagram we see how this happens with Ted, a man who does not feel sleepy at bedtime, but may feel sleepy at 6 PM or in the early half of the AM. He never feels well in the morning when he must get up and go to work.

Diagram V-13:	*Abnormal functioning of the Timekeeper of Sleep (**Zeitgeber**) in Ted's brain*

☼ → 👁 → 🧠 → Ž → 🕯 → ☢ → R$_x$ ↔ (⊡ Rx ⊡) ↔ ☯

| 1 | 2 | 3 | 4 | 5 | 6 | +7 | ±7' | 8 |

(1) Cycle of night and day sends a message through *(2) Ted's eye to* *(3) his pineal gland that then sends a message to* *(4) his Zeitgeber.*	*Somewhere along this route 1-2-3-4 something is malfunctioning and Ted is not enjoying normal sleep cycles: Ted is either* *(5) staying up late or (6) sleeping poorly, tossing and turning, replaying the day's events in his mind.* (7) Prescription of medicine may provide symptomatic relief and with a return to:

(8) balanced restorative sleep—hopefully. However, Ted needs to remember that this is a temporary treatment for a permanent problem (⊡ ⊡) which is still bouncing around erratically and just barely controlled by medicine. This is a way of dealing with the symptoms, but there is no known permanent remedy.

Here are some examples:

- Arleigh has always had nonspecific or variable sleeping problems which require him to have sleeping pills available but he does not need to take them every night—but needs to have them just in case of a "bad" night. This is common. Doctors believe it is due to temporary and minor, internal or external stresses.

- Some patients like Marla are naturally high-strung and anxious and may in fact suffer more than one anxiety disorder, such as social phobia, free-floating anxiety, recurrent stress disorders, other fearful states, and panic attacks. These cause her to be tired and anxious in the daytime. Marla often lacks the ability for "self-soothing" and is wound up every night at bedtime and cannot fall sleep. Fear of not sleeping becomes a form of nocturnal anxiety that is just added on to all the daytime sources of anxiety. Surprisingly, patients like Marla have much improved sleep just by the fact of treating the daytime anxieties and may or may not need regular sleeping pills.

- Dale: Then there is Dale who can have a normal night's sleep but his problem is that he is on a sleep cycle that is longer than 24 hours: he might be on a 26 hour sleep cycle so that he wants to stay up an hour later each night. (In reality, our bodies tend to be on a 24-25 hour cycle naturally: did the Earth rotate more slowly in the distant past?) Other patients like Dale may be on a 22 hour cycle, but at least they are tired at their bedtime in the early evening; they can add on two extra hours by staying awake with coffee. They rarely might need some stimulants to take on an "as-needed" basis.

Temporary Sleep Problem

There may be a temporary sleep problem that has had a recent onset and is not perceived as a permanent symptom. This can occur commonly in major depression, which is often characterized by new onset sleeping problems. Usually the sleep problem only began sometime around the onset of the emotional distress. (These cases of sleep problem are easier to treat: treating the original distressing problem will usually result in resolution of the sleep problem within a matter of weeks or months.) These patients are coming in mainly about the emotional distress and often will not say much about the sleeping problem—if at all—unless quizzed about it. It is important for the doctor to determine which kind of sleep problem is present because treatment of problems one and two are often quite different.

Both

The third possibility is that the patient has both a mild lifelong sleep disorder and secondarily a new onset severe sleep disorder from some new cause. So he has two problems to treat.

Sleep disturbance is common in depression and may be accompanied by either poor sleep or excess sleep. Sleep disorder may be the first symptom of a mood disorder. Manic-depressives who are taking regular medicines may begin to notice the slow onset of insomnia, which is a warning sign that a manic episode may be approaching. Prompt treatment of this symptom can ward off a manic episode. Sleep is sometimes thought of as one of the "psychic appetites", other psychic appetites are food and desire (sexual appetite or libido). If there are alterations in these appetites, then the patient might have a major disorder.

Sleep Cycle

Sleep occurs in regular cycles all night long, and dreaming occurs several times each night too as part of the sleep cycle. Since these cycles occur in the brain, they are all electro-chemical in nature. Thus, this electrical activity can be recorded as tracings which show the way the patient builds upon his sleep cycles each night. This is a tracing of our sleep cycle for the whole night and it can be quite long. We usually start out with slow wave sleep (SWS) and this is followed by REM sleep (Rapid Eye Movement). We continue to have a few or several cycles of alternating SWS then REM until we wake up in the morning (if we have normal sleep cycles). During REM sleep, we become activated and move around. Men may have erections during this time. Dreaming is normal and occurs during REM sleep. People who have disrupted sleep from any cause (stress or medications) remember more dreams each morning and feel that this is abnormal: remembering several dreams is abnormal, but having them, is not.

Animals have REM sleep, too. You can watch your dog having REM sleep: observe the heavy rapid breathing, twitching of muscles and eyelids.

Healthy Sleep ("sleep hygiene")

Sleep experts advise us that the best quality healthy sleep can be obtained if we all follow the accepted guidelines. Some of these are fairly obvious but should be followed by anybody who experiences a lot of sleeping problems:

1—Do not eat large meals near bedtime.

2—Eat no spicy or highly sugary snacks near bedtime.

3—Do not do strenuous exercise near bedtime.

4—Do not consume caffeine in the evening.

5—Alcohol at bedtime does not promote good sleep.

6—The mattress should be comfortable as well as the bedroom.

7—The bedroom temperature should be below seventy-five degrees Fahrenheit.

8—Do not go to bed angry.

9—Stay on a regular bedtime schedule, going to bed at the same time and arising at the same time.

10—Avoid napping in the daytime.

11—Reserve the bed for sleeping and go to bed only when it is bedtime. Do not lie in bed all night eating, snacking, and watching TV—plus, television affects brain waves adversely.

12—older patients feel better if they can read themselves to sleep.

Following these guidelines is especially important for patients whose main complaint is just a sleeping problem that is not due to primary emotional distress.

*　　　　　*　　　　　*　　　　　*　　　　　*　　　　　*

Treatment of Sleep Disorders:
The method of treating sleep disorders relies on "Sleep Induction".
Sleep Induction means causing sleep or knowing how to relieve disordered sleep. Sleep induction depends on doing something to our body. There are four usual methods for inducing sleep, which are chemical, biological, herbal, or physical induction. **Chemical induction** of sleep relies upon using "sleeping pills", also known as sedative-hypnotics. **Biological induction** of sleep relies upon putting a biological biochemical into our bodies that is normally present but in insufficient amounts. **Herbal induction** relies upon consuming substances not found normally in our body. Finally, **Physical induction** of sleep uses the external environment to trigger the release of internal chemicals ("hormones"). This sleep induction depends upon using something that is already in our body.
*　　　　　*　　　　　*　　　　　*　　　　　*　　　　　*

Chemical Induction ("Sleeping pills")
I have put this term in quotation marks because this is not how doctors classify sleeping pills pharmacologically. For the purpose of this book, it is most convenient to divide sleeping pills into:

- Addicting synthetic sleeping pills/Habit-forming (synthetic chemical)
- Non-Addicting synthetic sleeping pills (synthetic chemical)
- Addicting and Non-Addicting "natural" chemical induction, see *III-Herbs* below

Addicting/Habit-forming sleeping pills of pharmaceutical quality have been used for over a century starting with the first barbiturate that was made in Germany. Its inventor felt that the state of induced sleep was very calming like the Italian town of Verona so he named the drug "Veronal". As time went by other barbiturates were made and then other drugs whose chemical structure was inspired by barbiturates.

Over the next few decades, a lot of sleeping pills were invented and almost all were powerful, addicting and lethal in overdose (less than one month supply could be fatal especially if mixed with a lot of alcohol). These drugs are mainly of historical interest now and include drugs such as Doriden, Noludar, Placidyl, chloral hydrate, paraldehyde, Quaaludes, and also Thalidomide (not sold in the USA). So the search for safer sleeping pills became important.

Bromide salts also were popular but had various side effects (rash and itch).

Alcohol (ethyl alcohol) does occur naturally in our bodies but is not recommended as a sleeping aid. A couple of synthetic alcohols and aldehydes have been tried also.

In the next stage of development, a Swiss chemist took his cues from the Valeriana plant, which apparently has been used by Europeans for thousands of years as a calmative. He isolated one of the active ingredients and named it for the plant, "Valium". The number of fatal overdoses was vastly reduced with the use of these medicines. This was a huge improvement as far as patient tolerance and safety, but these drugs could still be fatal if taken in huge quantities with other sleeping pills and immoderate amounts of alcohol. Doctors made certain to limit supplies to once monthly and the suicide rate was much decreased. Soon, other Valium-like drugs were manufactured by making slight modifications in the chemical structure of Valium. These drugs are all habit-forming just like the parent drug, Valium. The issue of Valeriana and its addictive potential is debatable, but it is sold in American pharmacies without a prescription which implies tacit FDA-approval of its non-addictive status—at least for now. It may, however, be habit-forming.

The next wave of drug development produced a new group of even safer but still habit-forming sleeping pills such as Ambien, Sonata, and Lunesta. Lunesta is the only one in this group which is approved by the FDA for long-term treatment (more than a month). And the search goes on for new sleeping pills with new chemical properties.

Non-addicting sleeping pills (synthetic)

Most of these are sold only on prescription. These are all artificial chemicals that are manufactured in a chemical factory with the main distinction being that they are not habit-forming or—at least—non-addicting. The main subgroups include antihistamines, sedating antidepressants, Seroquel, and Buspar (see respectively in Chapters V-7, V-4, and V-11). The ones which are sold without prescription include doxylamine, meclizine, Benadryl, and Dramamine.

Rozerem is the first melatonin-active pharmaceutical intended as a sleeping pill—and, it is non-addictive. It must be taken every night for a couple weeks before its subtle effect appears.

Biological induction

These include "natural" substances that occur normally in our bodies already, but they may be insufficient because our bodies do not routinely make enough or the production has decreased in the senior years of life.

Melatonin is a natural sleep-inducing substance in our brains. A natural sleep cycle begins when our brain naturally releases a surge of melatonin each night. As our brains become older the production of melatonin may decrease; then it is harder to fall asleep. Other sleep problems may be related to working night shifts, changes of time, or of time zones. Melatonin is especially helpful for jetlag since Melatonin causes the brain to fall asleep normally and makes the brain go into a natural night of reasonably normal sleep cycles. Melatonin resets the *Zeitgeber*, so to speak. The pills are available without a prescription at retail pharmacies in various strengths: 0.5 mg, 1 mg, and 3 mg tablets. Start with a low dose and gradually increase up to a maximum of 9 mg. I have patients with chronic lifelong sleep problems who are now doing much better on a combination of 9 mg of Melatonin mixed with other types of sleep-promoting substances.

L-Tryptophan is also very helpful for starting natural sleep cycles. This also is a natural substance that occurs as part of the proteins of our body. It is an amino-acid. It had been widely popular in the 1980's as a natural sleep-promoter that also helps induce sleep. It was taken off the market for about twelve years because of one bad batch that was turned out once in one Japanese factory. The whole situation has been extensively studied (to be certain of no repeat episodes), and L-Tryptophan is now considered safe. It is back on the market and can be purchased without a prescription; however, some of the retail pharmacies may still be leery of selling it (fears of lawsuits). Check on the Internet and at vitamin shops.

L-Tryptophan in high quantities is also found naturally in turkey, bananas, and milk. Warming of milk tends to release more of the bound Tryptophan into free Tryptophan. Warm milk can be useful unless the patient is lactose-intolerant. L-Tryptophan can be combined for extra effect with the sedating antidepressant, Trazodone. L-Tryptophan starts the sleep cycle but may lack the complete effect of restoring a natural sleep cycle all night long. It is available as 500 mg tablets: take six to ten. A tiny carbohydrate snack may enhance absorption.

Herbal induction

Herbal products are sold without prescription in the USA which means that the FDA feels that the herbs do not pose the risk of habituation or addiction. However, there are reports that some of these can at least cause psychological dependence.

- Valeriana is a tranquilizing herb. (It contains a cornucopia of aromatic plant oils: iridoids and flavonoids (valerenal, valerenic acid, valeranone.)

- Belladonna is another tranquilizing herb that is a source of scopolamine and atropine. Some people develop a habit to this herb.

- Kava kava is sold as a natural tranquilizer in the USA but in its natural source-lands it is considered to be habit-forming like caffeine or nicotine.

- There are other weaker and less potent herbs that are slightly calmative but not habit-forming (passionflower, chamomile, and so on).

Physical induction by means of manipulation of internal biochemical substances to induce sleep

("Natural" Treatment)
- Formalized sitting medication (for twenty minutes or more) as practiced in the Orient can be very relaxing; this technique can be learnt as sitting meditation in meditation centers.

- Daily exercise (preferably aerobic) for a half hour helps to release various "hormones" and chemicals inside our bodies. These can be beneficial for a state of mental and physical well-being.

- Psychotherapy with a psychologist can induce subtle relaxation.

- Biofeedback can be useful. Learning relaxation techniques can be helpful.

- Soaking in a hot tub will help lower blood pressure which can be perceived as relaxing.

- Tension can be relieved by achieving orgasm (releasing a cascade of dopamine and other internal hormones).

- Phototherapy or spending time in the sun may be relaxing to some people.

- Manipulations of sleep cycles may also be helpful (go to bed two hours later every night for ten days,if possible, to try to reset your *Zeitgeber*.

* * *

▶Unfortunately, we still know so little about sleep: why we sleep, how we sleep, why we dream. This will continue to be a fertile area of research for many years to come. We spend 30% of our lives sleeping and still do not know what sleep is or why we sleep [so much]. Understanding and treatment of these topics may open up new vistas to us.

Chapter V-14

Generic Drugs

Background

From a proprietary viewpoint there are two types of drugs: the generic drugs and the so-called "branded" drugs. Branded drugs are also called patent drugs or "trade-name" drugs. The great pharmaceutical houses produce mainly branded drugs. Some of them also own manufacturing subsidiaries that may produce generic drugs with names similar to the branded names. Some of the generic drug companies make only generic drugs. Generic drugs are deemed to be equal (in strength) to the original branded drug. Generic drugs are also referenced as "generic equivalents". The generics have been approved by our government (FDA).

There are several groups involved here, all with their own agenda: drug company, FDA, patient, doctor, pharmacy, and HMO. The drug companies deplore the day in which their profitable branded drug becomes a cheap generic. They have recently devised all sorts of ways to renew a patent by introducing a new "delivery system" for their cash cow. The FDA has the task to oversee the production of generic drugs and is responsible for certifying that generics are equivalent to the original branded drug. If they err, then they may suffer public outcry. Patients like the idea that generics are so much cheaper, but they personally want the top-shelf product for themselves—but at generic prices. Generics often create a headache for doctors who are usually caught in the middle of all the generic brouhaha by virtue of being the prescriber. Doctors have an underlying and uneasy sense that the FDA is a large faceless bureaucracy, that the drug companies watch their bottom lines, and that both FDA and drug companies have a certain insouciance about the whole generic delivery system. Pharmacies are the middlemen and do not invite backlash except when they make "generic substitutions" as permitted by State laws. HMO's are very frugal and try to save pennies everywhere (savings of eighteen cents per month per million members is $210,000 per year per drug multiplied by ten prescriptions is $2,100,000). This is how the financial game of give and take plays out per each player's perspective. This is true "pharmaco-economics".

Drug Company's Viewpoint

The drug company's primary mission is to develop and market immensely profitable new drugs—so that part of the profits can be used to research the next new drug. The pharmaceutical companies spend upwards of a billion dollars to bring each new drug to market.

The drug company that invents a new drug for sale on the market is entitled to a seventeen year monopoly on this drug. Only that company may market and sell its new drug, thereby deriving profits from it. The drug company has only this window of opportunity to recoup its losses in developing and testing the drug and to make a profit that can be plowed back into research and development for the next novel drug. In some cases, the seventeen years have started to toll months or even years before the drug debuts on the market; hence, in most cases, the drug company practically has fewer than seventeen years to make its profits. The drug's debut may be held up for a number of reasons outside the company's control: more testing required by FDA, an unforeseen technical problem in mass manufacturing, an odd side effect reported anecdotally, some possible unexpected secondary long-term side effects showing up in lab animals or early human volunteers, and so on. Then the drug may come to market (in the USA)—or it may be withheld by the drug company for various financial or legal risk issues.

After the patent does expire, any other drug company can start making the drug and selling is as a "generic equivalent". Sometimes drug makers in foreign companies produce generics of a popular drug while it is still supposed to be under patent protection (in the USA). This is a violation of international law. These foreign companies may be "pirating" the drug then offering it for sale on the Internet, but not specifically in the USA. On the other hand, some of the low-volume branded drugs are never available as generic equivalents even though the patent has expired. This may occur in cases where the many complex steps required to synthesize the drug are beyond the means of a small generic drug company; or, in other cases, that the original drug was never well received and hence would not be worth the trouble for a generic company to make its own generic version. A third possibility is that other pharmaceutical companies invented newer, improved, and nearly-identical "me-too" drugs which are considered superior to the original drug for various reasons (such as: pricing, side-effect profiles, etc.). Again, there would be no financial incentive to copy the drug and sell it in generic form. You might not be surprised to know that some parent drug companies own a separate corporation, which is set up to make generic drugs. Some generic drugs are actually made by the parent drug company (why not? They can still make a [small] profit from it). The brand-name drug is going out the "front door" of the factory, so to speak, while the same drug is packaged differently (different colored pill) and is going out the "back door" of the factory, as a generic equivalent.

FDA Viewpoint

The FDA's primary purpose is to protect the consumer (You/Us, the patients). It does this by voting to approve (or deny) a new drug as being worthy of addition to the American pharmacopoeia. Doctors and pharmacies are expected to follow these regulations. FDA has a secondary relationship with the drug company in granting the seventeen year monopoly over the new branded drug. FDA is not involved in legal squabbles or malpractice suits, but is very involved in reviewing complaints (by patients, doctors, or pharmacists) about the new drug.

Back in the past when generics started to become more commonly available there was a lot of concern about the quality of these drugs and about the quality control, too. It did seem to be true in some cases that the generic drug was not so pure or so potent as the original trade-name drug. The FDA looked into this issue and had made some adjustments to regulations.

Patient's Viewpoint

The patient's primary goal is to take the drug and feel better. We want patients to feel comfortable with the nature of the prescription (say, for an antidepressant) and with the probability of getting a generic substitution that is equally effective.

In some cases, patients who were switched from branded drugs to generics could tell the difference. This seemed to be a bigger problem in the 1980's than now. I have had a number of patients who have alleged this for Stelazine, Prolixin, and other drugs. It should be pointed out that these patients were all started on the original branded drug and then later were switched to generic equivalents when generic drugs became available many years later (which is many years ago, now). These complaints created a lot of concern. The FDA now insists that quality control of generics is within acceptable range and that those pills are of equal pharmaceutical grade. FDA wants patients to feel comfortable with the generic drug effects and with the whole generic substitution process. This has usually been found to be technically true from a processing and chemistry viewpoint.

At the patient's request, however, a doctor can order that a trade name drug not be substituted with a generic. This will appear on the prescription as "DAW", "Dispense as Written" or "do not substitute", or similar phraseology (depending upon that State's pharmacy regulations). There is no guarantee what will happen when the patient arrives at the pharmacy. There will usually be a series of painful financial discussions among the patient, his HMO, and the pharmacy. Sometimes the doctor might be asked to intervene; however, the usual results are that contravening medical judgment seldom trumps financial savings.

Unfortunately, a patient may need to negotiate a choice of two or three prices: this is usually a financial transaction between him and his HMO. Fortunately, when he finally leaves the pharmacy, he will have the precise chemical in hand—just maybe not delivered in the anticipated form for the anticipated price. Here is an example of "pharmaco-economics" for Zoloft where the numbers are mere approximations in 2008 dollars:

Chart V-14: Zoloft 50 mg is the Branded drug Sertraline 50 mg is Generic Zoloft						
Generic pricing (estimate): 100 mg pills cost 60¢ each 50 mg pills cost 50¢ 25 mg pills cost 40¢		Retail price (self pay—no HMO)		Wholesale price (HMO coverage)		
		Zoloft $2-3	Sertraline $1-2	Zoloft ($50 per month)*	Setraline 50¢ each	
30 day supply of 30 pills (50 mg) 30 day supply of 15 pills (100 mg) (break big pills in half)	= =	$96 $56	$58 $41	($1-2)	50¢ 60¢	
Total cost to Patient		$96 $56	$58 $41	$50 tier 3 copay	$15 copay generic	
Total cost to HMO		----	----	$40?	$9	

Remember that the pharmacy will add a dispensing fee of a few $$ to each prescription, regardless of the quanity of pills in the bottle.

For example, he may want Zoloft 50 mg tablets. The branded Zoloft 50 mg. tablets from Pfizer may be charged as a "tier three" HMO medicine (provided that his HMO even offers such a tiered option), a monthly copay of about $50. Without insurance, the branded Zoloft would cost about $2-3 per pill. He might be charged as much as $96 for this prescription. He may be able to opt for thirty tablets of generic Zoloft 50 mg for $15 (the generic co-pay under a basic HMO plan). If he opts to save money and take generic Zoloft, his HMO, however, may force the pharmacy to give him fifteen tablets of 100mg scored tablets, which he can then break in half. The reason is that the HMO pays about the same price for 50 mg or 100 mg tablets—that is just the way the drug is marketed. Assume that the HMO pays fifty cents for whichever size pill, you can see that:

30 pills x 50¢= $15 (for #30 of the 50 mg pill), whereas

15 pills x 60¢ ≈ about $9 (for #15 of the 100mg pill)—plus dispensing fee ($12)

If patients could take advantage of the HMO's discounted price for bulk, the patient couild acquire a one month supply of Sertraline (generic Zoloft) for less than his copay of $15. but he can't, so he pays. We pay. We all pay. It never hurts to ask the pharmacy assistant for price quotes.

To demonstrate the thrift of HMO's, imagine that the HMO has ten thousand patients receiving generic Zoloft like this every day. Then the HMO can save a lot of money on just Zoloft alone: ($12 – $9 = $3 savings per member per month per prescription):

*($3 savings/patient) x (10,000 patients/day) x (365 days a year) ≈ $ **13, 900,000** !*
HMO saves over thirteen million dollars a year, just by splitting Zoloft generic tablets!

Remember, that the pharmacies add dispensing fees. HMO's calculate tiny savings (in pennies and dollars) multiplied times millions of patients per year. This adds up to big numbers.

Doctor's Viewpoint

The doctor's primary purpose is to practice medicine from the standpoint of pharmacology and physiology. Concerns about the color, cost, and relative size of the pills, as well as fussing with the HMO and the pharmacy about dispensing and pricing issues lie outside the doctor's purview and control (in most cases). I habitually prescribe some drugs by their branded name, knowing full well that the generic will probably be substituted at the pharmacy. Other drugs that I habitually prescribe by generic name will almost always be filled with the generic, although a few patients have paid out of pocket to have the branded drug dispensed. This is quite rare.

This practice of generic substitution usually cannot be countermanded any longer by the prescribing physician. I can write whatever you please on your prescription, but in the end, the "bottom line" is the issue. Many patients think that I can cause the HMO to charge patients generic prices for non-generic drugs. Doctors have no power over that—if we did, we would change a number of other HMO regulations, too! Most of the fuss over money occurs when a patient arrives at the pharmacy, and this fuss is between himself and his HMO.

HMO's Viewpoint

In the past, patients could go through an appeals process in order to obtain the original branded drug and not the generic equivalent. This is rarely possible nowadays with managed care and HMO formularies (approved drugs lists). The doctor can prescribe branded drugs, but cannot enforce this. Most HMO's will not permit this nowadays and some may refuse these requests outright. Others may permit limited substitution with maximum documentation. In some cases, many patients have complained about a certain particular generic as being sub-standard to the point that the HMO will be more amenable to this substitution. Some of the HMO rules may be decided on an individual patient basis and on an individual drug-prescription basis. Some may permit branded drugs at the patient's request—as long as the patient is willing to pay non-generic prices: this could include dispensing the branded drug as a "tiered" drug (probably thirty to sixty dollars). The HMO's seem to change their rules on a yearly basis. Obviously, this is a complicated minefield to maneuver—which is why doctors dread phone calls about prescription denials. Most of the problems stem from contractual situations between the HMO and the patient over which the doctor has no control whatsoever.

Pharmacy Viewpoint

(Generally speaking, this is the reseller's viewpoint, whoever that reseller may be—it often turns out to be the pharmacy wholesaler who supplies a regional chain of pharmacies as well as pharmacies.)

Each State has slightly different pharmacy rules regarding the dispensing of generic drugs, but in general, a pharmacy may legally switch any patient to a generic drug, once that generic drug becomes available on the marketplace (subject to any countervailing federal or local laws). The generic equivalent must first receive FDA approval. The order to prevent generic substitution usually cannot be enforced by the prescribing physician.

Thus, the pharmacy is within its legal rights to dispense generics whenever generics are available. Also, note that pharmacists have a legal right to refuse to fill any prescription for any reason. The usual case in Los Angeles is that the pharmacies refuse to fill a prescription because the prescription has been written for a drug which they do not stock regularly or the drug is so esoteric that the pharmacy feels this is not profitable for them to order one bottle of pills for one patient and then give coveted shelf space to a half empty bottle of pills that will probably go unused—unless my patient returns for refills. Pharmacy shelf space is precious. I have encountered this problem when prescribing Kemadrin, Abilify 2 mg tablets, Prozac in 5 mg doses, and so on. I usually need to call the pharmacy and assure them that it will be a regular monthly prescription for the same patient. The pharmacy will usually acquiesce, but sometimes they will still balk and will notify me that "their supplier does not have that drug in 'the warehouse'". This is usually the ring of finality and I tell the patient to take the prescription to a small family-owned drug store, which is usually much more accommodating than the huge chain retail stores which survive on volume sales of popular drugs and not on esoteric niche drugs. Another reason for which pharmacies might refuse to fill a prescription is when they suspect that the patient has stolen or altered my prescription in order to write himself a bogus prescription. A third reason occurs when an obviously intoxicated or aggressively drugged up person brings in a prescription for

Valium, narcotics, or amphetamines. Additionally, pharmacists in some jurisdictions are within their legal rights to refuse to fill an "objectionable" or morally repugnant prescription for a non-emergency condition. (e.g., "morning after" birth control pills).

My patients' reports suggest that the effects and quality of modern generics are about the same as those of trade-name drugs. The one caveat is that if a patient starts on a certain generic drug from a certain drug company, then she needs to continue on exactly that same medication from that same source. If you are stabilized on generic G from drug company X then the quality of that drug will probably remain the same—just continue to take G from X. Really popular generic drugs are often made by two or three competing generic drug companies, X, Y, and Z. Sometimes even the parent company of the brand drug is selling its own branded product as its own generic drug G. Some of the patient problems and complaints seem to occur when the local pharmacy P switches suppliers of generic drug G. Company Z may undercut company X and give the pharmacy P a better wholesale deal buying drug G in bulk. Then Pharmacy P starts to buy drug G from company Z. Some patients who are stabilized on generic drug G from generic company X can feel different if given Generic drug G made by generic company Y. Patients might experience a difference in efficacy resulting from this substitution. In this case, patients should request the pharmacy to continue filling the prescription with generic X instead of generic Y —if possible. Other than that, the generics seem to work quite well.

Other Viewpoints

Large hospitals may have their own dispensing agenda, especially if they are part of a large corporate structure.

▶Summary

- In calculating costs, remember that pharmacies add on dispensing fees (like a handling fee).

- Pharmaceutical products are an immensely expensive enterprise with gargantuan profits accompanied by financial failures and agonizing disappointments of all kinds.

- Doctors have no real control over federal guidelines or State Pharmacy Laws.

- The financial issues are really a business negotiation between the patient and his HMO—outside parties such as pharmacists and doctors have no control over the HMO and its fee schedules.

- Pharmaceuticals are a trillion dollar business!

Non-Prescription Medications
OTC and BTC
(Over the Counter and Behind the Counter)

Chapter Outline	Chapter Topics of Interest
OTC Diet Pills	Medicines with Psychoactive Side Effects
OTC "cold medicines"	Stimulation(diet pills and cold medicines)
DXM, Tylenol	Sedation (cold medicines)
Miscellaneous medicines	None (cold medicines, DXM, Tylenol)

Non-prescription drugs can be purchased without a doctor's prescription. These drugs are commonly referred to as Over-the-Counter medicines (OTC's) and Behind the Counter medicines (BTC). OTC medications are available in unrestricted amounts. A person could go into a drug store and buy every box of an OTC medicine. That is not true of behind the counter medicines, which the pharmacist will dole out in limited amounts over a certain time period, and that dole is recorded using the purchaser's driver's license, usually. A fair supply of OTC's is available. The OTC drugs often have little or no mood or mind altering properties. Behind the counter drugs may be toxic in high doses or may have mild mood and mind altering effects, and that is why access to them is controlled.

OTC drugs usually fall into three classes that are of interest to psychiatry: they either possess modest mood or mind-altering properties or they have no such properties but can affect prescription psycho-active medicines. The third class would be OTC drugs that are fatal in cases of "terminal depression" (suicide).

The OTC drugs with psycho-active properties are the so-called "diet pills" and "cold medicines". (The diet pills are also separately covered in Chapter V-18.)

Apart from these medicines, DXM and pseudo-ephedrine are both special cases. DXM is a benign non-addicting drug that can easily be "cooked" into heroin or morphine. Pseudo-ephedrine is a non-addicting "sinus medicine" that can easily be "cooked" into "crystal meth". The government has determined it will make these two drugs available for people with legitimate medical reasons; however, access to the two drugs is limited in order to prevent diversion into underground drug labs. DXM is available as a pure OTC cough medicine, but access to it is "chemically" controlled: it has been adulterated in such a way as to prevent its conversion into dangerous narcotics. Pure DXM is also quite expensive (see below in this chapter). Access to pseudo-ephedrine is legally controlled nationwide: it has become a behind the counter medication.

OTC Diet Pills

The diet pills typically contain ephedrine, caffeine derivatives, or PPA (phenylpropanolamine).

The popular additive in diet pills is often Phenylpropanolamine (PPA) which is structurally related to the drugs of the adrenaline family (also related to amphetamines). And like the drugs in this class, it tends to suppress appetite, which is the desired effect. Typical to drugs of this class, it also possesses undesirable side effects such as elevation of blood pressure, which in turn might have detrimental effects on the kidneys which is not a desired effect either. Apart from that, PPA can cause nervousness, insomnia, and repetitive behaviors called stereotypies (when the drug user needlessly and automatically repeats actions over and over again). If high doses are taken too frequently and for too long, then the patient could become frankly paranoid due to two properties of taking excessive amounts of this medicine: the medicine can exert a direct effect on the brain to cause paranoia; and, the drug causes insomnia and loss of sleep, which can make anybody batty.

Sometimes diet pills might contain ephedrine or pseudo-ephedrine (Sudafed) which are also in the adrenaline-amphetamine family of drugs and can have similar effects to those of PPA. These drugs are potentially somewhat toxic, and at high doses, produce a lot of restlessness and nervousness that are not really pleasant. Anybody who really wants to lose weight should enroll in a medical weight loss program.

The newest over-the-counter diet drug, Alli, seems to be perfectly safe and has none of these side-effects because it has no effect on the nervous system whatsoever. As a matter of fact, it is not even absorbed into the body.

OTC "cold medicines" (pills for breathing, "hay fever", and sinus problems)

Traditionally, these drugs have all had mood and mind altering properties due to their mechanism of action. The mood and mind-altering properties were either those of stimulation or of sedation. Consumers complained, and the race was on to find drugs that lack these side effects. The newer drugs such as Tavist, Claritin-Loratidine, and Cetirizine lack mood and mind altering properties while retaining respiratory effects. These drugs are not covered further here.

The "cold medicines" with psycho-active side effects are divided into two general categories, based on mechanism of action: stimulation and sedation. The stimulating drugs open the airways and shrink the size of the blood vessels going to the nose. The sedating drugs are the sedating anti-histamines.

Stimulant cold medicines

The stimulating "cold medicines"—apart from the desired respiratory effects—also have stimulating effects on the nervous system, which some people find unpleasant. These effects include restlessness, rapid heart beat, high blood pressure, insomnia, irritability, impaired judgment, confusion, and agitation. The typical one is PPA, listed in the beginning of this chapter and in Chapter V-18. Stimulating respiratory medicines typically available in cold remedies include: PPA, ephedrine, pseudo-ephedrine, phenylephrine. See Chapter V-6 and the paragraphs above in this chapter.

Sedating cold medicines

The sedating "cold medicines", on the other hand, are "antihistamines". Several are available without a prescription. These drugs are not particularly toxic (except possibly in the elderly) and can produce a state of drowsiness, which is not unpleasant—and in some cases, even desirable. If a person is sick with a cold, then he probably should stay at home and rest anyway. Besides helping cold and sinus symptoms, anti-histamines also increase appetite, dry out sinuses, and cause dry mouth. In higher doses, some of them can cause mild symptoms of urine retention, blurred vision, and slight constipation. In very high doses, they may cause a paradoxical excitation. At least the dry mouth side effect does remind patients to drink fluids. If one can stay at home to nap and fall asleep while watching movies, then anti-histamines sound rather good. If, however, the person has important business deals and work to do, the sedation definitely becomes undesirable. Typical anti-histamines are: Benadryl, chlorpheniramine, and brompheniramine. (Doxylamine, Dramamine, Bonine, and Antivert are also in this family but have different uses: doxylamine for bedtime sedation and the others, for nausea and motion sickness.)

Thus, they dry up sinuses, their desirable effect. The corollary to this is that they will also dry up other secretions such as tears, saliva, and stomach secretions, leading to dry mouth, dry eyes, constipation and hunger. This is a direct effect of their antihistamine activity. In the elderly, this drying effect can be harmful in the following conditions:

- eye problems ("closed-angle glaucoma")

- prostate problems (men)

- severe constipation ("obstipation")

- symptomatic stomach ulcers

- memory problems (forgetfulness and dementia)

(Doxylamine is typically used as a "sleeping pill" not a "cold medicine".) These drugs are quite popular and provide a lot of benefit for sinus problems and mild sedation at bedtime.

Narcotics: DXM

Narcotics are dangerous drugs and are controlled by the government. Their useful medical effects are to deaden pain, suppress coughing, and stop diarrhea. However, in slightly higher doses they can cause truly bad effects. They may deaden the brain's perception of pain, but they can affect the brain so much as to make people feel dopey and groggy. Narcotics may suppress coughing, but they may also stop us from breathing altogether. They may stop diarrhea, but in higher doses they can cause dizziness, nausea, and even vomiting. But the worst problem of all is that of extreme addiction.

DXM

The only narcotic available OTC is DXM, dextromethorphan. It is a narcotic with only one first-rate narcotic effect: it can suppress coughing very well. At higher doses it is less likely to stop breathing than the addicting narcotics. It is available in a number of cough medicines. It can be purchased in purified form, but the purified form has been adulterated so that it cannot be "cooked" into heroin and morphine in underground labs. It is available as Delsym® and Luden's Honey-Tuss®—neither one of these has any psychoactive properties. However, DXM can raise blood levels of Paxil and other medications. At least one person has died from overdose of Paxil and DXM.

Alcohol and Sugar

Some cough medicines contain beverage alcohol. I urge psychiatric patients to avoid alcohol. Ditto for recovering alcoholics and drug-addicts. Nyquil, for example,contains up to 25% alcohol!!

Original Contac®: the original formula that made Contac famous contained a mixture of real belladonna extracts. This was the most powerful of all cold medicines, as far as sinus-drying. Because of the belladonna extract, it also had delightful mood and mind-altering effects. They changed the formula years ago. If you should find this preparation somewhere in the world, then you must remember *not to mix it* with any of the following:

the old sedating antidepressants, Parkinsonian medications, or FGA (first generation antipsychotics).

Guidelines for combining cold medicines with psychoactive medicines

In the past, manufacturers sometimes tried to balance out sedation and stimulation by putting one of each chemical into a single cough syrup or sinus pill, such as combining phenylephrine and chlorpheniramine. Cough syrups are notorious for having different ingredients. This is called "shotgun therapy"—hopefully, at least one target symptom will be "hit". The reasons for shotgun therapy are several. One reason is that of convenience for the consumer to have four or five medicines in one preparation. Another reason is that the combination of small amounts of several medicines can overall have a large effect, larger than the sum of their small parts. In pharmacology this is called "potentiation". Another reason for shotgun therapy is that the government does not approve consumers to have purified forms of certain drugs (dextromethorphan, for example). Robitussin® is well known for marketing many different combinations of cold medicines. Robitussin Night-time Cough Cold & Flu contains a rational mixture of Tylenol, chlorpheniramine, phenylephrine, and DXM that should be (psychiatrically) palatable to most people.

However, I prefer that my patients with serious mental illness check with me before consuming OTC stimulants. These are my general recommendations for patients in active therapy taking psychoactive medicines:

- If you are taking **MAOI**, you must talk to your prescribing psychiatrist. You must not consume any of the stimulating "cold medicines".

- Manic-Depression, Bipolar, Schizophrenia, Psychotic Disorders: avoid any stimulating cold medicines.

- Major Depression patients: either low-dose pseudo-ephedrine or phenylephrine—unless you have high blood pressure, then eliminate all stimulating cold medicines.

- Patients taking **SGA** *antipsychotics* should consider using sugar-free cough medicines.

- Anxiety Panic patients: plain chlorpheniramine; avoid the stimulants: phenylephrine, Sudafed, Ephedrine, and PPA (phenyl-propanol-amine);

- Anxiety Panic patients: pure DXM cough syrup is acceptable unless taking Paxil or Luvox, in which case halve the dosage of the pure DXM cough syrup; another option is to avoid DXM altogether and use *Guaifenesin* which has no psychiatric effects. Guaiafenesin helps loosen up chest phlegm (expectoration). It irritates the stomach, which then sends a nerve signal to irritate the lungs to cough up phlegm.

Some people find this stomach irritation to be unpleasant. Check with your primary doctor: he might willing to prescribe Tessalon Perles®.

- Dementia patients: check with primary doctor. Drugs lacking any brain side effects are probably most desirable: Tavist, Claritin (Loratidine), Cetirizine, and Xyzal. The sedating antihistamines will worsen dementia and cause other problems too.

- Patients taking sedating antidepressants or any of the anti-psychotics (Chapter V-4) would do well to steer clear of Phenergan (Promethazine).

- If taking Geodon, Mellaril, or Serentil, then avoid Seldane and Hismanal (off the market in the USA now: cardiac risk)

These guidelines apply to relatively young and healthy people. Anyone with a complicated medical history should check first with his primary care doctor.

This is a listing of "cold medicines" and their typical side effects: stimulation, sedation, or none:

	Stimulation	Sedation	Minimal Side Effects
OTC or BTC	Pseudo-ephedrine Ephedrine Phenylephrine PPA phenylpropanolamine Caffeine derivatives	Chlor-Trimeton Chlorpheniramine Benadryl Dimetane brompheniramine	Tavist Claritin (Loratidine) Cetirizine
Available only on Prescription	Ephedrine Theophylline Proventil, Ventolin Brethine	Phenergan Codeine	Xyzal Tessalon Perles

Table V-15 "Cold medicines" and Psychiatry: contact your doctor about these

Tylenol

Tylenol is a very good medicine that has helped countless persons since its arrival on the market. It helps to diminish pain and fever but has no effect on inflammation. It has no psychiatric effects. What people do not realize is that Tylenol can be fatal in overdose. Even worse is that the fact that some impulsive people who are trying to make a statement—or just to get attention—by dramatically staging an intentional but non-lethal suicide gesture are often unaware of how dangerous this gesture might be. Despite the fact that the person was probably not really intending to die, the outcome may be fatal. And worst of all is the fact that the patient will die slowly from liver failure over the space of a few days and will be clearly aware of what is going on but powerless to stop his death that is imminent In the emergency room, I had seen a young man who had done just this thing, taking a goodly amount of Tylenol, because his girlfriend had jilted him. He recanted his desire to die, but nonetheless spent the next three days clearly lucid with his family and friends around him in the ICU while his liver deteriorated completely. It would be almost impossible to arrange an emergency liver transplant within two or three days. Be careful of this drug that is not quite as innocuous as you may think. Also see Aspirin below.

Miscellaneous Medicines

Aspirin
also called ASA (Acetyl-Salicylic Acid)
Aspirin has no effect in Psychiatry, but—like Tylenol—can also be fatal in overdose.

NSAID

(Non-Steroidal Anti-Inflammatory Drugs)
 Other OTC medicines are anti-inflammatory pills of the family of NSAID's, such as Motrin (ibuprofen) and Alleve (Naprosyn, naproxen). These drugs have no psychiatric purpose. However, these pills can raise lithium levels—which is dangerous. If you are taking arthritis pills from your family doctor and lithium from your psychiatrist, be sure to inform your psychiatrist about this so that he can follow your lithium treatment closely.

 You must remember that all [allopathic] drugs are chemicals and as such are poisons which are doled out in doses small enough to be therapeutic but not large enough to be toxic.

►Guidelines:

- Choose drugs with agreeable side effects or none (Tavist, Loratidine, Cetirizine)

- The elderly should not take *any* OTC drugs for *any* reason without consulting their primary doctor: stimulating drugs raise blood pressure and sedating antihistamines have negative effects on the prostate, glaucoma, and other conditions.

- DXM is a superior cough medicine containing a purified substance with minimal sedation, *but* it can interact with other drugs, such as Luvox and Paxil (raising the Paxil blood levels).

Chapter V-16

Drugs Dangerous and "Dirty"

*A "dirty" drug always has many unpleasant side effects such as
dizziness, drooling, trembling, constipation, and so on.
A "clean" drug has few unpleasant side effects.*

Clozaril and MAOI, are truly dangerous and potentially lethal whether used alone or with other drugs. These drugs are typically *not* first line psychiatric drugs and in some cases are drugs of last resort. I think of Clozaril as chemotherapy. A few drugs are reasonably safe for whole populations, but when they do cause a side effect, it is catastrophic-to-fatal. Some medications can be reasonably safe when used alone, but potentially dangerous in certain combinations. These latter drugs "do not play well with others". The decision to use any of these drugs must be discussed with your prescribing doctor. You need to learn about the risks and the consequences. In all situations, you must determine the risks and benefits of these drugs: find out the risks of taking the drugs and the risks of not taking it; and, understand the benefits of taking it versus not taking it.

In this chapter we have four types of dangerous psychiatric drugs:

- **Inherently dangerous** psychiatric medicines: these are **always predictably toxic and/or dangerous** and require constant daily and weekly monitoring by both the patient and health care professionals: *Clozaril, Nardil, other MAOI antidepressants*
- **Relatively harmless drugs when used alone**, but if mixed with other medications can **predictably** produce a lot of side effects and toxicities: *Luvox, Antidepressants, Mellaril*
- **Frequently used drugs with a predictable probability of annoying but rarely life-threatening side effects**: all the Antipsychotics
- **Safe Drugs that very rarely (unpredictably) are harmful or toxic/dangerous**: (In other words, drugs that cause few inconvenience to the vast majority of patients, but when they do produce side effects, they are **catastrophic**): *Serzone, Lamictal, Depakote, Lithium, Trazodone, Tegretol*
- **Pitfalls**: drug combinations to avoid

Inherently Dangerous Psychiatric Medicines

These are psychiatric drugs that by themselves cause a lot of constant annoying side-effects on every day of therapy (which we commonly call "dirty drugs"). These daily side effects are often unpleasant. Or, they may not cause any significant daily annoying side effects, but are known for causing one or many very serious delayed toxic medical problems. Or, it may be a dirty drug on every day of treatment plus having serious delayed long-term toxic effects. Examples:

Table V-16-a Dangerous Drugs

	Life-threatening	Moderately toxic	Mildly toxic	Annoying
Assume: Always	Clozaril MAOI**(not Emsam)	Xyrem		
Often			Luvox + other meds	Antipsychotics, MAOI
sometimes		MAOI** Psychostimulants	Old antidepressants Antipsychotics	Old Antidepressants Lithium
Rarely	SSRI + triptans* SSRI + other drugs*	Emsam, Mellaril	Lithium Chantix	Luvox used alone
Very, very rarely	Lamictal, Tegretol, Lithium, Trazodone	Depakote Wellbutrin		

* "serotonin syndrome" / "other drugs" refers to "other antidepressants" and Buspar
**MAOI = Nardil, Marplan, Parnate, Selegiline, but not Emsam—chapter V-6

Xyrem

This is GHB, the so-called "date rape drug". It has only one medicinal use: for rare sleep disorders. It is extremely dangerous and causes people to pass out in a matter of several seconds. The manufacturer recommends that it be taken after the patient is already comfortably situated in bed. Xyrem is not available at pharmacies, only through a special program.

Lithium

Lithium has some common daily persistent and annoying minor side effects which are not life-threatening but may lower the quality of life such as: thirst, hunger weight gain, shaking hands, and acne.

The worst toxic problem with Lithium occurs when the blood level of lithium suddenly increases. If the patient does not realize this and continues to take the medicine he can become severely ill, end up in the intensive care unit, and rarely succumb to the toxicity. The toxic level of lithium is not much higher than the therapeutic level and—worst of all—can rise suddenly when the patient is apparently just taking his regular dosage. The therapeutic blood level is usually in the range of 0.5-1.5 whereas the toxic level can occur anywhere above 2.0 (these ranges vary slightly from lab to lab). This often occurs because the patient has unwittingly changed his intake of water, sodium, and/or potassium or all three. Some common drugs can cause problems too such as "water pills" or anti-inflammatory "NSAID" pills (ibuprofen, naproxen, and others). This is the worst of all the side effects because it is a medical and a psychiatric emergency.

For this reason, all Lithium patients need to be schooled to recognize the early warning signs and symptoms of rising lithium blood levels: hand and arm trembling and twitchiness as well as diarrhea. Patients can review and reinforce their ability to recognize these symptoms at every office visit.

The reader can see from table V-16-a that Lithium appears in more than one category: there are two reasons for this; (1) Lithium can inherently be mildly toxic in certain patients, but in other individuals who are so disposed, Lithium may often be more toxic—this seems in part to correlate to the unique ways that each individual can react in the presence of any medication; and, (2) this is intended to highlight the unpredictable nature of Lithium in any person at any time.

MAOI

MAOI Antidepressant drugs can be very dangerous but can also be very effective. "MAOI" stands for "monoamine oxidase inhibitor"—see Chapter V-6. These drugs are almost never used anymore with the possible exception of Selegiline/Emsam. Any patient who takes these drugs will receive extensive counseling by the prescribing doctor. MAOI may interact with other prescription medications to cause serious side effects. The main dangers occur when MAOI's are mixed with certain forbidden foods—unfortunately, quite a few foods are on the list. The wrong food could cause a spike in blood pressure and—in exceedingly rare cases—a stroke.

Clozaril

Clozaril is a dirty drug known for causing epileptic fits, heart failure, and life-threatening infections. These infections can be rapidly fatal since Clozaril prevents the body from fighting off infections. Clozaril is ideally prescribed by doctors who are very familiar with all its problems. It requires weekly blood tests that can be decreased later to biweekly. The prescriptions need to be coordinated between the lab, the prescribing doctor, and the pharmacist.

Clozaril has many drug interactions also. it interacts with Luvox also, but this can be used to advantage. A small amount of Luvox can boost the Clozaril blood level without increasing the number of Clozaril pills taken.

I would suggest that anybody taking any of these drugs make out a chart of the advantages and the disadvantages. In the right columns put down the numerical value of the importance or detriment to you, the patient. You can acquire this information from your doctor and case manager. This is a sample chart of how to do it for Clozaril:

Risks of Clozaril	±	Benefits of Clozaril	±
One chance in 1500 of Serious Heart disease (fatal)		Ability to go out in public again, to visit and have friends, to go on "dates"	
Gaining weight		No longer thinking that food is poisoned	
Altered blood pressure		Better relationships with people	
Blood tests every two weeks		Possibly pleasant sense of sedation	
Seizures		Control of severe psychotic illness	
Life-threatening infections		No longer hearing scary voices	
Very complicated drug regimen many reactions with other Rx medicines			

V-16-b   Clozaril   (I have chosen Clozaril because it is a highly toxic and dangerous drug which can be highly beneficial for those few selected cases.)

Each chart can be customized by allowing yourself to decide how mental illness limits your daily activities and how much the medicine might lift those restrictions and give you a lot more freedoms. And balance it against the toxicities of the drugs. Your therapist, pharmacist, or case manager can help you with this chart. This is how a patient, Mary, filled out her Clozaril chart and learned that she feels a (+14) advantage for her to take Clozaril, but this is just a fictional example:

Risks of Clozaril	±	Benefits of Clozaril	±
One chance in 1500 of Serious heart disease (fatal)	-2	Ability to go out in public again, to visit friends And to have friends	+15
Gaining weight	-12	No longer thinking that food is poisoned	+3
Altered blood pressure (impotence)	-1	Better relationships with people	+10
Blood tests every two weeks	-3	Possibly pleasant sense of sedation	+1
Seizures	-6	Control of severe psychotic illness	+9
Life-threatening infections	-3	No longer hearing scary voices	+3
Complicated to use/drug reactions	0		

Totals are   (-27)   (+41) = +14

Mary may have placed great value on the possibility of finding a boyfriend. Male patients may be distressed by impotence resulting from the lower blood pressure caused by Clozaril.

Relatively Harmless Psychiatric Drugs—when used alone

These drugs when used *alone* might occasion few problems and are reasonably innocuous. However, when combined with other drugs, they can often become quite *problematic*. At the least, they will predictably cause many side effects.

Luvox, in general, interacts significantly with many other prescription drugs. This effect is especially problematic when a patient already takes several other medicines. For this reason, Luvox is not ideal for the elderly or for anybody taking a lot of different medications.

Non-prescription "diet pills" and psychostimulants should not be mixed with prescription diet pills and psychostimulants because of many possible side effects (not the least of which could be heart attack or mini-stroke). Examples of psychostimulants are: Amphetamines, Ritalin, Cylert, Provigil Nuvigil—chapter V-6)

Emsam is a MAOI antidepressant and is usually exempt from the dietary restrictions (at low doses) since the drug is absorbed through the skin and not in the digestive system. But even Emsam could cause MAOI-type reactions.

Chantix is indicated to help quit smoking. Some people can become very depressed while taking Chantix.

Wellbutrin has been reported to cause seizures, but this has not happened in my patients as far as I have been told.

Frequently Used Drugs with uncommon but predictable probability of annoying but rarely causing life-threatening side effects

Lithium

I have listed Lithium here for a second time because it is basically a "dirty" drug with a lot of annoying side effects. Patients who are well educated about the signs and symptoms of Lithium poisoning are good allies at this level of Lithium treatment. They know that excessive trembling hands and diarrhea are warning signs.

Lithium has a few common daily persistent and annoying minor side effects which are not life-threatening but may lower the quality of life such as: thirst, hunger weight gain, shaking hands, and acne; fortunately, most patients only need to deal with one or two of these side effects and it is rare for a lithium patient to have all of these side effects;

Lithium has two toxic side effects which might only appear slowly and gradually after many years or even decades of taking Lithium. These two toxicities are thyroid disease and kidney disease. Hopefully, a patient is not going to be afflicted with both of these simultaneously. These chronic toxicities usually evolve slowly. Appropriate lab test monitoring can usually give advance warning of these kinds of toxicities so that Lithium can be stopped before the toxicity continues to worsen. Men seem to have a slight proclivity for kidney problems, and women, for thyroid problems. The worst toxic problem with Lithium occurs when the blood level of lithium suddenly increases. If the patient does not realize this and continues to take the medicine, he can become severely ill.

Tegretol has a lot of side effects such as dizziness or slowness; it also can suppress the bone marrow thereby leading to a sore throat. Blood levels are available for monitoring the effects of Tegretol. In very rare cases if the infection worsens, it could lead to death. Very infrequently, Tegretol might overwork the liver or lower sodium levels in the body. Extremely low sodium levels might cause permanent brain damage.

Mellaril has been used commonly for decades and has been known to cause possible heart conditions. This has not been a common problem.

Reasonably Safe Drugs that very, very, very rarely and unpredictably are harmful, toxic, or dangerous, causing Catastrophic Effects

These catastrophic side effects are incredibly rare: they can be measured on the order of 1 in 40,000 patients (Trazodone) up to 43 per tens of millions (Serzone).

Serzone can cause total liver failure and this risk is greater if taking liver-stressing drugs as with Depakote.

Trazodone use in sexually active men might result in permanent impotence

Lamictal—fatal skin rash

Depakote—liver failure (children, usually)

Lithium—seizures and death

Tegretol—can suppress the bone marrow thereby leading to infections. In very rare cases the infection could worsen and be fatal. Tegretol might overwork the liver or lower sodium levels in the body. Extremely low sodium levels might cause permanent brain damage.

[Merital (Nomifensine)—fatal anemia (off the market in USA)]

Pitfalls—these are combinations to avoid or situations to avoid

Medical medications processed in the liver. Psychiatric drugs that are processed heavily in the liver and taken in high doses can stress the liver. If a patient is inadvertently taking a number of other medical medications at the same time as the psychiatric drugs, the liver can become overworked and start to fail. Example of such psychiatric drugs are: Depakote and Serzone, mainly. To a lesser degree some of the older antidepressants, Tegretol, and any of the antipsychotics might have this effect, too. Examples of such medical medications that are hard on the liver include Tylenol, herbs, non-prescription drugs, "cholesterol" drugs ("statin"), some diabetes pills, male/female hormones, and various antibiotics such as: TB drugs (Isoniazid and Rifampin), anti-fungal drugs, antibiotics (erythromycin, other "-mycins"), and various others such as Darvon. The primary doctors are usually checking blood tests on any of these drugs whether the patient takes pills from other specialist or not. The combination of one liver-stressing psychiatric drug with a couple of liver-stressing medical medications might stress the liver even more than the sum of the individual medicines.

OTC analgesic medications: There is a completely separate situation involving people who are called "analgesic addicts". They are "addicted" to taking excessive daily amounts of OTC pills such as Tylenol, aspirin, phenacetin, ibuprofen, and others. These pills are liver-stressing. Excessive intake of such liver-stressing drugs can damage the liver after months or years or decades (Yes, some people do this for decades before they damage their bodies). These drugs are OTC (over the counter) and sold without prescription, so that these "analgesic addicts" can purchase unlimited amounts of their "drug of choice". These people take such OTC drugs in maximum or excess dosage almost every day. This is a behavioral problem, but is not a true addiction. Apart from causing liver problems, these behaviors can also put patients at risk for kidney problems. Treatment consists primarily of talk therapy. There may be a passive death wish linked to a mild underlying depression. These patients resist psychiatric intervention.

Soma, a muscle relaxant, can be turned into Miltown/Equanil (Meprobamate) which is a strong habit-forming sedative that everybody was taking before Valium was invented. Valium is a lot safer than meprobamate which is almost never prescribed now. For this very reason, Flexeril is now a more popular muscle relaxant.

Codeine needs to be turned into a morphine derivative in order to produce pain relief and there are certain prescription drugs that block this transformation. If these drugs are taken with codeine, then the codeine is not turned into the morphine-like painkiller: this may explain why some patients report that codeine is useless for them. Codeine undergoes transformation in the (CytochromeP_{450}) 2D6 system. Any other 2D6 drugs can block the transformation; there are many of these. This is a list of only the psychiatry 2D6 drugs: Paxil, Prozac, Wellbutrin, Prolixin, Haldol, Mellaril, Trilafon. Tagamet is a common medical medication with 2D6 blockade. (see Chapter II-4) Hence, Vicodin has replaced codeine as the common minor narcotic pain killer (Darvocet may also be helpful for some cases).

SSRI

Tricyclic antidepressants and SSRI antidepressants are sometimes combined. Be aware that they will both raise each other's blood levels and the patient may be having side effects thus necessitating a reduction in one or both. In severe cases this could cause the so-called "serotonin syndrome" which is a medical emergency (trembling, fever, confusion). We rarely prescribe Serzone nowadays and thus we no longer mix it with SSRI antidepressants as this combination also might cause serotonin syndrome. SSRI's and "triptans" could cause "serotonin syndrome" requiring a visit to the hospital emergency room. The "triptans" are a large group of migraine headache pills such as Imitrex, Frova, and many others—they all have generic names ending in "–triptan".

Accutane and retinoic acids may cause depression (dermatology)
Interferon can cause a deep depression (hepatitis treatment)

Cigarettes

Cigarette smoking can lower blood levels of certain medicines (Zyprexa). This effect is not due to the nicotine, but rather to the "coal tars" in cigarettes.

Grapefruit

Grapefruit juice can lower blood levels of certain drugs, this is mainly a problem for the PI class of AIDS drugs (pharmacies will typically put a grapefruit restriction label on the bottles of these medicines). This effect is mediated by the (CytochromeP$_{450}$) 3A4 system. If this is a problem with psychiatric drugs, we can increase the dose, but then the patient would need to consume the same amount of grapefruit each day. If grapefruit juice seems to make your psychoactive drugs less reliable, then the easiest solution is to avoid grapefruit. The psychiatric drugs which might be so affected are: Aricept, Remeron, St.John's Wort, Buspar, Tegretol, Tricyclics (Chapter V-7), Provigil, Buspar, Orap, Viagra, Serzone, SSRI's (Chapter V-8) and drugs of the Xanax-(subgroup)-family(Chapter V-11).

Alcohol

Most importantly, alcohol is not healthy for the following reasons: it interferes with some medications, it depresses the brain, and it is hard on the liver, too!! (some people self-medicate with alcohol as if it were a minor mind-altering liquid drug).

Dextromethorphan (DXM) is an over the counter cough medicine that can be dangerous, especially when mixed with drugs such as Paxil: this combination has been fatal. Overdose on dextromethorphan can present with narcotic-like symptoms. (Chapter V-15)

Certain non-psychiatric drugs can interrupt the normal processing of psychiatric drugs leading to an accumulation of unprocessed drug in the blood: there are many examples so always be wary of adding a new drug to your already established daily regimen of medications even if it is not a prescription drug.

This chart provides some perspective on and counterbalance to the dangerous drugs. You can see that there are safe drugs, but they are sometimes less effective or less potent. The more dangerous and "dirtier" drugs are more potent but carry more risk.

Table V-16-c   Listing of drugs from safest to most toxic

Drug name	Untoward side effects	Poisoning / Overdose (OD)
SAFEST ↓↓		
Neurontin	Dizziness	- - - -
Prozac, all SSRI's and SNRI's***		
Atarax, Vistaril	Sedation, dryness	
Buspar, Trileptal	"Buzziness", sedation,	
Trazodone	Sedation, dizziness	(Very rare heart attacks)
Lamictal	Allergic rash	Fatal rash
Wellbutrin	Constipation, headache	Seizures
Cogentin group****	Drying of body	
SGA antipsychotics Abilify, Geodon Risperdal & Invega Seroquel	Metabolic syndrome* Low blood pressure	? Heart problems? Parkinson's Disease Metabolic syndrome*
Tegretol	Dizziness, low sodium	Serious infections (rare)
Zyprexa	Metabolic syndrome*	Metabolic syndrome*
Elavil, Ludiomil, All Tricyclics**	Excessive slowing & Drying of body	Fatal in overdose (heart failure)
FGA antipsychotics	Trembling, slowing	Parkinson's Disease
Depakote	Liver stress	Liver failure
Serzone		Total liver failure
Lithium	Thyroid and Kidney problems	Serious seizures Death in O.D.
Clozaril	Metabolic syndrome*	Heart attack, seizure, Serious infections
LEAST SAFE ↑↑		

*metabolic syndrome is: overweight, diabetes, high cholesterol plus high blood pressure

**Tricyclic antidepressants include Elavil, Pamelor, Imipramine, Desipramine, Doxepin, Vivactil, Surmontil, and (Asendin).
***SSRI's: Prozac, Zoloft, Paxil, Celexa, Luvox, Lexapro; SNRI's are Effexor, Cymbalta, Pristiq
****Cogentin, Artane, Akineton, Kemadrin

Pharmacology of Addiction
(See Chapter VI-1 also: Alcoholism and Addiction)

We all have the ability to experience pleasure and pain, psychosis and sanity, euphoria and dysphoria (the opposite of euphoria), and so on.

There are exceptions. Patients with alexithymia are not aware of their mood and do not have apparent mood reactions. Patients with damage to parts of the brain (temporal lobes and thalamus) do not have feelings—a few rare people are born this way.

These feelings of pleasure and pain are the sensations of the brain. These sensations are created when our "brain hormones" connect to their corresponding brain receptors; receptors are like "docking sites" or biological berths on the nerve cell. (chapter II-2.)

Brain Mechanics of Addictions and Alcoholism

The plant and animal kingdoms are intimately intertwined. We have adapted to plants as have they, to us. Thus, we—for one reason or another—naturally possess brain receptors both to our own chemicals and also those found in plants. These receptors make us feel good (usually). These natural receptors can be stimulated by our own natural internal "brain hormones" which are already inside us. Thus, we have access to our own internal animal-sourced feel-good brain hormones as well as access to those coming from the plant kingdom (external chemicals). Of the internal substances, almost all are quite small and simple molecules that are supplied from many sources. The only moderately sized internal chemicals are endorphins, enkephalins and anandamide—and, even at that, they are less complex than the plant-based (external chemical) substances. (Ānanda is Sanskrit for "joy, bliss".) The brain hormones connect with their corresponding receptors. These natural receptors can be activated by our own natural internal "brain hormones" which are already inside us and which our body crafts from our food sources.

Nature, Nurture, and Numbers

We all have different numbers of receptors. The number is probably determined by nature (our genes) yet may be altered somewhat by nurture (childhood environment and overwhelming emotional trauma). We are all likely feckless pawns of our genes to a certain degree. Our genetic complement determines how many brain receptors we possess. Our genes may also determine how many—or how few—internal hormones we have.

This is an example of one path that could lead to addiction:

☘Morphine is a narcotic that occurs naturally in poppies.

○Endorphins are natural internal narcotics that we humans can produce inside our own brains. (The word "endorphin" is shortened from "endo" and "morphine", meaning "internal morphine".)

❦Our brains have receptor sites to receive the endorphins. When the endorphins connect to their receptor site, this should produce a pleasurable experience.

- Some people have enough endorphins (○) and feel good naturally.
- Some people do aerobic exercise, which releases endorphins (○), and they feel good naturally after their activities (some stressors and also sexual climax can release endorphins).
- Some people do not have enough endorphins, for various reasons: they may not feel good. They may be cranky, irritable, depressed.

This can occur if a person has very few receptor sites (❖), if the person's brain does not make enough endorphins(○), or if the endorphins are rapidly depleted (as in depression).

Any one who eats poppy morphine ❀ might feel euphoria. Or, the person could feel depressed because morphine is also sedating.

Assume that Mary's brain has one billion receptor sites for endorphins. Assume that her brain makes enough endorphins. She should feel good most of the time. She is accustomed to feeling good after aerobics: this is because she naturally releases a billion endorphins that fill her billion receptor sites. She feels even better then. If she takes morphine, only a few of her receptors will be filled, and she may experience this as an odd or incomplete feeling.

Assume that Joe has a shortage of receptors and a shortage of endorphins: he may or may not feel good. If he is under enough stress, his endorphins will be released, but they will be used up quickly because he was apparently born with a shortage. After a while, the stress will make him feel bad. If he takes poppy morphine, he might feel better because the morphine is doing for him what endorphins do. But that good feeling will wear off and he will take more morphine in an attempt to feel better. This leads to addiction, and his thousandth dose may never feel as good as that first dose. He may continue in his addiction "chasing the high" that he felt with the first dose.

	Mary	Joe
Baseline		
Endorphin Receptors	❖ ❖ ❖ ❖ ❖	❖ ❖
Aerobics releases Endorphins	○ ○ ○ ○ ○	○ ○
analysis	Mary has an abundant supply of endorphins and receptors	Joe has few of either— He has few reserves
Early STRESS releases endorphins (sometimes extra)	○ ○ ○ ○ ○ + extra ○○ ❖ ❖ ❖ ❖ ❖	○○ + ○ extra ❖ ❖
Extended STRESS Body struggles to make endorphins fast enough to keep up with stress (some are smaller)	○○○○○ ❖ ❖ ❖ ❖ ❖	○ ❖ ❖
After stress: Mary recovers Joe does not	○ ○ ○ ○ ○ ❖ ❖ ❖ ❖ ❖	○ ❖ ❖
Back to baseline Endorphin receptors	❖ ❖ ❖ ❖ ❖	❖ ❖
Take morphine pill	⊛ ⊛ - - - - ❖ ❖ ❖ ❖ ❖	⊛ ⊛ ❖ ❖
Analysis:	Mary has an odd and "incomplete" feeling	Joe feels good
Outcome	Mary will return to aerobics For a "natural high"	Joe may resort to using more morphine

Table V-17-a   Receptors and addiction

The apparently paradoxical reason for this is that Mary prefers to get her own natural high from her own internal transmitters that will fill many of her billion receptor sites to capacity. A drug introduced from outside her body (morphine) does little to make her feel better. Joe feels better because all of his receptors get filled and this feels like euphoria to him. People like Joe usually have a severe deficiency of their own internal hormones, and have never felt euphoria until they try some drug. Joe may be lacking natural internal hormones if he has been chronically depressed, which can deplete his natural supply.

This is a direct quote from reference 5 (Stephen Stahl MD PhD) p.505"

"...in subjects who have only a few receptors for a given substance, taking that substance will not cause much of an effect at first, but the substance will become more and more rewarding as the dose increases. However, in subjects with many receptors for a given substance, taking that substance will be aversive [unpleasant] and they will not want to try it again."

Cross Addiction refers to being addicted to other drugs in the same category without ever having taken them addictively. An alcoholic can become addicted to Xanax, although he had never taken Xanax compulsively. The cross-addiction is controlled by GABA which is the receptor for both these substances.

►   QUESTIONS

One Addiction

Q: What is the probability of being addicted to only one drug? (in other words, of having a deficient number of only one receptor type)

A: This is not readily known. Some people do report being addicted to only one substance, but not to others. Older alcoholics state that alcohol is their "drug of choice", but are nevertheless wary of any prescriptions for addicting drugs like codeine.

Many Addictions

Q: What is the likelihood of being addicted to more than one drug? (in other words, of having a deficient number of two or more receptor types)

A: Some drug addicts report having one main "drug of choice", but having tendencies to other addictions. Other drug addicts report that they have two or more recognized "drugs of choice". These responses are hard to analyze scientifically at this time.

Of course, some drug addicts report addiction to all addicting drugs. The cause for all-addiction is under research. In these cases, we can include gambling, sex, and food as addictive behaviors, too because these activities can release and increase dopamine as well as other good-feeling brain hormones. Many compulsive behaviors seem to release chemicals that make people feel good. Male hormones feel good while driving sex, but the orgasm releases dopamine. Food-addiction can release digestive hormones and increase sugar levels (release of noradrenaline). Chocolate can cause mild euphoria. (see list at end of previous chapter on functional Brain Chemistry)

Q: Is it possible that one major receptor deficiency impacts several receptor addictions?
A: Yes: dopamine [5, 19] is a possible candidate.

Q: How is it possible to have a genetically controlled deficit in all receptors?
A: Unknown.

- Maybe there is one master gene that controls the quantity of all the receptors, but this is not so likely. That means that the master gene would give out equal numbers of all receptors to each person. Joe would have a deficiency of all, and Mary would have a normal amount of all. This seems far-fetched. If there is one factor that can cause this mass "pruning", it is likelier to be due to some force from outside the brain: emotional trauma or environmental stress that cause adrenal hormone chaos.

- Some research[19] suggests that **dopamine receptor** deficiency may be pivotal in addiction to alcohol, amphetamines, and cocaine.

- Opioid (Narcotic) addiction is probably more of a separate addiction, related to **opioid receptors**

- Marijuana habit may be a separate addiction, to **cannabinoid receptors.**

If people acquire fewer receptors through genetics, then they are basically set up for the risk of addictions—no matter what. (The only recourse in this case is to avoid all drugs and alcohol—especially if there is a family history of alcoholism and addiction.)

If people start with a normal number of receptors through heredity/genetics, but if childhood and environmental trauma prune out many receptors, then this would imply that addiction might be preventable. More research is needed. The absolute number of molecules docking at the receptors is as important as the percentage filled.

The following table summarizes some of the brain receptor sites, the internal chemicals created by the body that bind to those sites, some of the external chemicals derived from plants and other substances that people take, the effect of the chemicals on the body, and

Everyone's Everyday Guide to Practical Psychiatry

the symptoms of excess dosage. This table has a large amount of technical information, which you should not feel you must understand in detail. There will not be a test.

Table V-17-b   Receptors

Name or Type of Receptor	Internal Substance	External Chemical	Sensation	***Overdose*** *Excess results in:*
				Cause of death in gray
Opiate	Endorphin Enkephalins	All Narcotics (morphine)	Euphoria, passive state of Well-being, lack of pain	*Constipation, Coma, Inability to breathe*
Cannabinoid endocannabinoid	Anandamide	Marijuana (THC, mainly)	Relaxation, Insightfulness	*Agitation, loss of ambition*
Nicotine	Acetylcholine	Nicotine	Calm but alert	*Anxiety*
Acetylcholine	Same (Ach)	ACHEI[ACHEI]	Alertness	*?dementia?*
Dopamine	Dopamine DA	Amphetamines Cocaine Rx medicine*	Euphoria Activation Pleasure	*Psychosis*
Noradrenergic	Norepinephrine NE	Stimulants* & Anti-depressants	Energy, drive	*Frenzy, stroke ↑ blood pressure ↑↑heart rate*
Serotonin	Serotonin	Anti-Depressants*** Cocaine LSD	Focused calm, Anti-obsession Concentration	*Hallucinations Death from (serotonin syndrome)*
Valium site	GABA	Valium-like drug Valerian herb, Neurology drugs[N] Alcohol	Calmness and relaxation	*Addiction Loss of drive, Memory loss, Apathy, Coma Inability to breathe*
Glutamate	NMDA	Phencyclidine PCP	Analgesia, delirium	*Psychosis, muscle rupture, Seizures*
Alcohol (direct & indirect effects)	NMDA, GABA DA,opioids,NE Cannabinoid	Alcohol	Euphoria, relaxation, chattiness	*Visual Hallucinations, Seizure, death*
Muscarinic	Acetylcholine	Belladonna Alkaloids**** Jimsonweed and prescribed drugs	Dries bodily Secretions	*Amnesia, (fever) Visual illusions, Organ paralysis, Seizures, Coma*

435

Legend for table V-17-c

ACHEI—drugs for memory loss: Aricept, Exelon, Tacrine, and Galantamine
N—gabapentin, gabitril, pregabilin
*for a complete list, see the chapters on antidepressants and psychostimulants
such as Effexor, Vestra, Pristiq, Ludiomil, Cymbalta
****SSRI antidepressants and Tricyclics—see chapter on antidepressants***
**** this is a large group of various medications: (1-) scopolamine, atropine, hyoscine; (2-) Tricyclic antidepressants and FGA antipsychotics (see chapters on antidepressants and Antipsychotics); (3-) the old neuro-psychiatric anticholinergic drugs like Cogentin, Artane, Akineton, Kemadrin (4-) assorted medical drugs like Bentyl, and so on.

Our genes are in charge of much that we feel and become. Our genes affect how we react to drugs and herbs Genetics affects our brain chemistry which affects our behavior, and hence, our lives. (See also Chapter II-4)

▶Our nature and nurture make us who we are which in turn crafts our destinies—we can not escape that fact. Our greatest triumph in life indeed may be the ability to rise above this basal destiny by imposing self-willed control over our behaviors. Nowhere is this truer than in the flight into health achievable in Twelve Step Programs—by those who truly want mental, physical, and spiritual health.

Chapter V-18

Diet Pills

This topic has been mentioned in Chapter V-6, but I will reclassify the diet pills here for the sake of clarity.

- Diet pills are also called *"anorexiants"*—they cause anorexia (loss of appetite, hence loss of weight)
- *"Anorexia"* means "non-appetite" in Greek.
- The study of weight loss as a medical subspecialty is *bariatrics* (in Greek, "bar(y)-" means "heavy" and "-iatric" means "doctor").

Curiously, most of the world is worried about starving, while Americans are obsessed with losing weight after eating compulsively. The main ways of losing weight are ***chemical***, ***biological***, or ***psychosocial***. A fourth choice of hypnosis has not been effective.

Most people opt for the ***chemical***: they want to take a pill to correct this problem. This involves pills. The main function of diet pills is to cause weight loss by any method possible:

- The commonest method is to take a drug that suppresses appetite (ampetamines, Tenuate, Mazindol, Meridida, and other stimulants that may be available with or without prescription). Some of these drugs stress the heart. The ones which do so are available mainly on prescription; which implies (to me) that the prescriber should make certain that your heart is capable of taking these drugs; if you plan to take these drugs plus daily aerobic exercise, then you definitely need a cardiac evaluation.

- Some drugs help burn fat and preferentially build muscle (anabolic steroids). Most of these drugs have a lot of side effects, such as over-masculinization and aggression. Many are available on the black market. A few of the weaker ones are available OTC.

- Another choice is to take drugs that help burn fat. Fenisec is a European anorexiant that claimed to burn fat and supposedly clears fat in the urine. The other choice lies in the ability of a drug to act like lipase. Lipase is a "fat-burning" protein naturally in our bodies (pancreatic enzyme—see Chapter II-4). New drug research has been

437

funded to find drugs that have lipase activity either by acting like artificial lipase or by causing release of natural internal lipase. Stay tuned for any results from this interesting research.

- The less common method is to prevent food from being absorbed (Alli).

Biologic methods **can be:**

- Bulimic behaviors which should be treated by a psychiatrist.
- Burning fat by inducing a state of ketosis ("bacon and mutton diet": diets based on protein and fat)
- Exercise more so that more calories are being burnt than the intake calories from the diet. This requires self-discipline to exercise aerobically on a regular basis (daily). It also requires calorie-counting.

Psychosocial approaches also require taking action, doing activity (exercise), group support, calorie counting or self-administered carbohydrate restrictions, and a new philosophical approach to life in general:

- OA
- Weight Watchers and other such programs

In order to be successful, these types of programs need to involve a psychic rearrangement of the overeater's priorities.

Drugs to Suppress Appetite

The classic group of appetite-suppressants is from the group of norepinephrine and dopamine derivatives (see Chapter V-6). One of these is available without a prescription; the others are habit-forming drugs available only on prescription:

OTC—Phenyl-propanol-amine (PPA) is an amphetamine-like drug that was on prescription, but now is sold Over The Counter (OTC). It can cause agitation, insomnia, poor judgment, and high blood pressure. Soon after PPA became available OTC circa 1980, I saw a case of a young woman who had taken so much PPA, that the resulting high blood pressure had caused sudden kidney failure (she had bloody urine).

Rx—these are all sold on prescription and are controlled by the DEA:
Amphetamines of all types: Dexedrine, Benzedrine, Ionamin, Pondimin (Chapter V-6)
Tenuate—an older diet pill with stimulating properties.
Preludin—related to amphetamines with similar properties.

The next three are not related to the amphetamines:

Mazindol (Sanorex)—mildly stimulating

Meridia—mildly stimulating non-amphetamine diet pill: mechanism of action unknown

Topamax—is the only non-stimulant, non-addicting drug that can cause modest weight loss if taken over a long period of time—see Chapter V-12.

Drugs to Suppress Appetite and Increase Activity Levels

Amphetamines increase pleasurable activity (Dopamine activity) and suppress appetite in the brain. First, get cardiac clearance from your doctor!

Drugs to Promote Protein Gain and Fat Loss

The anabolic steroids increase muscle and protein levels and decrease fat deposits. These drugs are not generally appealing to women. If these steroids cause deepening of the voice, this could be permanent.

Human Growth Hormone (HGH) may also be useful.

Drugs to Affect the Satiety Center

The hypothalamus in the brain contains a "feeding center" and a "satiety center" which must be dealt with. The feeding center is the appetite center. The satiety center tells us that we are fully satisfied, food-wise. Anorexiants may suppress the feeding center. There are few substances to fool the satiety center into thinking that we are full and satisfied. There is a lot more to eating disorders than the hypothalamus.

The hormone leptin (yes, "lepto-" in Greek means "thin") can fool the satiety center into thinking that it is satiated. There is as yet no specific drug for this purpose, but research is progressing apace.

Drugs to Prevent Food Absorption

Alli is the OTC name of Orlistat (Xenical). Alli is to be eaten with fatty foods. Alli interferes with fat absorption and effectively prevents it from being absorbed, hence no fat calories are consumed. Carbohydrate calories, of course, can still be handily absorbed—and are. As a result, the fats leave the body intact and unabsorbed. This usually causes fatty diarrhea. You can find out what this is like before starting Alli by drinking three times as much olive oil as is normally present in your salad dressing. Always take along extra underwear or adult diapers if leaving the house.

Weight-neutral Psycho-Active medicines

A couple medications do not routinely cause weight gain, Vivactil for example. Moban is an old antipsychotic that tends to cause weight loss of a few pounds.

Vivactil—an old Tricyclic that increases activity levels slightly and does not stimulate appetite—see Chapter V-7

Moban—one of the FGA antipsychotics—see Chapter V-4.

Wellbutrin—in theory, should not cause weight gain since it is derived from Tenuate, the diet pill. Wellbutrin might cause a few pounds of weight gain in people who feel constipated by it.

Geodon—a second generation antipsychotic SGA—see Chapter V-4.

Psychiatric Drugs *Notorious* for Causing Much Weight Gain

Seroquel and Zyprexa; Thorazine and Mellaril—all in Chapter V-4

Sinequan, Remeron, and Elavil—old sedating antidepressants—Chapter V-7

Lithium and Depakote can cause modest weight gain, too.

What's a Girl to do?!
(boys, too)

The main problem with diet pills is that the pill is effective while being taken, but once the pill is discontinued, the weight usually rebounds to the same level or even higher. The best way to lose weight is to adjust your lifestyle for the rest of your life. Adopt new eating and activity levels and do the following:

- Do exercise (aerobic, if possible) for at least half an hour a day (check with your primary doctor first)

- Stop eating junk food and fast food: Lori Corbin, the food coach on the local LA news, suggests avoiding any container of food with over five ingredients and also avoiding any foods "that your great-grandmother would not recognize". I agree.

- Learn to count calories: calculate how many calories you burn each day and then increase that number by 15%

- Follow the so-called Mediterranean diet

- Re-educate your taste buds to delight in fresh fruit and vegetables and to abhor the contrived tastes of fast food and junk food

- Avoid products containing corn syrup, high fructose corn syrup .

Chapter V-19

"Two Hundred and Sixty Side-Effects"
Package Inserts Clarified (PI)
Adverse Drug Reactions (ADR)

Synthetic drugs are poisons that are therapeutic if taken in tiny amounts. This is not to say that herbs are any better—herbs can be toxic if taken in high doses, too. Any chemical can be toxic if taken in high doses. Salt and sugar can be tasty if taken in "low doses". What would happen to you if you ate half a cup of salt or two cups of sugar? Even water is technically a chemical. Some people with a disease called dipsomania drink so much water, that they can cause themselves serious bodily damage. Any chemical can be toxic or poisonous if taken in excess dose or in overdose. Synthetic drugs receive a lot of negative publicity in this regard while their naysayers ignore the hazards of our proclivity to dietary excesses of animal fat, sugar, salt, flour, and the dizzying array of all the chemical additives, colorants, food preservatives, and what not.

Usually, synthetic drugs cause few side effects—and ideally, none. The first weeks on one of these drugs can produce some side effects. These may be a couple common side effects or a couple minor side effects. After a while, the side effects may seem to fade as the patient begins to feel better and then even better.

Sometimes a patient may have common but minor side effects to the drug. A patient might continue to refer to these as "allergies" when in truth they are not allergies. I see patients who say that they are "allergic" to Haldol because it tends to make them trembly. This is not an allergic reaction. This is a common side effect of Haldol, which is a manifestation of its clinical activity. If this discomfort continues, then the Haldol needs to be changed to another medication. Trembling is not a life-threatening side effect such as a rash.

One big problem is that of allergic reactions (rashes) that appear within a few days of starting the drugs. These types of reactions are allergic reactions in which case the patient should stop the drug and contact the doctor. Continuation of a drug causing a rash or true allergic reaction can have fatal results.

Examples of symptoms present in serious allergic reactions are rashes, tingling of the body, gasping and having trouble breathing, or fingers turning blue. The antidepressants that I have oftenest encountered causing rashes are Vivactil, Prozac, Paxil, and Effexor. Rashes are commonest in the first days or weeks of treatment. The FGA Antipsychotics can make people's muscles rigid and stiff. If this happens, the eyes might roll into the top of the head or the person might stop breathing. This usually occurs after months or even years on the medicine, so it is not a true allergy, but it is certainly an Adverse Drug Reaction (ADR). And the person should not take that drug again without overwhelming proof of its medical necessity.

Sometimes, a patient will under very rare circumstances have a life threatening reaction, an Adverse Drug Reaction (ADR). This can be due to the way that the new drug interacts with the patient's biochemistry or due to the way that the new drug interacts with all the usual drugs that the patient is already taking. The term ADR implies that the reaction is life-threatening or fatal—not just a regular side effect.

Package Inserts (PI)

To inform patients about side effects of new drugs, pharmacies place package inserts (PI) into the bag of prescription medications. Package Inserts (PI) are the preprinted papers that you will receive along with your prescription medication. Drug stores stuff these papers into each bag of prescription drugs that you buy. The pharmacy believes that this long list of possible side effects acts as a disclaimer and also serves to shift responsibility onto the doctor to explain to the patient why he would ever prescribe such a drug. Package inserts (PI) contain long lists of possible side effects that any prescription drug might cause:

1   *might* possibly *cause or* possibly *has caused;* or,

2   has been scientifically verified to cause.

There may be NO DIRECT PROOF or evidence that the drug in question has ever caused these side effects !

However, the FDA has required all of these effects to be listed in the interest of providing too much—rather than too little—information.

The common major side effects are those that will be experienced by a significant minority of patients. These side effects may or may not be a reason to quit taking the medicine. The less common major side effects occur less frequently than the common ones. Minor side effects are even less significant. Rare side effects may be serious or mere medical curiosities. The dubious side effects are those which doctors do not encounter in the normal course of clinical practice. These may be side effects for which no discernible effect could occur based on the rationally known physiologic, biochemical, or pharmacologic effects of that medicine and the human body.

The FDA, however, requires that the drug-maker list any possible side effects that could have occurred during clinical trials. (When the drug is being tested "experimentally" on human volunteers, the FDA requires listing all symptoms experienced by volunteers during that testing period, a time span, which can last for weeks or months.) Thus, if a patient in clinical trials experiences a cold or flu, sunburns, muscle aches while trying a new sport, or reaction to trying some exotic food, etc., then all of those symptoms are listed also as possible side effects of the new drug when in reality there may or may not be any likelihood that the experimental drug is linked to or causing those symptoms. The FDA is willing to err on the side of caution because they want to be perceived as being good watchdogs. Additionally, we all know that if the drug has not been completely vetted, it may be harmful. Once the drug goes beyond the experimental stages and is released onto the public market, then a drug recall is costly for the drug company, embarrassing to the FDA and dangerous for us consumers. Despite all the data from the pre-release clinical trials, it is often the case that a drug's toxicity—if any—becomes well known once it is available to the public. That is when doctors really become acquainted with its everyday advantages and disadvantages and its truly common side effects. Hence, all the precautionary side effects listed on the PI are excessive in number and terrifying to patients who may not be aware of all the medico-legal posturing that is going on in the background. If a drug later turns out to have a toxic effect, then all the players start pointing fingers at each other: (FDA, drug company, consumer rights activists, doctors, the general public, plus the affected patients and their lawyers: "you should have done more research!", "you should have reported those side effects sooner!","you should control the greedy cheapskate drug company!", "You shouldn't prescribe new drugs without a track record!", and so on).

When in doubt, one can check in the PDR (Physician's Desk Reference) where these kinds of "hierarchies" of side effects are spelled out more clearly. The PDR is also useful for checking on pill colors and sizes. The PDR will break down side effects by type and frequency.

I like to review the common side effects with patients and warn them about any serious problems that might arise such as rash, liver stress, falling blood pressure, sexual dysfunction, and so on. Despite this preparation, some patients will call me frantically about the PI. Usually, reassurance is helpful.

Current PI System

These are the problems with the current system of PI's:

–Problem #1—The P.I. is so scary that a patient might come back two weeks later and say "I never even tried that drug you prescribed because it has too many side effects".
–Solution #1—skim through the P.I. while remembering that it is presenting the absolutely most catastrophic results. Look at the first three or four common side effects and then set it aside.

–Problem #2—the P.I. can upset suggestible patients such as Mrs. Smith who fear that they surely will have side effects—sometimes patients pre-empt the appearance of side effects by convincing themselves that they are already having the side effects.

–Solution #2—Most, if not all, new prescriptions will result in odd side effects for at least the first week: this is an accommodation period during which time most synthetic drugs will exert some side effects. This is a regular and usual occurrence. I always try to stress this to patients at the time that the new medicine is prescribed. This period may be likened to breaking in a new pair of shoes.

–Problem #3—some patients misunderstand the P.I. and come to believe that they will have *all* the listed side effects!

–Solution #3—read the first few listed symptoms on the P.I. The P.I. should try to list only the common side effects in extra-large print and the legion of other side effects can be listed in smaller or regular font.

–Problem #4—Mrs. Smith takes one pill and has a minor side effect after which she refuses to take any more medicine. But, I am not aware of this until her next office visit by which time she has already lost a couple weeks by not starting the treatment.

–Solution #4—Stay in touch and alert us to your own self-treatment decisions!

Adverse Drug Reactions (ADR)

Synthetic drugs do cause a lot of bad side effects, injury, and even death. An estimated 110,000 deaths per year in the USA may be due to adverse drug reactions (ADR's). These deaths may be a direct effect of poisoning by or severe allergic reactions to the drugs; however, it should be noted that among these 110,000 estimated cases, many are directly or indirectly due to pharmacist error, nursing error, or doctor error.

These are the common causes of ADR's and all are contributory in more or less equal proportions:

- extremely rare and unusual reaction of one patient to starting a new drug
- drug-to-drug interaction
- dispensing error in pharmacy
- dosing error by nurses
- medical prescription error by doctor

In extremely rare cases, a patient might have a severe allergic reaction to starting a new drug that she has never taken before. If you fear that you are having such an ADR and you can not reach your doctor, then have someone drive you to the nearest ER. Usually these allergic reactions are not life-threatening, just scary.

Drug-to-drug interaction errors occur when: (1) the patient is taking drugs from various doctors and forgets to tell all her doctors about her current medications; (2) her doctor is not aware that certain drugs should not be mixed; —or also likely, (3) the patient forgets to stop the old drug while starting a new drug intended to replace the old drug and ends up taking both drugs. If these are two drugs with similar activity, then it is like overdosing. More than once, somebody has continued to take Paxil along with Zoloft when given the Zoloft as a new drug meant to replace the Pasil.

Dispensing errors occur in the pharmacy. The pill may be dispensed in the wrong size. Or the names of the pills become confused. This might happen if two pills have similar names. For example giving out "Serzone" for "Seroquel" (this made my psychotic patient worse), "Thorazine" for "thioridazine", "Clonidine" for Clonopin (now written as "Klonopin") These instances—plus others—have all really happened to my patients over the years; visualize this then multiply by the total number of prescribing doctors in our country. This is one reason that I encourage patients to bring all their pills to the appointments (so that I can review the medicine bottles).

The pharmacist errors usually occur outside the hospital. If the patients fill all prescriptions at the same pharmacy, then the modern computerized system will alert the pharmacist to any mixture of incompatible drug, as long as the system is functioning normally. Patients who are running around to different drugstores can not get this kind of guarantee. Pharmacist errors in the hospital might be due to mixing errors where a specialized and unique concoction has been ordered by the hospital doctor (for example chemotherapies and intravenous medication mixtures).

Dosing errors: Nursing errors can result in the wrong medicine, the wrong dosage, the wrong patient, at the wrong time, or incorrectly injected, and so on. I remember a fatal case in which a patient wrongly received 20 grams of magnesium injection, which had been misread from its (fairly clearly) written form of 2.0 grams. Another error consists of giving two pills, mistaking the quantity of pills for the size of the pill (2mg.); mistaking one patient's pill cup for another or one patient for another, and so on. The national nursing shortage results in nurses who are overworked, overstressed, and distracted by events on the medical floor.

Nursing errors can be decreased by assigning the same nurses to the same medical service. This is quite useful in the hospital where patients with similar problems may be housed in the same ward. For example, the cardiology nurses become very familiar with cardiac medicines, especially on the cardiac wards, after heart surgery, and in the coronary care unit. Nephrology nurses become familiar with renal dialysis and kidney medicines on the nephrology ward and in the dialysis center. Specialty doctors focus on their own specialty medicines, so nurses should have this same opportunity. Unfortunately, this may not happen in general medical wards and in nursing homes where patients are all mixed together. These various patients may have various and different specialty doctors, but the nurses are expected to know all the specialty drugs and routines.

Nursing errors can occur inside or outside the hospital and in nursing homes. Pharmacist and nursing errors can be decreased by issuing outpatient medications in bubble packs. Doctor errors outside the hospital usually occur when the patient is seeing many doctors for many medical illnesses and is not using the same pharmacy for all the prescription pick-up and each doctor may be unaware that there are so many other prescribing doctors or doctor specialists.

Doctor error usually involves mixing the wrong drugs together or adding a new drug to a list of pre-existing drugs that the patient is already taking whereupon the patient may have a bad reaction to mixing (all) the drugs. In a fair number of these cases, the doctor would be able to avert a disaster HAD HE KNOWN all the medicines, herbs, and over-the-counter (OTC) medications involved in the patient's regular regimen. Doctors forget to ask and patients fail to report changes in medicines and non-prescription drugs that they are taking, such as: ibuprofen, naproxen; Benadryl (doxylamine, bonine, Dramamine); excess calcium pills which might prevent absorption of some drugs (Thorazine); St. John's Wort, Valeriana; guaranà, SAM-e, and diet pills. And worst of all perhaps is drug misuse of "O.P." pills (Other People's pills).

Doctor errors in the hospital might include ordering intramuscular injections (Prolixin, Haldol, Risperdal) for a patient without reviewing the fact that the patient is taking prescription blood-thinners (Warfarin, Coumadin, Plavix, Persantine). This can result in excessive bleeding.

Other Issues

In some cases, even patient lifestyle and foods may affect medicines. Regular use of alcohol can be a problem since alcohol does not mix well with medications. Cigarettes can decrease the blood levels of some medicines. A patient taking many antacids (calcium) can decrease absorption of certain medicines (Thorazine). Some medicines should be taken with or without food. Cereals rich in phytic acid and oxalic acid can bind to (chelate) calcium and magnesium and make the minerals less available. The doctor may not know this if the patient overlooks providing this information.

A lot can go wrong in the world of synthetic drugs—and yet, a lot can go right. Vastly larger numbers of people have been saved by these drugs rather than killed by these drugs.

However, of the 110,000 deaths from ADR's, many can be averted by relying on computers and electronic systems: electronic dispensing of pills, electronic prescriptions automatically faxed to the drug store, etc.; however, there is still room for human error here and there. In the case of electronic prescriptions the doctor may forget to have the computer write important information.

Unfortunately, we must remind patients that healthcare workers are human and will always try to avoid making many mistakes; at least there are a lot of checks nowadays on prescribing medicine. It always sounds like a "cop-out" but we will resort sometimes to reminding the public that "Medicine is an art and not a science" (until we can mandate routine genetic drug reaction testing). There should be enough scientific overlay nowadays to protect the public from most ADR's—yet it still happens. Pharmacies often have modern computer software that can alert the pharmacist to potentially harmful drug combinations—as long as Mrs. Smith is filling all her prescriptions in that one pharmacy.

▶QUESTIONS

Q: Why do prescription drugs have so many side effects?

A-1: Because these synthetic drugs are toxic in large doses—yet therapeutic, when taken in very small amounts

A-2: In reality there are not nearly so many side effects as those listed. The symptoms listed as side effects include the following:

1—The **common major side effects**, those which are routinely associated with that medicine, of which there are usually a handful;

2—The **less common major side effects** which doctors and patients regularly encounter in relation to that medication;

3—**Minor side effects**;

4—**Rare side effects**; and,

5—Many **dubious** [and unauthenticated] side effects.

Section VI
SPECIAL POPULATIONS

Superscript numbers refer to references and citations at the back of the book

Essay on Alcoholism
Drug Addiction and Prescription Pill Abuse

*"Alcohol gave me the wings to fly
And then it took away the Sky"* [8]

Introduction

Alcoholism, drug addiction, and prescription pill abuse are all different clinical manifestations of the same disease. That disease is called chemical dependence (or dependency). (For those of you who are gardeners, an apt analogy would be the difference/similarity between azalea and rhododendron.) Chemical dependency is a very common disorder in the developed nations or anywhere that these chemicals are readily available. It is a chronic progressive disease, that ultimately kills its victims much as diabetes does, but chemical dependence is more insidious because it is the only disease that tells its victims that they have no disease and thus are in no need of any treatment or any intervention by others. Not only is chemical dependence a personal disease, but it is also a family disease in the sense that it changes its victims as well as their loved ones and all those closest to them. It never gets better—only worse and worse—as time goes by. It cannot be cured but it can be treated and arrested before it causes death.

Wherever the words "alcoholic" or "alcoholism" appear in these next three chapters, the reader should feel free—in general—to substitute the terms "addict" or "chemical dependence/drug addiction".

Specifics on Alcoholism

Alcoholism often runs in families. It can affect the individual (the alcoholic) and the whole family. There may be many family members with a drinking problem. Individual alcoholics coming from these families seem to acquire individual alcoholism early in life.

Additionally, in alcoholic families, one often encounters the non-alcoholic family members who do not drink (much) or who do not become alcoholic, but they will nevertheless end up suffering from the family disease of alcoholism. (See chapters VI-2 and VI-3). These families with apparent genetic alcoholism can be very dysfunctional and have many family secrets (Chapters VI-2-3).

Some families have mild to moderate cases of individual alcoholism. These families might be less dysfunctional than families replete with alcoholics and might have only a few family secrets—or just one. The cause is probably genetically related.

Some families have no history of alcoholism and may have just one individual alcoholic at any given moment. It is not clear if there is a genetic cause or not.

And, some families may have no history of alcoholism at all, but may have a lot of dysfunction. These families may not have the genetics for the disease, or their ancestors had had extensive alcoholism and all died off from it while passing down the "alcoholic genes" to distant cousins but not to the index family. In this case, the dysfunctional but non-alcoholic family has passed down these behaviors as their legacy, which can happen. In these latter two families, however, do not be surprised to find other compulsive disorders such as overeating, fetishes, obsessive-compulsive disorder, and religious fanaticism.

People become addicted to alcohol by drinking too much of it. Use of beer or wine portends well as compared to young people who start off immediately with hard liquor straight up. But—once again—any drinker can become an alcoholic. People who preferentially drink wine (France) or beer (Germany) can still become alcoholics.

Alcoholism can start at any age: some alcoholics have started as children, many as teenagers, more as adults. It can start late in life, also—sometimes paradoxically rearing its ugly head and becoming a serious problem only in retirement. Compulsive adults who come to drink compulsively in adulthood, have often been obsessively focused on their careers and education and other activities, and only later in life, feel the ability to ease up and relax—and then their inborn compulsions can turn about to embrace alcohol consumption.

Traditionally, men have been in AA, and women, in Al-Anon—but that is changing in the modern world. Traditionally, alcoholic men were allowed to have their misadventures and rugged experiences while alcoholic women ended up shelterd in and by their families. Al-anon was a place to vent emotions and feelings, a seemingly alien experience to which men must learn to accustom themselves. More women are showing up in AA; and more men, turning to Alanon.

"Alcohol"—is the common and popular way of referring to safe but intoxicating beverage alcohol.

"Ethyl Alcohol"—is the **common chemical name** of consumable beverage alcohol; it is a term used by technicians, pharmacists, doctors, and chemists. Industrial grade ethyl alcohol is not fit to drink. Ethyl alcohol can be abbreviated in chemical shorthand as "EtOH".

"Ethanol" is the precise and **formal chemical name** for ethyl alcohol and suggests that the ethyl alcohol is of highest purity (100%) and appropriate for use in chemical reactions. This could be consumed but undoubtedly would be a very harsh experience. This is also a common way for physicians to refer to alcohol. This can also be written as "EtOH".

"EtOH"—is the typical medical chemical abbreviation for writing about drinkable alcohol in doctor's progress notes.

"Alcohols in General"—Chemists have identified tens of thousands of alcohols, but they cannot be used as beverages. Almost all are poisonous. Beverage alcohol is the second smallest alcohol by weight. The only smaller alcohol in the family of the alcohols is wood alcohol. The third smallest is isopropyl alcohol, rubbing alcohol.

"Denatured alcohol"—is ethyl alcohol that is still ethyl alcohol for industrial purposes but has been treated in such a way as to make it unfit as a beverage.

"Wood alcohol" is methyl alcohol. This causes blindness and poisoning. Home distilling can produce ethyl alcohol with varying quantities of methyl alcohol. Hence, one should be wary of "moonshine".

"Rubbing alcohol" is isopropyl alcohol. This is poisonous. This is not a beverage.

"Glycols" are "double alcohols" (potentially poisonous also). Ethylene glycol is antifreeze.

Alcohol is an Arabic word used to describe the liquid chemical which is commonly called alcohol (*al-kuHuul)*. This word comes from *KaHala* meaning "to smear or blacken" also related to *kuHlun*, antimony). One Arabic idiom concerns awakening with "kohled" eyes—with dark bags under the eyes—as a marker for hangovers. The cultural effects and social stigmata of alcoholism have obviously been well known for a long time.

Other consumable alcoholic liquids which are not considered beverages but which are taken internally for medicinal or culinary purposes may also contain drinkable ethanol, and hence by extension, also contain measurable amounts of alcohol and should be avoided by recovering alcoholics (examples are: cough syrup, Nyquil, vanilla extract, cooking sherry, European desserts and bonbons, or any elixir). The use of colognes by recovering alcoholics is not usually a problem (unless the colognes are taken internally). Alcohol can turn up unexpectedly in our lives, and the alcoholic in early recovery needs to be watchful and guard against these situations.

I am using the term "Alcohol" to refer to consumable alcohol.

I am using the terms alcoholism, drug addiction, and prescription drug abuse almost in free variation (as if they were all the same); however, there are some differences and where I have specified a certain disease, it applies especially to that disease but might be applicable to all three conditions. Even back in the 1930's, some alcoholics—"Dr. Bob", for example, the co-founder of AA—did abuse prescription drugs in order to further their drinking "careers" in the sense that they used the medications to avoid alcohol withdrawal or to induce sleep or to feel less anxious or less depressed due to alcohol. Dr. Bob Smith and Bill Wilson were the co-founders of AA. Notwithstanding, their primary problem was alcohol, and any additional medications were intended to prolong or accommodate their alcohol consumption. Obviously, people recovering from chemical dependence should avoid beverage alcohols, food-ingredient alcohols, elixirs, and addicting drugs—especially those drugs that are cross-tolerant with alcohol (addicting anti-anxiety drugs such as Valium, Xanax, Klonopin, Fiorinal—see chapter V-11).

Specifics on Drug-Addiction

Remember that alcoholism, drug addiction, and prescription pill abuse are three names for one disease, chemical dependence. Also remember that **habit-forming** chemicals (those that cause "habituation") get people into a habit, that is into a routine ritual occurring at regularly timed intervals. These people get the same effect from the same habit in the same way every time that they use the habit-forming chemical. **Addiction**, on the other hand, means that a person is already habituated and is moving beyond this phase to a condition in which he will gradually be increasing the dosage in an attempt to feel better, but the intake of more and more chemical simply results in more and more harmful side effects. Habituation can go on for years and years unchanged. I have patients who have been taking 1 mg Ativan at bedtime for twenty years; others, taking Xanax ½ mg twice a day for many years. In no case have they moved beyond habituation into addiction—but they could: that is the danger of these drugs. This is not to sanction habituation as a positive effect, because habituated people have side effects to the drug habit. I know because their families tell me so. But the patients do not note this because they feel OK and the habit-forming drug tells them every day that they have no habit and thus no problem. There are other patients who have increased their Xanax or Valium on their own up to double then triple doses and still feel anxiety, restlessness, racing thoughts, and sleeplessness. These patients are addicted.

This is the reason for which the government has controlled access to these drugs for the last century.

It is easy for anyone to become habituated or addicted to these drugs: sometimes in a matter of days, weeks, or months. Then the addiction is established. Unlike these drugs, alcohol is very low on the scale of habituation and addiction for most people.

Curiously, during Prohibition, possession of alcohol was a felony whereas possession of marijuana was only a misdemeanor. Even more alarming: narcotics were all sold without a prescription until the early 1900's when they were all placed under strict government control (Harrison Drug Act).

Addicting drugs are either prescription drugs or street drugs. Addicting prescription drugs are all controlled by the US government (the DEA, Drug Enforcement Administration). These are:

- narcotics (also called opiates or opioid drugs) the "minor" narcotics are: Vicodin, Codeine, Talwin, Darvon; "major" narcotics are: Percodan, Dilaudid, Suboxone, Demerol; and very major ones are: Morphine, Methadone, Fentanyl, Sufentanyl, and others

- tranquilizers (minor tranquilizers, anxiety drugs): Valium, Xanax, Klonopin, Ativan, Librium, Serax, barbiturates, old sedatives, Miltown

- sleeping pills: Halcion, Dalmane, Restoril, Lunesta, Ambien, Sonata, and others

- Xyrem® (GHB) a very dangerous drug used only for rare sleep disorders; GHB is the "date rape drug"

- Stimulants: mainly amphetamines, plus Ritalin, Provigil, and Cylert

- Medical cocaine elixir

Other addicting and dangerous drugs are also controlled by the DEA but they are not available to the public on routine prescriptions:

- Narcotics: heroin;

- GHB date rape drug

- LSD, mescaline, other hallucinogenic drugs

- Marijuana (except in California where it is legalized under State laws that are subordinate to and in conflict with federal laws)

- Stimulants such as cocaine, MDMA, MDA (ecstasy, "crystal meth")

- Tranquilizers such as Quāālude

- Miscellaneous.

I have listed the second group of non-prescription dangerous drugs, because these are all quite popular still on the street and in underground labs. There are many examples left unlisted.

We have established that drug addiction is essentially the same as alcoholism, assuming that alcohol is a liquid drug. So, what are the **similarities** between alcoholics and drug-addicts?

The answer is "Compulsions". They are all obsessed with alcohol / drugs and are compelled to use them. Alcoholics and drug-addicts are obsessed with their "drug of choice" and feel compelled to use it. However, there are some **differences between drug-addicts and alcoholics**:

The substance of choice creates some socio-economic and legal differences, but ultimately the outcome is about the same: illness, incarceration, or death:

- Drug-addicts are more likely to have criminal records, serious legal problems, and incarceration since drug possession is usually a felony; alcohol is legal and is socially sanctioned. Drug addicts might be likelier to have had personal contact with gang-members and drug-dealers. Alcoholics' legal problems often climax with a DUI, which is serious, too. Alcoholics can be sent to prison for vehicular manslaughter and other crimes committed while intoxicated or in a blackout. This is the legal peril.

- Drug-addicts necessarily frequent seedy and dangerous places sometimes to obtain their drugs: dangerous parks late at night, gang-members selling drugs on street-corners, police "stake-outs", sleazy drug houses, and so on. End-stage alcoholics may end up in sleazy bars where they can be robbed. This is the social danger.

- Drugs cost more, so are more likely to make the victim financially destitute sooner. However, alcoholics have their own financial woes due to poor judgment and overspending while on sprees. This is the financial hazard.

- Drugs can be more addicting: it is said that Crystal Methamphetamine, Fentanyl, and Crack Cocaine can render some users totally addicted on the first day of using that drug; alcohol is not very addicting for the vast majority of people. Many alcoholics drink for years before becoming dependent on alcohol. This is the psychic danger.

- Morbidity: "Crystal Meth" addicts and IV drug users are likelier to suffer truly serious illnesses early in the addiction: hepatitis C, HIV, endocarditis, stroke, heart attack, tooth loss, brain damage. These are catastrophic medical problems that can appear earlier in the drug-addict's "career" than in that of the alcoholic. In early phases of alcoholism, most of the drinkers can usually maintain or regain a state of usually good health or at least superficially good health for a very long time before succumbing to the inevitable suite of medical problems (cirrhosis, "wet brain", emphysema, internal bleeding, repeated physical trauma). As the drinking progresses, the alcoholics can also deteriorate physically. The alcoholics can then suffer the ravages of cirrhosis, emphysema, diabetes, and seizures at much higher rates than comparable non-drinkers. However, even sober alcoholics may be more predisposed to develop more serious medical problems later in life than do non-alcoholics; this will depend upon how long they were drinking heavily prior to sobriety. Alcoholics' chances of living to be very elderly are reduced as compared to that of non-drinkers. In general, even a history of inactive alcoholism seems to shorten lifespan in some patients. This is the longevity hazard.

- Mortality: although both alcoholics and drug-addicts have a number of premature deaths, sober alcoholics may have a better chance at living longer.

Compulsions

Obsessions are intrusive unwanted thoughts that keep on haunting a person until he finally gives in to the thoughts and performs a compulsive act. The only way to appease the obsessive thoughts is to give in and perform the **compulsion**, which is often more like a ritual. Failure to perform the compulsion creates unpleasant anxiety in the obsessive person until he performs his compulsive act. This act relieves the internal obsessive tension but not for long. In the case of compulsive hand-washers, for example, the main outcome is a chronic dermatologic problem (severely chapped and raw hands), whereas in chemical addiction the compulsion centers around an addicting mind and mood-altering chemical that must be consumed and allowed to work its biochemical effect.

Chemical dependence includes an element of compulsive behavior: drinking or drugging compulsively, in other words. The alcoholic is obsessed with alcohol and drinks compulsively to satisfy his obsession. The obsession takes the form of an internal biochemical entrainment over his mind. He is obsessed with performing the ritual to soothe the obsession. Unfortunately, in the case of alcoholics and drug-addicts, the compulsive ritual includes consuming an addicting chemical.

When the obsessions become too intrusive and are counterproductive and result in ritualistic compulsive behaviors that lack any benefit, then we can diagnose obsessions and compulsions of clinical significance. The litmus test is whether these thoughts and behaviors are beneficial or maladaptive and how much they detract from or intrude into the person's quality of life. In other words going to "happy hour" on vacation is part of the usual experience. Having happy hour from 6-10 PM every evening after work is maladaptive.

(This is an aside on treatment strategies: Since Alcoholism and the other compulsive behaviors have an element of compulsiveness—but are not diagnosed as Obsessive-Compulsive Disorder—there may be some benefit in using Serotonin drugs if the alcoholic becomes very anxious and somewhat depressed. Chapter VI-7)

Co-addictions

Many modern alcoholics are dependent on more than two substances such as cigarettes, caffeine, Valium and other prescription drugs However, alcohol can be identified as the main problem ("the drug of choice"). A lot of these "co-drugs" are intended to ease the pains of the alcoholism (while in withdrawal or in states of intoxication). Perhaps Valium is taken to soften the alcohol withdrawal symptoms until the alcoholic can obtain his next drink. Perhaps a stimulant antidepressant is taken in the morning to try to counteract the usual hangover so that the alcoholic can try to drag through the next workday. Apart from pills, nicotine is probably the alcoholic's most frequently abused "co-drug" nowadays. It is estimated that half of alcoholics smoke and that one third of smokers have an alcoholic problem. Cigarettes are still a big problem among alcoholics. Chemically dependent people nowadays can be alcoholics, drug-addicts, or alcoholic-addicts.

If alcoholics and drug-addicts do not get clean and sober then they will share these **commonalities**:

- deterioration of physical health
- deterioration of mental health
- lapse of judgment and of morals
- spiritual "bankruptcy"
- legal problems
- financial straits
- impaired personal relationships
- unpredictable occupational history

If you have occasion to visit an open AA meeting of alcoholics or an NA meeting of narcotics anonymous you might observe some other slight differences in the attendees : (1) attire (sports clothes, "suburban casual" [AA] vs. leather jackets, trendy hip fashion and biker gear [NA], (2) adornments (jewelry and watches in AA vs. body hardware and tattoos in NA), (3) general deportment of the members, (4.) use of psychoactive medicines (it seems that more NA members are taking more psychiatric prescription drugs than AA members—or at least more prescription drugs per patient), (5.) financial status (AA members might be more likely to be employed than NA members who might be more likely to be on SSD, worker's compensation, etc) and (6.) psychiatric diagnosis (NA members are possibly more likely to be diagnosed as "Bipolar"). Of course, these are only crude generalizations and might have many exceptions depending upon venue and other socio-eco-cultural factors.

History

The prehistoric **origins** of alcoholism are unknown, but alcohol consumption is known to have been present throughout written history. Six thousand years ago, the ancient Sumerians allocated a significant amount of their barley crop to the brewing of beer, one of their favorite pastimes, as is well attested in their art and written business records (in cuneiform on clay tablets). The ancient Egyptians enjoyed alcoholic beverages too. Many other cultures produced alcoholic beverages such as the Ancient Greeks. The use of alcohols or other intoxicants or hallucinogens may have played a major part in ancient religious rituals: the origin of this religious use is supposed to date to ancient prehistoric times (back to shamanism) which manifested in ancient times as trance-like rituals, the Eleusinian Mysteries of ancient Greece, the use of incense, and so on. When we were hunter-gatherers, we probably did not stay in one locale long enough to become involved in the technology of producing spirits. After we began to live in permanent settlements, this technology probably became widespread. Maybe alcohol-production is one of the main reasons that our ancestors decided to settle down. Speculation about such ancient uses of chemicals is far beyond the scope of this handbook.

As far as geography of alcoholism, it seems nowadays to be somewhat commoner in the Northern climates, such as Finland, Russia, Ireland, Vermont, Alaska and other such places, suggesting a possible relationship to Winter Depression. Alternatively, the proponents of another theory posit that early civilizations began in the hot climates such as the Middle East during the end of the last Ice Age. Many of those original alcoholics were winnowed out thousands of years ago due to social ostracism, executions, or premature deaths. Newer civilizations of newer genetic stock sprang up more recently in the northern latitudes. This is debatable. Maybe it is possible for anybody with enough misery and stress to buckle under pressure and seek solace in chemicals. Perhaps future genetic studies might be able to unravel all this by identifying genetic risk factors that govern the onset of chemical dependence.

Alcoholism encompasses a broad range of signs and symptoms some of which are present in some people at some times, and these are variable. Alcoholism is a chronic, progressive, and terminal disorder. It can start out with different symptoms which can vary from mild to severe. These signs and symptoms can have different onsets. If alcoholism is allowed to progress relentlessly and untreated, then it will always end up the same, as a fatal disease.

Classifications and Causes

There have been different ways of classifying alcoholism. In the past, alcoholism was classified based on drinking pattern or on onset age of drinking or on family drinking patterns or on other criteria. As far as classification by **pattern** of drinking, alcoholism was once classified as non-abstaining (daily drinking) or non-detaining ("periodic" binge drinking). After any alcoholic has been drinking for many years, these two patterns practically merge when the number of days of binge drinking out number the non-drinking says. As far as classification by onset, some people become frank alcoholics the first time that they ever taste alcohol; at the other extreme, some people drink socially for many years or even decades, before beginning a slow insidious descent into alcoholism. As far as classification by family patterns (classification by genetics), there are families where many members of the family have drinking problems: for example: both parents, the uncles, grandparents, and so on. Surely there must be a genetic component which is evidenced most strongly in these families. This would be an example of "genetic" alcoholism, although we might make a case that it is due to nurture not nature, i.e. growing up in an alcoholic family where everybody drinks. Yet in Europe where children routinely drink wine, the prevalence and incidence of alcoholism is perhaps not too much higher than it is in our country. This is an example of what we call heredo-familial disease. This term captures both aspects of nature and nurture and combines them into one classification. Nevertheless, there are families which only show one alcoholic in each generation or one in every other generation. This might be called sporadic alcoholism (occasional and random). Regardless of the family pattern or of the individual pattern of alcoholic disease symptoms, if alcoholics continue to drink for very long times, then they all reach a common endpoint where they are severe alcoholics with total damage to their bodies.

It is a truism and an everyday observation that end-stage alcoholism will result in severe deterioration of medical, emotional, legal, social, and economic status. Alcohol affects virtually every organ of the body. The lungs are sometimes spared except for the fact that half of all alcoholics also smoke and this combination results in total body devastation. The nervous system and brain are badly affected, too. The legal problems can be legion and seemingly unlimited: DUI arrests and public intoxication are only two of the commonest ones. Other legal problems are related to acts committed while intoxicated or in a black-out and can be any kind of impulse-related crime. An alcoholic cannot claim a legal defense of temporary insanity since he has always had the opportunity to control or quit drinking. Black-outs and intoxication also would probably not pass the Justice system's "reasonable man test" i.e. a reasonable man would not have drunk so much. Alcoholics become general social outcasts and end up spending time with other alcoholics which is not very socially healthy. Alcoholics spend a lot of money on alcohol consumption by going out to bars and nightclubs, making legal restitution, hiring defense attorneys, paying for medical and psychiatric care, paying for 28-day "detox" programs, and all other manner of spending while on sprees, binges, or while in a black-out. Unchecked and untreated alcoholism will thus reach an end-point with institutionalization, incarceration, or death.

As far as genetic causes, there seem to be genetic correlations for alcoholism, but the exact genes are not completely known and in cases where those genes might have been identified there seem to be numerous genes expressing variable presentations. This is under study.

As far as individual causes, one theory states that many people are potential alcoholics, but of course one can only become alcoholic by drinking alcohol. Some people have "alcoholic personalities" but have never tasted alcohol or had never drunk very much. They may behave as frantically as the alcoholic. This can be observed in families where several family members are alcoholics: the non-drinker(s) in the family seem almost as out of control as the practicing alcoholics in the family. These types of out-of-control non-drinkers can benefit from attending Al-Anon meetings (a support group for family members of alcoholics). Some of these potential members of Al-anon who carry the "alcoholic genes" can turn into alcoholics if they ever started drinking heavily.

The biochemical causes of alcoholism are unknown but are thought to be regulated by certain genes. It is not clear if genetics causes alterations in the bodies and brain of alcoholics; however, it is the most plausible explanation since we know that some alcoholics have at least one genetically-based biochemical difference. In certain ethnic groups, the drinkers may be unable to de-activate alcohol due to a genetic variation; this can be seen in the Oriental (East Asian) and Native American populations. This results in a medical condition in which the alcohol by-products accumulate in the body and become poisonous, resulting in "toxic" behaviors. Other biochemical studies have shown that chemically dependent people might have a deficiency of dopamine, the brain hormone that produces a sense of well being and euphoria. Alcohol and stimulant drugs can alter the levels of dopamine, thus causing an alcoholic to feel euphoric—then afterwards he feels dysphoric (the opposite of euphoric). He gets 'happy' then crashes (into a hangover). Some researchers have suggested that such an alcoholic, whom we can callSean, is "self-treating" his depression, but that is probably an oversimplification. If alcoholics get into recovery and still feel depressed, they can respond to a wide variety of very effective antidepressants and mood stabilizers, most of which have little effect on raising any dopamine brain levels and some may even block dopamine; yet, these medicines give the recovering alcoholic a lot of relief. Furthermore, a few antidepressants can raise dopamine levels, but there is no really convincing evidence that these drugs help to stabilize alcoholics. And in quite a few cases, dopamine-raising drugs can make people like Sean feel unpleasantly over-stimulated. Another plausible explanation is that there is originally no dopamine deficiency whatsoever in chemically dependent patients and that habitual drug abuse/alcoholism depletes the brain of normal levels of dopamine so that the observed low dopamine levels are due to the effect of addicting chemicals and not the cause of the problem at all. Low dopamine levels may be a side-effect of drug abuse and not the cause of it. A number of alcoholics are exquisitely sensitive to panic-anxiety symptoms and phobias. These are mediated by a brain "hormone" called GABA; alcohol also appears to act on GABA to produce a sense of relaxation and calmness. The role of dopamine, GABA, and other brain bio-chemicals is still under study.

There are also ethnic differences which are due to genetic variations. About 25% of Orientals (East Asians) and many Native Americans lack a liver protein (acetaldehyde dehydrogenase enzyme) that processes and de-activates alcohol. The lack of this enzyme results in the build-up of an intolerably high dose of a toxic alcohol by-product (acetaldehyde), which causes bizarre behaviors. In most people and in most alcoholics, this liver protein processes and de-activates alcohol, thus producing a reasonably pleasurable experience. But, the people who have this genetic "defect" will get very sick physically and mentally and will derive no pleasure from drinking. Instead, they will experience flushing, nausea and other symptoms as well as raging out of control. Despite this effect, some of these genetically "deficient" alcoholics will still continue drinking compulsively and with impunity. Whether or not this is a genetic "deficiency" or "abnormality", is debatable.

Interesting, there is a drug called Antabuse (Disulfiram) that can create these unpleasant and "abnormal" effects in anybody who has "normal" genetics for alcohol consumption. Antabuse is usually prescribed to be taken once a day every day. Anatabuse is intended to prevent or discourage alcoholics from drinking during the workday. If the alcoholic drinks on Antabuse, then he will feel ill with flushing and nausea. The effect is considered by many to be very unpleasant; nonetheless, some alcoholics continue drinking even while taking Antabuse. (anecdotally, the "antibiotic" Flagyl can also cause this Antabuse-type reaction.)

Physicians who are alcoholics or drug-addicts can be placed in jeopardy of losing a medical license. This can be a very cogent driving force to get their attention, since physicians are presumed to have one of the highest alcohol recovery rates of any subgroup. As far as chemical dependence in physicians, they are usually alcoholics, and rarely addicted to street drugs. Some take a lot of prescription pills on the side as a self-perceived treatment for either withdrawal or intoxication symptoms (as mentioned earlier in this chapter). This is nothing new: some of the founders of AA relied on prescription pills for sleeping, motivation, and anxiety control so as to be able to further their drinking "careers". The only result of using pills was to "lower their bottoms" (see later in this chapter, under treatment) artificially and put off the day of reckoning while in the meantime their addiction grew worse. Anesthesiologists often become addicted to Fentanyl, an anesthesia drug that they administer during surgery. This is the most powerfully addicting narcotic on the market (along with Sufentanyl). Veterinarians may become addicted to ketamine, an anesthetic. State medical boards allow physicians access to specialized peer-support recovery systems (special unlisted AA meetings for doctors only).

Perhaps every human is susceptible to chemical dependence, but some people have lower (or higher) thresholds of tolerance; perhaps everybody could become chemically dependent when exposed to enough mental stress over a long enough period of time.

Symptoms and Signs of Alcoholism

There are many ways of describing the symptoms and signs. Various organizations have published guides such as the CAGE questionnaire—there are many organizations with many lists of criteria. The common signs and symptoms are those that come from drinking too much and too often. At one time, organized medicine established a limit of two cocktails per day (how big is a cocktail?). The quantity does not matter—all that matters is the effect of the alcohol the person.

We all know the common signs—

- Loss of equilibrium (dizziness), upchucking, eyes rolling around in head, heavy eyelids, passing out, slurred speech, wobbly gait, sudden anger and yelling, plus puffy dark eyes, red nose and cheeks, and so on; and the common symptoms—

- blurting out silly phrases or naughty innuendos, laughing too much, poor judgment, sadness, moodiness, anxiety and panic, poor sleep, bad dreams, and so on.

The course and progression of chemical dependence is painful to watch. Family members get embroiled in the whole merry-go-round caused by this disorder while the whole roller coaster of the alcoholic's life will continue until the patient either hits his "bottom" or dies. Many families have spent enormous sums of money to lock up the alcoholic family member for a month or more, but to their chagrin, he will usually start drinking again when he leaves the treatment facility. Some codependent families have paid dearly for several prolonged residential treatments but with no success. The alcoholic will quit drinking ONLY when he hits his bottom, ONLY when he is sick and tired of it, and ONLY when he has nowhere else to go.

"You can lead a horse to water, but you can't make it drink". [8]

Any alcoholic determined to have sobriety can usually achieve this in the most successful way known for the last seventy years: by going to daily AA meetings (which costs no more than a dollar a day). If psychiatric medications are needed, these should be non-addicting and prescribed by a psychiatrist who understands chemical dependence. We can send the alcoholic to AA but we cannot make him get sober or make him want sobriety—only he can do that. And he will only do that in his own time and in his own way.

Diagnosis

Anyone can make the diagnosis. Usually the family is the first to know, as in the case of the secretive "closet drinker". In other cases, the alcoholic might display his alcoholism repeatedly in public in which case his probable diagnosis will be well known—or suspected, although he is later surprised to learn that everyone knew of his alcoholism before he did.

Usually the **loved ones are the first** to make the diagnosis. Alcoholism counselors will make this diagnosis too on the basis of excessive drinking and disruptive behavior. Unfortunately, the only diagnosis that really matters is for the alcoholic to make a self-diagnosis, and this is hard to do because alcoholism is one of the few diseases that tells the patient that he has no disease.

American Psychiatric Association diagnosis is based on: "*…needing more and more liquor, devoting more and more time to getting drunk, fear of going into withdrawal if alcohol is not available, allowing alcohol to interfere with the main areas of life: occupational, marital, financial, etc.…*" This is the diagnosis that I use.

Doctors of general medicine might make the diagnosis based on: abnormal blood tests (liver, platelets, blood sugar, enlarged red cells, cholesterol) flappy wrists, red nose and cheeks, bruises, repeat minor accidents and falls, frequent respiratory infections, yeast infections and venereal diseases, weight gain or loss, alcohol on the breath, and so on.

AA advises each person to diagnose himself and for example suggests:

"We do not like to pronounce any individual as alcoholic, but you can quickly diagnose yourself. Step over to the nearest barroom and try some controlled drinking. Try to drink and stop abruptly. Try it more than once. It will not take long for you to decide…get a full knowledge of your condition." (p.30 of the "Big Book of AA")

"…we have had deep and effective spiritual experiences which have revolutionized our whole attitude toward life, toward our fellows and toward…[the] universe…" [8-c] ("Big Book of AA")

Treatment Yes, Cure No

There is only treatment and no cure. The main treatments can be divided into spiritual and pharmacologic, the spiritual being by far the more effective since it requires the patient to make a complete re-evaluation of himself and of his behaviors, goals, and desires with the hope that he can resolve old grudges and gripes and can learn new ways of accommodating other people. These then are the available treatment:

- **spontaneous recovery**
- **spiritual (AA)**
- **spiritual (religious)**
- **counseling and psychological treatment**
- **reality-based treatments** such as repeat interventions and "**raising the bottom**"
- **pharmacologic**
- **aversive treatments** including the taking of Antabuse;
- **decreased cravings**, using Campral or ReVia—and a possible new approach called **harm avoidance** which is likely to be just this season's treatment du jour".

Spontaneous recovery suggests that a drinker can quit on his own. These may be "alcoholics" in common speech, but not by the AA definition. The very AA definition of alcoholic is that of someone who cannot quit drinking on his own. The next two paragraphs discuss the philosophical issues and semantics; the reader can skip this unless he is especially interested in these technicalities.

Spontaneous recovery is a common occurrence and regular feature found in many people who quit drinking. People often refer to "spontaneous recovery" as alcoholics who "quit drinking on their own". Some terminology needs to be qualified and explained, however. First off, we must quibble over the definition of what is an "alcoholic". Many people might be considered alcoholics, but many of these are usually heavy daily drinkers who have not "passed over the fine line", or they may be weekend bingers who have not yet "passed over the fine line". These people are alcoholic in the sense that they drink too much and too often. But they have not yet crossed over the "fine line". Once "over the fine line" is the usual AA definition of a true alcoholic: this is a person who has lost control of his obsession and compulsion to drink. He cannot quit drinking on his own, hence he could not spontaneously quit drinking on his own, hence a true AA-eligible alcoholic can not quit drinking (permanently) on his own and could never achieve a "spontaneous recovery". And even if he could, he would be "dry" not "sober". I have seen a number of these guys and they are miserable.

The official AA definitions are found on pp108-110 where they list the four categories of drinking husbands.

I follow these official AA guidelines in defining an alcoholic as a "full-blown end-stage alcoholic". However, I follow the APA guidelines for diagnosing alcoholics in my office for various reasons. Accordingly, recovery in AA is a sine qua non for defining these alcoholics. In other words, when the Big Book of Alcoholics Anonymous uses the word "alcoholic", this is in reference to someone who has gone beyond the point of being able to recover spontaneously. Unbelievable as it sounds, do please note that there are young adults who are already "full-blown end-stage alcoholics"—how this happened at such an early age is not quite clear, but it is true.

As far as the **spiritual** angle, some people are able to get sober on **religion** alone, but the success of this approach is estimated to be around 3% or less. Religious or spiritual programs might appear to have a higher success rate because regular church-goers may be more open to accepting a Higher Power; the congregation may also try to intervene early while the drinker is still in the throes of alcohol abuse but not yet crossed over to total alcohol dependence. The **religious** approach is probably truly more successful if the person appears to be a true alcoholic, but is merely a very heavy drinker.[8-a] This presupposes that he has not yet crossed over the bio-chemical point-of-no-return into alcoholism (crossing the "fine line").

More successful—and actually the only successful—treatment for full-blown alcoholics is **AA.** This program was originally formulated as six steps: [8-b]

1—Complete Deflation [of ego]

2—Dependence on and guidance from a Higher Power (choose any)

3—Moral inventory (writing and listing one's bad behaviors)

4—Confession ("witnessing"—perhaps "self-witnessing" is more accurate)

5—Restitution [righting wrongs done while drunk]

6—Continued work with other alcoholics (helping them to get sober).

However, some of the steps have been amplified and subdivided to turn six steps into the **Twelve Steps** which we know today.

AA did not appear suddenly from nowhere fully fledged. The tenets and approach belonged to a previous self-help program from the nineteenth century. These were the Oxford Groups, which stressed the need to confess one's wrongs publicly (by "witnessing") and to make amends to people whom we have been wronged. The Oxford Group was not a recovery group by modern standards. However, the Oxford Group did provide a platform upon which "Dr. Bob" and "Bill W" (Bob Smith MD and Bill Wilson) could craft a sobriety program—after some trial and error. Dr. Bob and Bill were the co-founders of AA, a movement which has saved untold millions of lives. It has been shown in many cases that the spiritual part of the program is the most important part—for, without a sense of reliance upon a "Higher Power", all the medicine in the world will offer very little chance of prolonged recovery. The spiritual aspect requires the alcoholic to revamp his way of looking at and responding to the world.

Alcohol counseling with an alcohol counselor can be very beneficial too. Or the alcoholic might have psychotherapy issues that would require him to do "talk therapy" with a therapist or psychologist. This is usually very helpful and commendable. Most recovering alcoholics have a number of counseling and therapy issues which need to be discussed with at least one trained professional.

Most alcoholics will not quit drinking until they are truly "sick and tried of being sick and tired" from alcoholism and have perhaps reached a curious state in which they can no longer get drunk but also can not get dried out. This uncomfortable state might be the last straw and as such offers a window of opportunity during which the alcoholic might become more tractable and more willing to seek treatment. At this brief moment he is "hitting bottom"—or at least the first of his bottoms. This is a fleetingly brief opportunity to coax him into accepting treatment. If he cannot be engaged into treatment at this point then he will at some point resume drinking until he hits a lower bottom. Once again, at that point there might be another window of opportunity. Unfortunately, some alcoholics never reach a bottom like this. Instead they will die from all the socio-economic and medical ravages of alcoholism which are too numerous to count. In these cases the "bottom" is death or, alternatively, death supervenes before the alcoholic hits his [first] bottom. Here are a series of bottoms. At each bottom (1), there is a chance to try to get sober. If that chance is lost, then the next chance will occur at the next bottom (2)—and so on, down until the last bottom (3) or death (4):

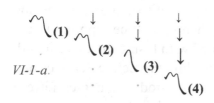

VI-1-a.

I had briefly had one patient, "Don", in his late fifties who had been in and out of AA, multiple detox programs, and residential settings since his early teens. During all those decades he usually could not stay sober but for a matter of weeks (or months) before resuming his drinking or drugging (stimulant street drugs). Once Don did stay sober for a couple years. Since he had started drinking in his teens, his personality style was still rooted in the teen years (yes, an alcoholic's maturity level freezes at the age of onset of heavy drinking—same for drug addicts). He started seeing me right after his favorite sponsor moved out of state. There was no real psychiatric treatment to help him until he was ready to quit drinking, that is until he finally hit his bottom. And he had hit many bottoms over and over. The worst bottom had not yet been reached. Don quit calling and I heard later that he had moved out of state to live in the city as his favorite sponsor. He had no serious medical problems.

This very brief case history illustrates all the following points: (1) Don had a serious case of "genetic" alcoholism—a real "alcoholic" family; (2) in these "genetic" type cases, the addiction seems much more intense and untreatable; (3) a 58 year-old person with minimal sobriety and onset drinking in early teens will act like a teenager while he is at the age to be a grandfather; (4) he enjoyed a socioeconomic level where there was not enough pressure placed upon him to quit drinking—an alcoholic will not quit drinking as long as someone is always going to soften his fall; (5) he had decided to turn his favorite sponsor into his Higher Power, which is not recommended, since a sponsor is basically just another recovering alcoholic; (6) mixed addictions with two drugs of choice are harder to treat; (6) an alcoholic will quit drinking only when he has hit his last bottom—wherever and whenever that is; (7) for some alcoholic-addicts, death is their bottom; and, (8) enablers can lead a horse to water, but they cannot make it drink.

Reality: Everyone—hopefully—has a level of despair or disability that they can no longer tolerate. One technique of formalized alcohol treatment teams is to "raise the bottom" artificially—this requires getting absolute and non-negotiable leverage against the alcoholic which is the only way to get an alcoholic's attention. Most alcoholics are only willing to admit that they have a problem when their life is in such a shambles that it becomes obvious even to them. This can happen with divorce, loss of job, loss of license, loss of family support, financial bankruptcy, many urgent trips to hospitals, legal problems/incarceration (DUI) loss of custody of children,catastrophic medical disease, and so on. Their "bottom" can be artificially raised in a number of maneuvers: refusing to fund their lifestyle; having child welfare take custody of their children; placing them on probation at work; placing them on legal probation in the court system or obtaining a TRO (temporary restraining order), confiscating their cars; garnisheeing their wages, making them wear electronic shackles, and so on. The treatment team may decide that the patient's right to practice law will depend on his full co-operation with the team; if not, then he will be reported to the State Bar. This is often effective with men who might be faced with losing their livelihood. As for women, the threat of having the treatment team notify Child Protective Services that the patient is an unfit mother and is recommended to lose custody of her child(ren) sometimes suffices to get her full co-operation. When they get to their [artificially raised] bottom, then they are willing to admit that they have a problem, and a window of opportunity for treatment will open. Some people may be ready to quit after a first or second DUI, some quite after a divorce, and some never reach their bottom which is so low that they die first. In these cases, the urge to drink (use drugs) is so strong that raising the bottom artificially has no effect whatsoever.

VI-1-b

In the previous example of Don, his bottom could be raised artificially if someone had some leverage over him—something that would help him make a flight from alcoholism into recovery. As it turns out, there was nothing seemingly that could have done that for Don, absent a life-altering spiritual experience. In other cases like his, try to imagine either raising the bottom at (3) or of a major spiritual revelation at (3). This is depicted in diagram VI-1-b. After this event, the alcoholic rises up to recovery (4) instead of descending into death. What are the directions to AA? *"Go straight to Hell and then make a U-turn."*

Pharmacologic treatment involves differentiating the treatability status of a drinker, and this can subdivide into a two-pronged approach also.

Treatability Status

In some cases, the patient is not a full-blown end-stage alcoholic by any means. Let's take a patient named Willy who might not be completely chemically addicted and falls into the alcoholic rubric of being a **"problem drinker"**; this is meant to suggest that Willy is reacting to problems in his life. This is a form of "self-medicating". The supposition is that he is using alcohol (or drugs) as a means of escape from some temporary major stress factor (the "problem" drinker's "problem"). Men often resort to this behavior since it allows them to show their otherwise suppressed feelings. This does not necessarily imply that problem drinkers like Willy will ever become alcoholic—unless he cannot quit drinking.

In some cases, the "problem drinker" continues to **drink routinely** because of an ongoing problem which has become permanent. This is popularly known as "self-medicating". This seems very ominous because regular drinking could lead to permanent alcoholism. Willy is becoming an habitual drinker. Willy needs to get into therapy right away to try to resolve this problem without using chemicals. Otherwise he could become a full-blown alcoholic. Of course, he could turn to compulsive gambling, sexual compulsions, or overeating.

Psychoactive medications cannot cure "problem drinking" either, but on the other hand, the problem drinker has not (yet) become a true alcoholic. The APA refers to the problem drinker as "alcohol abuse" (not "alcohol dependence", which is "true" alcoholism). AA refers to these cases as "heavy drinkers" (not having crossed the "fine line", hence not yet alcoholic—but getting close).

In the cases of true alcoholics, pharmacologic treatments cannot cure full-blown alcoholism and are only an auxiliary treatment to the main treatment which is regular attendance at AA meetings or some equivalent spiritual program that results in a "spiritual realignment".

Two-Pronged Medication Treatment Approach

A person may be given medicines to decrease his desire to drink or he may be treated for a separate mental health problem.

The patient can be given a drug which will **decrease his desire to drink** (Campral, ReVia) or decrease the pleasure from drinking by making him physically ill (Antabuse). However, the obsession to drink is usually much stronger than any medicine. Besides, he needs to be willing to take the medicine. If he shows willingness to take the medicine, then maybe the next move will be to have willingness to think about getting sober, and then later, having willingness to get sober.

He can also be treated for a separate **mental health diagnosis** such as Mood disorder or Psychosis—this approach relies on the usual psychiatric treatments. In general, people like this are referred to as having "Dual Diagnosis" (having a chemical dependence diagnosis plus a separate psychiatric illness) and these people need to have both conditions treated in order to give themselves the maximum chance at recovery; nonetheless, these patients have a harder time reaching equilibrium than patients who only have a chemical dependence diagnosis. They will have much trouble staying sober if the primary psychiatric disorder remains untreated. And they will definitely have worse mental health symptoms if they do not stop drinking or drugging.

The use of psychiatric medicines for alcoholics who have a second mental health issue apart from alcoholism itself is always a conundrum. Some of the "fundamentalist" alcoholics in AA advocate "natural" recovery and may reject the use of any mind-altering or mood-altering substance and may croakingly denounce these treatments while sucking up a pot of coffee daily and smoking a pack or two of cigarettes (brain researchers opine that nicotine is as addictive as cocaine). Psychiatric drugs can be helpful for recovering alcoholics under certain circumstances and with certain caveats:

- —use of addicting drugs must be avoided, especially amphetamine-like and valium-like drugs;

- —prescriptions must originate from a psychiatrist who really understands the pitfalls of relapse and the caveats of sober treatment. One favorite drug that is typically claimed not to be addicting is Klonopin; however, it is addicting, it is in the valium family of drugs, and it is a controlled substance (it is regulated by the DEA—Drug Enforcement Administration in Washington, D.C.); see Chapter V-11.

- —patient's diagnosis must be severe enough to warrant a prescription: people having a minor depression or adjustment disorder (chapter IV-3) should be referred first for talk therapy; and maybe after that, for medications;

- —prescriptions for major psychiatric medicines should be avoided in early sobriety—especially in the first month of sobriety. Alcoholics in early recovery are awash in sequential waves of strong and fluctuating emotions. Those cases need to have some length of recovery, otherwise psychiatrists end up treating transient and fluctuating symptoms caused by the early stages of sobriety. Each early phase of early sobriety corresponds to new waves of emotions that appear with practically the regularity of the tides coming in. Some psychiatrists become overenmeshed in treating each new "neaptide" or "ebbtide". All of these emotional alterations suggest the need to add on some other medicine as symptomatic treatment for the current emotional tide or to keep changing medications every couple weeks. This is not at all helpful to the patient who needs to be allowed have some firsthand experience with these feelings. Wait until a full-blown alcoholic has been sober for a while, otherwise the psychiatrist will end more confused than the patient about which symptoms need treatment. I commonly see patients who are more or less typical alcoholics in early sobriety who end up in my office with a bag of pills: anti-depressant, anti-anxiety, anti-manic, anti-psychotic pills and, of course, the perennial favorite—Klonopin again. New drugs are added every couple weeks to treat the side effects of the previous drugs that were supposed to treat the emotional tides. Newly sober people on Klonopin will start to have Klonopin side effects which are not recognized as drug side effects and seem to need treatment. And the Klonopin side effects have been mistaken for psychiatric symptoms for which he is now on permanent disability. The only exception regarding psychiatric medication in very early sobriety should be for somebody who is clearly manic or psychotic or suicidal—in other words, somebody who is having a psychiatric emergency (see psychiatric emergencies). These patients need to be medicated as soon as possible. All others should wait a reasonable amount of time. What's reasonable? If you relate well to your psychiatrist who is familiar with practical treatment of addiction, then the two of you can decide together.

Psychiatric drugs can be used but very carefully, and any chemically dependent patient who declines them on philosophical reasons should have his wishes respected.

Aversive treatments consist of treatment that gives the patient negative associations with drinking. Antabuse is a daily medicine that produces nausea in the presence of alcohol. These treatments are not a regular part of American psychiatric treatment for alcoholism. Antabuse is not perfect. Recovering alcoholics who are licensed professionals in a diversion program usually go to a designated person to consume the Antabuse on a daily record. The record of daily consumption is duly recorded by the administrator of the Antabuse. Examples of such licensed professionals would be airplane pilots, lawyers, and all licensed medical professionals (physicians, nurses, and so on). Some alcoholics have developed the ability to drink even while taking Antabuse, which is another reason that Antabuse has lost some of its therapeutic clout in the USA.

There is another new "treatment" called "**harm avoidance**" which is proposed by a small number of psychiatrists. This treatment requires the patient to take a medicine which will not allow him to feel a real "buzz" or euphoria from drinking alcohol; however, he is allowed to drink what and when he desires. The reasoning behind this method is that he will desire to drink less, because it does not produce a "buzz"; hence, he will drink less and not get out of control. This is "controlled drinking", which a real alcoholic can not handle, for when he drinks he always drinks too much for too long—regardless. This is part of the basic definition of alcoholism. This treatment requires the patient to take a drug such as Campral or Revia. There is not a lot of information on this treatment. Successful treatment is probably likelier in the cases of alcohol abuse rather than full-blown alcoholism. This is a novel and non-traditional approach to chemical dependence treatment, and there are gainsayers among the majority of alcoholism treatment providers.

Strategy of usual and customary psychiatric treatment:

First, determine if the patient is a full-blown alcoholic or not. This is simple: tell the patient to quit drinking until the next appointment; if he cannot quit drinking, then he most surely is an alcoholic. If he can quit drinking, then perhaps he has not crossed the biochemical point of no return (the "fine line") and is only a very heavy drinker and not yet a full-blown alcoholic.

Secondly, if he cannot quit drinking, then he is a real alcoholic. If he is full-blown and cannot quit drinking, then he should give some thought to beginning regular attendance at AA meetings.

In serious cases, if he might be in danger of serious withdrawal, then he might need a formalized and medically supervised detoxification in the hospital for a few days. People at high risk for serious withdrawal are those who have had D.T.'s or seizures, people with serious medical problems, a history of extreme daily amounts of alcohol (a gallon or more of hard liquor), a history of high daily doses of alcohol plus high daily doses of Valium-like drugs (20 mg or more). After detox he can attend AA which will provide answers to many of his problems much better than any pill. AA may also provide a "social milieu therapy".

If there were no real risk of withdrawal, then he can skip medical detoxification and go directly to AA meetings. Initially, he may be given a mild non-addicting sedative to help with sleep or anxiety. A few months after he has been in AA, and when his nerves are not so jumpy, it will be possible to discern which kinds of medicines—if any—that he will need: anti-anxiety, anti-depressant, other or none.

Thirdly, if the patient can quit drinking on his own, then it might be instructive to suggest that he try a couple AA meetings so that he will know where to find a meeting in case he resumes drinking and makes himself a full-blown alcoholic. Additionally, we would suggest some sessions with the therapist and a course of appropriate medications provided that there are any residual symptoms which need to be treated.

The usual prescription medicines that might be helpful are:

- for anxiety: Buspar, Atarax/Vistaril, or very low dose Sinequan;

- for depression and anxiety: an SSRI drug such as Prozac, Zoloft, Paxil, Lexapro;

- for irritability and severe insomnia: low doses Zyprexa or Seroquel briefly;

- for insomnia and depression: Remeron;

- for mild insomnia: Atarax, Rozerem, Desyrel;

- for mild detoxification at home: Depakote (or Tegretol);

- for mild-moderate detoxification at home: Librium and thiamine pills (Vitamin B_1), 100 mg. twice a day.

- avoid getting cross-addicted to Klonopin, Ativan, or Xanax (prescribed by well-intentioned family doctors)

Fatality: Lethality of Chemical Dependence

Indirect socio-physical causes of death:
Chemically dependent people often die from accidents while intoxicated and from various other problems. They can get involved with shady characters who are very dangerous; also auto accidents are certainly possible as well as falling or passing out in seedy locales or getting mugged, jaywalking late at night; getting lost in dangerous neighborhoods or driving the wrong way on the freeway or driving off a hillside; passing out in a blizzard and freezing to death; downhill nighttime skiing while in a black out; being battered from late night barroom brawls, and so on. These indirect causes can be legion, and the morning papers and evening news often detail a spate of these types of occurrences that the astute listener and reader may link to alcoholism.

Medical causes of death can include: falling down while very intoxicated, head injuries causing bleeding into the brain; choking on one's own vomit; unwitnessed and uncontrolled persistent epilepsy-like seizure caused by alcohol withdrawal; accidental excessive alcohol poisoning; vomiting blood due to internal bleeding; heart attack due to excess cigarette consumption while disinhibited on alcohol; nutritional defects and B-vitamin deficiencies; cirrhosis, pancreatic disorders with or without secondary diabetes, total brain impairment, free-bleeding and so on.

Emotional *causes of death*: most alcoholics stop developing normally at the age at which they start to drink compulsively. If the alcoholic started drinking as a teenager, then he will approach the world as a teenager even though he is now middle-aged. Emotional causes of death can include all the impulsivity and carelessness seen in youth.

Psychiatric causes of death: These are manifold and important and often manifest as suicidal behavior due to depression. Suicidal—and parasuicidal—behavior can be quite high among dry, sober, and practicing alcoholics. (Chapter IV-7) Suicide obviously refers to completing the act of killing oneself (overdosing, hanging, gunshots, crashing cars into trees, etc.). Parasuicidal behavior is risky careless behavior that could predictably result in personal death and occurs when the alcoholic is not completely suicidal but is very ambivalent about life (and death). This can take many forms: alcoholic diabetics who decide not to inject insulin; depressed patients who quit taking antidepressants; psychotics who quit taking anti-psychotic medicines; experimenting with death by taking a "small overdose" that is not fatal but results in a permanent physical or neurological defect, and so on.

Dry alcoholics may be depressed because they have no socio-spiritual basis, may feel alone (no AA group connections), or lack any philosophy about life and death (i.e. no solace in any program of spirituality or religion). They may feel socially isolated, divorced, and on bad terms with their offspring (because they did not work the twelve steps). This category might be overrepresented by alcohol abusers rather than true alcoholics. If they had never crossed the line into true alcoholism, then the complete AA program may indeed not speak to them: they are caught in a type of spiritual limbo, but may find some outlet to be able to cope with their situations: yoga, intense volunteerism, meditation, or anything that might make them feel whole again.

Practicing alcoholics often become very depressed about the hopelessness of ongoing drinking and all the perceived losses and failures in their lives, which might seem unsalvageable and irrevocable—including the failures at trying to get sober. They are at high risk when extremely intoxicated and maudlin. During these times, they are no longer inhibited by any fear of reality and may take intentional or accidental overdoses. Intentional overdoses occur with lethal intent when the person feels completely beaten by life circumstances and really has no desire to survive. Those who are truly intending to die, often use lethal means such as guns, hanging, or jumping from high places. They have probably been thinking or brooding about suicide for a long time prior to acting. Accidental overdoses occur due mainly to forgetting how much medicine they had just taken or annoyed that the first doses seem not to have "worked" rapidly enough, thus leading the person to take added pills to try to get a better effect. These people are not truly intending to die—they are just being careless and unsafe in monitoring their behaviors. Some of them do die, but a lot more end up surviving, and if the accidental overdose were sizable then they might end up with permanent mental or physical damage. I have seen two patients survive after shooting themselves in the head right through the brain; and, I have seen people die from trivial overdoses of prescription medicines due to the powerful additive effects of mixing certain medicines with alcohol (this is very true of Tylenol, too). Any of these types of behaviors warrant admitting a person involuntarily to a psychiatric hospital for a few days of observation despite the primary diagnosis of alcoholism. (Chapter IV-7)

Sober alcoholics can become depressed and suicidal too, but for different reasons—usually for the same reasons that the non-alcoholic might commit suicide: feeling hapless, hopeless, and helpless; suffering a deep melancholia; having prior history of severe depressions; failure to engage in or benefit from psychiatric treatment; overwhelming onus of genetic loading (a lot of depression, suicide, schizophrenia and alcoholism in the biological family of origin). "Fundamentalist" alcoholics may absolutely refuse to take any mind or mood altering medications. In effect, their actions tell us that they would prefer to die sober than live with artifical mood and mindset. Psychiatric disorders are very serious and should be treated appropriately: non-pharmacologic treatments are available!

Spiritual causes of death from alcoholism: Some alcoholics can curiously end up dying from a spiritual disequilibrium that I call "resentmentosis". They start to obsess over some trivial resentment from the past and it starts to gnaw away at them. They cannot let it go. "Resentmentosis" may indeed be the second or third leading cause of death in modern alcoholics (along with emphysema, pancreatitis, and cirrhosis). Resentmentosis is like drinking poison and hoping that your imagined adversary will die. This can happen to any alcoholic who might be in a "dry drunk". This can especially apply to alcoholics who never went to AA or to alcoholics who dropped out of AA and forgot what they had learned there. They are predisposed to a lot of obsessive brooding and sulking about unresolved issues (which can only be mollified by working the Twelve Steps); however, a lot of them are more willing to try anti-obsessive medications than to go (back) to AA meetings. They seem to be chronically plagued by a host of resentments against the whole world and may use the resentments as a reason to start drinking again. They are also expert at wallowing in self-pity: they have a bad case of the "poor-me's" or "pour-me's" ("pour me another drink"). The alcoholic believes that the self-pity and resentments are problems, which can only be cured by starting to drink alcoholically again: this is because the alcoholic's response to anything is to drink. Or in the alternative, we could say that they never got truly sober and so have no guarantee against future relapses due to the lack of any new-found form of personal spirituality. In these cases, the dry but not (yet) sober alcoholic might resume drinking. And in any case, a return to drinking –under any circumstance—can be lethal for any alcoholic (see above all the aforementioned causes of death).

So the causes of death in untreated alcoholics may range from psychiatric to physical and medical and even to spiritual. Alcoholism untreated is often fatal.

Outlook and Long-term Outcome

The common wisdom is that an alcoholic who does not quit drinking will end up either in jail, the hospital, or the morgue. Long ago, the main causes of death in alcoholism were liver cirrhosis and "wet-brain" (total alcoholic deterioration of the brain). Since AA was started, however, the number one cause of death among alcoholics is now emphysema: alcoholics apparently can quit alcohol but not cigarettes. Cigarettes have been noted to be as addicting as cocaine, whereas alcohol addiction is not usually nearly so addicting. Common contemporary causes of death in alcoholics are emphysema, heart failure, depression, diabetes/pancreatitis, and "resentmentosis" followed by cirrhosis and seizures. Some alcoholics suffer from significant depression and can benefit from mild anti-depressants. Some alcoholics will take these prescribed medicines and some will not. Some go on self-treating depression with coffee and cigarettes. The ones who wish to get sober "naturally" (without using any mood-altering or mind-altering medicines) may recover from depression and some may die from the depression—directly or indirectly. Depression can lead a person to suicide which is a direct cause. Others may expose themselves to dying indirectly from the depression: inattentiveness may cause accidents and falls, lack of motivation may jeopardize health in other ways. Nowadays alcoholics can end up receiving treatment for their problems and can live longer and productive lives than would have been imaginable seventy years ago (before AA became a formalized program of recovery).

Hard drinkers may have a spontaneous remission and quit drinking suddenly on their own; however, they are likely to go into a so-called "dry drunk" state which can be very unpleasant for the family. He may be "dry" but definitely not sober.[3]

►QUESTIONS

Q: When can an alcoholic go back to social drinking?

A: Usually Never. Some heavy drinkers like Willy are not full-blown alcoholics and may be able to decrease, control, or modulate their drinking. However, the true alcoholic has consumed enough alcohol to create a permanent change in his brain in the form of a "spiritual-mental lesion" such that he can never drink again with any sense of control. My viewpoint is that everyone is born with a certain sized empty vat that he will be allowed to fill up with alcohol during his life. Some vats may be huge, and others, tiny. After the person has used up all his allotment then he can drink no more lest he become alcoholic. Going over the limit causes alcoholism. The bottom line is that a person who never drinks alcohol will not become an alcoholic. Dr. Bob even points out that his own drinking was originally a "privilege that was so badly abused [by him] that its privileged status was withdrawn"(paraphrase from p.181 of the Big Book of AA).

Q: What will happen if the alcoholic does not hit his bottom?

A-1: Some people are such low-bottom drinkers that they die before hitting their bottom: death is their bottom or their bottom is lower than mortality;

A-2: Some people lack the ability to observe themselves as they really are and thus never self-diagnose (this is called lack of humility).

A-3: Some alcoholics naturally live their whole lives without hitting a bottom. In all three answers above, there is unfortunately nothing that anyone can do to help the alcoholic; the friends and family will need to understand this fact and avoid enabling or meddling.

A-4: Some alcoholics hold onto fatal secrets or have a lack of honesty or lack of willingness to be honest. They will take these secret facts or secret feelings to the grave rather than deal with them here and now.

These situations (A-1-2-3-4) need to be viewed as chronic and incurable—but not a permanent SSD disability! SSD mrely serves to validates all these perverse machinations.

Q: What is the best way to treat alcoholism?

A: The best way to treat ALL diseases is PREVENTION.

Q: So where is the alcoholic's "bottom"?

A: There are as many answers to this question as there are alcoholics.

If the treatment works well, then the patient can get sober; otherwise, he might go back to drinking. Or if he quits drinking but is not really sober then he can end up in a "dry drunk" state which is characterized by being cranky, resentful, irritable, needy and possibly aggressive. Twelve Steps programs have much less than a 4-10% chance of helping a chemically dependent person on the first time around (this percentage is only a "guesstimate" and would include people who are forced to go to AA as well as those members who go to AA voluntarily but have a few little binges afterwards). Notwithstanding, the Twelve Step program is the most successful (or least failure-prone) way of getting sober and staying sober. People can have "spontaneous recovery", but some of these who are true alcoholics will end up in a "dry drunk" which is not true sobriety.

Q: How could I prevent myself from becoming alcoholic?

A: If you never drink alcohol, then you will never become alcoholic.

This is exceptionally good advice for those who come from alcoholic families. If you come from an alcoholic family and never drink alcohol, then you will not become alcoholic—however, if you carry the alcohol genes then you could go directly into a type of "character defect" state that can be treated very effectively by your attending regular Al-Anon meetings.

Q: Why does he keep on drinking?

A: He has more addiction (to alcohol) than good judgment. He has not yet made his own self-diagnosis. He is afraid to face harsh reality without being medicated. Drinking has become a regular compulsion and also a form of escapism.

Q: How long will he keep on drinking?

A: Until he hits his "bottom". "Hitting his bottom" means that he gets so bad that even he recognizes that he has a drinking problem. Many families plead and implore their alcoholic to stop drinking. Over and over again, the families will bail him out of the morass of this problems. This only prolongs his agony and keeps him from reaching his bottom with the end result that he will drink for several more years before reaching his bottom. The kindest act is to avoid helping him so much (this action of helping too much is called "enabling"). Stop enabling him and let him hit his bottom as soon as possible so that he can get into recovery as early as possible.

Q: What if we do a family "intervention" and all sit around and tell him that he is an alcoholic?

A: He may take note of this family meeting, but it probably will not make him quit drinking— at that time; however, it may plant a small seed in his mind. He is likely to respond with anger, denial, rationalization, minimization and resentment. And the intervention group is likely to be a gathering of the same people who have individually been complaining about his drinking for a long time anyway. Simultaneously, he may feel special that so many care enough to come together on his behalf (remember the old adage that the alcoholic is an "egomaniac with an inferiority complex"!). Even if he does respond with anger, sarcasm, or resentment, he will usually end up saying something to the effect of "thanks anyway but I'm really capable of managing my own life right now [and I definitely don't need all of you to be bossing me around]". Alcoholism is the disease that tells its victims that they do not have a disease. Remember that the alcoholic is an "egomaniac with an inferiority complex"

"...Who is convinced against his Will is of the same Mind still..." [8]

▶Alcoholism is a compulsive disorder; it is the best known of all the compulsive disorders. The alcoholic is obsessed with alcohol: this leads him to drink compulsively. This form of compulsive disorder is reinforced by more than internal hormones: it is reinforced by an addicting drug, alcohol.

▶Alcoholism, drug addiction, prescription pill abuse, and chemical dependence are all the same actor but wearing different costumes and face masks.

▶Alcoholism is a permanent condition that can be arrested at a certain stage but it can never be cured with our current levels of technology.

▶Only a small percentage of alcoholics are able to "dry out" for long periods of time (15–25%); fewer than those attain sobriety or quality sober recovery (5-15% maximum); Many die from the disease in one way or another (with their deaths directly or indirectly linked to alcoholism).

▶Alcoholism is the only disease that tells its victims that they have no disease.

▶Alcoholism affects the alcoholic and everyone around him: it is a family disease.8-a (ref-8)

There are other compulsive disorders which can be amenable to Twelve Steps Programs: Overeaters (OA), "Shop-aholics", compulsive gamblers, Cocaine Addiction, Sex Addiction/Sex Love Addiction, Emotionals Anonymous, debtors anonymous (DA), CA (Cocaine Anonymous), Marijuana Anonymous, Crystal Meth Anonymous, and of course,

NA (Narcotics Anonymous). We are very lucky to be living in the hearth-land of Twelve Step programs where these self-help programs are readily available and have improved the quality of countless lives by relying upon non-pharmacologic treatment methods. Most of these programs are listed in the phone book (at least, in Los Angeles).

8-a (ref-8) pp.20-22, 108-13
8-b (ref-8) p.292
8-c (ref-8) p.25
3-   ref.3 p.788

Chapter VI-2

Essay on Codependence

So you love an alcoholic?
(So you love an addict?)

Codependence (or codependency) is a "situationship" (an unhealthy situational relationship) in which one person is obsessed with another person who in turn is obsessed with some force outside the relationship. The first person is the codependent—let's call her Helen. The second person in this case is Sean. Helen is the codependent, and Sean is the dependent. In our example, Helen is essentially addicted to Sean, and he is addicted to alcohol and cocaine. The codependent, Helen is over-enmeshed in the life and lifestyle choices of her husband, Sean, an alcoholic-addict. Helen obsesses over Sean all the time. She worries about what he is doing, where he is, and how he is. In a normal relationship, the two spouses should ideally be focused on each other mutually, but probably not to a point of pathologic obsessiveness.

Within the context of a marriage, wives are likelier to be codependents of alcoholic husbands, and husbands are likelier to be chemically dependent. Statistically speaking, Men are less likely to stay with an alcoholic or drug-addicted wife—unless they have decided to have an "open marriage" or a marriage of convenience. Women are likelier to stay with chemically dependent men. Women are likelier to have an alcoholic father, and women are likelier to divorce one alcoholic and marry another alcoholic. However, many men can still end up being codependents, just not in the classic alcoholic marriage stereotype. Codependence in men can occur when their children are alcoholics. Codependence occurs frequently in men of wives who are "shop-aholics" or "food-aholics". In many cases, the codependence goes unperceived by the men, unless they somehow end up in psychotherapy and become psychologically sophisticated. They cannot work on a marital problem in therapy unless they can identify what the problem is. Shop-aholic and food-aholic women tightly weave their pathology throughout their marital relationship and often control their husbands with sex and high calorie foods. Let's face it: as long as men are sexually satisfied, they are a lot less likely to squawk. And, of course there are shop-aholic men: three late-model cars, a vintage car, two motorcycles, jet-skis, a truck, a boat, and a big screen TV—all financed on credit payments. One could say that men shop less, but when they do, the cost of men's toys is much higher.

Psychiatrists do not typically treat these "situationships" and relationship issues directly—therapists often do this work nowadays. The primary treatment form is "talk therapy". However, it is important for me to know the source of the psychological distress. If the wife of an alcoholic husband is depressed because he has another woman and their credit cards are all "maxed out" in a community property State, then she should feel distressed. I need to know the cause—if any—of the psychological distress in order to treat it correctly. If all the distress is from the husband's antics, then the wife probably needs a small dose of a drug like Celexa and needs to start attending Al-anon. Many of these wives flatly refuse to attend Alanon. Some even want to be put on permanent disability! The treatment of these relationship problems is a lot different from that of recurrent major depression in a woman who has a wonderful life but who has unlucky genetics and biochemistry.

Helen is indirectly affected by alcohol and cocaine.

Helen is directly affected by Sean who is directly affected by alcohol and cocaine.

The behavior of Helen (a codependent person) is **indirectly** affected by alcohol and drug craving.

Helen		Sean		Alcohol
.2		1		0.

The behavior of Helen (a codependent person) is **directly** affected by alcohol and cocaine craving to the second degree of separation.

Status	2nd degree		1st degree		Ground zero
Role	Helen Supportive Enabler		Sean Alcoholic-addict		Alcohol & Cocaine The Obsession!
Diagnosis	Co-dependent		Dependent		Compulsion
Function	Indirectly Dependent on alcohol and cocaine ↔ & Directly Dependent on the alcoholic ↔		Directly Dependent on Alcohol-Cocaine	↔	Symptom of the Compulsive Disorder

VI-2   Co-dependency

I use the term "second degree of separation" because Helen, the codependent wife, has a primary dependence on the alcoholic-addict who in turn has a primary dependence on alcohol, thus giving Helen a secondary dependence on alcohol and cocaine. Any factor that affects alcohol or cocaine affects Sean directly, and Helen, indirectly. If cocaine shipments are interrupted by the DEA, then Sean will drink more and probably become angrier and more violent. If he has no money to buy alcohol, then he will go into withdrawal, which will make for a highly emotionally charged homelife. Sean, the alcoholic-addict craves alcohol and cocaine and they become his best friend and primary love-objects. He craves / loves chemicals more than he esteems Helen. This obviously interferes in the marriage between two people and becomes a marriage among a chemical power plus two people.

Actually, a codependent can be anybody (not just a wife and husband) who is in any kind of relationship with a person dependent on alcohol or drugs. The co-dependent can be spouse, parent, child, lover, and so on. Perhaps even an employer. Co-dependence refers only to an abnormal relationship with the alcoholic/drug-addict. If your relationship with the alcoholic is normal, then you are not co-dependent. Of course, if you are normal, then your normal response is not to put up with all the alcoholic's shenanigans. These are all serious conditions because people die all the time from being dependent and from being codependent. These are all role-playing and symptoms of a severe dysfunctional compulsive disorder.

Fatality and Lethality

for Sean

As already mentioned in Chapter VI-1, Sean can die from many causes: accidents, stabbings in an alley, shootings in bar-room brawls, heart attack from cocaine overdose, alcohol poisoning, HIV and Hepatitis-C from shared needles and promiscuity, drug deals gone wrong, accidental and intentional suicide, and so on.

for Helen

She is caught up in a dangerous game with Sean who is well known for car crashes, firearms, jealousy, paranoia, psychotic behaviors during black-outs, etc. He might become so enraged as to commit murder while in a black-out. Sean can become infected with Herpes, HIV, or Hepatitis-C and pass it on to Helen. Sean can get these diseases from promiscuity, intravenous drugs, and in other ways. Helen can get into a car with Sean when he is so impaired that the car crashes. Men like Sean are capable of assaulting their wives who try to sneak off to Alanon meetings: the alcoholic's stated concern is jealousy, but the real source of the anger is that Helen is taking action against his chemical dependence, in effect labeling him an alcoholic-addict—and that wrecks his self-esteem. Sean's stated concern is that she is either looking for a new man in Alanon—or worse, is sneaking around with another man while claiming to be at an Alanon meeting. Co-dependency is an abnormal state that has an abnormal focus on the abnormally chemical-dependent person. Helen responds abnormally to Sean's abnormal behavior, which in turn is fashioned by the alcohol—and by his abnormal alcohol cravings.

Normal people end their relationships with alcoholic-addicts or at least put severe limitations on them. The main reasons for which a normal person might end up staying in such a relationship are either because of being blood relatives, having young children together, or because of legal-financial commitments. Apart from that, most non-alcoholic friends will eventually distance themselves or entirely absent themselves from the lives of practicing alcoholic-addicts. Normal people will establish boundaries and not allow chemically dependent people to violate these established boundaries. Even blood relatives and legal commitments will not be enough to keep the normal person in the alcoholic's wake as they also proceed to remove themselves from the alcoholic's sphere of influence. The blood relatives stop seeing the alcoholic or tell him to leave. Sometimes they harass him enough about his alcoholism that he will want to leave. Or wives with small children will leave the alcoholic. Even legally committed partners will eventually dissolve the contractual relationship, be it spousal, occupational or professional. Or in the case of an end-stage alcoholic, the partners will just wait a little longer for the alcoholic to become really sick or die. People who are only legally bound to alcoholics and who are not from alcoholic families and not from grossly dysfunctional families may likely choose to bail out (dissolution of marriage or of commercial connections and contractual relationships), in many cases because they are emotionally healthy and find nothing of interest in maintaining a relationship with a chronic alcoholic. Perhaps they have a sixth sense which forewarns them that staying with an alcoholic would require a lot of extra footwork and chagrin. Which it does. Sometimes, one wonders if the codependent is hopelessly in love with or hopelessly addicted to the alcoholic.

Many wives of alcoholics come in for a visit and become argumentative with their therapist and psychiatrist. They offer up similar psychological defenses as vocalized by alcoholics themselves. These three main defenses are **denial, rationalization, minimization**, and so on. **Denial** that anything can be done or denial that there is a problem (of alcoholism). **Denial** that he is a real alcoholic: "Oh, he only drinks on the weekends". **Rationalization** that she is depressed naturally and that her bad feelings and anger have nothing to do with alcoholism. Or, she may **minimize** the whole situation, "Oh well, he quit drinking on his own four months ago". She does not understand that he is still an alcoholic whether he is dry (not drinking) or sober (not drinking and in a program of spiritual recovery). Many wives rebuff any suggestion that they should go to Alanon: "He should go to AA, that's his problem not mine". This is a failure to realize two things: that alcoholism is a family disease and that the family members who have chosen to stay with an alcoholic-addict are often as symptomatic as the chemically dependent person. If she intends to stay with him, then she will need Alanon. If she has no intention of going to Alanon, then the marriage will become as miserable as they both already are. Thus, the wife may yell at the therapist who is trying to help her, leave in a huff, and no-show for the next doctor appointment. The unfortunate truth is that a person like Helen who is so codependent, has her own suite of problems that need treatment in Alanon. That is her permanent mental condition. She can divorce him and never re-wed. she can remarry a non-alcoholic. The new circumstances do not matter, because she is still going to be an "alanonic" in the same way that Sean will always be an alcoholic whether he is drinking or not…a surprising number of Helen's find that they must return to Alanon after divorcing their Sean's—lest they jeopardize all their current relationships, including that one to the new non-alcoholic husband. What a drag! This is the unfortunate truth. Fortunately, Alanon exists today in the USA and is a viable treatment option that costs only a dollar.

These three defense mechanisms oftener than not, summarize the attitude of the alcoholic's wife, and she will not get better until she can acknowledge this simple fact. Some never do. Often she moves on and finds a new psychiatrist who will not force her to go to Alanon but who will put her on permanent disability so that she can stay at home and stew and fret over the alcoholic. She will have much self-pity and continue suffering the family disease of alcoholism. She will get the new doctor to prescribe prescription drugs which are not going to do anything—except possibly awaken her own latent alcoholic genes, if she happens to come from an alcoholic family (many women of alcoholic fathers marry alcoholic men). And then, she will always be having bad reactions to the drugs because the drugs can not cure untreated co-dependence! Not anymore than drugs can cure alcoholism. There are probably half a million women on permanent disability trying all sorts of psychiatric drugs and to no avail—this subjective sense of misery can go on for many years long after the alcoholic is gone. This is a great analogy to a medical-surgical condition: if treated at the right time and in the right way, it can put a patient on the road to recovery. If not, then the condition festers for years and begets new intractable symptoms, which are even harder to cure or treat. And, rarely do.

Remember the 3 *C*'s of Alanon: Helen did not *Cause* the alcoholism, Helen cannot *Control* it, and Helen cannot *Cure* it. (Helen cannot C*ontain* it, either—if you would like a fourth "C")

The family members who find Alanon will also find a kind of enlightenment in the objectivity of looking at their family situation. These are the lucky few who are willing to follow medical advice and not be so head-strong and defiant (which are—after all—alcoholic traits).

Alcoholism tends to cluster more in some families than in others. Thus, if you are in a family of alcoholics but not [yet] alcoholic, you should remember that you have the genetic risk, too. And people who tend to marry alcoholics tend to come from alcoholic families: the attraction seems undeniable. Among the blood relatives, there is the likelihood of common genetic loading. Indeed some potential Alanon members (from alcoholic families) skip the Alanon program entirely and go full steam into full-blown alcoholism after which they will try to get sober in AA and then stay sober in AA. If they can stay sober long enough, they may—or may not—identify Alanon issues in their lives that require attention, too. A small percentage of these recovered alcoholics will then avail themselves of the Alanon program and get "double sobriety" in both programs (called "double winners"). If they had just gone to Alanon first, then they could have avoided becoming alcoholics, thus retaining the privilege of being able to drink socially.

A number of our patients have or have had major relationships with alcoholics/addicts. This has left them and their behavioral responses permanently altered although our patients do not realize this because the behavioral changes build up gradually over years of living with a practicing alcoholic/addict. All too often these patients are still suffering from these perilous and scarring relationships years later and do not fathom it. They feel bad and unhappy and want pills and permanent disability (SSD). They do not wish to do the appropriate therapy which is to enroll in individual therapy with a therapist, group therapy with other emotionally handicapped patients, and group therapy in Alanon—the last of which they especially despise and resist. Here is a classic response: "I can't leave him at home alone for an hour while I go to an Alanon meeting—I don't know what he might do!"(this is a real quote) They want to take pills that will instantly ease all their bad memories. If there were such a pill then the governments would probably be adding it into the public water supply. These patients also want to sit at home all day on disability and wallow in self-pity, which are alcoholic behaviors and which the co-dependent often holds in common with the alcoholic. These co-dependent non-alcoholic spouses are acting like dry alcoholics; however, they cannot see this. The subtext of what the co-dependent patient is requesting is that she/he wants to take pills in the hopes that the alcoholic problem will go away. But it won't, and unfortunately it does not work like this. Whenever patients from alcoholic families are making these kinds of requests, we need to keep in mind that the codependent patient may share a lot of genetic material with the alcoholic-addicted family member(s). The *modus operandi* of the whole family is to resort to use of chemicals in times of crisis, which in an alcoholic family could be a perennial series of crises requiring constant mind and mood-altering substances in the form of Alcohol or of prescription medications. Often the co-dependent Helen might complain that Sean is "causing" her to "stress out". In reality, Sean can cause only what Helen will permit. Our perception of the whole world is in our minds. Re-orient your mind, re-orient your perceptions. An important lesson is that Sean must be truly powerful if he can control Helen's mind and "make" her "crazy".

If you really love an alcoholic-addict, then you must do these things:

1—detach with love: this means that you realize that you have control over only yourself and no one else; Remember the 3 C's of Alanon (Helen did not cause Sean's alcoholism, she can not control it, and can not cure it)

2—work on yourself: if you get straightened out in Alanon, then you can be of maximum help to the alcoholic (and yourself);

3—do not overact;

4—do not make yourself alcoholic or crazy!

5—Do not let the alcoholic make you crazy—or drive you to drink!

6—Make contingency plans for income, escalating violence, and lodgings.

Do it!!

▶*The alcoholic has his arms wrapped around the bottle,*

and you have your arms wrapped around the alcoholic!!

Essay on Dysfunctional Families*
R U the "Identified Patient" in your family?

Chapters VI-1 looked at alcoholism as a symptom of or disease marker in the dependent person. Chapter VI-2 applied some of these principles to the codependent. This chapter looks at alcoholism as a symptom or disease marker for the dysfunctional family, taken as if the family were just one unit or entity—like a corporation. The family is treated as if it were just one unit, an incorporate entity.

I am using this term "dysfunctional family" to refer to a group of people who feel connected by blood, marriage, or adoption—under adoption, I include godparents and very close friends who are viewed like cousins. There are several ways to focus on family dysfunction, but here I am going to confine my description of dysfunctional family to an "institution" that is set up to protect a family secret.

A dysfunctional family may have various outward appearances, but inwardly they are characterized by irrationality, non-systematized favoritisms, and clandestine maneuverings for power and money. Sounds like a corporation or bureaucracy, doesn't it? Other internal machinations include attempts to cover up family secrets, preventing the outside world and/or some family members from uncovering The Secret. Outward appearances correlate to corporate "images". Most dysfunctional families try very hard to look better than they are, and considerable psychological energy may be channeled into this endeavor.

If the dysfunctional family is large enough, each member may have a special role with a special title, much as corporations do.

The Secret

People have always had secrets. Families have always kept secrets. Governments have always kept secrets: good governments as well as bad ones. Secret-keeping may be necessary for the protection of the commonweal. Keeping secrets is like eating: a normal amount may be required for the survival of a family or society, but when the process becomes perverted, convoluted, excessive, arbitrary, and irrational, then secret-keeping becomes a psychiatric pathology. When the secret becomes a tangled web of deceit that materially harms societies or emotionally cripples family members for life, then the secret-keeping begets malignant consequences. Emotionally crippled family members often function way below their potential, and in doing so produce two more problems for society. The cripples end up being dependents on society rather than strengthening it, and they often produce the next generation of dysfunctional emotional cripples.

These malignant family systems typically cause psychic ruptures that appear in the form of psychological tumult, which must be minimized lest some persistently curious outsider try to ferret out The Secret. The barometer of the level of dysfunction is usually evidenced through behaviors of a so-called "identified patient"(IP) which is an inherent part of the dysfunctional institutionalization. The identified patient is the family member who is most distressed by the family dysfunction, whether this person knows The Secret or not—he/she usually knows of it or of its likely existence, but usually not of its depth or all its sordid details. The bellwether of the dysfunctional family is likely to be the "coordinator" or the "peacekeeper".

At the core of the dysfunction usually lies the family secret. The Secret entails shame. The Secret may be alcoholism, incest, sexual abuse, or some other immoral or illegal activity. The Secret must be protected and hidden at all times because revealing it could lead to problems. Examples of such problems are:

- disintegration of the family: the whole family is set up in order to protect The Secret, and if something happens to The Secret, then the family will be stripped of its mission: think of this family as an erratic and self-serving dictatorship in some small country that does not want to be toppled;

- legal and financial ruin: revealing The Secret can result in catastrophic turns of events from the legal and socio-economic viewpoints; if father is sent to prison for sexual abuse, the family is left without a source of income

- social ostracism: the Family loses whatever community standing it had

- psychological chaos: the psychiatric results for most of the family members are also burdensome, and many of them may end up on SSD instead of as productive members of society.

The purpose of the dysfunction is none: there is no inherent advantage to keeping The Secret, but families will do so doggedly, until confrontation outs it. The behavior that begets and feeds The Secret is invariably rooted in some offensive malignant compulsive behavior, e.g. sexual predation. The nature of The Secret is oftenest that of a taboo perhaps of a sexual theme: incest, for example. The cause, therefore, of The Secret is rooted in human frailties: lust, cupidity, gluttony, avarice, power-mongering, and so on.

Alcoholism is often the most noticeable symptom of the dysfunction. Alcoholism is the visible symptom (sign) of keeping The Secret, and not the true cause, as is often thought. However, alcoholism enables the perpetuation of The Secret because alcohol blurs memories, suppresses the barriers of morality, and lowers inhibitions about acting impulsively and compulsively. In many cases, active alcoholism is one of The Secrets. The dysfunctional alcoholic family—like the dysfunctional alcoholic individual—often believes that no one knows the secret, when in fact it is probably known by others, such as employers, in-laws, and the neighbors.

Origins

The origins of family dysfunction are lost in the mists of prehistory. Dysfunction is so prevalent worldwide that it almost seems to be institutionalized. No family is perfect and all have some degree of dysfunction, some more, some less. Families with minimal dysfunction have typical roles for each parent, child, and family member. Every [significantly dysfunctional] family has different roles, which need special descriptors, such as scapegoat, peacemaker, *Benjamin* (identifiable "favorite" child), "identified patient" (IP) and so on.

Characteristics

General observations about dysfunctional families:
- the dysfunction (or the proclivity for dysfunction) is most typically passed down trans-generationally (from one generation to the next);
- the identified patient is merely born into this situation and has little hope of changing the rules, unless he is a superhuman like Alexander the Great, who nonetheless had a well-documented and extremely dysfunctional family which he could not change either, so he went to live on a different continent;
- the identified patient has as much hope at changing the rules as you might have if you tried to change the rules of baseball—moving to a different continent would provide breathing space but no real solace or better treatment outcome: after all, the USA is at the vanguard in assessing and offering treatments for identified patients;
- in most cases the identified patient does not even know what a dysfunctional family behavior is since it is all that he has ever known—there has been no basis for comparison in his life;
- in functional families, there is a well-established hierarchy of roles and well-known rules of engagement. For example, the father might be the titular head of the family—although the mother may be the neck that turns the head ("My Big Fat Greek Wedding"). The children (and any other indwellers) usually have assigned and stationary places in the hierarchy—often even the family dog has a permanently assigned position in the family! Stability of the roles in the hierarchy allows family members to focus on other matters as performed from a platform of stability;
- dysfunctional families are often fragmented (not whole or complete): there may be different factions vying for power;

- since dysfunctional families are fragmented, outsiders are often involved as mediators or in other ways: family services, best friends, drinking buddies, pastors, unofficial "emergency" babysitters (mother made another suicide gesture in response to learning of her alcoholic husband's new girlfriend), and so on;

- rules of engagement must be learned and relearned because the rules may change from day to day;

- the identified patient (IP) is almost always marred for life; it is only in recent decades that Americans have devised Twelve Step programs to help people suffering from these problems;

- "Normal" people [those from functional families] who marry into a dysfunctional family may initially resist being role-cast, but almost inevitably will little by little be slowly drawn into the psychodramatic maelstrom and can be completely engulfed in it, also; however, people who marry into dysfunctional families probably have a predisposition for this kind of role-playing (that is, they are not totally normal), even if they marry the most nearly normal-seeming family member, usually the peacekeeper or coordinator;

- for the identified patient, recovery is possible, cure is unattainable, and damage is lifelong;

- the combined forces of the behaviors of the dysfunctional family and the Family Secret may coincide to make the identified patient mentally ill—in extreme cases, this can result in extreme mood disorders, suicide attempts, and possibly turning to alcohol for relief;

- the dysfunction can come to an abrupt and violent endpoint as in those cases we see on TV when someone (the IP perhaps) goes berserk and shoots his whole family—this could be described as a terminal Alanon event.

- The Secret usually begets smaller spin-off secrets—and all of these secrets need to be assigned dispositions as to who will cover them up and so on;

- There is no happy ending for these families—ever: no matter whether The Secret is ever outed or not.

- The family dysfunction will pass down to the next generation—regardless of whether The Secret has been outed or not.

- The dysfunctional behaviors (role-playing, assigning dysfunctional roles involuntarily, and keeping of lesser secrets) can pass down to the next generation without any alcoholism or sexual abuse.

Personal Symptoms

If you are born into the family and have known nothing else in your life, your point of reference is skewed. Direct observation, increased objectivism, or self-analysis may point you in the direction of the psychology section in the library or bookstore. Even likelier, you may end up in therapy when you are still young. Obvious clues originate from your own internal feelings and symptoms. If you are symptomatic, then try to identify the symptoms before taking an overdose, driving drunk, or being unacceptably promiscuous. Your family may be dysfunctional under these circumstances:

- If you are often aggrieved, depressed, or angered by the behaviors that you receive at the hands of your family members;

- If the sources and causes of these feelings of anger, depression, and aggrievement are clearly out of proportion to those in seemingly functional families;

- If you feel that *something* is not right in your life but are unsure what it is;

- If you have trouble forming romantic relationships;

- If you have trouble keeping relationships;

- If you have unexplained failures at life, such as poor grades (despite being smart) or frequent job turnover;

- If there is domestic violence in your family (whether you are the victim or perpetrator or not);

- If there are secrets in your family which outsiders must never know; (such as: Uncle Ben really died of "AIDS not of "cancer", father slept with youngest sister, mother is/was a "closet" alcoholic);

- If there are irrationally assigned taboos: no talking about Greta's high school field trip: this may not be a secret in or out of the family, but it is never discussed among certain persons in the family: there may be an arbitrary assignment of who may speak to whom about which taboo subjects and under what circumstances;

- If you have multiple visits to mental health professionals over the space of many years;

- If you feel overly sensitive or sensitized to family matters;

- If you feel that you were born in the wrong place at the wrong time; and,

- If they are not dysfunctional, then it certainly is likely that you are; if you answered "yes" to some of these questions, maybe you should do some on-line searches and think about making an appointment to see a counselor.

Role-playing

The identified patient (IP) is the one that is singled out by the family as the gadfly or "whipping boy"; the IP is that one who evidences a lot of "expressed emotionality". The dysfunctional family distracts attention from The Secret by refocusing outsiders on only one individual and his behaviors. The identified patient may be the easiest "mark" or may be adjudged to be the one person likeliest to divulge The Secret to outsiders. The identified patient has serious psychological repercussions caused directly or indirectly by The Secret—whether he **knows the whole secret, parts of it, or *nothing* of it**. Direct emotional repercussions are experienced if the identified patient is the abused or the victim. Indirect emotional repercussions appertain to the fact that the IP perceives that her/his sibling(s) who are being abused, are receiving more preferential treatment or "intimate favoritism" from the perpetrator/abuser and paradoxically yearns to be closer to the perpetrator without realizing the extra consequences involved. In this case, the IP is unaware that the favoritism is doled out in exchange for "services rendered". The process of "inferiorizing" the IP may be nothing more than the fact that the IP is of the wrong age or gender to be eligible for the "perpetrative favoritism". In indirect repercussions where the identified patient is not actively aware of the abuse, he/she may perceive that the abused siblings are receiving special treatment not accorded to the IP. This special treatment may also be given secretly so that the identified patient will not know about the special treatment at all. This prevents the IP from requesting the same special treatment for himself also, while not patently aware of the tasks for which the reward is given. This secret reward becomes an offshoot of The Secret. This is how many minor secrets arise and flow from The Secret.

The expressed emotionality of the **identified patient** is his reaction to being singled out as the least preferred family member. Whether the IP does or does not know why he is singled out is ultimately not important. The expressed emotionality of the IP serves one positive purpose because his emotionality distracts attention from The Secret; however, his distress is negative in that it attracts attention from outsiders. This could result in outsiders (County Family Services or Child Portective Services) delving around and possibly unearthing The Secret. The emotional shenanigans of the identified patient do create a risk that The Secret will be outed. The temporary solution may involve consciously seeking temporary ineffective treatment for the IP—perhaps find a child psychiatrist to diagnoses and treat the IP as ADHD. This maneuver can provide a lot of distraction and—best of all—it probably will not help the IP so much, but it may cure any secondary depressive symptoms that he has from all the family stress. But of course, the focus is still back on the IP. Now he has a "psychiatric disorder" that has no known cause. (Thus, it could not posibly be due to The Secret; hence, there is no secret for the County to delve around trying to find. Then, hopefully, county services will close the case—provided that it ever had come to their attention).

This creates stress for the **Coordinator** of the family who may or may not know the full extent of The Secret—he may be nothing more than the fall guy (patsy, shill), such as Halderman or Oliver North. Nonetheless, it is his job to try to keep the family relations stable without any alterations in this scripted psychodrama.

The **Keeper of The Secret** will obviously be under a lot of stress also, as if running down the field with the football. If The Secret is outed, then the Keeper will feel that she has failed her mission and will fall into an abject clinical depression. She will also be depressed by the aftermath of the outing of The Secret (see below).

The **Peacekeeper** who is always the central-most figure has to get busy trying to calm down the ruffled feathers of the identified patient who is the primary problem; then the peacekeeper has to unruffle the feathers of all the family members who have been secondarily upset by the identified patient's shenanigans. When the status quo is recast, then the peacekeeper can rest for a while until the next outburst.

In smaller families, the family coordinator and the Keeper of The Secret may be the same person. In some families, the identified patient may also usually be the scapegoat.

The **scapegoat** is the person who is indirectly—and often irrationally—accused of initiating or perpetuating the malignancy of The Secret.

Example: The identified patient could be the middle sister who is acting out because the youngest sister is being given more preferential treatment (because she is being "impositioned" by father [the perpetrator]). Eldest sister might be the peacekeeper, mother may be the main Keeper of The Secdret, younger brother may be the mascot and Eldest brother is made out to be a perpetrator or the primary perpetrator. It is better eldest brother be "publicly sacrificed" (incarcerated) so that the family will not be subjected to the catastrophic outcomes that would ensue were The Secret actually revealed, that father is the perpetrator (see below). The identified patient needs to be branded as "psycho" so that any of her allegations or guesses about the nature of The Secret will not be taken seriously by the authorities. If the family has enough money, it is wise to send the identified patient to some other State to live with a family member or better yet, sent to a very distant boarding school—hopefully on a different continent. The family might also decide to move to a different city or state.

Le Benjamin (la benjamine) means *"the favorite child (the youngest child)"*, (New Cassell's French dictionary). The Benjamin has this role for life—unless he/she does something very outré, which is very unlikely because the benjamin has a most honored role and would be foolish to relinquish it. The bestowing of this accolade may seem arbitrary because it often is.

The **Cleaner** may be the person who removes the daughter's panties or provides lubricant for penetration of boys and girls; launders the bed sheets after the victimization; provides an alibi for the perpetrator as needed.

The **Enabler** arranges the stage setting and facilitates the circumstances under which the victimization will take place: the Enabler may take the other family members out of the house while leaving the victim at home alone with the perpetrator—this could be in the form of shopping trips, baseball games, and so on.

Functional families produce a stage play that usually plays according to certain traditional norms.

Dysfunctional families produce an extravaganza that is truly a psychodrama in every sense of the word. Dysfunctional families have specific roles assigned to each family member. These are not the expected roles. In the following table, you can see the traditional roles in a functional family. Obviously, in smaller families, one family member may "wear several hats". Oftentimes, there may be only several roles and not all the dizzying array that I have presented herein below. The dysfunctional family has many roles, some of which are descriptive; the list can be extended, too.

(This is my own terminology)

Table VI-3-a Functional vs. Dysfunctional Families

Functional Family

Ground Rules are Known
Father
Mother
Eldest brother
Eldest sister
Brothers, ranked by age
Sisters, ranked by age
Grandparent(s)
Other kin
Family dog

Dysfunctional Family

Roles in Dysfunctional family	Person typically Fulfilling this role	Description of This "Job title"	Examples in Governmental Analogy
Dependent	Alcoholic	Molester	Dictator
Codependent	Enabler of alcoholic	Spouse	Vice-president
Perpetrator	Father, uncle, Grandfather	Molester	General of the Armies
Peacekeeper	Sibling	Placates everyone	Minister
Coordinator	Mother		Chief of Staff
Keeper of The Secret	Various		CIA
Mascot	Youngest sibling or member who is infantilized		Minor Celebrity (the "Vedette")
Le Benjamin	Favorite child, often The youngest child	Has this role for life	A royal; or "most favored nation"
Identified patient IP	One usually: Emotional sister Angry brother	Unjustly accused	Sam Shepard
Martyr	Mother		Minority Leader?
Scapegoat	Varies	He who loses at "musical chairs"	the Fall Guy
Enabler	Facilitates keeping The Secret at any cost		Political appointees
Other assorted relatives living in the home			Heads of lesser agencies
Other assorted relatives "staying" in the house			Populace
Non-family staying in the house: friends, lovers, perpetrators, and sundry abusers			Government Functionaries

Outsiders exerting Influence over the internal dysfunction			Allies and Foreign Embassies
the Wielders	The Inner Circle		The Cabinet
Outside agencies	Police, County, School officials		
the Excluders	The enforcement arm of the Inner Circle	Keep the Identified Patient off kilter but under their thumb	IRS, FBI who treat the IP as a "person of interest"
the Patsy the Shill	Take the rap for one-time offenses of the perpetrator		Halderman Oliver North
the Cleaner	Does the dirty work for the perpetrator and cleans up the aftermath		Garbage men
Bellwether	Official family spokesman		Spokesman
Black sheep	A distant satellite who is not really in the loop (which may not be such a bad role)	Is considered to be more than one standard deviation from the family's "norm" (whatever that is)	Ex-patriot
Maternalized eldest sister			Aide de Camp
In locō patris (person acting as the father)	mother's abusive boyfriend, live-in grandfather, uncle, eldest son, mother, angry step-father...	Empowered as Perceived authority Figure, possibly worse than the Perpetrator	Bureaucrats
Provocateur Provocateuse	An in-law who is insidiously drawn in		Immigrant
family dog	If there is one, it's uncontrolled and untrained		

After the identified patient moves out of the household, the excluders will continue to treat him in a very erratic way, at times seemingly amicably, at times, peevishly; and, at times they will break off communication for indefinite periods of time for unknown—or at least unstated—reasons. At this point, the IP may also end up being the Black Sheep, unless that role is already filled. This is part of the power-mongering. If the identified patient says or does something that might seem threatening, then he will be punished by temporary, partial, or limited excommunication. Unfortunately, the identified patient does not even know what innocent little remark that he might have said to warrant such erratic treatment. He is not likely to find out since dysfunctional families avoid open confrontation for fear that escalating anger will result in someone's inadvertently or expletively referring to The Secret. The temporary excommunication is sent out by the excluders to remind him that any worse transgressions on his part will be treated in an even more draconian manner (effective excommunication for years, perhaps?) Temporary exclusion is like a warning citation.

Perhaps the identified patient should not even care if the excluders exclude him permanently, but he does. This is a refrain at Alanon meetings. Unfortunately, most identified patients wallow along in the psychological mire for years. This is due to three reasons: they are sensitive people, they are often co-dependent, and this is the culture in which they grew up: to eschew it is to repudiate the first eighteen years of one's life and all those memories, good along with bad. They may go for counseling and discuss "auto-divorce" with the counselor, but the act itself can be scary: "sometimes something is better than nothing". In reality, the coordinator or peacekeeper will intervene and try to mollify the identified patient, since the abrupt act of "auto-divorce" would once again shine a bright spotlight on the family. Outsiders would want to know why the family excommunicated the identified patient or what had prompted him to take such a drastic action as to "auto-divorce" himself from the family. So, the identified patient is once again reeled in and left flopping around on the deck for a while, until impelled on to the next scene in this seemingly endless psychodrama.

One common technique used in the USA is that of moving to another part of the country, under the guise of graduate school or job opportunity. This can sometimes be a hallmark of dysfunctionality. A "visible sign" is what outsiders see. An "inapparent sign" is what insiders see. "Symptoms" explain the reasons for the behaviors.

Table VI-3-b   Markers for Dysfunctional Families

Visible signs and markers Seen by outsiders	Inapparent signs Seen by insiders	Symptoms (causes & explanations)
Frequent ER visits	Emotional abuse	Overdoses
Frequent visits by Police or county agents	Unexplained injuries	Drunkenness
Family moving to new City (too many people "snooping around")	Identified patient puts restrictions on personal contact with family (two hours per month)	The Secret is in danger of being outed
Identified patient moves far away	"Caller ID" on phone blocks callers	Attempting a "geographic cure"
Frequent bruises, cuts, Quarrels	Premature deaths	Moral & spiritual "bankruptcy"
Parking cars on front lawn	Passive-aggression	Anger, Alcohol
Loud music late at night	Defiance	Anger
Teenage pregnancy	Incest or not	Life Ambivalence
Fewer Grandchildren than Children	Prolonged role-playing (Benjamin for life)	Self-indulgence
Failing school grades	Poor concentration	Distractions
Involuntary incarceration	"Voluntary incarceration" (joining the army on the day after high school graduation)	Utter Desperation

Practically speaking, a person brought up in this dysfunction has adapted to it and will be repetitively drawn to it over and over again. "Auto-divorce" would result in the levying of extreme guilt—or of other manipulations such as production of shame, embarrassment, duress, or coercion. The status quo of the family dynamics must be maintained at a set level, a level set by the majority of the Excluders.

Table VI-3-c   Subtle Differences between the Scapegoat and the Identified Patient

	his suffering is	outsiders see suffering as
Scapegoat	<u>Objective</u> *(kicked out of the main house for being egoistic, harsh, rough , confrontational, or too" randy")* **"Your sisters are no longer safe around you! Get an apartment"**	<u>Subjective</u> *(angry drunk) "I'm as mad as Hell! I don't need you— or anybody!"* **"He's always had tantrums and bad behaviors—he'll never change for the better!"**
Identified Patient	<u>Subjective</u> *(expressed emotionality with Weakness of spirit and of convictions due to low self-esteem)***"Just pull yourself together so you can protect your sisters…Stop being so useless—get a job"**	<u>Objective</u> *(maudlin drunk) "Poor me! Why would anybody Love me, want me, or need me!"* **'He's always been whiney, he cried all the time when he was a baby. He'll never make it on his own—he's lucky to have us!"**

Explanation:

The scapegoat:

Assume that he is blamed unjustly in relation to The Secret. The family may issue innuendoes suggesting that he has been kicked out of the main house and forced to sleep in the pool house "just in case to keep his sisters 'safe'", when in truth he is not the perpetrator. Instead of dealing with this in a mature and functional manner, he acts out angrily and goes out drinking. That is his objective suffering. Outsiders see that he got drunk and maudlin and perceive that his suffering is coming from within him when in reality it is visited upon him by external agents (the Keeper of the Secret et al.). A less immature scapegoat would try to auto-divorce the family and move far away and try to go on with his life without them. He drinks because of displaced anger that he will not confront. He may or may not know about The Secret. He may have even been initiated by the perpetrator at some time in the past—either as a sexual victim or as an involuntary accomplice under the "tutelage" of the perpetrator. (How much would a ten year old boy really know about sexual mores—especially if he had only known amoral or immoral conduct since birth? And might have been plied with liquor or marijuana?) All men [at least, heterosexual] who have been childhood sexual victims are very emotionally distraught and are permanently damaged psychically. (I have heard a few gay men in this situation who shared that they did not find this act abjectly denigrating—but they are the exceptions.)

The Identified Patient:

He has inner pain because he knows or senses that something is not right. If he turns to the bottle for solace, it is to self-treat his symptoms (subjective component). When the family sends him to a 28-day Rehab, the outsiders perceive his pain objectively, as if some external treatment would cure his internal spiritual problem. He drinks because of spiritual digression, weakness, and fear of confronting the real issue—but not necessarily because of The Secret. He senses The Secret but may not know all about it.

Repercussions

Socioeconomic and Legal Repercussions caused by Revealing The Secret
Assume that the father is having incest with one daughter. Nowadays the penalty for that disclosure will result in the following repercussions:

- disruption and disintegration of the family;
- divorce;
- social castigation and banishment from the family;
- incarceration of the father,
- after which he will be forever on the list of sexual predators;
- the children may end up with a stepfather who is also a sexual perpetrator since dysfunctional women usually gravitate to the same kind of men;
- high costs of hiring a criminal lawyer for father;
- possible distress sale of the house and move to a poorer living situation (motel even);
- other associated costs

Psychiatric Repercussions and Consequences of Revealing The Secret

Many of the family members will probably end up seeking mental health treatment. The most severely afflicted (in order of severity from first on down) are:

1   the abused victim
2   the identified patient
3   the scapegoat
4   the martyr
5   the Keeper of The Secret
6   the Enabler

The psychodrama is now over…or is it?

More on Family Secrets

The family secrets are of two **types** and two **extents**: there are personal secrets and shared secrets; there are some secrets that are known to outsiders that are not known to insiders and some that are known to insiders and not outsiders. The mechanics of how these are established is usually beyond the control of the dysfunctional family, although they usually maintain the fixed false belief that they can control this; in reality, the locus of control is outside the family.

Table VI-3-d   Examples of Secrets

Types of secrets→ _____ Extents of secrets ↓	Internal secrets known only to family insider(s)	External secrets known to one or more outsiders
Solo and personal known only to the Secret-keeper	Kate had anonymous sex on spring break and later had an abortion using a pseudonym	Kate had a "three-way" on vacation
Shared between or among a subset of family insiders two or more	Kate's sister, Jo, had driven Kate to the abortion clinic	One of the two was the Mayor's son who had date-raped Jo the year before

Regardless of who is the abuser or perpetrator, there are certain factors which can represent the paternal contribution of the dysfunction:

- if he is alcoholic, then the alcoholism sets up a vicious cycle that keeps him seething;

- illegitimacy issues (" I think my sons look like my best friend and not like me");
- resentments.

Whereas these may be maternal contributions to the dysfunction:
- not blood relative;
- certain extreme behaviors of the offspring (in traditional families, the father's love is often considered "conditional", but that of the mother, "unconditional" whereas all bets are off in dysfunctional families);
- irrational decisions "just because…"

Socioeconomic and Legal Repercussions due to Revelation of The Secret

Despite best intentions, some outsider(s) may discern the nature of The Secret or may discover the actual Secret itself. This can disrupt the whole shaky scaffold that supports The Secret. These disruptions may out The Secret and end the whole elaborate protection system. Apart from outing The Secret, there are actions by certain family members that can jeopardize the integrity of The Secret without actually outing it. These persons are serious disruptors of the family dynamics and this is how they could jeopardize The Secret:

- if one family member voluntarily leaves the mêlée temporarily (prolonged residence overseas, "elective auto-divorce", or "parentectomy")
- if one family member involuntary leaves (incarceration or prolonged residence abroad)
- if one person leaves permanently (coma, death, etc.)
- if a new person (in-law) joins the family—that person needs assignment of a new role
- if the identified patient does something to attract a lot of kudos
- if the identified patient becomes notorious, infamous, or publicly sanctioned (in a very negative way)
- if any family members unexpectedly become alcoholics who in weakened moments may threaten to reveal The Secret
- then any of these events will cause a power shift that might jeopardize the keeping of The Secret.

For example, naturally sensitive may people turn to alcohol. Naturally oversensitive or emotional people may turn to alcohol. Naturally normal people subjected to severe family dysfunction may end up becoming alcoholics due to the whole process: they end up more sensitive. Innate alcoholics are very sensitive, also. alcoholism is normal in dysfunctional families, and usually the amount of alcoholism correlates directly to the number and severity of family secrets. Alcoholism is just a symptom of family dysfunction. Although the occurrence of alcoholism in any family can depend upon nurture (upbringing) and upon nature (genetics and birth status), the frequency of alcoholism is higher in dysfunctional families for a variety of reasons.(I am using "birth status" to refer to any physical problems at the time of birth [was the baby a breach birth or was the baby's head pulled out of the womb by a strong arm and forceps] and the rank in the family [eldest, middle, youngest child]). The severity of alcoholism is also more severe in dysfunctional families. For example, a reasonably normal family might have one heavy drinker who rarely gets out of control. the dysfunctiona family might have three alcoholic members who drink every day but do not usually have legal problems as well as two severe alcoholics who are always having legal and financial problems.

Table VI-3-e   Nature and Nurture compared by type Family

Nurture → (Upbringing)___ Nature↓ (birth status) (genetics)	Reared in functional Family	Risk of Alcohol Abuse	Reared in dysfunctional family	Alcoholism occurrence
1-Normal	Normal	very rare	Emotionalized/normal	rare
2-Sensitive	Sensitive/normal	rare	Emotionally crippled	possible
3-Oversensitive	Sensitive/oversensitive	unlikely	Emotionally crippled	likely
4-Alcoholic	Alcoholic	Likely	Alcoholic	certain
5-Psychiatric	"Stable" Psychotic	possible	Unstable Psychotic	probable

Explanation of Table VI-3-e:

1-) I am using "emotionalized" to refer to the fact that this child has been caused to become emotional on the basis of nurture alone. He had had no genetic susceptibility. You can see that if he had been brought up in a functional family, then he would have not even become alcoholic; the apparently stressful environment of the dysfunctional family has pushed himover the edge.

2-) Sensitive children are often described as "artistic" or intuitive. These children reared in a functional family may become accomplished artists, photographers, sculptors, humanities professors, directors, and so on. Those same children reared in a dysfunctional family end up on permanent disability.

3-) Oversensitive children are prone to having non-psychotic psychological problems, especially neurosis.

4-) Some people are born with extremely high chances of becoming alcoholic, on a mainly genetic basis: there are a lot of alcoholics on both sides of the family; the child fell in love with alcohol instantly the first time he tasted it (which often happens while he is still a small child). This is a regular genetic occurrence in dysfunctional families and would be considered probable and predictable. Genetic alcoholism in functional familes is less likely and would be considered "sporadic" (random) alcoholism, and probably has a later age of onset and overall follows a milder course.

5-) Persistent and severe psychiatric illness (PSPI), such as psychosis. PSPI is unrelated to any alcoholic tendencies—these patients turn to alcohol as a way of trying to dull the extreme agitation caused by the crushing frenzy of their wildly racing thoughts related to psychosis. Unfortunately, this form of self-treatment always ends badly for the patient. Statistical surveys suggest that well over half of these PSPI cases abuse alcohol (and/or drugs). Some of them may end up as alcoholics, too.

In all the above cases, children brought up in dysfunctional families are likelier to have more significant mental health problems as well as a higher risk of alcoholism.

PSPI brought up in dysfunctional families will lack any concept for normalcy and have no understanding of consistency. They may be so emotionalized, oversensitive, or neurotic that they can not even conceptualize what PSPI is, and so they have no insight into their problems. Without insight, they will deny that they have any problem. Thus, they refuse to take antipsychotics and become "non-adherent" with the prescribed drug regimen. They will have been forced to conform according to their dysfunctional family's fixed false belief system. Fixed false belief is the definition for delusion. Thus the PSPI child has been subjected to a social delusional system. On top of that, the PSPI child will also suffer from psychotic delusions that are related to his inborn psychotic illness and are a different type of delusion (psychiatric delusion). Hence, he will have a miasma of "social delusions" and psychotic delusions swirling about in his head, driving him mad.

Psychotic children reared in a functional family have a better chance of wanting to be adjusted to normal society and of having a reference point for how to achieve this and what is feels like. These are more likely to take their medications as prescribed ("adherence"), and to understand the reasons that they have psychotic symptoms (cognition without "projection") and to be able to express their opinion that they really have psychosis (lack of "denial"). They are more likely to seek treatment if they think that their psychosis is getting worse ("insight").

Child abuse is a serious felony because it ruins the life of the victim forever, causing her/him to be an emotional invalid for the rest of his/her life. As an analogy to child abuse, the system of castigating the identified patient is as equally devastating. The identified patient is tossed into an emotional Duat (hell) from which the only escape is auto-divorce of the family, death, or resolution by mutually engaged family therapy—the likelihood of having all the dysfunctional family show up voluntarily for a prescribed course of family therapy is very very very low. Perhaps in the future our legal system could develop a system whereby an identified patient could be given the option of leaving the dysfunctional family at any age and by his request at any age. This would be a modified and limited system of emancipation for minors under the age of sixteen.

Families, like other groups, play favorites. If a family has an unfavored child which they see as too sensitive (from their perspective), that child should be allowed the choice to live with another family. Blaming the child is absurd, since the child was born—through no fault of his own—into a family where he is destined to be out of step: for example a clumsy child born into a family of athletes, a neurotic child born into a family of extroverted politicians, or a gifted child born into a family that ridicules "eggheads". If the IP child and dysfunctional family are so out-of-step, then is it not better for the child to grow up with his own kind?

Treatment

"I'm tired of playing the role of Mordred!"

The first step is to admit that there is a problem.

Everyone who is symptomatic from being in the dysfunctional family may avail himself of treatments available today. The main treatments are individual therapy, group therapy, and a Twelve Step Program such as Alanon or Adult Children of Alcoholics. Medications may be helpful also, but are not necessary for recovery.

If you choose not to follow any of these suggestions, then the minimum that you need to do is to make amends to those who feel wronged by you. Or whom you feel that you have wronged. This is called cleaning off your side of the street. If you have done this, then this act should bring you some comfort, closure, and resolution. Whether you choose to cross that street again or jaywalk is a decision that you can make later. Maybe the other side of the street is further than it seems.

Sometimes the identified patient is galled that he needs to make amends to people who have equally wronged them. Remember that they are sick too—the IP and the whole family is symptomatic. The whole family as one unit is psychosocially ill. They are likely to remain sick because only a tiny percentage of dysfunctional family members ever make it in to recovery—most die with—or from—this illness. Maybe you should start going to a recovery program and hang around with people in recovery instead of dysfunctional family members whose behaviors are still on toxic auto-drive.

Additionally, high emotional stress can cause overeating, high blood pressure, and then heart attacks as well as other stress-related disorders that can hasten a person's premature demise. Recovery brings freedom. Live free before you die! Make a flight into health!

▶QUESTIONS

Q: Why so much energy poured into keeping The Secret?
A: the Family wants to keep The Secret as a secret because in many cases, the penalties for disclosure are severe and harsh and may result in litigation, incarceration, or even death. The whole family may be disrupted or destroyed: this is very traumatic for all the family members. They will all become as miserable as the IP and the whole family might end up disabled. The Secret is usually the main secret, but it also produces spin-off secrets, which must be protected, too.

Q: What is an identified patient (IP)?
A: It is the one family member that is oftenest blamed for almost everything (in really enormous families, there may be more than one identified patient, but even if there are, each one of them will have different roles or titles assigned, such as "identified patient who causes mother the most anguish" or "identified patient who is usually well-liked except when drinking". But typically, there is only one IP; the other candidates may adopt the roles of scapegoat and black sheep.

Q: Why do families have an "identified patient"?
A: Not all families do have an identified patient—this role appears only in significantly dysfunctional families.

Q: What is the purpose of the identified patient?
A: The identified patient serves as the repository for all the residual dysfunction. All dysfunctional families generate a lot of "psychic" waste, and this "waste" has to be

disposed of in some way so as to leave the favored children unscathed and firmly ensconced in their [artificially] assigned positive roles of beneficence. "Functional" families deal with the psychic waste in the following ways:

1   the person responsible for the disturbance is penalized for bad behaviors and not rewarded—in dysfunctional families, punishment may be given out to those least responsible in order to spare favored children or the actual guilty perpetrator or child;

2   punishment equals the gravity of the offense; in dysfunctional families, this is not true;

3   justice is meted out evenly;

4   gifts and assets are distributed per capita to avoid gross unfairness and so that each child receives an approximately equal share of beneficence.

Q: How will I know if I am the identified patient?
A: Is your role in the family abbreviated, altered, trivialized, attenuated, or minimized as much as possible? If so, then you are probably the identified patient in your family—or may soon be, if you step over the "invisible line" (excessive or inappropriate talking or asking about family taboos or closely held family secrets).

Q: Why doesn't the identified patient simply change the family?
A: The Weight of History and Genetics makes this option virtually impossible unless the family only has a couple members. Remember that the identified patient was born into this situation and was forced to conform to it. He is as much a victim as anyone else. the dysfunctional family refuses to change because it is like toppling a government: everyone will be scrambling for new roles while in the meantime the County workers may get involved if there is even a hint of child abuse.

Q: What is the purpose of all these strange-sounding dysfunctional roles?
A: The purpose is nothing more than to try to protect The Family Secret. It seems like such a huge production!

Q: So why should the identified patient even care if the excluders exclude him permanently?
A: Maybe he should not! This might be his chance to "auto-divorce" the family and make a "flight into health". (In Alanon, this is called "detaching with love"). If he did that, he would be at the first step in recovery. Unfortunately, most identified patients wallow along in the psychological mire for years. They may go for counseling and discuss "auto-divorce" with the counselor, but the act itself can be scary: "sometimes something is

better than nothing". In reality, the coordinator or peacekeeper will intervene and try to mollify the identified patient, since the abrupt act of "auto-divorce" would once again shine a bright spotlight on the family. Outsiders would want to know why the family excommunicated him or what had prompted him to take such a drastic action. So, the identified patient is once again reeled in again and left flopping around on the deck for a while until the next scene in this seeming endless psychodrama.

Q: How does this look and happen in real life?

A: Identified patients receive mixed messages, as well as confusing, arbitrary, and conflicting ground rules. These rules can change arbitrarily from day to day without any apparent explanation. The child becomes overly sensitized, stressed, confused, and then depressed (see chapters on depression). After all this, the identified patient is further castigated as if he were the runt of the litter or the omega-dog. Depressed people use up all their brain hormones trying to run their internal bodily systems and have no energy left for reacting to environmental stimuli (such as concentrating on homework or pleasurable pastimes). They become the human equivalent of the "rescue" dog whose reaction to all situations is to scrunch over with its tail between its legs. How can the identified patient ever be successful as an adult?! Those who might appear to be successful, are still performing well below their potential. Maybe the IP can squeak through law school or a professional school with marginal standards, but he could have achieved much more and at higher levels having come from a functional family.

The identified patient's viewpoint is trivialized as being overly subjective and "anti-majoritarian" (at odds with the "majority" opinion, and hence invalid). The Excluders rush to invalidate any of the identified patient's feelings. His/her feelings are treated as heresy since he/she is at odds with the fixed false belief system promulgated by the family propaganda machine—remember that the dysfunctional family has internal policies and politics and an external "image" to maintain. Just like a dictatorship!

Q: What is the main cause of the family dysfunction?

A: It has several causes:

1   primarily it is set up and to keep secrets, of which there are many types and these are never discussed—whereas, functional families tend to deal with these issues in a candid and open matter and avoid filing away unresolved secrets: after this process, the issue may lie dormant in the functional family, but at least the issue has been discussed to the mutual satisfaction of family members (hopefully);

2   a family which has certain taboo subjects may be dysfunctional, if the taboo is not rationally based;

3   also it is caused by lack of communication;

4   and also caused by tangential communication;

Q: How does the identified patient survive in the dysfunctional family?

A: He has two choices. He can say and do whatever the Excluders and Wielders want. Or he can socio-emotionally distance himself completely from the dysfunctional family, with or without a "geographic cure" (moving far away).

Q: Does the identified patient have any other common names?

A: This is the most technically precise term; similar terms in the common language might be "scapegoat" of the family, or perhaps "black sheep".

We all have different relationships with different people. The relationship between A and B is unique and so is that of B and C; A & C do not have a hybrid relationship of 50% AB and 50% BC. The AC relationship is unique in its own way.

Q: Is there relief for the identified patient who is still suffering?

A: Yes. Start attending a recovery program (such as Alanon). This is the most effective treatment. Individual psychotherapy is also helpful. Medications might be needed.

Q: so when does this all end? With the death of the perpetrator?

A: It never ends. It is trans-generational, which means that its characteristics are passed down from one generation to the next—perhaps latently (lying in silence) or patently (obvious to everyone).

Q: How will I know if I am dysfunctional?

A: Do you feel like Cinderella? Oedipus? Hercules? Mordred?

Q: How many dysfunctional families are there in the USA?

A: That depends upon the definition of dysfunction and upon whether one plans to include secret-keeping dysfunctional families or all dysfunctional families.

Q: Is there any hope?

A: Yes—see treatment.

Summary:

1   As you can see, the consequences of revealing the secret are dire.

2   The identified patient is permanently damaged. Whether or not The Secret is ever revealed, the psychological outcome for the identified patient is the same.

3   If the identified patient is responsible for revealing the secret, then he will also be

shunned by the family as a *personna non grata* to the nth degree.

4   If The Secret is revealed, then the dysfunctional family will wander aimlessly in a psychological wasteland. Their original purpose is gone. Their spent labor is not a marketable skill. What will they do now? Probably go off to marry into other dysfunctional families and get involved in some other dysfunctional relationships since these people repeat their same mistakes over and over again—unless they can get some serious professional help. They are creatures of habit whose habit is that of finding dysfunctionals.

5   Treatment is available in the form of group therapy programs such as Alanon; however, very few people ever avail themselves of this path to recovery; and,

6   Continuous emotional stress can cause premature death.

7   The preferred children may squawk about the IP's squawking, but they have never walked a mile in his shoes.

The psychodrama is now over…or is it?

If you are in therapy, keep on plugging away. Remember what happened when the Hobbits felt lost in the forest. They were actually on the edge of the forest. One of the dwarves climbed to the top of a tree that happened to be rooted on lower ground. His viewpoint afforded only a vast ocean of green leaves; had he climbed up a taller tree, he would have seen that they were already on the edge of the forest. Strive to climb the tallest trees!

Chapter VI-4

PREGNANCY
Psychiatric Drugs during Pregnancy
PMS

Pregnancy is a very exciting but stressful time for a woman, and it is much more so for those women who are taking psychoactive medicines. The main topics of this chapter are:

- Use of any psychoactive drug during pregnancy
- Different types and cases of psychiatric disorders in regards to need for medications during pregnancy
- Presence of major mental illness during pregnancy

These topics are medically complex and ethically challenging. Use of psychoactive medicines must be handled very carefully, for the sake of the baby.

Use of Psycho-active Drugs in Pregnancy

Some women are taking psycho-active medications for various diagnoses that are not those of Persistent and Severe Psychiatric Illness (PSPI). Possible diagnoses are for ADD, lifestyle alterations (weight loss, smoking cessation), insomnia, adjustment disorder, overspending, mild anxiety or minor depression. These conditions do not absolutely need to be medicated during pregnancy—except for smoking cessation, which is important for fetal well-being. On the other hand, women with PSPI may require use of major medications in pregnancy. However, these types of medications can expose the baby to risks of serious malformations, which will likely last for its lifetime. These malformations can be visible (physical deformations) or invisible (lifelong behavioral and/or emotional problems). The medicines might even result in premature delivery or stillbirth.

Different Types of Disorders and Cases Needing Medications

There are certain psychiatric **disorders** that are inherently mild, moderate, or severe:
- Mild disorders would include Adjustment Disorders, mild chronic anxiety, minor depression

- Moderate disorders would include Panic and Depression
- Severe disorders are Mania, Psychosis, Schizophrenia, Severe Depression

Women with mild disorders should fare well unmedicated during pregnancy.

Then there is a broad spectrum of **cases** that might or might not need medication during pregnancy. The cases refer to individual women. A woman could have a mild, moderate, or severe case of psychosis. If it were a mild psychosis, for example controlled well with Moban 5 mg a day, then treatment options during pregnancy are more flexible than the treatment of a woman with a severe psychosis. Severe in this case could either mean that she is so ill that she needs three or four major medications to control her or that she will immediately start to decompensate if she misses just a few days of medication. Mild cases of major depression can sometimes be treated with psychotherapy alone, whereas severe cases of major depression involve suicide gestures. Mild cases of mania may present as an energetic, dynamic, gregarious, and enthusiastic woman who has a sense of her limits and is able to maintain judgment. Severe cases of mania might be running naked down the street screaming in the wee hours. Please note that these three types of cases are somewhat variable.

These then are the basic cases and choices:

Mild cases may be able to forgo medications during pregnancy.

Moderate cases would include women who have major emotional problems but have a history of being free of symptoms for [long] periods of time between the "nervous breakdown" periods: these women might get by with some sort of manipulated decrease in the medicines such as:

- —taking a lower dose (or none) of the medicine during the risky trimester (various medications may be safer or less safe during certain trimesters);
- —using the medication as an on-and-off treatment ("pulse therapy") during the trimesters;
- —using the medicine only "as needed"; all of these options require a lot of cooperation between the psychiatrist and the patient with input/feedback from her husband/father-to-be.

Severe cases of women who have major neuropsychiatric disease and are continuously ill and always in need of medication: this third case is a difficult ethical and medical situation. Despite the anecdotal observations that emotional illness might slow down during pregnancy, it is important to plan for a possible emotional decompensation of the mother during or right after the pregnancy. Patients who have severe illness can decompensate quickly and become wild, violent, and irrational, thus exposing the unborn baby to (foreseeable?) physical damage and trauma and possible spontaneous abortion.

Major Mental Illness during Pregnancy

Pregnancy of a patient with major psychiatric illness is difficult at best. Patients who have persistent and severe psychiatric illness (PSPI) often become pregnant accidentally. Thus, the child had not been planned or wanted; indeed, in some cases the patient could be so psychotic as to be unaware of the pregnancy for a while. These cases usually do not receive regular prenatal care and the outcome for both the mother and baby can be unpredictable. Surprisingly, the babies of high risk psychotic mothers might be as healthy as the babies of very high functioning patients—although not usually. Obviously, a woman with PSPI will have a difficult pregnancy whether she is medicated or not. Oftentimes, these women do not take their pills regularly under the best of circumstances, so expecting extra diligence in pregnancy is expecting too much. Often they are single mothers. If they have had PSPI, they may also be alienated from their families.

An unstable mother might resort to using street drugs and alcohol to control her agitation. An unstable mother may forget to eat wholesome foods, to take daily vitamins, and to show up for obstetric appointments. Whether or not to medicate is a Hobson's choice that may require choosing the lesser of two evils. And, ultimately the parents-to-be need (if the father is available) to make an informed decision: whether it is better to be uncomfortable for a few-several months or possibly condemn the baby to being some sort of invalid for the rest of its natural life. Or choose an intermediate path of either taking the pills "as needed" (whenever she seems to worsen) or as "pulse" therapy (one week on medication followed by one week off, then back on again). The psychiatrist and obstetrician can provide input, but ultimately, you, the parent(s) must make the final decision.

The medical issues should center on preserving optimal physical health for the baby as well as emotional stability for the mother. This is also a serious ethical issue: whether the mother should remain completely sane and medicated during pregnancy while exposing the unborn child to possible poisoning or whether the unborn child should be spared the peril of neuro-psychiatric drug poisoning while the mother might be exposed to the risk of having seizures, profound melancholy, or psychotic breakdowns.

Trimesters

Different activities occur in the unborn baby at different stages in the trimesters:
1st trimester—is a time for laying out the cell layers and general organization of the organs in the fetus as it progresses from embryo to fetus;

2nd trimester—is a time for brain structure to take shape; and,

3rd trimester—is a time which is critical for growth of the fetus and further functional development of the nervous system and other organs.

In many cases, different psychiatric medicines will produce worse malformations in a certain trimester but perhaps not in the other trimesters. This is another strategy to consider if an expectant mother MUST be medicated during pregnancy. See Table VI-4-c.

The three trimesters of pregnancy can be a biochemical minefield and there is still much to learn about prescribing drugs in pregnancy because information on drugs in pregnancy only trickles in anecdotally. Drug companies do not run clinical trials on pregnant women in our country for the obvious reasons: responsible mothers would probably not participate and the drug company would be wading across an ethical minefield. There will be isolated reports that such and such a drug was given to a certain patient during pregnancy and the outcome will be noted. This is the usual source of this information. Some researchers try to collect this type of random information on isolated pregnancies where the mother had chosen to take such and such a drug during pregnancy or had accidentally taken it or had been forced to take it. There was one large study done in France. The Republic of France did a large [retrospective] study some years ago, which consisted of looking back at individual women who had been so sick that they had to take psycho-active medications during pregnancy. This study, of course, was haphazard and none of the women had been in a formalized and controlled research study. The researchers looked at the obstetric records of approximately five thousand women who took anti-psychotic major tranquilizers during pregnancy (now referred to as first generation antipsychotics, FGA's, chapters V-4, also see IV-1). There was a modest increase in minor defects such as cleft palate or cleft lip (which can be treated with plastic surgery), but otherwise the rate of birth defects was not much more than that of pregnant women who had taken no drugs during pregnancy. By the way, all these anti-psychotics in the study are on the usual "C-list" of table VI-4-b. And all these drugs are the older drugs that have been around for decades, the so-called FGA's (see Chapter V-4 on antipsychotic medicines). Since these drugs have been in use for upwards of half a century, there is now more experience with them and with their possible side effects so that psychiatrists can feel some comfort level if prescribing FGA's in pregnancy. The other goal of this French study was to find out if the children grew up to have behavioral problems or major mental illness as adults. This is harder to assess since these children inherited 50% of their genes from a psychotic mother and many were also reared by a psychotic mother (nature plus nurture both working against the children).

I have devised chart VI-4-a as a general guideline regarding whether or not to medicate.

Genetics

Whether to medicate mildly-to-moderately ill women is a quandary. Genetics may trump this vexing quandary anyway. Even if the mother foregoes all medicines for the sake of the baby's health, we need to recognize that she can pass on her genes to the baby, thus making the baby more vulnerable to developing major neuropsychiatric illness despite the total lack of all medications during pregnancy, regardless of all the best medication decisions.

Moreover, people with severe mental illness have altered blood levels of all types of biochemicals and hormones: cortisol, for one example. It has also been suggested that the blood of an unmedicated and mentally unstable mother might contain such alterations. This is in the blood that flows through her body and then into the womb. Conversely, a medicated and stable mother might not have sufficient levels of these aberrant chemical messengers (to deliver to the baby's blood supply and its developing brain), resulting in a healthier baby.

Breastfeeding and Postpartum

This needs to be decided in advance. Mother's milk confers more immunological protection to the baby than that from any other sources. However, the greater likelihood is that of no breastfeeding. Psychiatric drugs pass into breast milk and then into the baby.

Patients with mild diagnoses might be able to breastfeed for a few months then switch to other sources. Those with moderate and severe diagnoses should not plan on breastfeeding.

Patients with mild cases may or may not need to resume the medicines soon after the baby is born. Patients with moderate and severe cases should not plan on breastfeeding.

In the postpartum period, all women are susceptible to postpartum depression or postpartum psychosis—even those without any psychiatric history. Look to your family history for clues: were your mother, grandmother, sisters, and aunts prone to serious postpartum psychiatric problems? If yes, then this increases your odds of the same. Postpartum depression is more common than postpartum psychosis.

The mildest cases of postpartum depression are called "baby blues" and often do not see a psychiatrist. The usual cases of mild to moderate postpartum depression in previously "normal" women start gradually after the baby is born and start to build up symptom-wiss within a few to several months. These cases will usually need some minor antidepressant. Plan on not breastfeeding from this point on. Patients with long histories of depression may likely come down with postpartum depression.

Patients with pre-existing psychotic disorders are all at high risk of getting ill after the baby is born. The original psychosis might come back with the same symptoms or worse. This can be treated with standard antipsychotics or ECT, if necessary. All cases of preexisting psychosis should not plan on breastfeeding at all.

Other factors that aggravate the risk of postpartum disorders are stress-related: sleep deprivation, single motherhood, financial problems, lack of family support, and so on.

Table VI-4-a shows general predictions of outcome for both mother and baby as a function of taking or not taking medications during the pregnancy.

Table VI-4-a Psychiatric Status predicting Need for Medications during Pregnancy:

Maternal Status	Medications Used	Outcome for the Baby	Outcome for Mother
Mild case in Mother	1-no Rx drugs used during pregnancy→ 2-limited/few pills→	1-"natural" outcome; did baby receive the genes for psychiatric diseases, anyway? 2-Probably safe for baby	a)No Diagnosis —or— b) "baby blues" after baby is born
Moderate Case in Mother	1-no medication Used in pregnancy→ 2-minimal amount of medicine ___→___ 3-moderate amounts of Rx medicines →	1-Probably safe—Even without Rx drugs, could baby receive blood-borne hormones from mother, anyway? 2-Probably safe: benefits probably ___ outweigh risks_____ 3-variable (unknown or unknowable risks	a) Probable "baby blues": need for mild depression treatment --and/or-- b) Possible Psychotic illness after baby is born (need for anti-psychotics)
Severe Case in Manic, Depressed or Psychotic Mother	1-no drugs used in Pregnancy→ - - - - - - - - - - - - - - 2-moderate amounts of medicines are needed (risk to baby increases) - - - - - - - - - - - - - - - 3-High doses of Rx drugs needed (highest risk to baby)→	1-psychotic/manic or violent mother: risk of spontaneous or traumatic abortion? - 2-Visible Deformities in baby? Treatment is likely necessary - 3-Invisible Malformations? Future or current behavioral/emotional illness?	Probable psychotic Illness or Psychotic Depression after Baby is born

The expectant father should come in with the patient to see the psychiatrist at least once. The father-to-be can often provide a lot of helpful background information on the patient's baseline behaviors. Ethical and medical decisions should be primarily made by the couple while guided by the doctors.

Drug Safety
Pregnancy Drug Categories (A, B, C, D, X)

Some women who really need to be medicated during pregnancy need to be aware of the level of safety or of danger that is inherent in their current medications. For this reason, the FDA has drawn up some general guidelines regarding drug safety during pregnancy. This next Table VI-4-b gives some general idea of the rating of your current medicine. For example if you must be medicated during pregnancy and are currently taking a "D" or "X" rated drug, then at least you might have the chance to "upgrade" to a "B" or "C" rated drug during part or all of your pregnancy with the option to return to your usual medication after the baby is born.

The FDA has devised a rating system for drugs in pregnancy: the A-list drugs are known to be safe in pregnancy. "D" drugs are risky. "X" drugs are very toxic in pregnancy and should be avoided. "B" and "C" drugs are intermediate between safe "A" drugs and the "D" or "X" drugs. However, it should not be inferred that all the drugs on the B-list are completely safe; some of them are not necessarily known to be "good" in pregnancy—so far, they are just not known to be "bad". The letter grades should not be misconstrued to coincide exactly with medication quality and safety—but it may be.

Drugs on the "A-list" are known to be safe in pregnancy (but no psychiatric medicine is on the A-list). "B" or "C" class drugs may have made those lists due to lack of negative data rather than to proof of safety in pregnancy (or they may actually be known to be safe). Try to avoid "D" drugs and do definitely avoid "X" listed drugs during pregnancy.

CATEGORIES A, B, C, D, X (established by the FDA)

A—No psychiatric medicines are on the A list.
B—three psychiatric drugs are on the "B" list: Buspar, Ludiomil, and Clozaril. Clozaril is the only anti-psychotic/anti-manic that made the list. It is hard to imagine Clozaril being on the B-list and some references place Ludiomil on the C-list. Attributes of B-list drugs are:

   i.) either safe in animals even at high doses (but human studies have never been done); or,

   ii.) in the alternative, a drug can get on the B-list by being safe in humans but causing possible birth defects in baby animals.

C—Drugs which can cause birth defects in animals at high doses but have never been formally studied in humans—this includes many psychiatric drugs (most of them). The drugs have not been formally studied in humans because this is highly unethical and would endanger the baby.

D—Drugs which cause birth defects in humans at normal doses: Paxil and Lithium, as well as some of the epilepsy drugs that used by both psychiatrists and neurologists. (There is some current debate about downgrading Zoloft to the D-list [from the "C" list].)

X—Drugs that are often lethal to or causing catastrophic birth defects in baby humans and/ or in animal pups.

In the chart below, please note that the B-rating may mean that the drug is safer than a C-rated drug *or* that the B-rating may simply mean that there is not as much information available on the B-rated drug and if that information were available, then perhaps that drug would be demoted to the C-list rating too.

Table VI-4-b These are the five FDA pregnancy drug categories where "A" is safest during pregnancy and "X" is very dangerous. "B" is presumed safe, and "C" is not usually toxic. "D" should be avoided, if possible.

A	B	C	D	X
				XXXXXXXXXXXX
Folic Acid			Herbs??	
		Wellbutrin	St. John's Wort?	
Vitamin B-6	Ludiomil	SSRI's*(Prozac, Lexapro...)*		
		(except Paxil)	Paxil	Alcohol
		Effexor		
Synthroid		MAOI's(Nardil,		
		Marplan,Parnate)		
??Tryptophan??		Strattera,Ritalin		
		Dexedrine,Provigil		
	Clozaril	Ionamin		
		Trazodone		
		Serzone		
??Midrin??		Doxepin	Pamelor,Elavil	
		Desipramine	Imipramine	
		Asendin		
			Librium,Valium	
	Buspar	Atarax,Klonopin	Ativan,Xanax	
		Meprobamate	Serax,Tranxene	RESTORIL
	Meclizine	Tegretol,Trileptal	Tegretol-1st trim.	DALMANE

	Benadryl	Lamictal,Lyrica		
		Neurontin	Seconal	
	Tylenol	Haldol,Inapsine	Lithium	
	Flexeril	Orap,Compazine	Valproate	
	Imodium	Trilafon,Prolixin	Triavil	
		Mellaril,Loxitane	Dilantin	
	Caffeine			
	Sudafed	Zyprexa, Seroquel		
	Tavist	Risperdal		
	Novolog	Soma,Robaxin	Nicotine	
		Codeine	Methadone	
	Pepcid	Axid	Talwin	
	Zantac	Cogentin,	Dyazide	
		Symmetrel	Atenolol, Inderal	
	Maalox	Urecholine		
	Famciclovir	Acyclovir	Aspirin	

SSRI's = Prozac, Celexa/Lexapro, Luvox are C-list SSRI's; Paxil is D-list, Zoloft is now C but might be demoted to D.

Guidelines for and Notes on Dangerous Drugs:

1—Paxil is an SSRI antidepressant drug that was recently demoted to category D from category C. Some of the other SSRI drugs are now being scrutinized. Some people who have gone back and run other statistical studies on Paxil opine that the D-rating may not be totally deserved. Others predict that Zoloft also might be demoted to D-list from the C-list. There is a lot of anecdotal information on Prozac in pregnancy and it is not unfavorable.

2—Some drugs are safe in certain trimesters but toxic in other trimesters. (see table VI-4-c)

3—in Germany, the herb, St John's Wort, is treated as a prescription medicine because it is known to cause birth defects if used during pregnancy. Nonetheless it is still sold in the USA without a prescription (buyer beware).

4—The Europeans still remember the Thalidomide tragedy from half a century ago. This drug was not approved by the FDA. Thousands of European babies were born severely disfigured (limbless) but survived. This drug has been off the market since then. Its only use now is for the treatment of Leprosy and it can be dispensed only in Leprosy colonies. The FDA can conjure up the memory of this European tragedy to counter complaints from doctors and drug companies regarding the FDA's strict policies and vigorous vetting procedures.

5—Lithium can cause heart defects in babies.

6—Some drugs for Bipolar condition cause major malformations: Depakote, Tegretol.

7—Alcohol, cigarettes, street drugs are all bad for the baby. Relatively heavy drinking during pregnancy can cause Fetal Alcohol Syndrome (FAS) which can result in permanent defects and especially mental defects. Smoking affects the baby and should be avoided. Babies born to cocaine-addicted or heroin-addicted mothers go through drug withdrawal as soon as they are born. Also try to avoid caffeine.

8—What about all the chemicals in our food? And in the soil and air? These have yet to be studied extensively.

9—herbs are dried plants that contain hundreds or thousands of chemicals. Beware.

DRUGS with MIXED RATINGS in PREGNANCY *Table VI-4-c*				
drugs on this list can be riskier in one trimester than in others				
		T R I M E S T E R		
NAME of DRUG		1st	2nd	3rd
NSAID DRUGS:				
Aleve, Naprosyn		B	B	D
Ibuprofen, Motrin		B	B	D
ALCOHOLIC DRINKS				
Social drinking		D	D	D
Heavy alcoholic		X	X	X
Tegretol		D	X	X
MEPROBAMATE		C	D	D

BETA-BLOCKERS				
Inderal, Propranolol		C	D	D
NARCOTICS used	Oxycodone	B	B	B
in low doses or only	Vicodin	B	B	B
occasionally	Methadone	B	B	B
	Talwin	C	C	C
NARCOTICS used	Oxycodone	D	D	D
in HIGH doses and	Vicodin	D	D	D
Daily	Methadone	D	D	D
	Talwin	D	D	D

►QUESTIONS

Q: Why do we not have more information on drugs in pregnancy?

A: In order to have high quality statistical information about this subject, the FDA and the drug companies would need to design clinical trials to compare known drugs to placebo in the usual clinical testing format. First of all, the FDA is not going to design a test where a hundred pregnant women will receive placebo versus a hundred pregnant women who receive the investigational drug. Secondly, [hopefully] no mother would be likely to volunteer to be in such an ethically challenged study. Thirdly, the drug companies would not want to incur the [legal] expenses of such a test (at least not in the USA).

Q: So what is the advice for pregnancy?

A: Answer:

1—Discuss your case with your obstetrician.

2—Discuss your case with your psychiatrist or neurologist

3—If you have a mild case it would probably behoove you to forego the use of some of these drugs for at least during the first and second trimesters. A couple of these drugs are safe in the first and second trimester but not in the third.

4—Consider switching to drugs on the B-list.

5—Avoid St John's Wort, herbs in general, and drugs on the D-list and X-list.

6—Avoid taking [unknown] herbs or any herbs without safety information from the FDA.

7—Consider ECT (Shock treatments for severe cases—this treatment is safe in pregnancy as the electricity runs between two electrodes in the mother's brain and none of the electrical charge reaches the baby's brain); usually these treatments are given every other day for two-three weeks and then stopped when the patient feels better. The effect should last for at least a month. In patients with severe mood disorder or thought disorder it might be wise to give a "booster" treatment once a month after the initial treatment in order to keep the mother feeling better for the duration of the pregnancy.

7—Consider phototherapy: The use of phototherapy may be very effective for mild cases of depression. As a matter of fact, it is so effective that bipolar patients have switched into a manic sate while using a Light-Box. The only cost is that of buying a Light-Box from one of the manufacturers (few hundred dollars).

8—Most Importantly: *Be well informed!*

9—Drugs on the C-list must be evaluated in light of the advantages and disadvantages of taking it or not, and this can be a difficult decision.

10—Psychotherapy and massage and biofeedback can all be helpful. Psychotherapy can be as useful as medications for at least one-two days after each session—weekly psychotherapy may be quite palliative for mild cases.

General Guidelines

Are you feeling overwhelmed with so much decision-making possibilities? Most people would like some sort of written instructions which they could review, revise, or discard. So I will make a list for you.

This is my personal opinion:

- In general for everyone: Try to avoid all synthetic and exotic herbal chemicals: no drugs or herbs (including tobacco) or alcohol for all three trimesters Herbs contain hundreds if not thousands of chemicals and have not been assigned any ratings by the FDA. If you want to use herbs in pregnancy, then beware.

- Mothers who have severe neurological or psychiatric conditions such as severe manic-depressive illness or a severe psychotic illness will need to take some form of rational medication treatment.

- Mild cases of depression or anxiety: try to avoid any drugs: use phototherapy, psychotherapy, massages, biofeedback, insight meditation, take time off work to relieve the stress that causes the symptoms. Psychotherapy can be as effective as pills, but the effect only lasts for one day and must be repeated perhaps twice a week at least—a small price to pay for a healthy baby.

- Moderate cases of depression or anxiety—try the suggestions in the above paragraph, then consider any medications on the Category B list: Buspar, Ludiomil, Benadryl.

- Moderately severe cases: consider drugs on the C list, preferentially SSRI antidepressants. Not much is known about Luvox and Celexa/Lexapro. Avoid Paxil (also known as paroxetine or Pexeva). Zoloft is being scrutinized closely to see if it too should be demoted to join Paxil on the D-list, but Zoloft demotion does not seem too likely at this time. Prozac is likely the best choice for the main reason that it has the most experience of being taken in pregnancy. The reasons are that it has been on the market the longest and it is/was the most widely prescribed of all the SSRI antidepressants. Hence, Prozac has been used by countless millions of women—some of whom became pregnant unexpectedly while taking it. And some of whom opted to continue taking it during their pregnancies. The same story is found for major tranquilizers (antipsychotics)—the drugs with the longest track records are Prolixin, Trilafon, Stelazine, and some other of the first generation of antipsychotics FGA's).

- Severe to very severe cases: Try Clozaril or ECT (Shock treatments); one other tactic would be to admit yourself to a psychiatric hospital. Being in a controlled environment can have soothing effects too, allowing yourself to get away from outside stress while letting the nurses guide you slowly through your daily routines and letting them medicate you on an "as needed" basis only, as this might reduce the overall exposure to medicines. The negative side of "as needed" drug usage is that there will be no stable blood level of the drug.

- Actively suicidal: Brief Clozaril Therapy (25-50 mg a day for a two weeks trial).

As the severity of symptoms increases—and in all severe cases—the likelihood of needing medicines also increases. Women with a long psychiatric history would gain more benefit from being medicated since they should be able to function better during the pregnancy and afterwards. They would be able to rest, relax, stay nourished and focus on the baby.

Self-scoring Table

Here is a general chart VI-4-d that might be of some help with general guidelines: give yourself scores based on these scales. For example, if you were mildly depressed for one year after graduating college and spent that time drinking and drugging, and are not married but have a lot of sisters who are very involved in your life, then score yourself with $1 + 0 + 3 + 4 + 2 = 11$ total: expect a fairly good outcome. (This chart is just a contrived and general scoring system and is not based on extensive statistical data.)

Table VI-4-d   Self-Scoring table

	1 Mild cases	2 Moderate	3 Moderately-severe	4 Severe
Psychiatric History	None	Little	Some	Persistent
Psychiatric Hospitalization	None	None	Once	Multiple
Alcohol-drugs	No	Socially	Enough	Excess
Major Medical Problems	No	Few	Yes	Yes
Husband status	Attentive	Present	Aloof	Absent
Family support	Much	Good	Fair	Dysfunctional
Suicidal...? *	None	Ideas	Gestures	Overdose(s)

*See Chapter IV-7 for Suicide terminology

Assign 1-point if you are in column 1; and   2 points in column 2 and so on.
| | | |
Fairly Good   10-15   Good Outcome score: under 10
Not stable   16-20
Risky   21-24
Catastrophic   25-28

In Review:

- Table VI-4-a shows who might not need to be medicated

- Table VI-4-b shows where each drug lies within the table of safe drugs in pregnancy.

- Table VI-4-c shows that some drugs are safe in one trimester of pregnancy but can be dangerous in another trimester—this might be of benefit if planning some sort of off-and-on "pulse" therapy during pregnancy.

- Table VI-4-d shows a possible scheme for self-scoring to see where you fit as far as risk group

- Table VI-4-e shows how drugs receive their ratings in relation to animal studies and to human studies, keeping in mind that some of these drugs have earned their ratings based on animal studies and information on human babies is still lacking by and large.

Tactics and Strategies

So now you are armed with:
- An arbitrary and general scoring system
- Category rating charts, and
- My opinion

You still need to discuss this issue with:
- the father of the baby (if he is involved)
- your obstetrician/midwife
- your psychiatrist, psychotherapist, or psychologist

These then are the tactics and strategies you should try:
- Changing drugs according to trimester;
- Resorting to use of non-pharmacologic (and non-herbal) treatments;
- Scheduling too many doctors appointments rather than too few;
- Hiring extra domestic help during pregnancy;
- Avoid junk foods, fast foods, cats, and polluted areas;
- Get plenty of rest and any kind of activity or recreation that makes you feel good;
- Stay close to mother, sisters, and expectant friends;

Then you can make a decision and perhaps you should plan psychiatric resources during the pregnancy one week at a time, always planning for the next week in advance but realizing that the plan could be subject to change.

Addendum for Especially Interested Readers

If you were wondering how the FDA compiled its chart and wanted to know all the details, I have shown the basic process herein below. The FDA studied pregnant animals and compiled systematic information on other mammals. Then the FDA collected sporadic isolated information about human pregnancies that had gone forward with medications during pregnancy. This second source of information is obviously not systematic.

Table VI-4-e   FDA Pregnancy Category Ratings: This is how drugs are assigned their ratings. If a drug has known characteristics—as in the cases of "A", "D", and "X" listed drugs— the outcome is well known. An "A"–list drug is known to be safe to humans. Characteristics of the "B" listed drugs are fairly re-assuring, whereas those of the "C" listed drugs are equivocal. "D" and "X" should be avoided whenever possible!

	Human Studies done	HARM to Baby outcome	Animal Studies Done	HARM to Pup outcome	Risks to Human Baby
A	Yes	**NO**	---none---	------	None apparent
B B	Yes ---none---	**NO** ------	Yes Yes	yes no	no (low) risk to human baby unknown (low?) risk to baby
C C	---none--- ---none---	------ ------	Yes ---none---	**Yes** ------	Possible risk to humans* --no information available—
D	Yes	**YES!**	---none---		Moderate risk to baby
X X	Yes -----	*¡Severe!* -----	----- Yes	----- *..Severe..*	Dangerous/lethal Likely dangerous

*Unknown risk to humans, but drug is dangerous to [other] mammalian offspring!

This is how to use the table: Assume you are taking Prozac for the last six months and you become pregnant.

- ~You can look up your status in table VI-4-a
- ~You can look up your risk factor severity in VI-4-c
- ~You can look up Prozac in table VI-4-b and you will see that it is category C:

- ~You can check what "C" rating really means by looking at above table VI-4-e: this C-rating

May have two meanings:

 i)-that no human studies have ever been done in pregnancy, and

 ii) no animals studies were done, or if animal studies had been done, then the pups were harmed.

> Once More, this is a review of the roster of pregnancy safety classes of psychiatric drugs:

A: Drugs—no psychiatric drugs

B: Buspar, Ludiomil, (Clozaril)

C: some SSRI's, Doxepin, Desipramine, Tegretol, Trazodone, Lamictal, phenothiazines (the old first generation antipsychotic drugs)

D: Paxil, (Zoloft, too perhaps?), Alcohol, Lithium, Elavil, Pamelor, Imipramine, Depakote, Dilantin, Ativan, Xanax

X: Dalmane, Restoril

Stay in touch with your obstetrician and psychiatrist.
May you stay well during pregnancy and have a happy healthy baby!

Addendum on PMS

PMS is the older term, "premenstrual syndrome". It is now called Premenstrual Dysphoric Disorder or Late-Luteal-Phase Dysphoric Disorder. The last two names are the newer names. As you can see, both incorporate the word "dysphoric". Dysphoric describes how people feel when they have dysphoria. Dysphoria is the opposite of euphoria. In general, dysphoria means feeling miserable and cranky. *Dorland's* mentions "*excessive pain, anguish, agitation, disquiet, restlessness, malaise*". PMS is the easiest term.

Several of the antidepressants can be helpful, and some are FDA-approved for treating PMS.

(see also Chapter V-8) Paxil, Zoloft, and Sarafem (Prozac, really) are approved for treating PMS. This is usually a low-dose treatment. Often the treatment is taken for only ten-fourteen days per month. If there is an underlying depression, then the treatment can be taken every day. Apart from these approved medications, other antidepressants might be helpful when given "off-label".

Chapter VI-5

Essay on
CHRONIC PAIN

Pain is a sense of discomfort and is mainly perceived by the patient—hence, it is a symptom (see Chapter I-4). Pain can be classified by sensations that can vary from patient to patient. Pain has a number of different levels of **duration, intensity, location, characteristics, causes, and tolerance**. **Duration** can last from one hour to a lifetime. Surviving a major illness may involve living with uncomfortable side-effects or tolerating various pains during the treatment or even after the disease has subsided (as in Shingles). In many cases of long-term pain, the pain symptoms can be as unique as is each patient and his medical history. **Intensity** can range from mild to severe to "the worst ever"; doctors usually will ask the patient to classify the pain on a scale of one to ten, ten being the worst. Pain **location** can be in one small spot ("right there on my abdomen"), a region of the body (left foot), a system of the body (glove and stocking areas of both feet and hands), or the whole body (past history of massive burns all over the body). **Characteristics** describe how the pain feels: is it heavy pressure, or stabbing, or burning, or gnawing? Which factors make the pain worse? Or better? **Causes** can be from external injury, internal organ changes, infections, cancer, parasites, and so on. Different patients have different **tolerances** to pain: some people can tolerate a lot and some, none. Actively psychotic patients feel almost no pain. Patients can be hypnotized to feel little or no pain. Sitting meditation can reduce mild pain sensations—as can certain non-addicting medicines (Motrin, Naprosyn). Pharmacologic and psychiatric treatment, of course, will also need to be tailored to that particular patient. Duration of pain is almost as important as its intensity, and in long-term pain cases, these two are usually intertwined—from a treatment viewpoint.

Typical short-term pain occurs after surgery or after breaking a bone. This is usually treated with narcotics for a short while. Psychiatrists are not involved with short-term pain. Psychiatrists are involved specifically with long-term pain. **Location** is not typically a focus of treatment unless it involves some symbolic area of the body: women after mastectomy, men after prostate or genital surgery, an athlete with bone cancer of the leg. In these cases, psychotherapy is perhaps more important than medications. **Characteristics** may not be a focus of treatment, unless they are constantly changing. Pain with greater **intensity** will require higher doses of medication usually. **Causes** of pain may also have symbolic meaning to a patient. Psychotherapy once again may be helpful, and some people may need religious counseling also if they perceive the cause as originating from a Higher Power. Such examples might include HIV in a man with no known risk factors. Psychologists might help patients with questions of "why bad things happen to good people". Religion might be helpful for issues of "Why me?" However, in general, most chronic pain patients merely have chronic pain without all these complicated qualifiers. As far as **tolerance**, the pain is not tolerable, otherwise, the patient would not be referred to a psychiatrist.

Psychiatrists approach pain treatment by thinking in terms of the **duration** of pain since we are almost always called upon to treat only long-standing pain (and not short-lived or intermediate pains). The duration of pain can vary a lot, such as short-lived pain, long-term discomfort, and long-lasting pain (chronic pain). This chapter focuses on duration of pain: treatment of chronic pain of all kinds.

Duration of Pain

Short-lived Pain

This is the pain that occurs right after surgery; this kind of pain will normally last for a short period of time. It is usually treated with narcotics for a brief time and in most cases, the pain eventually disappears in a predictable time frame. It can also be felt initially after a serious injury or broken bone or the passing of a kidney stone, and other such sudden medical events. Short-lived pain does not involve the psychiatrist.

Residual Pain

Some patients will have an injury or medical condition requiring physical therapy or surgery or both. After medical or surgical treatment, the patient may improve significantly, but not completely. He may be left with a residual pain that continues to be mildly annoying. Psychiatrists may become involved in some of these cases. The causes of this pain can be physical or mental:

- physical pain can be due commonly to three sources: some residual scarring due to having surgery; chronic progressive medical problems; and, medical errors,such as surgical sponges left in the body. Physical pain as such can be a minor but permanent physical (not mental) alteration inside the body due to the surgery itself which has resulted in physical changes inside the body such as **internal scarring**, etc. In these cases, the patient is often not happy, but—as patients—we need to remind ourselves that surgery has cured a major condition but left a minor discomfort. In ancient times, this major condition could have killed us, but now we survive. Period. And these treatments were not even readily available then. But, now we are kept alive as a result of the operation which leaves us with a residual minor discomfort. Nowadays, at least there are systems of compensation for some of these cases such as settlements and permanent disability—not to mention the availability of mild pain-relieving medicines. A patient named Elsa has a long-term medical condition, which is **arthritis of her whole body**. The arthritis gets worse each year. The Arthritis has caused progressive backache. Then the arthritis caused a second back problem: a new but localized back pain that she had tolerated for five years while it continuously worsened. Then she had back surgery. The localized back pain is better, but during those five years, the arthritis was causing progressive deterioration in her whole back. That back ache (from arthritis) is still present and has grown worse over five years, but there is no surgical treatment for that problem, which is a diffuse ache and not a localized pain At least, the painful condition caused by arthritis was successfully treated, although the arthritis continues to make her whole body ache worse each year. The third possibility is that some **object** (surgical sponge) has been left inside the body accidentally. This is an extremely rare cause of this kind of discomfort.

- mental anguish by the patient who had expected 100% curative results, and who has been cured surgically but left with mild residual pain—these patients obsess over the surgeon or the surgery itself so that they become emotionally afflicted and conflicted;

Chronic Long-lasting Pain

This is a pain that originally had a known cause, but has taken on a life of its own independent of the original hurt. In many cases, the original hurt seems to have disappeared while leaving a long-lasting pain in its wake. The most typical of these pains are backaches and neck-aches (lower back pain and upper back pain); these pains might involve the spinal cord, which is an area of potential discomfort partly due to our habit of walking upright. Backaches and neck aches can often be traced back to an episode of heavy lifting or physical trauma (whiplash), but this pain persists indefinitely long after the normal person would have recovered from the symptoms of neck-ache or backache. This type of pain persists and never gets much better because of a number of factors. In years past, this pain was treated with narcotics. Then treatment philosophy changed and doctors decided not to treat this kind of pain with narcotics; however, in recent years medical treatment has completely swung around and come back to using seriously high doses of very powerful narcotics for this kind of pain. In some cases, it is not really clear if major narcotics are beneficial or not: long-term use of high doses of major narcotics has a tremendous effect on mood and thought as well as causing severe constipation and risk of addiction.

From a psychological viewpoint, most of these people become habituated or addicted to narcotics and then begin to show all the psychological traits of untreated drug addiction such as resentments, anger, projection, denial, poor judgment, and lack of perspective. (See chapter VI-1). These psychological traits are often the reason for psychiatric referrals.

Other Chronic pains

These may start with a seemingly innocuous event or even a non-event and might appear to have come from nowhere, such as walking across the living room. These pains even appear while the patient is at rest. Pains of this nature will be seen by all the usual doctors and medical specialists, and in many cases a real cause can be found, such as kidney stones, gall stones, fibroids, benign tumors, polyps, rheumatoid inflammations, orthopedic problems, unusual headaches, and so on. There are many causes of these kinds of pains, and most will be found to have a known cause, which hopefully is treatable. Among the hundreds or thousands of these cases, however, there will always be a few that defy current diagnostic abilities. Some of these kinds of pain will end up as long-term pain. Those cases for which no known cause can be found are usually sent to see psychiatrists. This does not mean that they are "crazy"—it just means that psychiatry is the last (or next-to-last) resort, treatment-wise (with high-dose narcotics being the last resort). The subtext is that current medical science cannot cure you, and you will need psychological comfort because there is no known cure; and, also because you will have to re-train yourself to live with the chronic pain. Psychiatry is known for using a number of non-addicting drugs that are not real pain-killers, but can indirectly help with the biochemistry of pain management. Therapists can provide emotional support during this difficult transition time, too. Thus, psychiatry has something to offer in terms of ongoing emotional support and in terms of medication management without using narcotics.

Headaches can become a chronic pain but usually not. There are many potential classifications for headaches and treatments for headaches. Understanding and treating headaches is quite complex, and there are doctors who specialize in the treatment of headaches.

Another type of chronic pain occurs with fibromyalgia, which is not well understood. There are rheumatologists and also specialists who see many fibromyalgia patients. There is an ongoing attempt in the medical community to learn more about this condition. There are a few psychiatrists who specialize in fibromyalgia pain treatment.

Chronic terminal pain of a fatal illness

This is the pain of a terminal illness, usually associated with cancer pain, but can apply to other slowly progressive fatal illnesses. As the fatal disease progresses, the pain may worsen. The fatal illness is slowly destroying the body, and so the pain will continue getting worse. These patients should be given whatever they need to control the pain because: (1) they have real pain (2) the pain will continue to get worse (3) there is no need to worry about long-term addiction, and (4) we have the medicines available to help these patients. Any available medicine should be used: Ritalin, Narcotics, Valium, etc. In the past, some doctors opined that cancer patients should not be totally medicated so that they could have "meaningful" conversations with their families (while writhing from agonizing pain, no less). The philosophy on this topic has changed dramatically in recent years. Currently, we want patients to have whatever comfort they need. As a result, California has mandated that all practicing physicians receive training on this issue. The cancer patient should be able to collaborate with everybody on his treatment team regarding medicines, comfort levels, and overmedication. Nowadays these patients are usually enrolled in a hospice program.

"Phantom pain" is another kind of discomfort which is an ongoing sense of limb pain in a limb (leg usually) which has already been amputated.

The nervous center of pain perception lies in areas of the brain. The psychiatrist becomes involved because some psychiatric medicines have biochemical activity in those brain areas and coincidentally can effect pain control. And psychiatrists are most familiar with neuro-psychiatric medicines of this type.

Chronic Pain is defined as a long-lasting kind of pain that never gets better. This really seems to be a different kind of pain from short-lived pain. Most people have short-lived injuries, which heal up normally within a reasonable period of time. A small group of people do not heal, and they continue to have aches and persistent pains that go on and on. There are other kinds of long-lasting pain (such as fibromyalgia) which seem to appear slowly and without any apparent causation. The causes for these kinds of pain are not well understood; the sense of pain perception is believed to lie on the sides of the brain (parietal cortex). In the early stages of chronic pain, most doctors will prescribe the usual medications such as Ibuprofen (and other drugs in this class) and non-addictive muscle relaxants (such as Flexeril) and then later may resort to using Valium (as a muscle relaxant) and minor narcotics (like Darvocet or Vicodin). If the patient still has persistent pain, then the primary doctor will usually follow one of four courses of action (depending upon the nature and significance of the injury):

1—Follow-up visits with primary doctor to continue seeing the patient and trying different combinations of muscle relaxants (Flexeril, Soma, Robaxin), minor narcotics (Vicodin), drugs like Ibuprofen (Naproxen, Toradol, Voltaren, and others), as well as Ultram;

2—referral to a medical specialist such as a rheumatologist;

3(4)—referral to a Pain Management Unit; or,

4(3)—referral to a psychiatrist (some patients see us first before resorting to the pain clinic).

Some patients become indignant about choice #4 and refuse to go to see a psychiatrist, believing that their suffering is being belittled or given short shrift. It seems to them that their primary doctor is diagnosing their pain as psychiatric rather than physical. This is not true.

Types of Chronic Pain

Mechanistically, we can look at four possible **types of chronic pain** (from a drug-responsive viewpoint):

- **Chronic Progressive Pain:** This is an ongoing **physical pain** or physical evidence of pain which is documented by lab tests and/or X-rays (diseases such as spinal canal stenosis, cancer pain, rheumatoid arthritis etc.). Not only are these known to be real physical injuries that are visualized by X-ray (CATScan, MRI), but also these diseases are chronic and progressive, possibly life-threatening conditions that will only get worse with time. Doctors are concerned with making these patients as comfortable as possible for as long as possible. Some of them may even opt to enter a hospice program. The primary treatment team for these kinds of chronic pain usually involves pain specialists, oncologists, and internal medicine specialists all of whom are prescribing anti-pain medications: there is usually no need to consult psychiatrists in cases of chronic progressive pain. If the treatment team discerns a secondary or independent psychiatric problem then the patient may be referred to psychiatry since in these situations psychiatric treatment may be helpful as a secondary or add-on treatment. Psychological support may help with the different kinds of discomfort in these diseases. Probably the most important reason for referring these patients is not for prescriptions but for **counseling with a therapist** in case the patient might have any unresolved psychological issues. A therapist can do a few sessions of therapy focused on spiritual belief systems and the issues of immediate concern surrounding issues of the chronic progressive disease.

- **Chronic Controlled Pain:** This is **perception of pain** that occur in **diseases which are known to cause discomfort**, such as tingling or burning sensations (like diabetic foot pain or Shingles). However, these are diseases that really do not show up on the usual medical tests (X-rays can be normal) and which may not really be considered chronic progressive terminal illnesses, but rather a long-term but non-progressive pain sensation. However, there is definite evidence of the known primary disease (blood sugar in Diabetes, tell-tale skin lesions of Shingles, for example), and the known primary disease usually is known to be accompanied by some sort of controlled pain. In these cases with normal X-rays, there is no exact evidence that correlates to the severity of the pain. In other words, we cannot look at an X-ray and see total bone destruction. We must take the patient's interpretations of his symptoms as the main evidence. Psychiatric drugs can help people cope with this kind of discomfort.

- **Chronic Functional Pain:** Let's take a patient named Carl. This type of pain can occur in patients like Carl who have an unknown pain: pain of unknown cause or duration. This type of pain centers around the belief in the fact that Carl perceives pain despite the lack of abnormal X-ray findings or any abnormal lab tests. (The lab tests seem "normal"). Carl has no severe medical condition known to present with chronic pain. There is no documented painful fatal illness as in rheumatoid arthritis or any diagnosable chronic continuous pain source as in shingles. In fact, there is no known cause of the pain at all. Moreover, the pain often behaves in ways that do not conform to any known medical model of anatomy or physiology. The pain might migrate around the body erratically hurting in different places at different times in a vague manner that is not diagnostically suggestive, and the pain may have indescribable intensity. The pain might be accompanied by medically incongruous explanations about the agents that might worsen it or improve it. Carl is a good candidate to see a psychiatrist because he most likely has an underlying depression (or somatic disorders). Chronic depression makes pain feel worse, and chronic pain makes depression worse.

> Depression ↩↪ Pain

Fortunately, patients like Carl may have a fairly good response to antidepressants. We call this "functional" pain: this means that it functions like pain but has no known cause or structural explanation (no anatomy).

- **Low Pain Threshold** patients have a **high sensitivity to mild pain**, a pain that would be mild or low-grade in most people. People with a low-threshold to pain experience a mild pain as being moderately severe and a moderate or severe pain as being excruciating. They may unflinchingly rate the pain as "11" on a scale of "1" to "10" where "10" is assigned as the worst pain ever. Such a patient seems to have her nervous system "wired" in this oversensitive manner. Since that is the case, then she too can benefit from calmative psychiatric medicines because her pain sensing areas of the brain (and nervous system) are probably "over-reactive". This is the class of patients who have long histories of multiple problems with medications, but can often derive a fair amount of relief by combining several non-addictive medications in very low doses. Typically, this patient comes from the family doctor because she has already acclimated to minor narcotics and has become dependent on them. These patients are typically addiction-prone, and the real problem is in weaning them off narcotics onto a non-addictive neuro-psychiatric medication. They will quickly acclimate to minor narcotics (Vicodin) and minor tranquilizers (Valium) and become dependent on narcotics and habituated to Valium. The use of addicting drugs in these patients will quickly set up a cycle of ever escalating pain by two possible mechanisms.

In the first scenario, the low pain threshold will be calmed by Vicodin for a while (habituation), but her brain will require larger than average doses and will become accustomed to these doses and require more, leading to addiction. In the second scenario, she will overreact to any slight perceived or imagined pain and she will quickly take a "preventive" dose of Vicodin for pain that she fears *might* occur in the next half an hour whereas a reasonable person would adopt a wait-and-see attitude about remote medicating of such a possible pain. Low threshold patients are so sensitive to low doses of pain and so afraid of feeling any pain that they would prefer to take medicine in anticipation of any possible future pain and can not tolerate waiting for any pain that *might* arise. In this sense, she is impulsive and somewhat dramatic in action. Although from her viewpoint, she is being pro-active instead of reactive. When dealing with narcotics, proactive decisions are likelier to lead to addiction. Narcotic habituation can be common, going from Vicodin to mid-range narcotics and eventually ending up on major narcotics such as Oxycontin, Morphine, or even Methadone. Eventually, none of the narcotics help much anyway. In a sense, she is like a "pain hypochondriac".

VI-2-a This is my summary explaining similarities and differences of the types of pain:

Underlying illness	Type of pain*	Lab tests X-rays	Pain outcome
A-Chronic progressive	severe progressive (+)	(±/ ±) (biopsy±)	likely fatal
B-Chronic controlled	moderate-stable (+)	(– / ±)	not fatal
C-Chronic functional	Variable-chronic (–/0)	(0)	not fatal
D-Low Threshold	slowly progressive (±)	(±)	Addiction

*(+) shows actual known pain source.

Examples

A)-Cancer or Rheumatoid Arthritis: X-ray evidence (+) and blood test evidence(+) are both present.

B)-Diabetic Nerve pain of feet: X-ray (−), but sugar is (+) in urine and blood.

C)-Functional Pain (Backache):   X-rays and lab tests usually non-specific (0) and do not show "hard evidence" of back disease.

D)-Low-Threshold /Low Pain: impulsive behavior (0/±), otherwise no "hard evidence"

In the early stages of chronic pain, the pain sensation travels in the nerves up to the brain and is constantly bombarding the brain with pain signals for a long time. These pain signals force the brain to process the type of pain and see what it is. It often turns out to be just the same old signal coming from the same place in the body with the same message. After weeks of this bombardment the brain becomes weary and is using up its chemical hormones (serotonin and norepinephrine, for example) dealing with the constant incoming pain signals which by now are routine rather than urgent. Eventually the brain is depleted of these chemical hormones needed to react to and process this information. Then the brain enters a fragile and fatigued state similar to that of depression (just imagine what it would be like to have somebody constantly pinching you day and night for a long time).

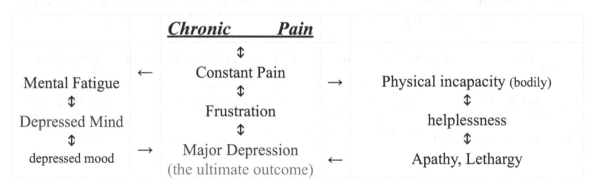

VI-2-b   *In chronic pain, all roads lead to brain fatigue and depression*

Chronic pain can involve many parts of the body including nerves, joints, and bones. Most common are complaints of backache, neck ache, and headache because the spinal cord is very vulnerable to aches.

Chronic pain patients do not work for various reasons: some cannot physically work, some believe that they cannot work, and some fear that they cannot work. So, they stay in the house and brood about the pain. The best way to get better is to do something or have a part-time activity: do craftwork, for example. Antidepressants can help people to become more motivated to do anything that they can.

The pharmacologic treatment of chronic pain is complex and depends upon the experience of the psychiatrist more than almost anything else. Willingness of the patient is about equally as important. Patients who like narcotics do not want to quit the narcotics; and, they do not want to see any psychiatrists. However, their treating doctors have told them that the narcotic usage is veering toward addiction and the narcotics will be tapered off—despite much protestation by the low threshold pain patients. When they find themselves forced to see a psychiatrist, they usually arrive with a negative attitude and lack of interest in any treatment using non-addictive medications. Furthermore, by the time the patients are seen in psychiatric consultation their situation has usually deteriorated further. Some patients are referred directly to the Pain Management Unit and do not ever see a psychiatrist. If a patient is sent to see a psychiatrist, this visit will usually be the intermediary step between the internist and the Pain Management Unit. And often other medical specialists are visited during this period, too. The psychiatrist is thus an intermediary step along with the other specialists. This serves as acknowledgement that this pain treatment is actually for pain treatment and not for psychiatric illness. The patient should try not to let this psychiatric consultation upset him. This is often the usual flowchart for these chronic pain patients:

#1 Primary Care Doctor	(#2) ⇨ specialists ⇨	(#3) ⇨ pain clinic
Family Practice Internal Medicine	Psychiatry, Sports Medicine Rheumatology, Physiatry Physical Therapy, etc	Pain specialist

Treatment

The course of treatment often centers on the nature of the pain-control as well as on the characteristics of the pain itself.

Patients who have *fatal illnesses* will need escalating treatment for escalating pain due to the escalating fatal illness. They will need to have pain control reviewed often. This is one case where pain control should be administered proactively and not reactively: stay on top the pain control and always stay ahead of it. Patients who experience good control and stability on their pain medicines will be able to continue on those as provided by the primary doctor—unless there is an increase in pain or apparent loss of pain control in which case they will be sent to see some specialist.

Patients with *functional pain* (cases without any positive lab tests or significant diagnosis) will likely be sent to see a neurologist or other specialist, at which time a few of them might be found to have an unusual medical condition. However, a lot of these will lack a known diagnosis and will then be referred back to the primary doctor who in turn will send the now-confused patient to a psychiatrist. At this point, she may resort to traditional treatments (see below). The primary doctor may also sense that the course of treatment is skewed and that psychological issues are involved and may just send her directly to the psychiatrist at which time the primary doctor may preface the referral with the statement that there will be no more narcotic prescriptions unless she does go to see the psychiatrist. Unfortunately, if this decision is made years after she is dependent on (habituated to) narcotics (Vicodin often), then a visit to the psychiatrist might not be fruitful since she is already accustomed to the drugs and is uncomfortable without the drugs and reluctant to make changes or to disrupt what she feels is a state of semi-stability.

- —Patients with the *chronic progressive* fatal illnesses may go directly to the pain clinic or see specialists first. They may also choose to go into hospice care.

- —Patients with the *chronic controlled* cases will likely see specialists.

- —Patient with *chronic functional* pain are very likely to see specialists.

- —Psychiatric referral is highly likely *for low threshold* pain patients. referral can be "leveraged" by the internist's refusal to continue prescribing narcotics.

- [E)—a fifth category would be malingering or factitious disorder (not discussed here).]

Needless to say, the treatment of chronic pain is an art not a science since there are no blood tests to measure narcotic blood levels and few—if any—lab tests to measure pain levels directly. There is little objective evidence (few signs). The treatment of chronic pain will rely upon subjective reports from patients (symptoms) and upon intuition and experience of the treating specialists and doctors.

Some patients will choose to "go out of network" (for treatment) at this point, being thoroughly disgusted with medical science. They will seek alternative treatments such as yoga, herbals, and acupuncture. The combination of these three remedies may indeed be helpful, especially if all three are used together and provided that the patient is able to set aside prejudices against the use of traditional treatments instead of always turning to Western Medicine for drugs, drugs, and more drugs. Patients would need to re-think treatment plans, understand the subtleties of these remedies, and gain a belief that these remedies might help—and have faith in the belief that these might help. The main hindrance is that patients of modern Western Medicine demand instant improvement and immediate relief. They are not prepared to take on a new way of life where treatment response is measured in months and years instead of minutes and hours. Thus, they sabotage their own health by being "minutes wise but years foolish". Alternative treatments may help some people— otherwise we could not have survived for all these millennia.

Some of the medications commonly used by the psychiatrist are: Neurontin, Elavil, Cymbalta, and Effexor. There are a number of other treatment options and sometimes the real treatment ends up by finding the correct mixture of a few correct medications in the correct amount (which can vary from impossibly tiny amounts to really high doses) and which only time can tell. Unfortunately, many chronic pain patients may have only a partial response to psychiatric medications: maybe feeling 35-50% better at most which is below the success rate for treating depression in general. This can be an unfortunate outcome and serves only to highlight the fact that we still have much to learn about pain and its management.

PATHWAYS to ADDICTION via medications in progressive order:

Use ⇆ Misuse⇆ Abuse⇆Habituation ⇨⇨ Overuse/Dependence ⇨ Addiction.
  (⇆ *indicates reversible state; but* ⇨ *indicates one way only with no return*)

When patients are using narcotics, these progressive stages (above) are always as much of a focus of attention as in the pain level itself.

 ⇨"Habituation" means that a person needs to take the same dose to receive that same relief *and* that the drug does need to be used on a regular basis.

 ⇨"Addiction" means that a person needs to take higher doses just to get the same effect—and often the patient is taking higher doses than prescribed, and the doses are taken more frequently than prescribed.

Patients with **chronic progressive** fatal diseases may use progressively more medicine as pain rises and the disease progresses (anxiety levels will rise too). This is usually habituation:

A:_____

Dosage of pain killer goes up with time often in tandem with the constantly increasing pain levels too. But this is not true addiction since the pain medicines are keeping pace with the pain and its source.

Chronic controlled cases may or may not be taking narcotics.

Chronic functional pain patients may or may not be taking a combination of psychoactive and narcotic medicines. Sometimes these patients may take an extra dose "as needed": this is not really a problem unless it starts to resemble early stages of addiction.

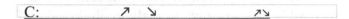

C:

D.) low pain threshold patients are often taking narcotics to which they become habituated or addicted:

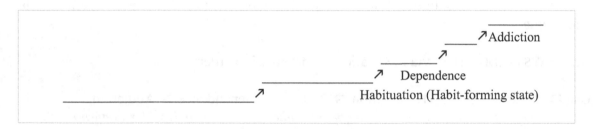

_____ ↗ Addiction

↗

_____

↗ Dependence

↗

Habituation (Habit-forming state)

Other kinds of Patients sent for Psychiatric Evaluation

There are other kinds of patients sent to the psychiatrist for pain evaluation. These are not really pain patients at all, but they are presented here for the sake of completing the chapter.

Malingering occurs when the patient knows he is pretending to have pain and he knows what the reason is (to get narcotics, to get out of work, to get out of jail, etc). These are not even medical patients. The biggest tip-off is that their signs of pain can be easily disproved by a neurologist; also, any medical doctor (including psychiatrists) will find that malingerers' stories do not ring true and that their symptoms do not conform to any known anatomical relationships.

Factitious Disorder occurs in patients who have deeply-rooted psychological problems which have not been addressed in therapy. This patient causes illness in herself but does not know what the reason is (she is reacting against a terrible childhood trauma of some sort). So she is knowingly creating her signs and symptoms which may sound halfway genuine but factitious patients are usually very "needy" psychologically speaking. The self-induced medical problems are a way to seek sympathy and concern from their primary doctor. The primary doctor will eventually come to understand their unmet emotional needs and also realize that his treatments are not producing predictable results. He will then caringly (hopefully) refer her to mental health specialists. She may have emotional symptoms which will immediately take center stage while the bodily symptoms fade away. She also will have an odd way of modulating her moods—over which she has no voluntary control. This will differentiate her from malingerers. A very famous type of this disorder is Munchausen's Syndrome.

"Somatic" patients in some ways resemble chronic functional pain patients but also resemble low-threshold pain patients. Somatic patients differ, however, in three ways: (1)- if there are pain complaints, then most of these complaints are rooted in real physiology and anatomy; (2)- most of the symptoms focus on many generalized organ systems; and, (3)- pain complaints will partially improve with psychiatric treatment. Somatic patients are overly concerned about all their bodily sensations in general, and any pain concerns are incidental. Usually they focus more on discomfort or concern over the normal range of normal bodily functions rather than pain as a primary concern. They often have a multitude of variable and odd pain symptoms. But—unlike low threshold pain patients—somatic patients can have some success with psychiatric medicines but never really get better than about 40-50%. The patient may have anatomically and physiologically realistic pains including all sorts of generalized body sensations. She seems to be overly sensitive to nerve impulses arising from all parts inside her body whereas low threshold pain patients experience oversensitivity based mainly only on the musculo-skeletal system, and their pain is perceived to be coming from sources outside the body.

Hypochondriacs are a different diagnosis: these people are afraid that they might get sick. They overreact to the smallest sensation. Chronic pain is not typical of their condition.

VI-2-c   Different types of Chronic Pain Patients

Illness	self-induced	Is cause of pain known to patient?	Real reason for / cause of Pain (pathologic process)
A) Progressive	–	Yes	Catastrophic illness
B) Controlled	– (?)	Yes	Medical illness
C) Functional	slightly-partly	Not really	depression/helplessness
D) Low Threshold	(somewhat) (±)	(needs someone to take care of him/her) (±)	Addictive/dependent personality or co-dependent
E) Malingering	Yes (+++)	Yes (+)	Has a personal agenda: –to avoid jail, punishment, fines or –to obtain money and entitlements
F) Factitious	Yes (++)	No (–)	unmet needs from childhood
G) Somatic	not really (±)	No (–)	overly sensitive to sensations from inside their bodies
H) (not a chronic pain patient) Hypochondriac	no	No	dependent personality Unmet childhood needs

►QUESTIONS
___

Q: Why should a chronic pain patient continue seeing the psychiatrist?
A: This is because certain psychiatric drugs are effective for treating chronic pain. Psychiatrists are most familiar with using these non-addicting drugs on a long-term basis. Psychiatrists can manage the side effects.

Q: I have seen all these specialists including neurology, rheumatology, etc. and now I am more confused. Why can't they diagnose the cause of my pain?
A: The apparent answer is that medical science does not know what to do next except send you to a psychiatrist, the specialist of last resort for many patients.

▶Chronic pain is very annoying, uncomfortable, or debilitating. It decreases the quality of life substantially, reducing earning potential, sociability, and self-esteem

▶Chronic pain effects on the human brain are not unlike those of depression—and can often have a partial positive response to antidepressants.

▶Chronic pain can improve with medication, physical therapy, and a part-time productive activity. So do it!

Behavioral Disturbance in the Elderly
Nursing Homes and Dementia

Dementia is a chronic progressive fatal brain deterioration usually following a course of several years, its length depending upon the type of dementia. The dementing process can start in one region of the brain and then spread to other areas of the brain. The region in which the dementia starts will dictate which early symptoms show up first. There are different kinds of dementia: Alzheimer's is merely the best known dementia. The first symptom in Alzheimer's is usually loss of short-term memory. The disease is named for Alois Alzheimer who described the behavioral problems and brain changes a hundred years ago. Other types of dementia start in other parts of the brain. The early symptoms of those dementias will correlate to which brain area is first affected. Eventually, all the dementias will have a common outcome of total brain deterioration.

Genetics

When adult children bring in their parent, they often note that some one else in the family has had "Alzheimer's" (although in some cases it might have been another type of dementia such as vascular dementia or alcoholic dementia). The frequently asked question is regarding their own risks of becoming demented in later life. As far as genetics, there are two answers. Firstly, there are specific types of Alzheimer's that are transmitted genetically, these being related to any one of three chromosomes 14, 19, or 21. These can be readily transmitted as dominant traits, meaning that most/all blood relatives have the gene for the trait. A second type of Alzheimer's can cluster in families. Having family members with this form can put a person at some risk: identical twins might have a 40-50% of both having the sporadic form and 8-50% for fraternal twins. Having non-twin siblings with it is a lower risk, perhaps 2-20%. Having any relative with Alzheimer's can increase your risk about eight-fold.[3] The genetics are complicated and the percentages vary depending on the genes and families studied.

The risk of developing Alzheimer's increases the longer we live. It can start as early as age 30. People with Down's Syndrome can routinely acquire Alzheimer's dementia after age 35. Cases with strong family inheritance can occur earlier in life: Persons with both dominant genes can get this disease at an early age, perhaps in their 40's or 50's. It can appear in the 60's, and its risk rises quickly with age, no matter how long a person might live.

Researchers suggest that the number of elderly Americans will continue to increase due to advancing medical technology and treatments. That technology is becoming costlier and costlier from year to year as are the newer treatments. Nursing home care is already costly and will probably continue to rise due to increased federal regulations and litigation issues. More and more elderly will need care each year. The tax burden may become enormous or the federal government will have to change fee structures, reimbursements, and regulatory oversight. Or the government may establish less restrictive residences such as "Board and Care" homes or provide financial support to families to keep their elderly at home.

Common abbreviations used in this chapter:
- ECF: extended care facility (nursing home)
- SNF: skilled nursing facility (nursing home)
- ADL: activities of daily living (ability to dress, groom, toilet oneself, etc.)
- IADL: instrumental activities of daily living: food-shopping, driving locally, doing light housework, cooking simple meals, handling money, walking on stairs and outdoors, and *taking correct pills on time*
- UTI: urinary tract infection (a common cause of delirium in the elderly)

Hospitals and Residential Placements

Some patients with dementia become aggressive and combative and may end up in a geriatric psychiatric ward (of a hospital). After the person is stabilized, he may be able to go home and live with family members or he may go to a regular nursing bed in a SNF. If he continues to be erratic and aggressive, he may need to go live in a SNF (ECF) with a locked unit. These locked units are reserved for patients who have serious behavioral problems. These behavioral problems might be from a *lifelong history of psychiatric illness* or from *new onset* of serious behavioral problems.

People with *lifelong histories of severe psychiatric illness* may often become demented in their old age, and then they too might need to be placed in a SNF or ECF. Many of them occupy regular nursing beds while stable on their usual psychiatric medicines. Some of them may deteriorate so much from the chronic psychiatric condition plus the advancing dementia, that they too may need to be in a locked unit of a SNF. This would mainly refer to schizophrenics and manics. We refer to these as "chronic" patients. Chronic psychiatric patients rarely survive into old age because severe psychotic illness usually shortens a person's average lifespan by ten to thirty years. Schizophrenia and Mania occur with high rates of suicide, poor personal care, and major medical illness. But, some of these "chronic" patients can survive into their 60's and 70's and, they are likely to get dementia, perhaps due to the fact that they have impaired brain function already. When "chronic" patients do develop a dementia besides their original psychiatric illness, their original schizophrenic and manic behaviors can be even worse and more disinhibited. This can result in violent outbursts, agitation, and socially inappropriate sexual behaviors.

Sudden onset of serious behavioral problems in elders without known past psychiatric history can include: inappropriate sexual advances (men and some women too), hypersexuality, chronic intrusions into other patients' rooms possibly accompanied by petty theft, responding to delusions, and other unacceptable kinds of acting-out. Sudden onset is usually the result of a stroke, in which case the psychiatric symptoms will remain static—unless the person has a second stroke that results in further psychiatric deterioration.

New onset of serious behavioral problems in elders without known past psychiatric history can include fixed false beliefs that they are being harmed in some way, such as: being poisoned by pills or by the heating system or having all their money stolen. They lose the ability to control themselves socially and can also have angry outbursts or sexual impulses.

Other medical problems that might cause an elderly person to have sudden onset or new onset of behavioral problems and need to stay in a locked unit of a nursing home are sudden onset of new psychosis late in life, worsening dementia, or deterioration of a chronic lifelong psychiatric illness.

Common reasons for psychiatric visits to a nursing home

I am frequently called to go to nursing homes of which I service about twelve on a regular basis and another fifteen or twenty in outlying areas of Los Angeles County. Usually the patient is suffering one of a few diagnoses common in this population: psychosis, adjustment disorder, depression, or worsening of dementia. A less common cause is delirium. Many of these SNF visits are requested because the patient seems psychotic and federal guidelines demand that psychiatrists see patients with these apparent problems. If the patients are not psychotic, then they are usually agitated or angry about some issue which could range from medical problems, behavioral problems, or social problems. Medical problems could include undiagnosed pain and infections (UTI), and if medical problems worsen, the patient might become delirious. Behavioral problems could be due to worsening dementia, amorous attachments to other incompetent patients, or claims that roommates are stealing from the patient. Social issues may concern being confined to or being placed in a nursing home along with feelings of betrayal. Other problems may be situational which the nursing staff may solve by re-orienting or re-directing the patient; and, other issues may actually be rooted in the reality of the current environment and situation.

Anger comes from various sources such as loss of control, betrayal, family refusal to care for patient at home. Depressive reactions coming from various sources: loss of intimacy, loss of control, loss of home and beloved pets. "Adjustment disorders" come from the stress of being placed in a new situation. Medical problems are frequent such as UTI, other infections, or inability to express pain symptoms. Worsening dementia may be due to lack of stimulation. There may have been a pre-existing depression or serious psychiatric disorder. Often there may be problems with roommate(s) or a dislike for assigned nurse or current room assignment. Some people get a SNF-induced psychosis such as hallucinations and paranoia. Moreover, there may really be a reality-based problem such as seeing real ants in the room at night or that the room temperature is not comfortable.

Patients often have an emotional reaction when they first arrive in a SNF. If they are demented, they get upset because they do not recognize their surroundings. If they are depressed but not demented, they become much more depressed because they know where they are. These reactions can be of anxiety, agitation, or worsening of depression; the symptoms that appear depend upon the person's baseline personality. This reaction is considered to be an "adjustment reaction" and is diagnosed as an "adjustment disorder" (this is a real psychiatric diagnosis and in fact is a condition that any of us might have in reaction to unpleasant events). This is a new diagnosis to add to the current diagnosis of depression or dementia. This "adjustment disorder" will usually play itself out slowly (in two to four weeks) as the patient becomes more accustomed to the new routines of his new residence and accustomed to being among a group of peers including the "intimacy" of having one or more roommates. This is a normal reaction for most people. However, most patients having this adjustment disorder do not require a psychiatric visit at all since the patient will learn to adapt to a new environment within a few weeks. Some adjustment reactions may drag on for months and turn into a real depression, but hopefully, not. We humans are—after all—highly adaptable.

This adjustment reaction can occur in a dementia patient or in a fully aware patient. Remember that the typical dementia patient may have a poor memory and may forget events of yesterday—or of even a few minutes passsed. From the viewpoint of a dementia patient (patients with short-term memory loss), she goes to sleep one day in one place and then the next morning awakens in a SNF. Imagine how scary that could be: not remembering where she had been and not recognizing where she is. She feels disoriented and does not recognize her new surroundings. She has an anxious adjustment disorder which can be accompanied by a lot of agitation initially. After a few weeks, she will usually calm down as she becomes attuned to the new routine (as well as can be expected). The other case is that of the fully aware patient: she recognizes that she has been transferred to a SNF and realizes that her worst fears have come true. She usually will calm down as she learns the new routine. Different SNF's have different tolerance levels for adjustment disorders, depending more on the staff's reactions rather than on the patient's: some SNF's will call for an immediate psychiatric visit, others will wait a week to see if the behavior resolves, and some of them solve it in-house by behavior management. If the psychiatrist is inveighed upon to prescribe a medicine, then it will only be needed for a couple weeks. The best treatment is re-orientation and re-direction by the staff with occasional doses of Ativan. If there are residual behavioral problems, then the psychiatrist can be called.

In the case of the fully aware patient, she understands the significance of this placement: that this might be her last residence and she will never be able to return to her pets and home. These patients may go from a depressed adjustment disorder to a frank depression, which seems to be a legitimate response when facing exposure to a sudden life-altering change of this magnitude. This reaction usually is diagnosed (initially) as a depressive adjustment reaction. It may progress into a major depression which will then need to be treated with antidepressants.

Legal Issues

Diagnosis of dementia means that a patient will no longer be a competent adult which means that he will lose his right to drive a car and will need to have a **legal guardian** who will be in charge of his "person" and/or of his "estate". There are a number of common-law and statutory guardians. Similar terms are [21]: guardian, protector, preserver, or conservator. "Conservatorship of the person" refers to making accommodations for the patient's physical well-being: such as medical care, housing and so on. "Conservatorship of the estate" refers to paying bills and budgeting monies on behalf of the patient.

DNR status and Living Wills need to be established at the appropriate times. A living will is a legal document that the patient creates before he becomes incompetent (demented). This usually is an expression of how much life support he wants to receive in the case that he might have a fatal illness. DNR status means "Do Not Resuscitate". A dementia patient who "codes" (has a heart attack) would likely be in a [worse] vegetative state after revival from a code.

Common Behavioral Problems and Psychiatric Issues in Nursing Home Patients:

- *Dementia*
- *Delirium*
- *Depression*
- *Adjustment Disorder*
- *Psychosis*
- *Miscellaneous behaviors*

The vast majority of these disorders can be treated at the SNF without transferring the patient to a locked psychiatric hospital. Each change of housing further disorients the patient. It is preferable to treat the patient in the SNF (after all, it is an institutional environment with nurses in attendance). Depression, delirium and worsening of dementia are the disorders most likely to need psychiatric evaluation.

Dementia

Alzheimer's dementia may progress slowly with just its typical symptoms described below.

In the usual case of Alzheimer's Dementia, this is what may happen in the earliest stages:

- Loss of short-term memory that appears in the form of forgetfulness: such as forgetting new names and dates—the memory problems will worsen and become more obvious to everybody

- then loss of higher functioning such as handling money, writing checks effectively. and loss of etiquette, grace, and social restraints

- as the disease progresses to mid-stage, there will be further deterioration of mental abilities and logic, as well as abnormal sleep, pacing, trying to elope from home and getting lost in the neighborhood

- then there is loss of ability to bathe and feed himself and he will classically fight off all attempts at bathing; he begins to crave only sweets and likes to be driven around in cars which seems soothing

- then he starts to sleep a lot and shows repetitive activities and repetitive mouthing of apparently meaningless sounds (like hooting or cooing)

- eventually, there is loss of bodily functions, swallowing, and rolling over (this only further increases the risk of developing serious bed sores)

- and finally, he loses even the most primitive neurological abilities and enters a "vegetative" state of non-responsiveness (sometimes not even wincing when pained) after which he will have loss of brain function involved in swallowing—and then later lose the ability to breathe on his own.

This stepwise deterioration in functions in old age mirrors the reverse pattern by which he learned functions gradually in going from toddler to child to teenager to adult. In the downward progression, the patients show "retrogressive" deterioration: the last learned tends to be the first lost (this is why dementia patients should not drive a car or run a business and this may be why they like sweets and riding around in cars). The last learned skills are sometimes the first to be lost.

Alzheimer's with Depression

Alzheimer's may often present with a depression as the disease progresses. This is treated as an elderly depression.

Alzheimer's with Psychosis

Alzheimer's may also present with psychotic features. One of the most common behavioral problems is yelling and screaming all night while hallucinating. This is not healthy for the patient because he gets no sleep. His roommates and neighbors do not get restorative sleep, either. This is treated as an elderly psychosis. Many family members do not want their loved one to receive antipsychotics for various reasons. Unfortunately, if they refuse the antipsychotics and the patient continues to be aggressive, disruptive, and psychotic, then the SNF will instruct the family to take their loved one to another institution. SNF's have a zero tolerance for these kinds of psychotic behaviors. See the treatment section below.

In psychiatry, we code Alzheimer's Disease as both a neuropsychiatric condition as well as a medical condition.

In the last stage, the patient no longer responds to people, pain, or any stimulus, and has completely lost his personality and identitiy. At this point, some family members opt to have the patient kept alive artificially by inserting a feeding tube so that the nurses can shove rich nutrient liquid into the tube. The patients stare blanklyinto space in the daytime. Patients spend the whole night trying to rip out the feeding tube, and this requires that their hands be tied to the bed. Sometimes the family even wants the patient put on a respirator (breathing machine). The question now should be, whom are they saving? Doctors and nurses usually think that the use of feeding tubes and respirators is not appropriate for the following reasons:

- the patient has no brainpower or personality left: there is nothing left (to revive);

- this is a natural outcome of Alzheimer's and cannot be cured at this time;

- this is the ultimate outcome of any disease or even of life itself;

- this is an unwarranted expense that will not gain anything;

- the patients have no idea what is going on—tubes are being shoved into their bodies: this hurts and scares them; and,

- the patients probably would not want it either. This is why it is important for *everybody* to draw up proper documents while still lucid , competent, and in good health. Yes, that means you, too. Your family doctor and lawyer can assist you with this process.

There are actually several types of Dementia, and the most commonly known dementia is Alzheimer's Dementia ("Dementia of the Alzheimer's type" is the proper term). Other types are vascular dementia , alcoholic dementia, Lewy Body Dementia, Fronto-temporal/ frontal lobe dementia, dementia pugilistica, and mixed dementia. Most dementias are a chronic progressive disease that is usually fatal within a number of years. Different types of dementia may have differing early symptoms but they all end up at a similar final pathway. Vascular dementia is about as common as Alzheimer's dementia.

These are the less well-known *dementias:*

Frontal Lobe Dementia starts in the front of the brain which is in charge of judgment and decision-making. Astute family members will know that there is something wrong but perplexed by the fact that these patients still have excellent short-term and long-term memory. That is because memory function is not so dependent on the front of the brain. These patients are notorious for having no ambition, no motivation, and seemingly can never make a decision. They sit and lie around all day completely aware of their surroundings and remember what is going on, but can never take the initiative to do anything, start any new projects, or finish any old projects. For example, Alzheimer's patients have no idea what to do with a blank check whereas frontal lobe patients may know know all about the check, but refuse to pick up a pen much less write on the check. For them to write out one check could take days, weeks, or months, whereas the Alzheimer patient might readily grab the check, write nonsense all over it, and then tear it into pieces which he throws down the garbage disposal or angrily throws at his caregiver.

Vascular dementia is due to cardiovascular problems such as high blood pressure, high cholesterol, and heart disease. These patients can typically have a stroke or a "mini-stroke". Each time that a heart patient has a stroke, she may lose part of her mind. This loss can result in physical disability (weak right arms or legs) or mental disability. So, this dementia progresses with sudden obvious downward lurches. Each stroke brings a new disability. If there is sudden onset of memory problems or strange behaviors, then it is likely due to a stroke or a mini-stroke (and not Alzheimer's, for example). The mental changes depend upon the part of the brain where the stroke happened. Thus, the resulting mental problems can be memory problems, excessive anger, total lack of motivation, or—in the worst cases—a psychotic symptom.

The psychotic symptom consists—like most psychotic disorders—of some fixed false belief or of seeing imaginary things. Stroke patients with one psychotic symptom may be aware that the symptom is not realistic but can not stop obsessing about it—unlike psychosis in schizophrenia where there is total loss of contact with reality. Stroke patients know that this is a new symptom and it feels alien to them, but they can not ignore the symptom. They usually have just one new symptom appear. This symptom may be something totally new for the patient, an unpredictable behavior that she has never had before. Or, the stroke may release her inhibitions and expose a personality trait that she has aleways had, but is now no longer able to control or suppress.

In the first case, let's take Margie who has been psychologically "normal" all her life. Later in life, she has developed heart and blood pressure problems. She takes several heart pills and blood pressure pills.. She is stable enough that she sees her primary doctor for these prescriptions and has only been to see the cardiologist a few times in as many years. One night she goes to sleep perfectly fine, and the next morning she awakens with a fixed false belief that she must go to Miami, Florida, to find her mother (who is by now deceased and never lived in Miami, but in Jacksonville, and only as a girl). Margie will become angry if people disagree with her, and she might suddenly decide to leave home without a suitcase, hail a cab to the LAX airport and buy a one-way ticket to Miami. She may get into an argument with the airline because she refuses to pay for the ticket, and they will call airport security who calls the family to come pick her up and take her home. She continutes to insist on going to Miami and becomes argumentative with the family, too. It is highly likely that she had a vascular stroke affecting an area of her brain. The good news is that the stroke caused no physical problems like limping, but the bad news is that this fixed false belief (delusion) is permanent. Furthermore anti-delusion drugs work well in "natural" delusions but not so well in stroke-caused delusions. To make matters worse, there is no FDA approved drug for this purpose, and the FDA has labeled all the anti-delusion drugs of increasing the risk of heart disease if given to elderly people with this type of condition. The adult children find this information on the Internet and refuse to let her take any anti-delusion medicines yet continue to demand treatment for the delusion. This is a case of a new onset of a symptom that did not correlate to the her past or her natural personality. These anti-delusion medicines work equally in men or women.

In the second case is Norma who had always been very popular with the boys and had been married four times, surviving each husband. She had been a swimsuit model and was Homecoming Queen. She has had a similar set of medical events as Margie above. In Norma's case, however, her latent coquettishness is no longer suppressed and she has become sexually seductive towards older men whom she meets. This behavior has gotten her into social trouble on numerous occasions. This behavior apparently has always been a part of Norma's personality. She had been able to control these urges until the stroke removed her inhibitions, so that now she acts and thinks according to her real "default" mode. She may need similar medicines to those of Margie. If this happens to elderly men, we give them a very low dose of the female hormone, progesterone, which controls them perfectly. This is not FDA approved but has its origins as a once standardized treatment for sex offenders, so there is experience with it. Once again, his family or guardian needs to give consent. Obtaining consent is usually not a problem: I am somewhat reluctant to give this as a prolonged treatment, but I have had family members request that the treatment be continued. Once the hormone stops, these men will once again become satyrs (overly sexual), a beahavior which SNF's will not tolerate.

Stroke-induced psychotic symptoms can be treated with some success by using anti-psychotic medicines. That is the good news. The bad news is that anti-psychotic medicines were designed and approved for use in real psychotic psychiatric patients with diseases like schizophrenia. Thus, these drugs may *or may not* help the stroke patient's psychotic symptoms. The proper diagnoses are "Psychotic Disorder due to a Stroke" and "Vascular Dementia".

Alcoholic dementia is caused by decades of brain damage from alcohol. Alcohol kills brains cells with every drink. Thirty years of alcoholism can cause serious brain damage. In the past, end-stage alcoholism and alcoholic dementia were diagnosed as "Wet brain" and sent to an asylum. (This is now called "Wernicke-Korsakoff" disorder).

Mixed dementia means that more than one dementia is diagnosed in the same person.

Head trauma can cause a dementia-like illness.

This may happen soon after the head trauma or may not show up for years. Another name is Closed Head Injury (CHI). This can happen after any injury: car accident, falling down, and so on.

This can also happen with professional boxers, years after their professional careers have ended. It is a delayed dementia. A special term is reserved for this type of dementia, *dementia pugilistica*. I have had three professional boxers with this disorder. This dementia seems slightly different in two ways: all three men had significant jealous delusions (jealous of their wives seeing other men) and the disorder seemed to descend into a level corresponding to the mid-stage of Alzheimer's and then not progress so typically below that as in Alzheimer's. In this prolonged phase it seemed to mimic a vascular dementia.

Delirium

Delirium occurs rather suddenly when the patient becomes quite disoriented and has bizarre behavior or sees strange objects, especially late at night (visual hallucinations). This is usually caused by the sudden appearance of a medical disorder, often due to an infection, especially Urinary Tract Infection (UTI) or pneumonia. Oftentimes the delirium can occur in a dementia patient, which makes the diagnosis more difficult since it seems as if the dementia has suddenly worsened. Dementia also occurs with visual hallucinations—but in dementia the visual images increase slowly and become worse gradually over a period of time; they usually start for a while in the middle of the night every night and progressively advance to include most of the dark hours of the day and night. The two likeliest causes of suddenly worsening dementia would be a mini-stroke or an infection. Delirium can be a serious disorder and requires vigorous treatment (which is to correct the medical cause of the delirium). A mini-stroke would require different additional treatment approaches. There is no specific treatment for delirium since it is caused by some other medical event. In other words, the correct treatment is to treat the medical disorder which has caused the delirium. Delirium, by definition, has psychiatric symptoms, but is not a true psychiatric condition such as schizophrenia is. Psychiatrists do not typically see a majority of the delirium cases.

Depression can occur frequently in nursing home patients. There are several sources of depression. Some people have had major depression previously before they became elderly. Although they may have been free of the depression for years, any tumult like placement in a SNF could cause another major depression. Other people may acquire a first episode of major depression late in life due to various causes: the aging brain, socioeconomic problems, divorce, grief, loss through death, bankruptcy, and so on. Older adults cannot bounce back so easily from these problems as can young adults and may develop a first-time major depression. Even though the depression is under medical supervision, any further deterioration in health necessitating a SNF placement can aggravate the underlying depression and it may need higher doses of antidepressants or other medications. Some people with manic-depressive illness may have only had mania during their adult lives, yet they can also have a first episode of major depression under these circumstances—these can be suicidal depressions. Still other people have a depressed adjustment reaction to SNF placement, but gradually come out of that episode in a few weeks. (Also see the chapter on Depression).

Adjustment Reaction is diagnosed when the patient is suddenly placed in a nursing home (against his wishes) and is upset and anxious and depressed. This will usually subside after a month. The adjustment is usually that of a depressed adjustment, but sometimes anxious adjustment can be seen also. (see the beginning of this chapter)

Psychosis can occur also. This is less common. Patients may think that the staff is trying to poison them or they may develop paranoia about roommates or some of the other patients. They may claim that their possessions are being stolen—which is often reality-based and not delusional. Nocturnal hallucinations may occur. These are usually visual hallucinations. In some cases, these may be early signs of dementia, and in other cases, the correlation is less clear.

Miscellaneous behaviors occur occasionally. Hypersexuality is rare, but sexually inappropriate behaviors occur with frequency. This usually just requires redirection or a room change. In some cases, residents re-enact their adolescence. Other kinds of social behavioral problems typical of group living may occur.

Treatment

Treatment from the psychiatric viewpoint involves medications. This is why psychiatrists are called to the SNF. Other treatment modalities are important such as behavior modification and social interventions, but these are undertaken as part of the nursing treatment plan and are arranged in-house.

Medicating Dementia/Alzheimer's disease

There are five medications on the market approved for treatment of Alzheimer's dementia [and vascular dementia]:

- RAZADYNE/REMINYL (GALANTAMINE)
- ARICEPT (DONEPIZIL)
- EXELON (RIVASTIGMINE)
- COGNEX (TACRINE)
- NAMENDA (MEMANTINE)

These medicines have a claimed benefit in improving memory and daily functioning and do so—for a while. The benefits are usually more apparent to the family than to the psychiatrist. In their favor is the fact that patients taking these drugs do show improved numerical scores on memory tests. On the other hand, the drugs may not really be so effective. Studies have shown that the use of these medicines can delay placing a loved one in a SNF by 6-12 months thus allowing her to stay home with the family longer (if that is really what the family wants). These medicines cost upwards of $140 per month and some insurance plans may cover some or all of them. In contrast, staying in a SNF costs thousands of dollars per month.

Delirium

Treatment of Delirium (as previously mentioned) requires identifying the medical cause of the delirium and correcting that medical problem. UTI is a common contributor to delirium in the SNF. The psychiatrist should not even be routinely called to see a delirium—unless it is a confusing clinical presentation.

Depression is often associated with deterioration of the brain in dementia. Remember that the brain function is deteriorating; the brain areas controlling mood and emotion may also deteriorate, and the patient may have decreased level of "brain hormones". Also, all patients are aware to some degree that they are deteriorating and this gives them a sense of depression. Also their living situation often changes, thus posing new challenges which result in an "adjustment disorder with depressed mood". Another possibility is that a mini-stroke has caused a sudden worsening of a mild depression. Current treatment uses standard antidepressant drugs in half doses or even one-third doses. Preferred drugs are Lexapro and Zoloft, but any may be needed, depending upon the whole medical history. Avoid Luvox and Tricyclics (Chapter V-7).

Adjustment Disorders: occur when a person has a reaction to a new situation. It may take the form of anxiety or of depression or mixed symptoms of both. Its presentation depends on two factors: the patient's baseline personality style and the circumstances that resulted in SNF placement. At any rate, these reactions will hopefully clear up within a couple of weeks or months although in some cases the recovery can be much larger. The psychiatrist may prescribe treatments as for anxiety or for depression as above. Short-term use of Ativan may be helpful.

The adjustment disorder usually resolves itself after a month. If a depressed adjustment disorder persists and morphs into a depression, then the patient will need standard treatment for depression. A prolonged anxious adjustment disorder is less common and will often respond well to very low-dose Buspar. (Generally speaking, Ativan should be used short-term only for anxiety.)

Psychosis: symptoms of Agitation, Delusions, and Hallucinations

Symptoms of Psychosis are one of the main reasons that that psychiatrists visit the SNF. Psychosis is certainly the most important reason for a psychiatrist to visit the SNF. The SNF doctors can treat depression with antidepressants and anxiety with Ativan, and the nursing staff can treat patients with behavioral modifications; but neither these doctors or nurses are in the best position to treat a psychosis. These psychotic symptoms are usually part of the Dementia, in other words the diagnosis under treatment is *Alzheimer's with Psychosis*—or psychosis present in another type of dementia. Psychosis poses treatment challenges. Anti-psychotics and anti-manic medications are the current standard of treatment but are not really FDA approved for use in Dementia but these drugs are approved for use in Psychotic states: there is no FDA approved drug for agitation, hallucinations, and delusions in dementia. Since the psychosis is probably caused by the dementia, we try to treat the patient's psychotic symptoms since there is no real targeted treatment for the underlying [cause of the] dementia. Some patients experience so much brain deterioration that they seem to become psychotic in the sense that they are no longer observed to be in good contact with reality. On rarer occasions, the patient might be taking some medical medication that causes the psychosis, in which case the dementia is not causing the psychosis (such as steroids and digoxin, as well as Parkinson's drugs and other stimulants). The usual standard treatment is an antipsychotic, either a first generation antipsychotic, FGA, or a second generation one, SGA. (Chapter V-4)

The so-called atypical anti-psychotics, SGA, might double the risk for a mini-stroke, but this opinion is based on only four clinical trials where normal-acting Alzheimer's patients were compared to psychotic Alzheimer's patients. The normal-acting group was not receiving any antipsychotic. Those of you familiar with statistical analysis will see that this is a flawed conclusion. The FGA antipsychotics are given in very small doses. These can cause Parkinsonism, but the chances of this are not great because these side effects appear after many years and the elderly are exposed to only tiny dosages.

Sometimes when I start a psychotic SNF patient on an antipsychotic medication, the family calls hysterically because they went on-line and found out that Haldol (FGA) might cause Parkinson's or that the "atypical antipsychotics" (SGA) might cause diabetes or stroke. They assume that we have no familiarity with the primary drugs of our specialty and that they have discovered something of which we were unaware. All the antipsychotics can have long-term risk at any age group, but the percentage of these reactions occur much later in therapy—and a dementia patient who is already psychotic does not really have a "much later" timeframe. Sometimes I suggest that the overexcited family members research antipsychotics on-line and let me know which one seems more appealing, so that I can prescribe it. The family needs to orient itself to three salient facts: All these drugs are toxic, dementia is fatal, and the SNF will not keep a screaming patient. Oftentimes, when the SNF nursing staff is caught in this situation, they will send the screaming psychotic patient to a psychiatric hospital by ambulance in the middle of the night. This results in further confusion and disorientation for the patient. Additionally, the hospital will medicate the patient with antipsychotics, anyway. If the family forbids giving antipsychotics in the hospital, then the family could become liable for a large part of the whole hospital bill. Thirdly, the original SNF usually refuses to take that patient back under any circumstances, so the patient ends up "warehoused" in a psychiatric ward awaiting transfer to a second-choice SNF. Then the patient is shuttled off to some other SNF where he is disoriented again and none of the staff knows his background information. And he will definitely end up in a different SNF because hospitals will not keep these patients long-term.

Miscellaneous: Inappropriate Sexuality:

It is not extremely rare to encounter hypersexual men in these placements. An effective treatment is a very low dose of the female hormone, Provera 5 mg. The ethics of this are debatable, but it produces excellent results. The only change is that he becomes appropriate. This is not my favorite treatment, but often the nurses and family implore me to keep him on this treatment. In the case of sexually explicit women, the primary intervention may be done by nursing: moving her to a different ward. If not, she may need a low dose of a mild anti-psychotic or anti-obsessive medication. Male hormones will only serve to make these women more sexual. Treatment-wise, these are difficult situations, but once again, do remember that SNF's have zero tolerance for these behaviors.

Treatment Strategies in Summary

The medication treatment of dementias is based solely on symptoms: anti-anxiety pills for anxiety symptoms, anti-depressants for depressive symptoms, anti-manic or anti-psychotic for bizarre, manic, or uncontrolled psychotic behaviors. The doctor prescribes according to symptom and not according to the underlying cause, dementia, because dementia currently has no cure and no specific treatment either. There is no one specific treatment for each condition, much of it depending on the patient's physical condition, mental and spiritual conditions, medical diagnoses, significant psychiatric problems in the remote past, the patient's drug formulary (the drugs that the HMO will allow), the psychiatrist's philosophy and experience, and so on. Some of the usual and commonest drugs are: Lexapro, Zoloft, Trazodone, Remeron, "memory pills", Depakote, Buspar, Risperdal, Ativan, and Haldol. Although there are five FDA approved dementia drugs on the market, these drugs do nothing for new onset psychiatric symptoms. These drugs help restore some memory functions and IADL's.

The diagnosis and treatment of nursing home patients will continue to evolve. One of the most salient problems that I see is the "institutionality" of the nursing homes: some of them seem uninviting and depressingly institutional. Patients seem to be arranged there in an impersonal setting basically waiting to die—and no matter how psychologically impaired they might be, they mainly seem to sense the utter finality of this place that is their final stop in life. Many must be ruminating about the fact that they have ended up there despite their expressing wishes to the contrary for most of their lives. For a steep price, a less institutional setting can be acquired, but this is financially out of reach for many Americans and will probably be even more unattainable if the future government is overwhelmed with such a huge disabled and invalid population—which at this time seems quite likely, barring any series of catastrophic pandemics.

Perhaps the best treatment of all would be the use of familiar-style modular nursing home units where the patients and staff live and function together in a family-style environment accompanied by a couple cats, a small lapdog, and parakeets. Some institutions are turning to this method apparently with positive results and feedback and are finding that it costs only a little bit more for such a pleasant setting. I shall look forward to visiting those places!

▶QUESTIONS

Q: Will the Vascular Dementia patient continue to deteriorate like an Alzheimer patient going slowly downhill until the end?

A: No. If there are no further strokes or mini-strokes, then the patient's mentality should not deteriorate [so quickly]. The likeliest cause for further deterioration is more strokes and min-strokes.

Q: What are the chances of a second stroke or a cascade of mini-strokes in Vascular Dementia?

A: Quite likely, unless the patient can avoid all the risk factors for a second "vascular event".

Q: Are there any patients who do not have a second stroke?

A: The elderly with known risk factors are likely to have a second mini-stroke. Risk factors are: high cholesterol and high blood pressure (or erratically high blood pressure that spikes frequently).

If the patient is young or middle-aged and had a first stroke due to excess cocaine, "crystal meth", or diet pills and has since now entered twelve steps treatment and has eliminated risk factors then this patient has a better chance of avoiding any strokes for a longer time. This would, however, require lifestyle enhancements, such as regular exercise, weight control, dietary restraint, and control of cholesterol and blood pressure.

Q: So, then, will our parent go on to have memory loss like that seen in Alzheimer's disease?

A: Usually this is so—if the dementing process involves memory areas of the brain.

Q: What is the difference between elderly behavioral disturbance and elderly psychiatric illness? A: I usually use "behavioral disturbance" for patients who have never before seen a psychiatrist in their lives or are having adjustment disorders or situational reactions which strictly speaking are not real psychiatric illnesses but more of a temporary reaction. I usually reserve "psychiatric illness" for those who have had intermittent mental or emotional problems throughout their adult life or are now quite psychotic or delusional or severely melancholic. Usually the difference lies in the number, strength, and kind of psychiatric medicines required: Lexapro for a mild depression; whereas a severe case might require treatment with Risperdal, Depakote and Remeron.

3-ref. 3 pp. 726-7, 2524-6
21- ref. 21 pp. 277 & 632

Chapter VI-7

Impulse Disorders
Impulsivity and Compulsivity

These are some definitions from: *Dorland's **Medical** dictionary:*

- "Impulse" is a "sudden uncontrollable desire to act";
- "Compulsion" is "an irresistible impulse to perform some act contrary to one's better judgment or will".

    Just for comparison, these are the definitions from *Black's **Law** Dictionary:*

- "Impulse" is a "sudden urge or inclination; thrusting or impelling force within a person";
- "Compulsion" is "objective necessity…forcible inducement to the commission of an act…"

The medical dictionary equates an impulse to a desire, whereas the law dictionary equates impulse to impelling force (impulse and impel are the same word roots). Psychiatric experts define impulse as an impulse… Then the medical dictionary defines a compulsion as an impulse—at least this one agrees with the p*sychiatric experts* [3] who offer these definitions:

- Impulse Control Disorders are the "failure to resist an impulse, drive, or temptation to do something or perform some act that is harmful to the person or others" (p.1409).
- Compulsion: "uncontrollable impulse to perform an act repetitively" (p.539).

These definitions all seem a little weak to me; and these are the supreme sources for defining these terms! Seemingly, these are disorders which we have trouble defining and yet we all know what they mean. I have nothing better to offer except my own comments on these two psychiatrically important subjects.

Impulsives

By my definition, people with impulse disorders (whom I call impulsives) are those who are quick to get upset whenever something disagreeable happens to themselves. They typically react without thinking. They seem to have little control over their reactions or over any assaultive behaviors that might immediately ensue. It appears that they lack the ability to stop their angry impulses from bursting out. This does not, however, excuse the behaviors medico-legally (unless the courts find evidence of an "irresistible impulse").

The causes of impulse disorders are not well known. The current theory—which seems rather weak—is that impulsives have a real and inherent lack of ability to control themselves. This lack of ability may come from at least one or more sources: nature, nurture, adverse events during pregnancy, and cultural expectations (societal norms). Causes from nature are presumed to be genetic. Some boys (and girls) are just born with unpleasant behaviors. Causes from "nurture" refer to having a bad childhood in abusive homes. Abused children may grow up to be abusing adults and pass these behaviors down to the next generation, and so on. There are also maternal factors that should not be ignored. Many bad things can happy to a baby in the womb: smoking, alcoholism, street drugs, malnutrition, promiscuity, as well as maternal infections such as viruses and venereal diseases can cause problems. If a mother falls down hard or is abusively hit, this can cause damage. As far as cultureal expectations (societal norms), in some societies, joining youth gangs can be normal [3(p.661)]. This could also depend upon one's definition of a "gang"

Teenage boys normally congregate, and any of these are technically a "gang". This theory of "cultural expectations" seems rather weak because it offers some casual observations but no real biochemical explanations or evidence of genetic underpinnings. Theories notwithstanding, the reality is that impulsive people can be violent and unpredictable.

Impulsive personality styles usually start at a very young age and remain as permanent personality traits. The intensity of the styles might gradually wane with time. Provided that the patients live that long. By the very nature of the condition, there is a certain amount of associated fatality because impulsive people are risk-takers. Injuries and death are part and parcel of these personalities by the very definition of impulsiveness. People with extreme forms of these personality styles often run aground of society and its laws. They may perish in their teens and twenties. Compulsive Disorders often seem to worsen with time. Impulsivity seems to exist along a spectrum ranging from never-impulsive to almost-always-impulsive:

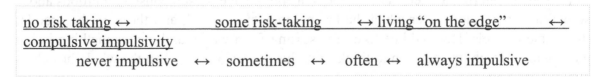

no risk taking ↔   some risk-taking   ↔ living "on the edge"   ↔
compulsive impulsivity
            never impulsive   ↔   sometimes   ↔   often ↔   always impulsive

Some people are natural born risk-takers and impulsively act out whatever comes into their minds. Often without studied purpose, they will simply leap into some activity that could be perilous. On the other hand, some people are very restrained and aloof and rarely take risks. Indeed their idea of taking a major risk might be a two week cruise across the Pacific Ocean or investing in the stock market. The average person is not a big risk-taker as a child. However around the time of puberty, teenagers—especially boys—will become much more ambitious, reactive, and impulsive. Accidents are the number one cause of death of teenage boys. This behavior gradually tapers down within a number of years. If it does not taper off, then it could become a genuine impulse disorder—especially if the risk-taker becomes "addicted" to the adrenaline rushes from risky and daring behaviors.

The usual kinds of impulse disorders are not violent. These four diagnoses include:

- Kleptomania: compulsive stealing, usually from stores, and often in a ritualistic way: these may be useful, non-useful, or unneeded items, the importance is that the item is a token in the ritual.

- Compulsive gambling

- Hair-pulling (possibly with eating the hair)

- Self-mutilation: cigarette burns on the body, superficial cutting of skin (a prominent symptom of Borderline Syndrome, Chapter IV-6 (Self-mutilation also occurs during extreme psychosis and in the very rare Lesch-Nyhan Disease—but differs from a merely anxious compulsion)

These following two impulse disorders, however, are violent and endanger other people:

- Pyromania: This is Arson.

- Raging and Explosive Anger ("road rage") as exhibited repetitively and habitually as part of one's basic behavior

Compulsives

The compulsive behaviors of OCD (Obsessive-Compulsive Disorder) is believed to stem from an internal anxiety state. In OCD, a compulsive person constantly broods about something (obsession) over which he has no apparent control, and the more he broods, the worse he feels. He could be free of obsessing for a while, and then something in his environment might trigger him to think about his obsession, and then the whole brooding cycle starts again.

These broodings are called obsessions. The more that a person obsesses, the more pressing the obsessions become. The obsessive anxiety is a pressure that builds up like steam. In order to relieve the anxiety of the obsession, the OCD patient needs to complete an anxiety-relieving act. This is his compulsion. This cycle of obsessing and releasing anxiety with a compulsive act is repetitive. Psychiatrists call this the ritual and neurologists sometimes refer to it as a "complex tic". Whatever it is called, it releases the pressure that has built up from the obsessions.

Obsessions are intrusive unwanted thoughts that keep on haunting a person until he finally gives in to the thoughts and performs a compulsive act. The only way to appease the obsessive thoughts is to give in and perform the compulsion, which is often more like a ritual. Failure to perform the compulsion creates unpleasant anxiety in the obsessive person until he performs his compulsive act. This act relieves the internal obsessive tension but not for long. When the obsessions become too intrusive and are counterproductive and result in ritualistic compulsive behaviors that lack any benefit, then we can diagnose obsessions and compulsions of clinical significance. The litmus test is whether these thoughts and behaviors are beneficial or maladaptive and how much they detract from or intrude into the person's quality of life.

I like to differentiate OCD from Obsessive-Compulisve personality (OCP) and just plain obsessiveness. OCD is obviously a disorder. Briefly speaking, OCP is like a hard-core workaholic. Obsessiveness is the conscious ability to force oneself voluntarily to be responsible. This is not OCD and perhaps a minor version of OCP, but is not pathologic; indeed, these are responsible and dutiful people who make themselves perform excellently. A little obsessiveness is beneficial since it propels a person to do what needs to be done now and not to put it off until later. It would be an understatement to say that obsessiveness propels medical students through the rigors of medical training and law students through the gamut of legal training. In these cases, obsessiveness helps people to keep up with schedules (or even ahead of schedule), to plan ahead, to show up on time consistently, and to plan ahead for putting up with a lot of perceived adversity. This behavior is then adaptive and beneficial, and most medical students do not suffer from OCD or a serious case of OCP, either.

Table VI-7-a	OCD	OCP	Obsessiveness
Self-Control over his action?	No Involuntary	No Involuntary	Yes Voluntary
Resulting Actions	Repetitions Rituals	perfectionism, hoarding, stubbornness, stinginess	High Achievement Excellence, Success
character	overanxious	rigid workaholic	responsible, dutiful
Purpose of Action	Relieve stress	Control	Success in life
Flexible-changeable?	NO!!	likes his daily routine and forces it on others	Can change in order to excel/succeed

The reader can see from Table VI-7-a, that these three obsessives are really quite different, although there can be a spectrum, too. Some people with OCP might be a little OCD, or some medical students might be closer to OCP than just mere obsessiveness. Some people might want control, success in life, and stress relief. Other combinations are possible.

Obsessions and compulsions are thought to be related to altered serotonin levels in the brain; the evidence is empirical (based on experience and casual observations) in the sense that serotonin-activating drugs help suppress the obsessions and hence decrease the need to act out the compulsions. Examples of the symptoms of obsessive-compulsive disorder are many but include such behaviors as:

- —constant obsession with germs, resulting in constant hand-washing so that hands become dried out;

- —leaving home and returning home two minutes later to check and see if the doors are closed and doing this several times, resulting in tardiness in arriving at main destination;

- —certain meaningless rituals (or at lest meaningless to onlookers). Performing the ritual gives emotional relief to the patient (reduces stress and ánxiety). (See Chapter VI-7.)

Obsessions		Compulsions
Did I turn off the stove? I think I checked it 5 minutes ago but I can't remember—I should go back and check it...	→	Go back once to check
	←	Go back twice to check
I know I checked it 10 minutes ago, but I was so anxious	→	Going back every 5 minutes
About going back to check it that I can't remember	←	"I forgot if I checked it..."
If the stove was on or off...	↔	
		and so back and forth
(remember that OCD is a type of anxiety disorder)		

VI-7-b   OCD (Obsessive Compulsive Disorder)

There are some OCD patients who mainly have the persistent obsessive thoughts and almost never act on them (obsessions without compulsions)—usually because the compulsion is dangerous or socially repugnant or downright illegal. These obsessions can build up for a very long time. If these patients become sufficiently disinhibited (by alcohol), then they might act out—usually with devastating consequences.

The kinds of Compulsive Disorders are several: OCD is well-known (Obsessive-Compulsive Disorder). Alcoholism is a compulsive behavior. Over-eating, over-shopping and over-spending (cluttering and hoarding) are also compulsive behaviors.

Try to think of alcoholism in this compulsive light. After alcoholics have been drunk and done something socially unacceptable or repugnant, then they feel great remorse, and start to have two obsessions: one obsession about what they have just done (remorse anxiety), and a second obsession about what they might do next if they get drunk again (anticipatory anxiety). As the day wears on, they will then have a third obsession of where to get the next drink (next-drink anxiety). These are the past, present, and future anxiety obsessions. Since alcoholics are obsessed with putting the liquid drug alcohol into their bodies, then they have an ever-present obsession with alcohol. Unlike OCD patients who do not take chemicals, alcoholics rely on an addicting chemical. Thus, their present obsession is also their addiction anxiety. There is great likelihood that they will do another repugnant act while drunk and thus perpetuate the cycle of past remorse anxiety needing present treatment amidst uncontrollable anticipatory anxiety of what they might do next, in the future, when they drink again.

Remorse anxiety occurs after a black out. A hard-drinking alcoholic while very drunk can have black outs for which he has no memory on the next morning An alcoholic may wake up the next morning in a strange place with a strange person. Or after he comes to, he might notice that his car's front bumper has a big blood-stained dent on it. Just think of all the anxiety that accompanies the morning after a black out! After routinely going through these cycles, alcoholics end up with multiple sources of anxiety: remorseful past memories, present addictive anxiety, and future anticipatory anxiety, as well as unremembered blacked-out past happenings and their possible present or future repercussions.

OCD patients know that their OCD symptoms (or alcohol cravings) are alien. Impulse patients do not think about this at all. Compulsive people can resist the temptation for indefinite periods: minutes, hours, years. They have internal control that will eventually let down its guard.

Impulsive people cannot resist the temptation and give in to almost immediately. Alcohol can further lower inhibitions in all impulsive and compulsive people. Alcohol can make compulsives impulsive, and impulsives, explosive.

Diagram VI-7-c   *Impulsives and Compulsives*

Disorder	External Trigger▶	Internal Source or Cause of Anxiety	Self-control	Resulting Behavior Problem
Impulsive 💣	**External Stimulus** 🌐▶	**Lack of INHIBITION** 1-genetic factors 2-maternal factors* 3-bad childhood (abuse) 4-cultural norms ▶→	–<u>None</u>– *no Internal Defenses* ▶→	**Immediate** (angry speech or bad deeds) 🗣💣
Compulsive 🔒🗝🔓	**External Stimulus** 🌐▶	**OBSESSIONS** from an unknown Cause ▶→	–<u>Yes</u>– ↻ Natural brakes ↗	**Delayed** (Rituals) 🕐 ⇤
	-or-	*Internal Stimulus* ↰☐⇢☐⇢☐		
Alcoholic Compulsive 🍸 *Diagram VI-7-c*	**External Stimulus** 🌐▶ ↯	**OBSESSIONS** over: 1-PAST deeds (<u>remorse</u>) 2-PRESENT situation: (Alcohol <u>addiction</u>) 3-FUTURE in general (<u>anticipatory anxiety</u>) ▶ →⇉	–<u>Some</u>– ↘ ⇒ ↪ ⇈ ⤵ *Weak Internal Defenses*	**Impending** ❗ (Loss of Control over Behavior) 🚓
	-and-	*Internal Cravings* ⇢☐⇢☐→⇉		

⇢ *is a weaker driving force than a solid arrow*

☐ *obsessions and ideas percolate around in a person's mind without causing action*

▶ *a stress factor from the environment*

⇤ *action is blocked in all directions*

? *outcome of actions can be unknown (?) or "exciting" (!)*

() *a number of repetitive acts is likely*

Impulsives: *a negative environmental stimulus can set this person off and he has little control over his behaviors*

*(maternal factors could include adverse events occurring while the impulsive patient was in the womb: maternal factors such as smoking, drinking, street drugs, poor nutrition, promiscuity, and infections such as viral or venereal disease)

Compulsives: *can be stimulated from the environment or just from inside themselves; they have ritualized behaviors such as checking that the door is locked, the stove is turned off, and a thousand more. Presumably, they have an anxiety disorder (OCD) of unknown causes. They can put off their rituals or "divert" them (⋯→) for brief while or for a long time. Until they do perform their ritual, the obsession is going around and around in their minds (⟳)*

Compulsive Alcoholics *can be set off by the environment; or if they see people drinking alcohol nearby, they can receive a powerful desire to drink (⚡) that sets off their internal cravings. The cravings to drink can be put off for a certain period of time, but the cravings increase in intensity (⇉) until the obsession to drink is compulsively realized.*

The actual causes of impulsivity and compulsivity are unknown. Compulsives will come forward and join in clinical trials because they are uncomfortable with their compulsions. They are often desperate for treatment. Impulsive people, on the other hand, do not routinely come forward voluntarily. Some researchers argue that impulsive disorders are closely linked to compulsive disorders. Compulsives can upon occasion demonstrate impulsivity in their compulsions. And, some impulsives can be compulsive about their disorders, too.

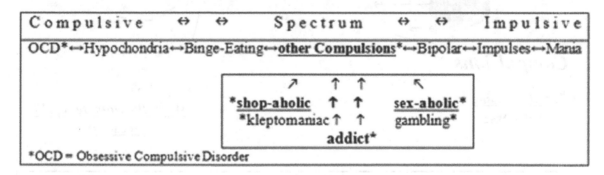

Figure VI-7-d Compulsive-Impulsive Spectrum (Hollander and Wong)[26] showing that shop-aholics are slightly more compulsive, whereas sex-aholics are more impulsive(Other Compulsions)

Diagram VI-7-c shows that Obsessive-Compulsives are relatively the most compulsive, and that Mania and "Personality Styles" (especially Antisocial Personalities and Borderlines) are relatively the most impulsive. The whole point of the diagram is to show that even very impulsive people can have a small amount of compulsive behavior and vice versa,

Impulsivity, Compulsivity, Impulsive Compulsivity

Impulsivity is a sudden desire to something without any warning and despite known hazards. Impulsivity might give the risk-taker a thrill or an adrenaline rush (like bungee jumping). The suddenness could be over the space of one second or a couple hours.

Compulsive behavior is a constant nagging desire to perform an act. This occurs when the person has a long-standing inner desire (obsession) to do this act. That inner obsessive desire nags and gnaws at him internally until he performs that compulsive act. Once he had done the act, then he feels calm and relieved. Impulses arise suddenly, are discharged, and then are gone. Unlike an impulse, a [compulsive] obsession is always present to some degree. Either an outer or an inner trigger will cause it to grow and grow until it can no longer be denied, and the obsession pops up as a compulsion. Performing that act will relieve him of his inner tension. A compulsion is the follow-through of an internal obsession.

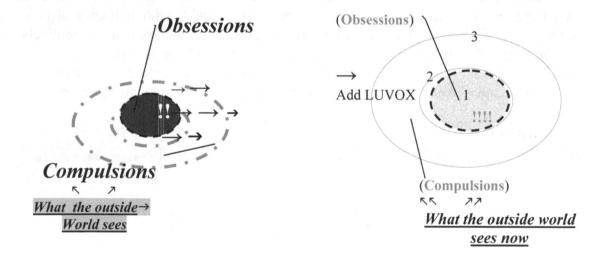

| Diagram VI-7-e-(i) | | Obsessions and Compulsions | | | Diagram VI-7-e-(ii) |
| Before Treatment | → | → | → | → | → | After Treatment |

In this diagram we can see that the obsessions ("!!") are inside and drive outwardly seen compulsions ("→") which come streaming out of him in the form of checking, counting, and other

rituals. An example of this is an obsession about being dirty: the compulsion is constant hand washing which can be so compulsive that the person's hands become very chapped—perhaps to the point of needing care from a dermatologist. Other obsessions center around safety. In safety obsession, an OCD patient is constantly checking the lock on the front door or constantly checking to make sure that the stove is turned off. Another compulsive behavior occurs when a person drives over a speed bump or tree bough and thinks that he ran over an animal or a person. He needs to drive back and re-check that—and may need to drive back a couple times to reconfirm his first impression. With medication, the intensity of the obsessions can decrease a lot (black to light gray), the compulsions will stop (arrows stop) compulsions diminish a lot (black to gray).

These patients may well be "serotonin-sensitive"; they could benefit from drugs that raise serotonin levels because such drugs:

1   *can suppress some or all the core obsessions, shown as action "1" above;*
2   *can decrease the obsessional driving of the [ritualized] compulsions, "2";*
3   *might help the patient exert some voluntary control to suppress and prevent the compulsions from externalizing and being viewed by the "outside world", action "3" above.*

In diagram VI-7-f we can see that the obsessions are always down there brooding and stirring about, eventually bursting forth as a compulsive act or ritual. Impulses can erupt suddenly without forethought and can be provoked by some internal factor ♥ or some outer stress ▦.

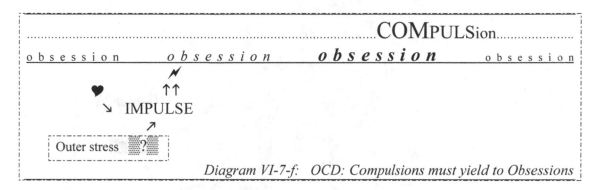

Diagram VI-7-f: OCD: Compulsions must yield to Obsessions

In this next diagram VI-7-g, we can appreciate the following:

- *A central lack of brain dopamine makes Joe feel miserable and restless. (symptom)*

- *A central lack of brain serotonin (presumably according to current theories) allows Joe to brood   and worry and obsess. (symptom)*

- *This obsession can only be relieved by Joe's acting out the obsession which then becomes Joe's compulsion. This act is a physical sign that alerts us to the fact that he has an unchecked obsession.*

- *The compulsion serves no real purpose but once it is acted out, then Joe will feel relieved.*

- *Rings of adrenaline are released when stimulated by an (external) impulse.*

- *The diagram also shows that this person is not "centered". A serotonin drug can sometimes "re-center" the person.*

- *Impulses are not the central issue but can be major problems with devastating results.*

- *Chronic anxiety is shown by the blank spaces between gray rings.*

- *Joe is full of internal anxiety and is drowning in an ocean of anxiety that surrounds him,*

- *Joe is stumbling over other psychiatric symptoms such as adjustment problems, social phobia, and self-medication with alcohol (or drugs).*

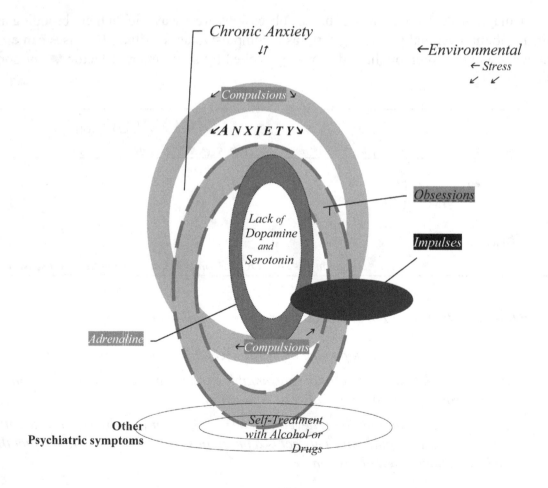

Treatments

Impulsivity

Impulsivity Treatment needs to be preventive, and it can be individual preventive treatment (pills), group therapy (men's group), or group protective preventive treatment ("extra-societal isolation"). Impulsive patients rarely refer themselves for treatment for no reason. They usually come in only when they are in trouble at work, at home, or with the courts. They are also often disappointed to hear that impulsivity is not a legal defense. There is little in the way of specific treatments.

As far as medications, the anti-epilepsy drugs (AED's) are sometimes helpful to tone down the intensity of the impulsivity. This would include notably Depakote as a first line but "off-label" treatment. Sometimes Buspar can be helpful for the anxiety. If the impulsivity is accompanied by significant aggression ("road rage") and so on, then Zyprexa might be helpful. For insomnia, use of Vistaril is rational.

Some patients with impulsivity are very explosive, intense, and emotionally always "on the edge". They need to stimulate themselves with impulsivity because they feel "under-aroused". Raising their serotonin levels might make them worse. (Consider drugs like Depakote or Zyprexa). These people are "serotonin-resistant".

Some impulsive people have a lack of inhibition in the sense that they blurt out embarrassing statements, perform miscued acts without forethought, and so on (this can also be found in ADHD and Tourette's). They always seem anxious and restless in social situations because they are completely aware of what they will do, and yet seem powerless to stop themselves from acting and speaking impulsively. They may well be "serotonin-sensitive"; they could benefit from drugs that raise serotonin levels because such drugs:

- can suppress some or all the core obsessions;

- can decrease the obsessional driving of the [ritualized] compulsions;

- might help the patient exert some voluntary control to suppress and prevent the compulsions from externalizing and being viewed by the "outside world";.

- compulsivity can be a personality trait, personality style, or full-blown Obsessive Compulsive Disorder (OCD). The difference depends basically upon the number of symptoms and how disabling they are.

CAVEATS: Do not give these following drugs to impulsive people:
- stimulants such as amphetamines or Ritalin will stimulate the aggression and make it worse

- sedatives in the Valium family will "disinhibit" the impulsive person—he will become less inhibited which means that he will have even less self-control (provided that he had any to start with); this caveat applies to Klonopin and all Schedule IV sedative-hypnotics.

Group therapy may include required attendance at men's anger groups or AA or other types of court-approved treatment.

"Extra-societal Isolation" amounts to incarceration for repeat offenders (recidivists). Incarceration for repeated impulsive violence is not necessarily an indictment of the characters of impulsive people, but rather an acknowledgement that they lack self-control over external events. Since there is no specific or highly effective treatment, a controlled environment becomes a rational treatment. Hence, external events are controlled in prison and their symptoms will not harm others.

Avoidance of chemicals that are known to cause or aggravate aggression is important. The two best known causes of aggravated rage are alcohol and body-building drugs (steroids, and others).

Compulsive Disorders: OCD

It is observed that drugs which restore balance to serotonin levels in the brain have a therapeutic effect on obsessions, usually by suppressing the obsessions so that the compulsions need not be heeded and sometimes by decreasing the obsession and blocking the compulsion. Beneficial drugs include Anafranil, Nardil, as well as Luvox and other SSRI drugs.

Since Alcoholism and the other compulsive behaviors have an element of compulsiveness—but are not diagnosed as Obsessive-Compulsive Disorder—there may be some benefit in using Serotonin drugs if the alcoholic becomes very anxious and somewhat depressed.

OCD is conceptualized as a serious anxiety disorder that responds rather well to the following types of medications with:

- strong serotonin activity: Anafranil, Luvox, Nardil

- moderate serotonin activity: Paxil, Imipramine, and others

- mild serotonin activity combined with other pharmacologic effects: Zyprexa, Seroquel, Abilify, Geodon, possibly Loxitane

Hair twisting and pulling (or eating) is a common type of impulsive behavior seen in the suburbs. (It is called trichotillomania).

Compulsive Alcoholism—whether it has these compulsive features, the treatment has been elaborated in Chapter VI-1.

Compulsive Overeaters, Over-spenders, Debtors (clutterers and hoarders): there are Twelve Step meetings available as well as a trial of serotonin drugs (which may have varying degrees of effectiveness).

▶**QUESTIONS**
_____

Q: When does impulsivity become a psychiatric disorder?

A: When the impulsivity is causing an abnormally unbearable amount of stress in the person's life. Also read the chapter on Insanity as Medical Defense

Q: Are there any medical treatments for impulsivity?

A: No. A number of medicines might be helpful but there is none specifically designed to treat this problem.

▶Obsessions drive the compulsions.

~Impulses interact with obsessions.

▶Other peripheral problems can be environmental stress issues.

Impulsivity, Compulsivity, and Relating to Reality

This is a special small section on verbalizations regarding the telling of untruths, falsehoods, fibs, prevarications, white lies, and so on.

Honest person...little white lie (fibbing)....Sociopathic liar.......Impulsive liar.....Compulsive liar
....(4)............(1)................(2)................(3)..........

(1)-**sociopaths** (antisocials) and personality disordered people will tell lies to get what they want. This is not a thought disorder, it is just plain chicanery, grifting, and swindling. It is premeditated, deliberate, and intended to extract undeserved goods from others.

(2.)-Another condition is impulsive lying. Although most people tell little fibs sometimes, and these fibs are impulsive, that does not make us (compulsively) impulsive liars. Some people are compulsively **impulsive liars**. This is a personal problem for them, and support groups have been set up for them. When faced with a reality, they want to appear better off—or more authoritative— than they are and impulsively will rapidly blurt out a white lie without much forethought and with so much confidence and conviction that they seem totally believable, probably due to the quickness of the blurted out claim. These are entirely plausible events but are known to be untrue to the impulsive liar. The claims are credible to the listener.

3.)-Beyond impulsive liars are the **compulsive liars** who have a psychological problem. They love to tell grandiose, incredible, and highly embellished stories that have no real purpose apart from entertaining themselves and their listeners who in the normal course of hearing the tall tales realize that much of the incredible story is fabricated and could not possibly have really happened. These compulsive liars do not have a real ulterior motive apart from that of ventilating a kind of internalized frustration which serves as a type of "psychic catharsis" (mental cleansing) and is a way for them to relieve this gnawing internal compulsive desire. After they have their say, they feel better but yearn to spin more long yarns that will go on and on—the psychological mechanism resembles that of other compulsive behaviors, such as compulsive sexuality, shopping or gambling. They like to go on and on until they feel relieved. The proper term for the compulsive liar is "pseudologia phantastica", which means fantastically false speech! Baron von Münchhausen had this compulsive problem, although the psychiatric syndrome named after him is rather different—see chapter on chronic pain.]

(4.)-"Selective Tale-tellers": Some people like to exaggerate their importance, or indeed have grand ideas of where they fit in the scheme of the universe. They do this to impress others. Their stories have a sizable basis in reality, but they build up the good parts of the story and eliminate any annoying detracting details. This is essentially a personality trait of grandiosity. It can occur in people who have narcissistic traits.

5.) Late-stage alcoholics appear also to make false statements. Alcohol consumption has caused multiple memory lapses or losses. This can happen in two ways: either the alcohol destroys some of their memories or they have no retrievable memory due to blackouts. The mind strives to fill in blanks to account for the memory blanks. In a third possibility, they mistakenly retrieve memories from a non-black-out evening and substitute that memory as if it were a registered memory from the black-out night.

6.) People with serious brain disorders may lose contact with reality. They may unwittingly fabricate all sorts of false statements and false realities, which they believe to be true. This can happen in delirium, schizophrenia, mania, psychotic depression, and dementia (like Alzheimer's dementia).

Chapter VI-8

HIV and the Brain (AIDS)
(HIV is a Chronic Brain Infection)

Introduction

Let us start out with quotes from Kaplan and Sadock:

"HIV is a lethal neuro-medical disorder...No other epidemic of the 20th century has been associated with as much social stigmatization and political interchange as has HIV...HIV tends to produce disease in the central nervous system (brain)....",
Kaplan and Sadock, p.1644: these are other various quotations from their book:

1   *CAT scan studies [of the brain] have revealed cerebral atrophy (brain shrinkage) in the majority of AIDS patients (p.1673).*

2   *Rates of depression rated as 25-35%, "in majority of [HIV] cases, "with some studies suggesting that in the majority of cases, the first major depression preceded the likely date of seroconversion [turning positive and getting the HIV diagnosis]", p.1660.*

3   *All types of neuropsychiatric symptoms can appear: mental slowing, impaired memory, in-coordination (clumsiness), personality changes, irritability, mental and behavioral abnormalities causing mild impairment of work and activities of daily living...(p.1671).*

4   *Decreased performance on IQ tests is usually related also to slow performance (p.1674); decreased performance from HIV is also often noted in other neurological tests, such as mathematical impairment, which is one of the earliest neurological problems (early detection with the "Paced Auditory Serial Addition Test", p. 1675).*

5   *Visuo-spatial abilities may decline (hand-eye coordination problems): problems in copying figures, completing drawings, p.1675.*

6   *Poorer scores on memory tests, and "complaints of difficulties with memory are ubiquitous [most HIV patients experience symptoms of memory problems, possibly*

575

from bradyphrenia ("slow brain")] p.1675.

Some authors have determined that the prevalence of Depression in HIV disease is the same as the rates in non-HIV gay men and injectable drug-addicts (*4-14%,* Dr. Rabkin). Other authors have concluded that there is more Depression in the HIV population than in non-infected groups.

POINT

Dr. Rabkin's study* shows that:

"The majority of HIV-infected people with current depressive disorders have a history of depression that [precedes] HIV infection, and depression is not correlated with disease stage, T-cells...or HIV medication...." Rabkin PhD, Judith, Depressive Disorder and HIV Disease, 1995).

MIDPOINT

"...25 to 35% [are depressed]...but a majority might have had depression prior to turning HIV- positive" (Kaplan and Sadock)

"Depending on how depression is defined and on the population being studied (teens, adults, men, women, gays or lesbians, and drug-addicts or not), the prevalence of depression has ranged from **10-50%.** *Even if the lowest estimates are accurate, depression remains one of the most common conditions seen in...HIV." Capaldini MD, Lisa, and Harrison MD, George. "Overcoming Depression,* San Francisco AIDS Foundation, *Winter 2003-004,www.thebody.com The Complete HIV/AIDS Resource.*

COUNTERPOINT

About 5% to 10% of the general population gets depressed. However, rates of depression in people with HIV are as high as **60%***..." AIDSinfonet.org, October 14, 2008.*

HIV as well as some of the medicines used to treat HIV can affect brain function. Memory problems, confusion, slowed thinking, problems talking, changes in mood and behavior and other problems can greatly affect quality of life and complicate HIV treatment. Some of these problems can be improved or reversed with treatment." Womenshealth.gov: www. hhs.gov, March 4, 2009.

"A diagnosis of HIV/AIDS usually precipitates some form of an...inter-personal crisis. When the person who has HIV/AIDS is a doctor, the... distress is compounded...Adding to the psychosocial distress of physicians with HIV is their inability to utilize the existing supports of community-based organizations." The Journal of the International Association of Physicians in AIDS Care, Volume 2, No. 11, November 1996 © Michael Shernoff.

AUTHOR'S Observations and Commentary

Psychiatric havoc wrought by HIV/AIDS can be overwhelming or even insurmountable in some cases. In the insurmountable cases, death by suicide or by parasuicidal behaviors was not rare at the beginning of the epidemic (1980's-1990's), but has been slowly replaced by a smoldering sense of hope in the last decade and a half—ever since the initiation of the use of HAART (Highly Active Anti-retroviral Therapy). Notwithstanding, the commonest psychiatric disturbances still seem to be anxiety and depression, followed in third place by medication side effects.

ANXIETY Issues

There are many sources of Anxiety:
- anxiety about death and dying;
- anxiety about abandonment by friends and family;
- anxiety about being alone (as in "not in a relationship")
- anxiety about self-esteem issues;
- anxiety about social stigmatization;
- anxiety about being a possible vector of contagion;
- anxiety about trying to start new (amatory) relationships
- anxiety about getting a second equally bad relationship-related disease such as
- herpes, Hepatitis C, and so on;
- low self-esteem from muscle wasting in chronic HIV; and,
- anxiety about physical defects caused by Protease Inhibitor drugs, resulting in further self-esteem (and vanity) issues.

The anxiety about death and dying is less than it was at the beginning of the epidemic when life expectancy was quite short. Young and middle-aged men had to deal with wills and trusts and other legal documentation deemed necessary by a responsible person who was expecting to die soon. This whole psychodrama was well documented in the movie *The Living End*.

Anxiety about abandonment and loss of relationships. When a person first announces his HIV-positive status to friends and family, there are sometimes unexpected responses: some will feel more nurturing and caring, some may withdraw, some may be outraged and cancel all connections to the HIV sufferer, and some may have not much one response one way or the other.

Becoming a modern leper is not likely to be an esteem-bolstering happenstance. Social and occupational stigmatization still happens nowadays, albeit at a more surreptitious level [than in the movie *Philadelphia*, 1993].

It is difficult to forge a new relationship armed with the knowledge that this is in effect a fatal venereal disease. Anyone who tries to enter a relationship with an HIV positive person is at high risk of contracting a fatal disease. However, it has been noted that a small percentage of Northern Europeans have resistance to the virus: they lack the necessary "docking site" on their T-lymphocytes, and thus the virus cannot infect them. Contrary to all the odds, I knew a young woman who was in a relationship with an HIV-infected ex-IV-drug addict (heterosexual). A couple years into the relationship, he was retested and was negative; she then left him!

Another odd case is that of a young man who had had an apparent "false" positive test for HIV, and after taking the HAART (Highly Active Anti-Retroviral Therapy) medications for some years, his labs were so good that he had himself re-tested and discovered that he was no longer HIV-positive. He then sued his former treating doctor! The whole point of these stories is that no venereal epidemic has so devastated a country [USA], since half a millennium ago when syphilis appeared in Europe resulting also in much sociologic chaos.

The anxiety of HIV seems to fluctuate, at times culminating in mini-panic states that often resolve within days. Usually, the best treatment is group therapy, individual psychotherapy, and SSRI antidepressants: if he is already on antidepressants, then continue the same dose or adjust it slightly.

DEPRESSION Issues

There are many sources of Depression associated with HIV and AIDS. These are the main Depression groups:

- Pre-existing Depression (which may include additional depressive symptoms as in A and B below):
- Depression related to the physical presence of the AIDS virus lodged in the brain and any physical damage that it might cause to the brain;

- Depression related to adjusting to a new life situation with serious revision of life plans and goals from a "five-year plan" to a month-by-month plan (in many cases);

- General Apathy that is defined as *"lack of feeling, emotion; indifference" (Dorland's)* varying degrees of loss of interest in life and one's surroundings and diminished concerns about the well-being of oneself or of others.

- Depression related to side-effects of the many new medications,

- Distress about the costs of medicines (as much as $5,000 per month),

- sense of stigmatization and fear of public recognition at the pharmacy; and,

- Grief and bereavement related to deaths and funerals of friends.

Discussion:

Pre-existing Depression: Most cultures of the world persecute gayness and may censure it with imprisonment or death. Little wonder that gay teenagers are tormented about being gay; at first, they may internalize the perceived hatred that society has for them—in other words, they take this socio-emotional miasma into their thought-life, and may start to hate themselves for involuntarily being members of one of the most hated minorities in the world. This is called ego-dystonic homosexuality. "Ego-dystonic" refers to having negative emotions about a subject: a person is at odds with his ego. Gay teenagers begin to understand that they will need to work much harder to reach personal goals. Adjustment to life will be much harder than for their heterosexual counterparts. Fortunately, gay men are able to bond tightly to each other and form support systems. Some teenagers become dysthymic (miserably unhappy) about this whole process and situation as they then begin to appreciate that their lives are not going to be "normal" in any way. This is called a depressive adjustment reaction. (This can even cascade into a suicidal depression.) This reaction can be common in and throughout high school years. It should resolve upon entering college and finding a new support group, the gay family. If this sad depressive reaction persists for years after high school and through college, then it is most likely a permanent minor depression ("secondary dysthymia"). Gay men who are already dysthymic (depressed chronically) will likely develop a second type of depression upon learning that they are HIV-infected. This will probably be a major depression superimposed upon the dysthymia. Previously non-depressed gay men who turn HIV-positive may develop a depressive adjustment reaction, secondary dysthymia, or major depression. Any of them may be likely to self-treat depression symptoms with alcohol. Hopefully, the situation will be just an adjustment reaction and resolve with time. As recently as fifteen years ago, the HIV diagnosis was a death sentence, and death usually ensued apace. Nowadays, HIV diagnosis is perceived as a chronic manageable condition, and young gay men seem to be throwing caution to the wind, as evidenced by a high prevalence of "bare backing" (sex without condoms).

Depression related to a chronic incurable brain infection. This subject has been debated for years. Different studies show some similar and dissimilar conclusions. There is usually little debate that a chronic infection of the brain must have some neuro-psychiatric symptoms.

Depressive Adjustment Disorder can occur whenever a person reacts to a life-stress event with depressive symptoms, such as sadness, disappointment, and the specter of multiple losses: loss of life, reputation, social status, love, money, goals, ambitions, dreams, jobs, aspirations, health, friends, lovers, and homes. Who wouldn't be depressed?!

Medication side effects of AIDS drugs plus a number of other drugs, which might need to be taken with the AIDS, drugs either to prevent secondary problems or secondary side effects.

- Some of the primary AIDS drugs have different side effects in different patients: this is just what happens in the general population, too. Some cardiac patients can tolerate one drug that others cannot. Sometimes, the specific AIDS drug must be taken due to certain individual case differences. Some of the HIV medicines can cause liver and/or pancreas damage, anemia, and permanent foot numbness. HIV positive patients who are in a Twelve Step program may want to avoid any drug compounded as an elixir (containing measurable amounts of alcohol). Viracept can cause mania.

- Secondary drugs are used to prevent problems that commonly occur as complications in AIDS (like Bactrim for Pneumocystis pneumonia) or antifungal medicines. Some people have nausea from Bactrim or Sporanox.

- "Side effect" drugs are used to try to counteract the unpleasant side effects of any HIV medications which must be taken and for which there is no substitute available. Such drugs might be used to prevent diarrhea, headaches, foot pain, and so on.

- Side effects from necessary psychiatric medications

FATAL HIV-AIDS PSYCHIATRIC CONDITIONS:

These are all rapidly progressive and lethal. They all have serious neuro-psychiatric symptoms.

Fatal Neuro-psychiatric condition *caused directly* by AIDS virus: ARDC (Dementia)
"In full-blown AIDS, the brain infection becomes overwhelming and causes a Dementia. This is also known as ARDC, AIDS Related Dementia Complex. It may happen in 20-40% of AIDS patients. ARDC is usually a preterminal event: expected survival rate after ARDC is diagnosed is quite short, possibly as little as six months. Hospice placement may be advisable.

ARDC is a much more aggressive and lethal dementia than Alzheimer's Dementia or post-Stroke dementia".

These quotes are from "AIDS Dementia Complex", Project Inform January 2007, (www.thebody.com):

"While it is clear that HIV can cause serious nervous system disorder, how it causes ARDC is unclear: Three recognized stages of ARDC:
Early stage symptoms: slowing of actions and thoughts, depression, mild loss of coordination, memory problems, irritability;
Middle stage symptoms: muscle weakness, general apathy, and further decline in all the early stage symptoms;
Late stage symptoms: psychotic, manic, bedridden, and spastic."

Fatal Neuro-psychiatric conditions *associated with* AIDS

PML (progressive multifocal leukoencephalopathy) This represents the re-awakening of a virus that is already in the brains of normal people (polyomavirus). Non-HIV patients have natural immunity; AIDS lowers immunity to the virus. It is a dire diagnosis with at least half so affected expected to live not much more than six months.

Brainstem lymphoma: Lymphomas are cancers of the lymphatic system (the AIDS virus likes to hole up in lymph cells). These are very difficult to treat and are obviously accompanied by a lot of neuropsychiatric symptoms. (The brainstem connects the brain to the rest of the body. Brainstem disease is as bad as a short circuit of an electrical system.)

Cancer: spread of AIDS-related Cancer to the Brain (from some other part of the body where the cancer originated as an "opportunist").

Fatal Brain Infections caused by infections other than the AIDS virus: for example, herpes, Toxoplasma, and others.

Considering all the neuropsychiatric disorders and socio-economic stigmatization, it is amazing that 100% of the HIV population is not psychiatrically handicapped. And there are still many people who believe that there is no connection between chronic HIV infection and behavior!

Chapter VI-9

Men's Issues

♂

Men's issues will of course discuss male sexuality. Specifically, the topics in this chapter focus on these arenas of concern:

- Effects on sex from mental illness (and from alcoholism and drug addiction)

- Effects on sex from psychiatric drugs (specific drug effects)

- Psychiatric effects of non-psychiatric medications on sex

- Impotence

- Treatment of premature ejaculation

- Prostate

- Fetishes

- Misogyny

Table VI-9 Men's Issues

Mental Illness Effects on sex	Effects on sex from psychiatric drugs (*extra vocabulary is in italics*)	Names of such drugs
-	**Anorgasmia**—having no orgasm (regardless of desire)	SSRI-SSNRI
-	**Delayed ejaculation**—unable to have an orgasm in a "timely" manner	SSRI-SSNRI
-		-
-	*Ejaculation*—sudden expulsion of semen	-
-	**Erection**—fully satisfying erection (Viagra, Cialis, Levitra)	Viagra et al.
	—partial erection is not satisfying	(BP pills**)
Psychological	*Flaccidity*—weakness, laxness, softness (penis)[11]	various
impotence	**Impotence***—lack of sexual power in the male	Mellaril
	(with or without desire) Mellaril, Serentil	Serentil
-	**Libido** = desire to have sex (with or without ability)	Wellbutrin
Loss of Libido	**Loss of Libido** = no desire to have sex	(Tagamet)
-	*Orgasm*—"Apex of sexual excitement"[11]	stimulants
-	Premature ejaculation—coming to orgasm too soon	-
Hypersexuality	**Hypersexuality**—above normal sexual activity	Prednisone*
-	*Satyr (satyriasis)* "excessive sexual desire in the male" (see	Male hormones
-	*nymphomania*)[11] beyond Hypersexuality	stimulants
-	**Priapism**—"persistent abnormal erection...pain and tenderness"[11]	Trazodone
impaired	(surgical emergency that could lead to permanent impotence)	-
judgment		-
-		

prednisone and male hormones are all steroid hormones—this family of drugs can cause increased or decreased feelings

**BP pills are "blood pressure" medicines (non-psychiatric drugs are in parentheses)*

****there are different types of impotence: from drugs, from diseases, neurological, or psychological*

Mental Illness: Effects on Sex

First off, please remember that psychiatric patients have a higher rate of venereal disease than the general population, because their mental illness may allow them to do impulsive acts of poor judgment. Psychiatric patients are more likely to use alcohol and drugs than the general population (self-treating?). Alcohol and drugs are notorious for activating people to do impulsive acts because the alcohol and drugs reduce judgment and remove inhibitions. These men often have **impaired judgment** regarding sex, sexuality, and choice of partners. So, venereal disease is common in this group.

(These are examples of venereal diseases: Syphilis, gonorrhea, CMV, herpes, Chlamydia, and others. Venereal diseases are often called STD, sexually transmitted diseases. Hepatitis-C is a real risk in the drug-addicted population. It has many means of transmission, and intimacy of all kinds is a risk for hepatitis-C. Sexually active men can also acquire NSU (non-specific urethritis) also called NGU (non-gonorrhea urethritis)— this can be caused by various germs NSU is not nearly so dangerous as the other STD's, but it is still a men's health issue..)

The first arena is the effect of mental illness on sex and sexuality.

Bipolar men are often sexually active. When men become hypomanic (mildly manic and euphoric), they become preoccupied with activities of all kinds. This we call this **hypersexuality** if it is severe enough. They can be very promiscuous and seem to be tireless.

Alcoholics can be promiscuous because of impaired judgment and loss of inhibitions. Perhaps worst of all, alcoholics can have promiscuous sex in a blackout and not even remember it the next day. Male *drug addicts* have several pitfalls in the sexual arena. Firstly, they can be extremely sexual and desirous while high on stimulants. They can also feel very romantic on marijuana. Sex on hallucinogens is a "unique" experience. Male drug addicts spend a lot of money on narcotics, both for themselves and for their girlfriends. This puts them at risk of venereal diseases. As a result, they often have no money. If going into extreme withdrawal, they may do anything necessary to get their drug of choice, which includes hustling and male prostitution. This puts them at greater risk of venereal diseases.

Depressive men usually lose desire in all pleasurable activities. They may have altered choices in food, pastimes, and companions. They may not eat or eat little; or, overeat in an attempt to feel a sugar rush. They stop weekend activities. They put off social encounters with their buddies, or tell their wives to take a message, often shunning any telephone conversations with anyone. This is **loss of libido**.

Specific Drug Effects on Sexual Functioning

Anorgasmia and delayed ejaculation are typically associated with the serotonin drugs (SSRI, SSNRI) which are: Celexa, Lexapro, Luvox, Paxil, Prozac, Zoloft as well as Effexor, Cymbalta, and Pristiq. There is no specific treatment for this: Buspar, Viagra, Periactin, and Wellbutrin have all been tried, with little success. This is not a feature of treatment with Serzone or Buspar (Trazodone is not recommended for sexually active men due to the possibility of Priapism—see table).

Erections will not be affected by: Wellbutrin, Buspar, stimulants, (or Serzone)—erections might even be enhanced. These following drugs are unlikely to cause much effect: Lithium, Depakote, Lamictal; Risperdal, Zyprexa, Invega, Abilify, Geodon; Neurontin, Trileptal. These antidepressants may not cause much inconvenience: SSRI, SSNRI, Vivactil, Desipramine, Pamelor, Asendin, Ludiomil. The following drugs can have variable effects: Seroquel, the rest of the Tricyclic antidepressants (Elavil, Sinequan, Surmontil, Tofranil), and first-generation antipsychotics (FGA's)—except Mellaril and Serentil that will prevent erections.

Impotence will definitely occur with Mellaril and Serentil.

Libido / Loss of Libido is not a regular feature of psychiatric medications since these medications are supposed to restore people to some sort of baseline feeling state.

Hypersexuality can be caused by stimulants (rarely excessive Prozac).

Priapism can be caused by Trazodone. This is very rare, but when it happens, it is a medical emergency requiring possible surgery. The surgical outcome might result in permanent and total impotence. I do not give this drug to men unless they already have permanent impotence, and even then the situation needs to be discussed with the man.

Non-psychiatric drugs that disturb sexual functioning

Some of the non-psychiatric drugs that psychiatrists use may cause psychiatric side effects as well as sexual dysfunction. Inderal, a drug for performance anxiety, would fit in this category, if a man were to take it every day, which is not likely. In that case, I would switch him to Atenolol. Atenolol can also be used every day to help control panic attacks and generalized anxiety disorder.

Another category of medications might deter a conscientious person from seeking to achieve full sexual satisfaction—this might occur in cases where the man is taking a drug for a fatal illness, AIDS, herpes, or hepatitis. The very knowledge of having these diseases might deter a (sober and unselfish) man from seeking complete personal sexual fulfillment. Interferon for hepatitis treatment can cause depression.

Premature Ejaculation

Premature ejaculation means that the man comes to orgasm too soon. This could be too soon by his own standards, or those of his lover, or both. This condition usually can have a negative effect on a marriage. Unfortunately, this is usually part of the way that that particular man is wired. In other words, this is the way he is. Some relatively normal men have this effect mainly when they are nervous, and their performance can return to baseline, when they feel more comfortable; although their spouses might think that baseline is usually not long enough.

The FDA has never approved a drug for this purpose. The makers of Paxil are trying to get approval for a drug called dapoxetine, but approval was rejected once. Nonetheless, there are a number of medications that are very effective, even if they are not officially FDA-approved. These are the newer medications (SSRI-SSNRI antidepressants—see Chapter V-8). Notably, Paxil and Zoloft. Other drugs with a lesser degree of this effect are Lexapro and Effexor. Please note that "normally" functioning men consider these side effects of delayed ejaculation to be annoying. The pharmaceutical industry likewise lists these sexual changes as (unwanted) side effects. But, the side effects are a boon to men with premature ejaculation. (Some normally functioning men are unaffected—or at least undeterred—by these side effects and go about their business as normal.)

The way this works is that the drugs tend to delay ejaculation in all men. A man with a two minute limit can extend longer. A man with a usual fifteen minute limit may expand to perhaps the better part of an hour.

Treatment of premature ejaculation typically requires only low doses of the so-called SSRI-SSNRI medications. Typically, the man needs to take enough medicine to maintain a low blood level, such as one half-one dose every day or every other day. Then the man can take a bigger dose a couple hours before sexual activity. This is practical information not found in the textbooks. Assume three men named Joe, Mike, and Jimmy:

- If Joe has premature ejaculation almost at the moment of penetration, then he will need to take at least 20 mg Paxil (or 50 mg Zoloft or 50 mg Effexor) every day. A couple hours prior to sex, he can take an extra dose.

- If Mike has only a mild case and he has endurance of a few minutes, then he can probably get by with 10 mg of Paxil every day or every other day, and take 15 mg about an hour and a half before sex.

- If Jimmy can last up to eight or ten minutes, but there is pressure on him to have extended stamina, then he could probably take 5 mg Paxil every day or other day and then 10-20 mg about two hours before sex.

- If any of these men take the "booster" dose an hour or so before sex, he will first feel a surge from the antidepressant effect itself which enhance his libido. The ejaculation will be delayed because he has maintained a regular blood level. A few hours after taking the booster dose, the man is going to feel a loss of desire whether he has ejaculated or not. The initial enhancement feeling is the antidepressant effect; the delayed ejaculation is a sought-after side effect, and the loss of libido is an undesirable side effect. Timing can be everything, and these three men may need to fiddle with the dosage on their own. Men who feel that the erection does not last until ejaculation should go to a sex shop and purchase a "cock ring" to maintain erections.

- Flaccidity and Impotence: if Joe has both problems, then he can ask his doctor about medications such as Viagra, Cialis, Levitra. Anyone of these three men can also go to a sex shop to buy a "cock ring"—this simple device (technically, a kind of partial tourniquet) will prolong erections in duration, quantity, and quality without causing any anatomic or functional damage.

- And yes, the SSRI drugs can be taken with male hormones and Viagra et al—but only in severe cases and under doctor's supervision.

Impotence

Paraphrasing Dorland's dictionary, 'impotence is a lack of power, chiefly sexual power, in the male; it can be loss of virility' (loss of manhood or manliness). Impotence can be caused by medications, psychiatric disease, nerve problems (neurological), psychological issues, alcohol and drugs, medical illness, surgical complications, or by unknown factors.

Possible causes of impotence:

- Unknown causes
- Psychological
- Psychiatric illness
- Alcoholism and drug-addiction
- Impotence caused by psychiatric drugs
- Impotence caused by non-psychiatric drugs that do have psychiatric side effects (Inderal)
- Neurological diseases (various)
- Medical diseases (diabetes)
- Surgical complication (pelvic surgery: bladder, prostate, rectal cancer, penile cancer)

(the last three are not discussed here in any great extent)

Other modifiers on impotence include whether it is:

- Selective (occurs with certain persons) or non-selective (occurs with everyone)

- Temporary (usually happens once per lifetime) or permanent (irreversible disease)

- Partial impotence or total impotence (partial impotence would be partial but unsatisfying erections)

- Constant or intermittent (off-and-on)

- "Extra-nocturnal" Does not happen at night in sleep (in other words, the man has erections during his normal sleep cycle)

All sexually functional men have erections with REM sleep each night. If a man awakens with an erection in the middle of the night or in the morning, then he is not functionally impotent. But if this same man cannot have erections in the daytime, then there are other factors at work, usually psychological, medication-related, or caused by alcohol and drugs. Some of these are examples of selective impotence. For example, truly impotent men (severe diabetics) do not have erections at night. Temporary impotence can happen and is not serious—it may even be a subconscious warning sign. The man may have fallen out of love with that partner or he is afraid of pregnancy. Some men will have partial erections alternating with flaccidity. This could be a sign of poor blood circulation (quit eating animal fat!). Full erections can alternate off-and-on with partial erections and complete impotence. Often a sign of aging; however, if he is a young non-obese man, then he needs a medical evaluation.

Every man will typically have one episode in his life when he is impotent for no apparent reason (*unknown* factor). This usually lasts a couple or few weeks, then goes away, usually never to return. In hindsight, it might have been due to some psychological problem that went unnoticed. This is a good example of temporary impotence.

Apart from these unknown factors, some men have an episode of *psychological* impotence, which is often due to rather obvious problems within his relationship. He may be angry because she keeps on eating and gaining weight. She may be running up the credit cards every month. Perhaps she is a "trophy wife" and has many apparent suitors. The man may hate his mother-in-law who came to live with them. Perhaps the man is having an affair and has no further interest in his wife. Any number of factors can be involved here. The treatment or resolution of each of them may be simple or complicated. If you are such a man who cannot solve it on your own, then perhaps you should see a (male) psychologist.

Psychiatric illness by itself does not cause physical inability to have sex, unless a specific part of the brain is affected. Schizophrenics fear intimacy. Paranoid psychotics are often too suspicious to have sex, in general. Extreme depressives have no desire for any pleasurable activities. Anxious men are too unfocused and distressed. Obsessive-Compulsive men do not achieve orgasm because they obsess about orgasm, germs, performance, or something else.

Alcoholics can often be randy while intoxicated and then selectively impotent the rest of the time. Alcoholic men in early recovery report increased sexual desire and ability, possibly due to restoration of physical health and restoration of REM sleep cycles. Drug-addicted men may be over-sexed while high on stimulants (cocaine and amphetamines) and may be partially or selectively impotent the rest of the time.

Psychiatric drugs that are notorious for causing impotence are Mellaril and Serentil. MAOI antidepressants (Nardil) cause this, too. These older drugs are not in use very much anymore, and even when they were, most men refused to take them. When the drug is stopped, the impotence recedes.

Non-psychiatric drugs that can cause impotence include blood pressure pills and Tagamet. The complicated chemistry of blood pressure pills results in low blood pressure and hence, inability to keep the penis engorged with blood. Psychiatrists sometimes prescribe certain blood pressure pills for psychiatric purposes. Inderal, for example, is used to treat "performance anxiety" on an "as-needed" basis. If used daily for years for blood pressure, Inderal can cause depression, strange nightmare, and partial temporary impotence. After these medications are stopped, the impotence should disappear. Atenolol lacks these side effects and can be used as-needed for performance anxiety instead of Inderal.

Neurological conditions can cause impotence in numerous ways. *Medical disease* is also a cause of impotence, notoriously serious diabetes. This becomes a permanent impotence. *Surgical complications* can result in impotence. This could include any surgery in the pelvic area, such as radical prostate cancer, bladder surgery, rectal surgery, or removal of penis for penile cancer. Mental health professionals can offer supportive therapy in these cases.

Treatment of Impotence

Psychological and unknown causes should seek therapy with a psychologist. Men with known medical causes, which can be remedied with Viagra, Cialis, or Levitra, should avail themselves of these treatments as long as there are no diseases or medications that would prevent use of these drugs. For partial off-and-on impotence, go to a sex shop and purchase a "cock ring". A man could also check in his city to see if there is a sex therapist or sexologist (specialty doctor). Yohimbine can raise blood pressure and has variable results. Male hormones might be helpful, but this would require thorough medical and psychiatric evaluations. If due to a psychiatric illness, then have the underlying disorder treated, after which you can see if the impotence has improved. Alcoholics and drug-addicts with problematic erections, need to get clean and sober.

Prostate

Urine leaves the man's bladder in a long tube called the urethra—the urethra goes from the bladder, passing through the prostate and through the whole penis: you can see the end of the urethra as the hole in the tip of the penis. In its trajectory, the urethra travels through the prostate like a road going through a tunnel. When the prostate swells in size, it can squeeze shut the urethra, mimicking a rockslide inside the tunnel. The tunnel becomes obstructed and not too much can go through it. This is called obstruction: urinary obstruction. This is a primary symptom of prostate problems. Urinary obstruction can also occur due to a diseased bladder. So, urinary obstruction has two causes, one due to the bladder and one due to the prostate. The symptom seems the same to a man, and only his doctor or urologist can be sure which is the cause.

Urine retention is the main symptom in both bladder and prostate problems. Other symptoms may also occur such as pain on urination, frequent urination, and hesitating to urinate. Once again, consult your doctor or urologist.

Psychiatry does not focus on the prostate. Psychiatric medications do not affect the prostate directly. However, psychiatric medications can affect the bladder and cause symptoms of prostatic obstruction. Typical causative medicines are the older drugs, such as all the Tricyclic antidepressants and the FGA antipsychotics (first-generation antipsychotics). There are two treatment options: change medicines or try Urecholine tablets. Discuss this with your prescribing doctor.

Fetishes

Some men find sexual excitement in "accessories". Men who go out in public dressed as women but unshaven and hairy are "cross-dressers" and are mainly heterosexual: women's clothing rubbing against their bodies is their fetish. The French poet, Paul Verlain, liked to wear his wife's shoes: that was his fetish. There was a young man who was excited by dressing up and wearing only a big diaper. Some fetishes include partial suffocation. There was a young man who had a girlfriend, and in secret he had a Lesbian intimate who would strap on a rubber phallus in order to give him "profound" experiences. There can be so many types of fetishes. Also, watch the uncensored version of the film "*Los Amantes*" (a true event in Spain).

Misogyny is Greek for "woman-hater". "*In some men the inability to ejaculate reflects unexpressed hostility toward women.*"*(Kaplan & Sadock p.1309)* These men would have libido without desire for the partner. Start therapy with a (male) psychologist.

Factoids

1   Men may experience a headache immediately after orgasm. This is called "post-

coital headache". It is not serious. If you are truly worried about having a brain tumor, then ask to see a neurologist in order to allay your fears.

2   Men typically have erections with each cycle of REM sleep every night. The average man would have five or six REM cycles for each night of sleep.

3   Men with medical impotence do not ever have erections during the day or during REM sleep; Men with psychological impotence (impotence due to nervousness) do indeed have erections during sleep.

4   Episodes of psychological impotence can occur normally at least once in a man's life. The episodes usually last only a few weeks then resolve, unless the psychological stress is ongoing in which case the best treatment is to see a psychologist. If there is no known ongoing psychological stress and the impotence has lasted well over a month and a half, then an appointment should be made with the family doctor. (We actually call psychological impotence "psychogenic").

5   In the past, men could be left permanently impotent after invasive prostate surgery. The less invasive surgical treatments reduce this risk of permanent impotence. The newest technique of laparoscopic prostate surgery apparently has even less risk of impotence. (Visit Urology at Cleveland Clinic website.)

In conclusion, we can see that many men's issues that were once beyond treatment are now amenable to treatment just in the last few decades. Talk to your doctor and avail yourself of these remedies.

VI-9-b Chart of Sexual Dysfunction

	Desire-Libido*	Erections	Stamina	Ejaculation-orgasm**
Zero-none	Depression Antipsychotics	Impotence Medications Diabetes, etc	Depression Old age	Medication effects Medical-surgical problem Anxiety, Misogyny
Weak	Depression Antipsychotics	Medications Blood Pressure Anxiety	Depression Medication	FGA antipsychotics** Anxiety
Moderate	Wellbutrin			
Strong	Stimulants Steroids, Bipolar Marijuana	Cialis, Levitra, Viagra	Stimulants	(sexual fetishes)
Prolonged	Hypersexuality Satyriasis	Priapism Trazodone	Stimulants Steroids	
Abnormal Problematic or Variable	Schizophrenia Alcohol-Drugs Lack of Desire	Alcohol-Drugs Psychological Impotence	Alcohol Drugs	Premature Ejaculation Relationship Issues OCD***

*I have combined these here in this table. Libido refers to having lustful feelings; desire more properly references attachment to a certain person, act, or event
**for psychiatric purposes, we will assume that ejaculation and orgasm co-occur (exceptions may occur with some of the FGA Antipsychotics: ejaculation without orgasm)—otherwise consult Urology textbooks
*** OCD: Obsessive Compulsive Disorder

This chart shows which sexual dysfunction might be associated with which disorder. For example, if you are a younger man with on-and-off impotence, but strong erections with Viagra, and you wake up in the morning with erections, then you might have psychological impotence or side effects from drugs and alcohol.

Medical Illnesses Masquerading as Psychiatric Disorders
Minerals & Hormones

Minerals

Sodium, potassium, calcium, and magnesium are important minerals found in every cell of our bodies. Our bodies need these minerals in order to maintain health and to stay alive. Like all chemical minerals, however, we can be poisoned by too much sodium, potassium, calcium, or magnesium—and medically compromised by too little. Therefore, our bodies maintain rather strict controls over the levels of these salts in our bodies (in health). Any significant imbalances result first in sickness and then in death. For example, if levels of these salts in our bodies increase or decrease abnormally, then we can die from heart or nerve problems. These are approximations of the amount of imbalance that we can tolerate:

- Sodium 6-11% variation in levels
- Potassium 25% variation
- Calcium 15-30%
- Magnesium 40-70%

If sodium levels drop, then a person seems to have depression with symptoms of lethargy, confusion, even stupor. Obviously, doctors need to know if this is depression or low sodium levels. If it comes on rather suddenly within a day or two, then it is probably not psychiatric. If sodium levels drop even further, this will cause permanent brain damage, progressing on to seizures and death.

If sodium levels rise too much, a person will exhibit a change in behavior and can become weak and irritable. He can have seizures or go into a coma.

Low potassium can result in fatigue, weakness, partial paralysis that might look like catatonia (a psychiatric condition in which people do not move or talk). Too much or too little potassium eventually ends with a heart attack.

Calcium excess can show up as apathy, "fatigue, depression, mental confusion, anorexia" [10]. (Anorexia is weight loss from loss of appetite). Death is cardiac. Low calcium levels can look like agitated catatonia in which patients act spastic and make strange facial expressions (grimacing). When I was an intern, one of the other psychiatry residents was called down to the ER to see such a patient, whose behavior the ER staff interpreted to be psychiatric. They were told to do a quick calcium level, and the patient did indeed have low calcium. These low calcium behaviors collectively are sometimes called "tetany". Death can occur from paralysis of the breathing muscles or from cardiac causes.

Table VI-10 Four important minerals: abnormal levels can look psychiatric

	Magnesium Mg^{++}	Calcium Ca^{++}	Sodium *(natrium)* Na^+	Potassium *(kalium)* K^+
Common Household Use	Antacids Cathartics (laxatives)	Antacids	NaCl Table salt	KCl* Salt substitute*
Current Medical Use	In pregnancy ("eclampsia") Heart disease	Prevent Osteoporosis	Normal saline Intravenous fluid	Cardiology Internal Medicine
Excess	Sedation. Weakness	Apathy, confusion, Anorexia, depression	Apathetic, weak Catatonic, irritable	
Deficit	Spasms	Manic agitation	Brain swelling Confusion	Fatigue weakness

(there are many salt substitutes containing potassium; for example, Morton's Lite contains sodium, potassium, calcium, and magnesium—plus iodide.) Ask your doctor before using! In table VI-11, we see that K $^+$ and Na$^+$ both have one (+) positive charge. Magnesium and Calcium have two plus charges (Mg^{++}, Ca^{++}). They have no specific use in psychiatry but imbalances of these two metals can present with symptoms that may look like psychiatric symptoms. See chapter on Lithium V-10

Low magnesium levels often occur with low calcium. They both have similar symptoms. High magnesium levels are usually due to taking too much magnesium by mouth, as in laxative abuse, or eating too many ulcer tablets. High magnesium levels result in sedation, muscle weakness, paralysis. Death can be from paralysis of breathing muscles or from an extremely slow heart. Excess magnesium can be fatal. When I was an intern, I witnessed the fatal outcome of a medical error resulting in injection of 20 mg of magnesium sulfate into a patient (instead of 2.0 mg).

Hormones

Thyroid hormone imbalances can masquerade as psychiatric disorders, although this is rare nowadays with modern lab tests and family doctors who slavishly check thyroid levels of all patients. They do this because thyroid disease is common nowadays and is easy to diagnose early by simple blood tests. High thyroid levels make people act manic—anxious, hyperactive, restless; patients do not sleep or eat much. Low thyroid levels make people seem depressed: they gain weight, feel unmotivated, and sleep a lot. I always check to make sure that patients new to me have had their thyroid blood test done by the family doctor. When a new patient comes to me I check to see if thyroid tests were done. If not, then I order these lab tests. I have only had one patient slip through this screening process somehow. I was treating her for depression for a few months, and the clinical course did not jibe. In reviewing her initial lab tests, I discovered that no one had checked her thyroid levels, so I did. She had low thyroid and went back to her family doctor. Nowadays, psychiatrists are much likelier to see thyroid patients who are not feeling well on the thyroid pills—they feel either too hyperactive or too lethargic from the medication, but their lab tests are "normal".

Steroid Hormones

These can cause a whole legion of possible psychiatric symptoms: psychosis, anxiety, irritability, insomnia, depression, even suicidal depression. This can happen with young men who abuse steroids of all kinds—many steroids are sold without prescription in pharmacies across America. The prescription steroids can cause this also, notoriously male hormones that can cause raging and *Prednisone,* which can cause mania or depression.

Male hormones in excess can cause agitation, aggression, and hypomanic behavior. This is usually due to using excess amounts of testosterone derivatives in pill form or in injections.

Low testosterone levels can make men pudgy, apathetic, and unmotivated. This can be seen with certain prostate cancer treatments and with Tagamet. These prostate treatments may act to suppress male hormones, and men might even get "hot flashes" as do women in menopause. Steroid treatments that emasculate men, can make men feel listless and un-spirited. Tagamet interferes with the production of male steroid hormones in the liver.

Female hormones in alternating levels can produce numerous symptoms such as depression, irritability, and moodiness with fluctuating moods throughout the day.

Adrenal Glands

The adrenal glands produce a specific **steroid hormone** called *cortisol*, which can be affected by any kind of stress, including psychiatric illness. *Cortisol* can also result in psychiatric symptoms if cortisol levels are too low or too high. Low cortisol is called Addison's Disease (supposedly President Kennedy had this). Symptoms are fatigue, weakness, and weight loss. If the adrenal glands produce too much cortisol, this is called Cushing's Disease. The symptoms of Cushing's vary and can include most psychiatric symptoms: psychosis, anxiety, irritability, insomnia, depression, even suicidal depression.

Infections of the Brain

HIV—this is covered in Chapter VI-8

Syphilis

If early syphilis (also called *Lues*) is not treated, it may incubate many years in the brain and cause serious neuropsychiatric illness later in life: mania, psychosis, depression, agitation. Dementia is the most common outcome.

Lyme Disease

This can be associated with chronic levels of high anxiety, which are hard to treat with the usual anti-anxiety agents, sedating antidepressants, antipsychotics, or epilepsy drugs.

Neurological Disorders

Dementia—see Chapter VI-6

Strokes can involve a sudden discharge of blood leaking into a part of the brain. That blood clots and occupies space, as if it were a (tiny) tumor. Stroke can also occur if the blood supply is suddenly cut off to a certain part of the brain (in which case, that part of the brain receives no oxygen and "suffocates" then dies). Regardless of cause, the "stroked" part of the brain is usually permanently damaged. If the stroke occurs over the speech center of the brain, then the person may be left wordless. If it occurs over the part of the brain that controls the left hand-arm, then that person will not be able to use his arm. If the stroke occurs in certain psychiatrically sensitive areas, then it can result in a permanent psychotic delusion. This is a major reason for referring stroke patients to psychiatry. This delusion usually remains the same and sometime the patient even knows that the delusion is alien and irrational but can not stop obsessing about it. This is not like schizophrenia in that there is usually just one symptom that is permanently fixed in the stroke patient's mind—unless he has a second stroke. (Schizophrenia is a constant lifetime illness enwrapped in multiple changing psychotic symptoms.) Unfortunately, stroke delusions often do not respond so well to anti-psychotics as does "natural" schizophrenia. Patients with stroke delusion are more consumed with obsessing about the delusion than reacting to it, which they realize is a delusion. They seem to be vexed—not so much by the delusion—but that they cannot get it out of their minds. This obsessive quality is harder to treat and may or may not respond well to anti-obsessive drugs. I had one patient who did well with Luvox (anti-obsessive), but this is an exceptional outcome. (Sometimes anti-obsessive antidepressants can aggravate any psychosis.) see chapter VI-6

A stroke may also cause depression which usually responds adequately to antidepressants and similar drugs.

Temporal Lobe Epilepsy(TLE) patients can have mood disorders and/or thought disorders. The temporal lobe of the brain is a focus of much psychiatric activity and research.

In general, the term "Epilepsy" means that there is a scar (or something) in a part of the brain. That scar can cause unexpected epileptic fits. There are as many kinds of epileptic fits as there are parts of the brain to be scarred. If the scar is located in a part of the brain that controls muscular activity, then we can see evidence of the epileptic fit because the patient loses muscular control and falls on the floor. What the reader may not realize is that any scar anywhere in the brain can cause any kind of neurological or neuropsychiatric behavior imaginable. A scar in the "laughter center" can cause fits of laughter: this is called *gelastic* epilepsy (*gelastic* means "laughing"— in Greek). The temporal lobe controls thoughts, moods, psychiatric behavior, so that when this part of the brain is scarred and produces a fit, TLE patients will have strange thoughts and sensations, like hallucinations, that may not be visible to observers and will not climax in falling to the ground.

Neurologists treat TLE, and TLE patients can be stabilized with modern epilepsy drugs.

Even when TLE patients are not having fits, they still have more psychiatric illness than the non-epileptic population. They are also prone to moodiness. They have more psychosis, but their psychotic symptom presentation is not schizophrenic. They may seem to have a mixed mood and thought disorder. Some classic cases of stabilized TLE patients demonstrate an amazing obsession to write down everything that they can think of ("hypergraphia"). Then they bring this material to psychiatric appointments. They may also appear a little bit distractible because they may be taking three major classes of neuropsychiatric drugs: epilepsy drugs, antidepressants, and antipsychotics.

M.S.

M.S. is multiple sclerosis, a progressive brain disease that often has psychiatric symptoms, mainly depression, sometimes euphoria, or rapidly alternating between happiness and weeping. (remember that M.S. may affect the temporal lobe of the brain as above in TLE) Sometimes first-time patients might come in because of loss of vision in an eye or dragging a foot. These early patients may also feel a vague sense of depression. Most of the cases I have seen were of M.S. with depression. M.S. changes with time, so that any psychiatric symptoms may change too. The usual antidepressants work well.

There is a whole specialty of Psychiatry that is involved in these medical, neurological, and "medicalized" issues: Consultation-Liaison Psychiatry. These are the psychiatrists who stay abreast of all the psychiatric aspects of medical illness and medical aspects of psychiatric illness. These specialists are uncommon and usually found in large hospitals where they interface with internists and surgeons regarding psychiatric issues of medical-surgical patients.

Section VII
PSYCHIATRY and the LAW

Superscript numbers refer to references and citations at the back of the book

Chapter VII-1

Psychiatry and the Law
Lex dura sed Lex

(the Law is harsh but it is the Law)

Psychiatry intersects with the legal system more than any other branch of medicine—with the exception of pathology. However, pathologists' cases are often deceased, leaving psychiatry as the branch of medicine that is oftenest involved with the legal rights of (live) patients. We become embroiled in the machinery of the legal system as a result of our patients' behaviors or occasionally of our own behaviors. All doctors practice medicine and we also practice psychiatric medicine. However, unlike "regular" doctors we must not only first practice medicine but also then fulfill three other aims as well in order to practice successful psychiatry:

- Practice medicine (psychiatric medicine)
- Protect society from our patients
- Protect our patients from society
- Protect our patients from themselves

As a result, psychiatry is involved in many legal issues. These legal issues are spread across a seemingly contradictory and broad spectrum ranging from protection of society from psychiatric patients to preserving the rights of individual psychiatric patients to depriving patients of their civil rights guaranteed by the US Constitution. This forces psychiatrists to become paternalistic, to which patients—and society as a whole—react with ambivalence. Ambivalence seems to permeate American perception of psychiatry as a whole. Psychiatry's legal maneuverings can be proactive or reactive: planning for future events or responding to past events. Psychiatry is called upon to try to predict future events (violence) and when these events never come to pass, psychiatrists are not regaled, but if these future events do come to pass, then psychiatrists are vilified. The legal maneuverings of psychiatrists can be self-serving (expert witness in tort cases) or selfless (child custody testimony).

Another way of looking at the spectrum of psychiatric involvement in the legal system is by classifying our participation as voluntary, involuntary, or obligatory involvement. Voluntary involvement usually results in monetary compensation for us, whereas involuntary involvement usually means punitive actions against the psychiatrist, especially as punitive monetary damages in the forms of fines and penalties. These are called civil damages when we are forced to pay fines and penalties. Sometimes the punitive damages are of a criminal nature, which can send a doctor to jail or restrict his ability to practice psychiatry. The outcome of a criminal punishment ultimately amounts to a civil damage by restricting his ability to earn income. Obligatory involvement refers to the fact that we must follow State Laws and regulations of the State Medical Board as well as following federal guidelincs: DEA (Drug Enforcement Administration) and CMS (Medicare-Medicaid) guidelines.

Voluntary Participation in the Legal System

(Usually results in payments to the doctor)

Doctor-patient relationship

This relationship is essentially a legal contract whereby the doctor agrees to give the patient "usual and customary" treatment and whereby the patient agrees to pay the doctor for medical services. This contractual relationship begins when the doctor has initial contact with the patient—typically in person (hopefully not by phone or e-mail). This legal contract could commence with a phone call, but this avoids the proper way of making a diagnosis [in person] which should occur as outlined in table I-4-a. This is why a doctor tries to avoid speaking with prospective patients by phone, unless the doctor is in a kind of practice where telephone advice is sanctioned as "usual and customary" medical practice (as in telemedicine). There are cases where a single phone call was construed as the beginnings of a doctor-patient relationship, but this would be rare. Thus, initial telephone contacts are with the office staff and not with the doctor.

Participation in a typical doctor-patient relationship is voluntary for both the patient and for the doctor. The doctor—as well as the patient—can stay in the relationship or leave it. He can leave it in several ways.

If he has an employment contract with an agency (corporate, non-profit, or governmental), he can resign from the position, quit it by giving a few months notice (usually three months), be fired, or not have the employment contract renewed. In these agency cases, the patients ("case load") "belong" to the agency and not to the doctor. Reassigning these patients to a new doctor is the legal responsibility of the agency. He just leaves when he is legally released from the employment contract.

If the doctor is in private practice then he will try to maintain enough patients to keep his business open. He will not want to lose any patients until they are ready to leave. And he will certainly not want to discharge any patients prematurely, that is he will not want to tell them that he can not see them anymore. Telling them this amounts to rejection of the patient and is extremely traumatic. However, under extremely unusual circumstances, he may be obligated by ethics—or forced by law—to transfer a private patient to another psychiatrist. Worse, he may not be able to tell the patient why, and the referring psychiatrist cannot divulge this either to her new patient. The reason is almost always an ethical dilemma or personal complication. He may sense that the patient has fallen in love with him—or the patient may simply tell him so (likely). Maybe he has fallen in love with the patient (less likely); or, there is some interpersonal conflict. The doctor finds out that the patient is dating his family member (Meryl Streep made a movie about this: she had to refer her client to another doctor). A female psychiatrist may feel threatened by a male patient and refers him to a male doctor. There are many possible reasons why this transfer of care might be necessary.

(See Chapters I-5, I-6, I-7)

However, under no circumstance can a doctor simply tell the patient that he will never see her again, announcing the current visit to be the last visit. This is "abandonment" and is illegal. He personally must continue to provide basic supportive care until the private patient is transferred to a new doctor. This can happen quite quickly since psychiatrists have a professional network that can facilitate such transfers. Abandonment will be avoided, but there are often ongoing abandonment issues that the patient will experience regarding the former psychiatrist. Oftentimes, this new issue needs to be addressed with the new doctor.

Although the doctors are voluntarily involved, the patients may be voluntary or involuntary patients. Voluntary patients can leave whenever they want, and involuntary ones cannot. The vast majority of the patients in a doctor-patient relationship are voluntary patients. Involuntary patients are "referred" by the court system. They are court-ordered to see a psychiatrist. They may have had domestic violence, they may be on parole, or they may be sex-offenders. The psychiatrist is responsible for sending reports to the judge and there is no confidentiality: whatever the involuntary patient says or does, should be reported to the court.

Psychiatrists working voluntarily within the legal system:

These are psychiatrists who are working on a legal team testifying either for plaintiffs or for defendants in court. Forensic psychiatrists serve as expert witnesses in court and describe **criminal** behavior to juries. The forensic psychiatrist will interview the criminally insane patients and explain the mental illness to the jurors. Forensic psychiatrists can also serve as expert witness in **non-criminal** cases (torts and civil cases) where they can give assessments of mental suffering of litigants who are suing a corporation for faulty products and services (product liability cases).

Involuntary Participation in the Legal System

(may result in monetary fines, legal sanctions, or incarceration for the psychiatrist)

The risk of litigation increases the cost of practicing medicine. However, the malpractice rates for psychiatry are still relatively low—when compared to specialty surgeons. Psychiatrists who also administer ECT (shock treatments) pay an additional hefty premium for doing ECT. The vast majority of doctors are good and conscientious and do not desire any bad outcomes. Errors can occur in any profession. Fortunately, most doctors have been so well trained that they can practice medicine carefully under adverse conditions. One lawsuit can be devastating for a doctor—even if he wins the case. There are special support groups for doctors involved in lawsuits.

Psychiatrists as targets (defendants) in legal cases where the psychiatrist is being sued by a patient or by a patient's family. These are some of the commonest reasons for suing a psychiatrist

Wrongful Death lawsuit: this usually involves suicide or homicide:

Suicide: if a patient commits suicide, then the psychiatrist can be sued for not preventing it; however, the family of the suicide victim may need to prove that the psychiatrist was negligent (providing substandard care) or reckless (worse care than negligence). It is a fact of life that psychiatric patients are likely to try to commit suicide as this is part of their illness, so the family needs to demonstrate that the psychiatrist acted wrongly in some way that is outside the "usual and customary" community standards for psychiatric practice. Even if the psychiatrist did give standard care, he may likely have to make monetary compensation of some sort

Homicide: **(a)**—if a psychiatric patient kills some specific person **intentionally** (boss, spouse, parent, etc.) then the psychiatrist can be sued for not medicating the patient correctly or for not preventing this or for not warning the victim beforehand: Besides being sued for wrongful death by homicide, the family can also sue the psychiatrist for failure to warn the intended victim. In many cases, the psychiatrist and family may already be aware who the intended victim was—the family needs to show that the psychiatrist acted badly, negligently, or recklessly. **(b)** if a patient **accidentally** kills somebody then a lawsuit might be brought also (example: a manic patient is not well controlled on his lithium and drives around corners too fast and hits a pedestrian at random). Even if the psychiatrist did provide standard care, he will likely need to make monetary compensation.

Injuries: If a patient injures himself or another person (not a fatal injury), then the psychiatrist might be liable to pay for the medical expenses incurred by the injured person (plus other damages perhaps).

Adverse Treatment Outcomes

Drug reaction or drug side effects are other significant causes of lawsuits; however, in most cases a drug reaction can not be predicted—or at least not yet, although this technology may be coming soon. Drug reactions usually fall into a few main categories:

- Allergic whole body reactions and allergic skin reactions (which can be life-threatening);
- Permanent Parkinsonism caused by psychiatric drugs; and,
- claims that new SGA antipsychotics cause diabetes

Restraints It is possible that patients can sue for being incorrectly restrained or having an adverse result from being restrained (being tied down while violently psychotic)
ECT: adverse outcomes from ECT (shock treatment): memory loss, broken bones, anesthesia reactions.

*Romantic and physically **intimate relationships with patients**.* This should be obvious to everybody that doctors are not supposed to seduce their patients or sleep with them. This applies to all medical personnel who hold a state license: therapists, psychologists, et al. The doctor holds a lot of power over the patient so that the relationship is not a mutual one between peers. Also the doctor would no longer be able to maintain objectivity about the patient's treatment which would often result in the patient receiving "skewed" treatment.

Failure to diagnose. Patients can claim that the doctor did not diagnose correctly, resulting in the wrong treatment, or that the doctor missed a diagnosis entirely. This is harder to prove in psychiatry than in general medicine, but still can happen:

Involuntary admission to a psychiatric hospital. Patients can sue if the doctor sends them involuntarily to a psychiatric hospital (against their will) for three days. As long as the psychiatrist has carefully documented the reasons why, then this is not an easy case for the patient to win. In cases where the doctor finds a reasonable medical probability of needing hospitalization, then this can be justified, especially if there is concern that the patient is unpredictable, dangerous, disorganized, or confused.

This three day cooling-down period may prevent death: it may avert an accidental or intentional suicide or homicide; it may bring to light the patient's desire to kill some specific person. In the case that the patient is somewhat mentally ill and homeless and seems to lack the wherewithal to find shelter and food, then this hospital stay could be justified also in order to protect the patient from himself.

Unusual Circumstances

Denial of consortium refers to cases where the two spouses have been separated involuntarily. This could be a legal claim if one of the spouses has been involuntarily institutionalized.

Alienation of affection occurs if the mental health professional is perceived as dividing two legally wedded spouses. A classic example is that of seeing a married man with his mistress for couples therapy: his wife can sue for alienation of affection (if she finds out about this couples counseling).

Abandonment (see above)

Medicare Fraud

Fraudulent overcharging of the government is another way that doctors can become embroiled in legal problems. This occurs when a doctor is overcharging the federal government for treating Medicare patients. The sums of money diverted can be measured by five, six, or seven digit numbers usually. This is really serious as it involves violation of federal statutes. Most of these federal investigations are usually triggered by egregious and massive diversion of monies over significant periods of times. Doctors who are convicted of Medicare fraud will have numerous legal and financial problems. Legal problems will involve being charged with violation of federal law and may likely incur one or all of the following punishments: the doctor can be sentenced to a federal prison, the doctor will have to pay fines and penalties, and furthermore the doctor will have to make restitution (pay back the money which was stolen from the government). This can cost a lot of time and money. Moreover, since this is a federal felony, the medical board will suspend the doctor's medical license so that he can no longer practice medicine legally in the State of licensure. Beyond that, the doctor will not be able to see CMS (Medicare-Medicaid) patients anymore or work in a clinical setting where CMS patients are served or if he does, he will be practicing under the supervision of doctors who retain the rights to see CMS patients).

There are some rural areas that are so desperate to have a family doctor, that some of these restrictions may be waived and the doctor might be allowed to resume working under a binding contract with the National Health Service or a Locum Tenens. (the government estimates that we have a shortage of 17,000 primary care doctors in rural areas)

*Miscellaneous and not professionally related: C*onviction of any *felony* can jeopardize a doctor's career and medical license. The reasoning is that persons of criminal bent should not be practicing medicine. Of course, psychiatrists can have other legal involvements that have no bearing on his ability to practice medicine and do not limit his medical license. Such examples are traffic violations and divorce.

Obligatory Participation in the Legal System

Licensing, compliance, insurance:

We need a State medical license in order to practice lawfully. Compliance refers to obeying all the rules, regulations, and guidelines established by the government, medical boards, and insurance companies.

Some aspects of obligatory participation may be semi-voluntary in the sense that the psychiatrist sometimes can opt out: we can opt out of Medicare-Medicaid and accept cash patients only; we can limit patient access to her own confidential medical chart; we can refuse to prescribe controlled narcotics to patients; in some States, we can practice without malpractice insurance ("going bare"), but that would be highly unusual.

Mandatory reporting: there are two situations in which the psychiatrist must breach confidentiality with a patient, or in other words, there are two communications that are not confidential . Firstly, any licensed health professional who learns of child abuse is legally bound to report it immediately; ditto for elder abuse. Secondly, the doctor must report confessions of murder to the police; murder—like child abuse—is exempt from the confidentiality rule.

Signed Release of Information

When patients apply for certain jobs, they may be required to reveal any psychiatric history—failure to mention this to prospective employers is considered dishonest. If you sign a release of information for us to divulge the contents of your confidential psychiatric chart then we will do so. If you want any information "filtered", then you need to let us know in advance that you want details to be minimized, unless the elimination of these data would result in illogical and inexplicable results in your care. In this case, the requestor would request clarification. And then we would need to confer with you on the next step. Oftentimes, the employers will be satisfied with a brief one-page summary of diagnosis and treatment dates. However, if you are applying for positions requiring security clearance or something of that ilk, then they will probably want the whole chart Xeroxed and sent to them. A government agent might come to the office and have me read the chart to him.

Subpoenas and Depositions

A subpoena from a judge compels a doctor to disclose the requested information in the medical chart. This may play out in several ways: the doctor may be forced to appear in court; he may be forced to bring the medical record to court; he may be forced to allow lawyers from the defense and plaintiff to look over the whole chart by coming to his office to see it; he may be forced to Xerox the whole chart and mail it to lawyers. Lawyers may come to his office and have a mini-court session in the office with interrogations by both defense attorneys and plaintiff attorneys, which proceeding is recorded by a court stenographer who accompanies the legal teams (this is a deposition).

Whoever is named in the subpoena is supposed to reveal the contents of the medical record. In certain cases, the office manager might be under subpoena and not the doctor. She may refuse to Xerox the chart and send it. If the doctor is under subpoena, he may refuse to send the chart or to cooperate with the request for various reasons. Whoever does not obey the subpoena is technically in contempt of court and this can have dire ramifications.

This is how it usually plays out. I am having a great week and suddenly a sealed subpoena is hand-delivered. Terror! The subpoena may request that we Xerox the whole chart and send it to lawyers in which case I need to read the whole chart to make sure that every "t" is crossed and "i" is dotted. Not uncommonly, the subpoena is for the chart of an inactive patient and we might have to request that the chart be sent to us from its storage site in Iron Mountain, which can take a couple weeks. Rarely, the chart is missing altogether which is calamitous, but we tell this to the court because it is the truth. The trial may go forward without this evidence if we say that it is missing. In the usual case, we Xerox the chart and send it to the lawyers. Sometimes, the lawyers can not interpret our handwriting and request to come over to interrogate us verbally at which time they will also ask us to tell them our impressions of the case and other information that may not be in the chart. Appearance in court is rare—but horrible. We have to cancel all our patients for the whole day and wait around in the court until an indeterminate time of the day. Then we take the stand, and the lawyers grill us—it can be very unpleasant since we speak "medicalese" and they speak "legalese".

Obligatory reporting to the Secret Service and clandestine services.

Not practicing in D.C., this issue has only come up once in my career when one of the Presidents came to Cleveland to give a speech downtown. The Secret Service came to the nearest tertiary care center (St. Vincent Charity) which was the nearest ER. It also happened to be the site of the regional Psychiatric ER. We were requested to disclose the names of any psychiatric patients who had expressed negative feelings toward the sitting President.

Psychiatrists and Drugs

1—Prescribing of regular prescriptions (Rx) requires only a State medical license.

2—Prescribing of scheduled drugs (Controlled Substances) is controlled by a federal drug license. The federal drug license is issued by the DEA (Drug Enforcement Administration). Access to scheduled drugs is controlled by the government because the drugs are addicting and some are also classified as dangerous.

a—Addicting Drugs are schedule two through five C-II—C-V (Valium, Vicodin, Demerol);

b—Addicting drugs which have their own special control mechanisms: the narcotic Suboxone requires its own special DEA license;

c—Dangerous drugs which are still available on written prescription but have especially restricted and tightly monitored prescribing control: Thalidomide, and Xyrem. These may be more dangerous than addicting: the tranquilizer Thalidomide caused catastrophic birth defects (but is used in leprosy treatment) and Xyrem is the infamous "date rape drug" which is used for treating Narcolepsy;

d—Dangerous drugs are scheduled C-I (LSD, Ecstasy, heroin, Quaalude, marijuana and others): some of these are not necessarily highly addicting (LSD); No doctor is permitted to prescribe these without a special [research] license; these are not FDA approved for use in humans. They are forbidden drugs.

e—"Abandoned Drugs"—these are drugs which were once marketed here in the USA and are legal here, but they do not produce enough profit to make it worthwhile for anybody to go on selling them here: Parsidol, mecamyalamine, Serentil, and so on. (You will need a written prescription so that you can order them from abroad.)

Confidentiality: psychiatric records are kept under double lock and key and are thus subject to double confidentiality (remember the Water Gate break-in?). Medical records about AIDS are also kept under this kind of confidentiality.

Patient access to her own chart. Many patients have read something about the HIPAA regulations which assure patients that they can know what is in their confidential charts.

This may be true indeed for medical and surgical patients, but it is often not in the best interest of psychiatric patients. We can decline to let the patient read her own chart verbatim which is acceptable legally under HIPAA as long as we provide her with a letter outlining the highlights and important aspects of her treatment.

People making this request are usually the ones who are least likely be served well by reading their own charts. These requests seem somewhat outré because: (1)-we are basically writing down what you tell us; (2) if you want to know your diagnosis, then we will be glad to discuss it with you; and, (3) we are aware of this eventuality and use succinct and specialized terminology which can really only be readily understood by those of us in the field who know how to "read between the lines", anyway. We will gladly Xerox your whole chart and send it to your new psychiatrist (but he is barred under federal law from re-releasing these records to any third party, i.e., his new patient).

Dangerous Patients

Patient aggression against a psychiatrist is another situation in which doctors interface with the legal system. This can include threatening or stalking the psychiatrist (for various reasons).

Some patients who are truly ill may become obsessed with their psychiatrists and may start stalking him or her. These are usually dangerous and psychotic patients so the psychiatrist may be in considerable danger. The psychiatrist will need to take appropriate steps to safeguard his life, including such actions as obtaining a TRO (temporary restraining order). Sometimes the patient imagines the psychiatrist as a focus of anger or romantic love or the patient is very needy of constant attention, or obsessed for some other reason.

Forensic psychiatrists or psychiatrists who deal with criminals may be exposed to a lot of danger also. This can happen in the case of an incarcerated gang member who wants some special treatment from his prison psychiatrist. Failure to comply could bring down the wrath of the street-loose gang members onto the psychiatrist or his family. Hopefully, the State government will seal the state's personnel records on prison psychiatrists.

Some psychotic patients who stalk psychiatrists may also kill the psychiatrist. This happens a few times each year in our country.

Dissident psychiatrists practicing in dictatorships can be punished by their government and can even be caused to "disappear" (this happened to at least three psychiatrists during the "dirty war" in Argentina in the 1980's). During the Cold War, Soviet psychiatrists were forced to diagnose political dissidents as obviously psychotic. These dissidents then received injections of long-last major tranquilizers (antipsychotics).

Under unusual circumstances, a deranged family member might kill a doctor if his loved one died or was maimed in some way that the family member imputes to be the doctor's fault. Psychiatrists might be killed by psychotic husbands of suicide wives (surgeons also can have this kind of bad experience with psychotic husbands in cases of catastrophic surgical outcomes).

Most doctors try to avoid coming into contact with the law if at all possible.

IV—Ethics

The word "Ethics" comes from Greek and means "morality, custom, character, temperament" [27]. Dorland's dictionary defines it as "the rules or principles which guide right conduct; the rules or principles governing the professional conduct of physicians". I envision ethics as the way I would like to be treated. Unethical behavior might not be illegal by State laws—but this behavior could become legislated as illegal in the future. A fair amount of unethical behavior is illegal or is at odds with the policies of the state medical board.

The use of non-standard, unusual, or idiosyncratic treatments (therapies) could be considered unethical in some cases but not necessarily in all cases. Patients should be given a choice of treatments and notified in advance if a treatment falls into this category. On the other hand, some patients are seeking out treatments which are novel or not "usual and customary". Some patients might have various reasons for this: recommendation by a friend, interest in novelty, desperation after having failed several other therapies. I think that it is important to alert patients to their various treatment options and to the expected risks and benefits. Psychiatry has had its share of "novel" treatments: "recovered memories", "primal scream", SAM-e, and so on.

In the case of elder patients going into their "dotage" or becoming "senile" (starting to have memory or judgment problems), it is important to find a balanced medium where they can be protected from possible indirect harm to themselves or others while trying not to deprive them of their autonomy (civil rights). Some of the murkiest ethical decisions concern the elderly who come in with younger unrelated neighbors or helpers who *seem* to be acting for the benefit of the elder patient—these may be lifelong friends or new acquaintances. In such cases, the elder is often childless or widowed. I do not allow these relationships to usurp the patient's rights. I ask them to come back for a number of visits while I try to acquire background information. Are there any blood-relatives anywhere— and if so, who and where? I usually insist that the elder patient begin working with one of our therapists who will provide an extra set of ears and eyes and is usually very capable of ferreting out the extent of the relationship between the elder and the "friend". In some cases, this friend may be the lifelong best friend of the patient's only daughter who recently died of breast cancer. The patient and friend may be bonded not only by a lifelong history but also now by grief. The two of them may have been very close for decades. In other cases, somebody from the neighborhood may accompany the elder patient, perhaps a casual acquaintance for only the last couple years—or perhaps the next-door neighbor who has a pertinent interest in keeping the patient from leaving the gas stove on and blowing up the whole house. Or to prevent the patient from summoning the police to the neighborhood by frequently calling 9-1-1. The next-door neighbor's personal interests may be at a practical level. This level of community involvement is admirable, but does not necessarily entitle a neighbor to the legal rights of a relative.

And then, there are the neighborhood opportunists who should not be entitled to have control over the patient's property. The opportunists often think that they are going to gain control over the patient's home and money, but we try to expose them and their agenda. The real legal morass here is where the opportunist has already cajoled the elder patient into signing legal documents. If we had never seen the patient before the signing, we can not attest to her mental abilities at that time—but we can make an educated guess. These cases are best left for the County to sort out: elder abuse and fraud department followed by assignment of a county-appointed conservator/guardian.

Some inappropriate and unethical activities by psychiatrists would be accepting exquisite gifts from patients, socializing with patients, bartering or trading services (psychiatric care exchanged for coiffure, free car washes, catering the doctor's daughter's wedding), and so on.

▶Psychiatry routinely has more interaction with police and courts of law than most other branches of medicine—except for pathologists—just by the very nature of what we do. Our intersections with the law are so frequent and ubiquitous, that there is an extra two-year program for psychiatrists who wish to follow a career path in legal psychiatry (forensic psychiatry fellowship).

Insanity as Medical Diagnosis and Legal Plea
Insanity as the Inability to Control our Behaviors
Criminality and Psychiatry

Psychiatry intersects the legal domain when a person's behavior flagrantly violates community standards. Such behavior could be immoral, illegal, criminal, or forbidden. Psychiatry considers criminal behavior to fall within a spectrum of "anti-social" behaviors, where "anti-social" means "against society". Many of the perpetrators of criminal acts are "anti-social" in the sense that their behaviors are against society—against the laws, morals, and codes of conduct of the society in which they live and which laws the perpetrators are presumed to know, having grown up in that society. Anti-social behavior is any act that jeopardizes the commonwealth of that society. There is a whole spectrum of anti-social behavior, ranging from one-time offenders to constantly repeating offenders (recidivists). There is no known medical cure for these anti-social behaviors (*Clockwork Orange*, notwithstanding). Notably, psychiatry has very little to offer in the ways of treating or controlling this condition and even diagnoses it by re-stating the condition using Greek and Latine terms ("anti-social", "sociopath", or "psychopath"). (The only known physical means of or medical remedy for controlling anti-social behavior is by means of a brain lobotomy, which is no longer in use.)

A one time anti-social act could be committed by a teenager named Andrew. He might not necessarily have a psychiatric condition. Who among us has never done anything naughty? Let that be the person to cast the first stone. "Anti-social" is not a psychiatric illness that relieves Andrew from facing the legal justice. Somewhere along the line from naughtiness to mischief to sin and then on to crime, society imposes incremental restrictions or boundaries beyond which he must not go or else the legal system will cite him or punish him:

carelessness ↔ mischief ↔ "wrong crowd"	↔ repeated bad choices ↔		misdemeanor ↔ felony
When to punish? here? ↑ or here?	↑	?	↑ yes ↑ here for sure...↑

As far as carelessness, occasionally, a schizophrenic or a manic-depressive will be so psychotic (or manic) that he may witlessly run out of a store with unpaid merchandise. Even in this case of a well-documented long-term psychiatric illness, it would be difficult to prove that a patient was mentally incompetent unless the psychiatrist had actually witnessed the act. The psychiatrist can provide a reference letter to the court, but the legal system may judge the patient guilty of shoplifting, regardless of any such letter.

"Mischief" may be a part of the impulsivity of adolescence. Mischief may be part of impulse disorders, such as kleptomania. These impulses are not excusable by the Laws (unless there is hard evidence of an "irresistible impulse"—see below). Not one of these is excused by the law on the basis of being compulsive or impulsive: Kleptomania, Oniomania (compulsive shopping), Dipsomania (compulsive drinking), and Satyriasis (male sexual compulsive), and Nymphomania (female sexual compulsive).

The repeat offenders—psychiatrically speaking—can perhaps be grouped as obsessive-compulsives, career criminals, or " 'good kids' who just fell in with a 'bad' crowd"—or somewhere along this spectrum.

Shop-lifting might be confined to a very brief period in a person's life (impulsivity) or it could be a long-standing problem (compulsivity). These are two different conditions: the brief time-limited shop-lifters who have suppressed psychological problems and are impulsively "acting out"; and, the compulsive shoppers.

Brief time-limited shop-lifters are acting out some suppressed emotionality. They usually have a lot of therapy issues that go back to an unhappy childhood or fractured relationships (for which they may still be blaming themselves—and hence, may feel that they are in need of punishment). Their ways of dealing with these suppressed emotions are manifold: often by self-injury, drinking, sulking, exercising, brooding, or going on any kind of spree (shopping, over-sexing, drinking, and so on). A desire for self-punishment may emerge as well as a need for a thrilling distraction for which shop-lifting temporarily provides a relief. This is not likely to be chronic as it probably is not the patient's self-treatment of choice. They know that petty theft is punishable, but savor the riskiness and in some cases they relish the attention, be it negative or not. These people may have psychological problems but they are still liable for their actions—and they know it, too. Middle-aged women are often found in this group: they may be single or in a loveless marriage. Sometimes teenagers and young adults engage in these activities for the thrill of the risk of being caught. This is impulsive shop-lifting.

In other cases, there is a second and different category of patients who are compulsive shoppers ("oniomaniacs"). They derive great pleasure from shopping and this activity may release "brain hormones" that reinforce the activity. These people are like modern-day "pursuit trackers". They track down sales, "stalk" garage sales, and so on. The spending of money is by itself exciting and that is merely compounded by the acquisition of stuff: these are usually women who like to vaunt their conquests the way that hunters and fishers talk about their game. These compulsive shoppers may be out on a spree or "on a run" and simply run out of money or have overcharged their credit cards to the point that they know it will lead to an argument with their husbands. So they continue their shopping addiction without paying for the merchandise. These can be impulsive decisions that are merely superimposed upon a long-standing compulsive disorder. The underlying compulsion has been present for a long time and will continue so until the patient enters a twelve step program for debtors, clutterers, and shoppers anonymous. Shoplifting is just an extension of their form of pathologically compulsive shopping—they have just run out of money! This is one of the subtypes of obsessive-compulsive disorders. These may be conditions of interest to psychiatrists, but such a diagnosis will not relieve the patients of legal consequences.

Then there is a distinct category, that being the career criminals who make a living by going against society. They are considered to be people with an "antisocial personality disorder" if their condition is mild to moderate. If it is moderate to severe we call them "sociopaths". The severest among these are the so-called psychopaths (old terminology). These terms are in common use among psychiatrists, but you may not find them described exactly like this in modern textbooks. The less horrific are the antisocial personalities who have a life-long career of deviousness, trickery, chicanery, petty theft, grifting, duping, and conning other people. They may limit themselves to mischief and misdemeanors and may not be physically confrontational at all, but are still liable for their illicit actions—and they know it too. Psychiatrists do not normally see these people ever—unless they come in for some additional and treatable condition such as depression or adjustment disorder. Anti-socials will never come in primarily for treatment of antisocial behaviors—unless sent by their defense attorney. The attorney is trying to find some psychiatric condition that would be a defense in court. Antisocials do not have a profound psychiatric illness that would excuse them from legal repercussions. The true sociopaths are worse yet and are usually the hardened career criminals, such as gangsters or mobsters. Felonious recidivism (repeat offenses) is their way of life. They have severe sociopathic disorder for which there is no known psychiatric cure—or exculpation, either. And, the worst of all the antisocial disorders are the psychopaths who would best be typified by dangerous stalkers and serial killers. Psychopaths have profound psychiatric illness which is incurable and not really treatable—their behaviors can sometimes be toned down or reined in by major antipsychotic drugs; however, if they do not believe that they are sick, then they will not take these drugs on their own after release from prison. And most of them will not take these medicines willingly. These are often the cases that need to serve out a lengthy prison sentence either in a regular prison or while in a forensic psychiatric hospital (a kind of high-security psychiatric penal institution). Like all severe personality disorders, sociopaths gradually "burn out"—or better yet, "burn down"—with aging. Psychopaths are extremely dangerous. Psychiatry has very little to offer all these anti-social people except for powerful anti-psychotic medications (which they are probably more likely to give to their victims than to take for themselves).

The word "insane" comes from Latin* and means "unhealthy" in the most general sense of the word. This word "insane" has certainly come to have the specific meaning of genuine mental illness in modern English. However, insane is usually used in "legalese" to be synonymous with mentally ill whereas modern medicine does not use the word "insane", instead opting to use terms such as "mental illness" to describe psychiatric disability of any kind.

Insanity as a concept has many interpretations. For all practical purposes, insanity is the inability to control ourselves: our ideas, our speech, our actions and behavior. This is a behavioral state in which involuntary impulse trumps voluntary control. Ultimately, if we all live long enough, I believe that we will all become "insane" in the sense of no longer controlling ourselves or of wanting to control ourselves; by saying "live long enough" I am suggesting that this behavior might occur only at age 120 or 130 years in some people. Most people do not reach that point in their lives. By saying "insane" I refer to the point in life where people are no longer interested in controlling themselves, no longer able to control themselves, or no longer recognize the difference between self-control and dyscontrol (poor control). At some point in life, a lot of people lose the ability or the desire to control themselves—this can be seen in elderly patients who have never had any psychiatric symptoms for the first seventy or eighty or ninety years of their lives. They gradually lose the ability or desire to control their thoughts and actions. As a consequence, they will do whatever they please and think, when and where they please. They might well say whatever pops into their minds without the benefit of the overriding censorship [of the Freudian "superego"] that governed their behaviors before senility commenced. They may or may not be entering into mild dementia. Sometimes, the basic personality comes to the fore absent any dementia. Thus, the fine line between "sanity" and "insanity" becomes blurred.

These types of senile disinhibition are often accepted by the average citizen to be a possible part of the aging process; however, when this inability to control one's self occurs in young people, it attracts a lot of attention. This behavior is considered abnormal and disordered (pathological) in young people. It is then diagnosed as schizophrenia, manic-depression, delusions, or similar diagnosis. And the patient is referred to a psychiatrist. The timing of the onset of this loss of self-control seems to have certain peak ages: at earlier ages from puberty into the early thirties (ages 16-30[+]); and, in elderly patients.

Criminal Behavior and Violence

Criminal behavior is a product of personality style: it spreads across all cross-sections of society. Schizophrenics and manics may be prone to psychotic behavior but they are not necessarily prone to violence. Violent behavior is dependent on personality, not on major mental illness.

One current theory advanced by psychiatric researchers is that of "spectrum disease" which suggests that all these manic and psychotic disorders are governed by one underlying pathology, but that its appearance in different patients depends on a number of variable factors such as genetics, environment, and upbringing. Renegade genes could be causing the driving force for the insanity and other rogue genes could be involved in producing the apparent and observable variety of symptoms. We also know that some genes are timing genes that can turn on and off at different ages through the span of our lifetime. This timed turn-on can occur with well-known medical problems such as high cholesterol, which can often have its genetically-predetermined onset in middle age.

Not Guilty by Reason of Insanity (NGRI)

The legal theory of this legal defense began in the 1800's and has percolated through the courts since then. This is a ploy initiated by many defense attorneys in criminal cases. The accused is sent to see a Court-appointed psychiatrist who may or may not diagnose the accused with a mental illness such as mania or schizophrenia. However, even if the accused person has a long history of severe mental illness, this diagnosis rarely releases a patient from legal liability in criminal trials. Being adjudged NGRI requires passing strict legal tests of being totally psychotic at the time of the crime. The following psychiatric diagnoses would probably never qualify for the legal remedy of NGRI : Personality Disorder, Sociopathic Behaviors, Depression, Adjustment Disorder, Drug Addiction, Alcoholism, and so on. These diagnoses could be mitigating factors (resulting in a lesser penalty) but not exculpatory (relieved of penalty). A smaller percentage may have a pre-existing mental disorder of schizophrenia, but this may not be exculpatory, either. Andrew who suffers from chronic schizophrenia is certainly entitled to enter a plea of NGRI, but then his attorney must prove that he was so psychotic at the time of the crime that he did not know the difference between right and wrong, or was suffering from an "irresistible impulse". This "irresistible impulse" must conclusively be proven by the defense attorney: only about 0.1% of these types of NGRI pleas are ever adjudicated (settled) in the defendant's favor, even when Andrew has a qualifying schizophrenic diagnosis.

As far as Schizophrenics are concerned, Andrew is no more likely—or less likely—to be a sociopath than you or I. Most schizophrenics know that they have a severe mental illness and that they need their medicines and even feel much better while taking their medicines as prescribed. If Andrew had committed a crime while psychotic, he will be held accountable, and he knows all this, too.

If Andrew had not refilled his medicines or was not keeping appointments with his psychiatrist, then he was "non-adherent" (not taking his medication on a regular basis). If his psychosis acted up during this time, then he may be at fault because he was not doing what he was supposed to be doing in order to prevent the foreseeable actions of un-medicated schizophrenia (a relapse into unacceptable behaviors).

On the other hand, there are some schizophrenic patients unlike Andrew who refuse to acknowledge that they even have a psychotic illness. This is "denial", as in they deny that they have a problem.

This is a personality "defect" with a certain amount of egotism (narcissism) and assumes a lack of humility on their part. Assume that the definition of humility is "the ability to see ourselves as we really are." Then they refuse to admit that they are schizophrenic despite overwhelming evidence to the contrary: multiple hospitalizations for hallucinations and runs-in with the police. This is their egotism. Admitting that they have a severe mental illness would be a huge blow to their ego. Also, narcissistic people resent authority (other than their own) and resent authority figures "dictating" orders to them. They resent the fact that someone does not share their opinion that they are superior and flawless human beings. These schizophrenics have two big problems: schizophrenia (an Axis I diagnosis) plus personality disorder (an Axis II diagnosis). These are the ones likeliest to have trouble with the police.

Similarly, stubborn patients want to make up their own treatment plans to the exclusion of medical advice. Some stubborn patients may resist medications on "philosophical" grounds. Examples are: they reason that their lives are already damaged by schizophrenia, so taking chemicals is just a weak "crutch"; or, that the medicines cause more damage than the disease; and some like to debate the causes of schizophrenia, pointing out that since psychiatry does not know the specific cause(s) of schizophrenia, then there really is no specific treatment.

These above types of patients are in denial and will never take their medicines correctly, and will always be out of control until they "burn out" sometime in later life. In actuality, sometimes they "burn down" and not out. Chronic denial patients cannot be cured with medicines—ever. If these types of schizophrenics also have antisocial tendencies and continue to deny that they have a mental illness, then they will continue to refuse medications and hence will repeat crimes. There is no apparent societal advantage to setting these people free before they have served their full sentence, be it in a regular jail or in a psychiatric prison.

And in a fourth category, sometimes diligent (adherent) patients will feel really good for a couple years on their medicines, then think that they are cured or start to forget to take their pills. They will eventually relapse and have an unpleasant episode. In some cases, obtaining the medicines is difficult. In other cases, the most diligent of patients will be tired of drug side-effects and quit the pills.

The fifth category is patients who are very diligent (adherent, compliant) who take their medications as indicated, but still have a break-through episode that the medicines somehow failed to prevent. Schizophrenia is like diabetes or heart disease: sometimes it can aggravate despite being well-treated. These patients are very well-meaning and would be most deserving of a medical excuse for any resultant psychosis.

There is also a tiny percentage of schizophrenics who do have good insight, good judgment, good adherence to psychiatric treatment, and do acknowledge that they have a mental illness. If there is some extenuating reason why they have not been adherent with their appropriately prescribed antipsychotic medication—that there is some circumstance beyond their control—then they might qualify for a plea of NGRI provided that they have been very compliant for many years, do have good insight, are willing to participate in their treatment plans, do show remorse, and can pass the "irresistible impulse" test. Under certain rare circumstances, they might be eligible for the application of the NGRI defense.

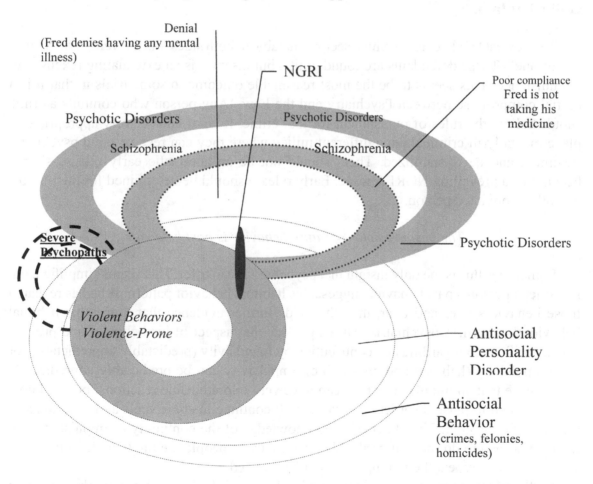

Diagram VII-2 NGRI This diagram shows that of all Antisocial Behaviors (crimes), most are committed by Antisocial Personality Disorders. And about half of these are violent

crimes. There is little overlap between ASPD and severe mental illness. The large gray ring shows all psychotic disorders, and schizophrenia is a smaller group within all psychotic disorders (white circle). The most common reason for psychotics/schizophrenics to get out of control is by not taking their medicines for any of several reasons, the most common and dangerous reason being due to denial (Fred denies he has any psychotic disorder that needs to be medicated in the first place). Of all these cases, only a tiny sliver of defendants (perpetrators) may be eligible for a legal plea of NGRI. The heavily dashed ring of severe psychopaths refers to serial killers and criminals of that ilk who are very violent, very antisocial, and whose behaviors take on monstrous proportions of a psychotic intensity— they are in a special category.

Guilty but Insane

The newest legal device—which seems palatable to both sides—is the verdict of "Guilty but Insane". These defendants are found guilty, but insanity is an extenuating (excusable) circumstance. This seems to be the most reasonable outcome to some trials in that it is a partial compromise between Psychiatry and the Law. 'Any person who commits a crime should follow the rules of punishment for that crime. It is, of course, very appropriate to place mentally ill criminals in a different milieu where they can receive good psychiatric treatment and be re-stabilized. There should not be an automatic early release simply because of a prevailing NGRI defense. Early release should be determined for them as for any other convicted person.

...The best predictor of future behavior is past behavior...

Sometimes this is the only insight that psychiatrists can offer. This seems simplified, but it is true: a person's past behavior suggests his habitual behavior pattern. If he has repeated those behaviors over and over, then that adds further evidence that that is his habitual behavioral pattern. A psychiatrist can emphasize that aspect of his behavior and provide some clarification regarding any contribution by impulsivity (predictably unpredictable) or by compulsivity (habitual and predictable). Impulsivity can be predictably unpredictable in the sense that an impulsive person can have very unpredictable reactions; but we know that he has an impulse disorder and that he will continue to show signs and symptoms of this impulse disorder. This diagnosis and knowledge of the continuity of impulsivity and its habitual nature do make it predictable. Compulsive people are predictable in that they will continue to repeat their compulsions unless treated.

Furthermore, manics and schizophrenics have habitual symptoms in the way that they have psychosis or mania. When schizophrenics become ill again, they go back to having the same delusions and the same hallucinations—they do not change or develop new symptoms. For example, psychotic jealousy about his wife is going to be the same symptom every time that a jealous man becomes psychotic: he will not suddenly change to another kind of delusion and will not start to have hallucinations of pink elephants. A bipolar who always starts new business venture while manic, will continue to follow that pattern, although with each manic episode, the costs of the venture may increase—he will not suddenly switch to manic preaching on the downtown street corners, or to irrepressible hypersexuality and promiscuity, so on. People will remain true to type, usually.

As such, these habitual behaviors emanate from the person's underlying personality style; this style does not change throughout life.

Some schizophrenics and manics can change their attitudes with therapy. If this happens, the outcome is that they become more adherent to medication schedules and doctor visits—and they also learn to recognize early symptoms of a relapse before the relapse overwhelms them. Additionally, they learn from past relapses that the ultimate outcome is unpleasant and they will have to deal with the aftermath of their behaviors when the whole episode is over. And lastly, they decide to be willing to learn that although being manic is highly pleasurable, they gain insight that mania may not be worth the trouble when balanced against the ensuing depressions.

What goes up, comes down.

▶QUESTIONS

Q: Is antisocial behavior a psychiatric illness?

A: Not exactly. We call it Antisocial Personality, which technically makes it a psychiatric diagnosis, but it has no known specific causes or treatment. This is true of all "personality styles".

Q: If I lose the ability to control my behaviors, then am I crazy?

A: It would depend on the frequency and intensity of dyscontrol (loss of control):

- If mild and occasional, a person could be seen as "neurotic" or "eccentric"

- If moderate and more persistent, it could be seen as a type of "Nervous Breakdown";

- If continuous but reversible, it is treatable;

- If constant and severe, it is truly grave and serious—it could become permanent.

When these behaviors impact any sphere of our lives (work, home, leisure) to various degrees, then they should probably be treated before they have the chance to progress further to the constant and severe stages. Progression is always a possibility.

Q: Is it possible that genetic variations result in peak onsets in different ages? Is it possible that timing genes are involved?

A: This will be a fertile area for research in the coming years.

Q: Am I becoming "insane"?

A: If you still have the capacity to process the concept of a diagnosis of insanity and you can contemplate the complexity of what this means, then you probably may not be—or at least not yet.

▶ The legal system seeks justice (not necessarily truth), is subject to political manipulation and pressure from society; jurisprudence also seems like a "soft science".

▶ When medically oriented doctors (psychiatrists) and lawyers meet in court, they both speak different languages, "medicalese" and "legalese",

---

* *"Insane" as a Latin word implies a broad range of dysfunction, often assumed to be mental illness; but, in Latin it can also mean "maddening, outrageous, ridiculous, extravagant, monstrous, inspired," ... (New College Latin & English Dictionary by John C. Traupman, PhD)*

Chapter VII-3

Going to the Psychiatric Hospital

This chapter gives a brief and general overview of admissions and stays in psychiatric hospitals. There are three basic types of psychiatric hospitalizations in the USA: free-standing, Governmental, or part of a General Hospital.

"Free-standing" hospitals provide only psychiatric care. This usually amounts to a conglomeration of psychiatric wards "under one roof" (under one administration). These hospitals afford more privacy because they are usually somewhat isolated and specialized. You will not bump into your neighbors who are visiting their new grandchild, and so on. The disadvantage is that these hospitals have no real provisions for a full range of medical emergencies. Medical doctors come to visit patients in these hospitals and may even have a dedicated office on-site. Any serious medical emergency requires that the patient be sent to the nearest general hospital by ambulance. Conveniently, the larger of these free-standing institutions do provide on-site ECT ("shock treatments").

Governmental hospitals are run by counties, cities, states, and the federal government. Large counties often have a designated county hospital to which all indigent patients go for treatment. Very large cities might have such an institution also. Most States run state hospitals which are intended for two types of patients: long-term chronic persistently and severely ill psychiatric patients and forensic patients (criminally insane). The federal government has federal prison hospital prisons, but most notable the VA system. States with very small populations might not run state hospitals but contract out with free-standing hospitals to see State patients.

General hospitals often have a psychiatric ward as part of their suite of services. These types of hospitals are familiar to you. They typically have an ER, an intensive care unit, and operating rooms. The advantage of this location is that emergency medical treatment is just down the hallway. These are preferred settings for geriatric psychiatry units and for medically ill patients. General hospitals are fun and exciting locations for psychiatrists who are more biologically or medically oriented or who have very ill patients.

Admission to a Psychiatric Hospital

What it Means

It may mean being put in a psychiatric hospital against one's will. There are two ways to get a bed in a psychiatric hospital: Voluntarily or Involuntarily. If the psychiatrist allows a person to sign voluntary admission papers, then it is a tacit acknowledgement that the patient has enough wherewithal to realize that he is in a severe emotional crisis. But nowadays HMO's (in California) will not pay for a voluntary admission—only for involuntary. However, PPO's usually will pay for both. A voluntary admission can sign into the hospital—but can also sign himself out voluntarily. An involuntary patient is deemed to be so sick as to need hospitalization against his wishes. Psychiatrists usually certify how sick involuntary patients are. Criteria for being this sick include: suicide, homicide, psychosis, and "grave disability" (see below).

VOLUNTARY

A patient can admit himself voluntarily by having a conscious feeling that he is experiencing so many symptoms that he wants to be in a safe place. HMO's usually do not pay for voluntary admissions as they feel it to be an unnecessary expense. HMO's reason that the symptoms can just as well be treated at home or in the doctor's office. Voluntary patients may realize that they are in crisis or—worse—are having a psychiatric emergency. In some cases, the HMO voluntary patient (in crisis) and the admitting doctor can reach a conclusion that the crisis should really be upgraded to an emergency. This will be covered by your HMO. However, if your HMO looks back later and decides that you were "just in crisis" and not "emergent", then the HMO will often not pay for the admission. The HMO will send the bill to those involved in your admission—usually you and the admitting hospital and its doctor.

INVOLUNTARY

The second way for a person to get into a psychiatric hospital is to be put there against his will, involuntarily, by having a psychiatric emergency. In this case, a psychiatrist will fill out all the paperwork—unless the police or some other qualified certifying agency has already filled out the paperwork, which can be an extensive amount of paperwork in some States. Basically, this paperwork deprives a citizen of his civil rights for a brief period of time (This includes separation of a married couple, "loss of consortium"). Children and adults who are already wards of the court (such as adult mentally retarded or elderly Alzheimer patients) can be signed into a psychiatric hospital against their will if the guardian wants it so. If the guardian/conservator does not want the patient in the hospital, then the psychiatrist can still sign in the child or ward. The guardian may later sue the psychiatrist, but at least the psychiatrist was trying to preserve a life.

The main reason that guardians and conservators oppose involuntary admissions against their wishes is usually encountered in cases of Alzheimer patients whose adult children are reluctant to deplete financial assets. Parents of children under eighteen usually oppose involuntary hospitalization by the emergency psychiatrist for totally different reasons: the stigma of being in a psychiatric hospital, or the negative experiences that the children might encounter there, or meeting up with other kids who are even worse.

Psychiatric Emergencies

Nonetheless, psychiatrists are duty-bound and legally obligated to admit anybody—voluntarily or involuntary—to a psychiatric hospital if that person is probably having a psychiatric emergency. The four situations that constitute a psychiatric emergency occur when a person is:

- homicidal
- suicidal
- actively psychotic
- "gravely disabled": a person is so disorganized or so mentally incompetent that he cannot independently care for himself and there are no community resources immediately available to fulfill this mission—or such similar wording (depending upon State laws).

Homicidal Persons

This is a very dangerous group of people who can include former criminals, stalkers, sexual predators, jilted lovers, ex-patients, alcoholics-drug-addicts, political dissidents, disgruntled employees, and so on. These people will not voluntarily show up requesting treatment since they believe that the problem lies with the source (or target) of their anger. These people certainly will not accept any medical or psychiatric treatment voluntarily—although they make a pretense of being treated if a felony is hanging over them. The most effective treatment is usually that of a legal remedy: incarceration and temporary restraining orders. It is very difficult to get these patients to take any medicines unless adverse legal consequences can be brought to bear. In some cases, long-lasting injections can be given: three antipsychotic medicines are available in the form of long-acting injections; also some sexual predators in the past have agreed to take long-acting female hormones (Depo-Provera) to tame their sexual urges. Sometimes a combination of medical, psychiatric , and legal treatments can be effective—but only if the patient has incentives to get better (such as supervised visitation rights with his children, return to his job, other incentives plus the threat of a long incarceration if he relapses). How many Psychiatrists does it take to change a light bulb? Only one, but only if the light bulb really wants to be changed.

In case of doubt, always try to have a potentially homicidal person sent involuntarily to a psychiatric hospital for a few days of observation. During this time, any/other potential victims can be warned, and the seriousness of his threats can be investigated. This also gives the treatment team time to observe his baseline behaviors and discern if he has violent propensities. His legal, medical, and psychiatric records may be accessed during this time. If he has a long history of violent crimes, then the court system should take custody of him. If he has an unusual and rare medical problem that might predispose him to bad judgment, tantrums, or impulsivity then he is a "med-psych" case and will need further observation. If he has a long psychiatric history, then it most desirable that he be kept in the psychiatric hospital involuntarily. Some preliminary probate court hearings are held in the psychiatric hospital and sometimes they may be held in the courtroom to which the violent patients must be accompanied by sheriff's deputies.

If there is still a lingering doubt after a few days of enforced observation, then he should be recommended for a prolongation of his involuntary hospitalization and observation period (for about two more weeks). Of course, the legal system might opt to observe him during this time in their own institution and they may transfer him there. The important decision is to detain him until there is reason to believe that he is no longer a danger to society.

The famous Tarasoff case in California helped to establish the law (case law precedent) for dealing with dangerous patients. That law states that if any mental health professional reasonably believes that his client/patient might be on the verge of killing somebody then that professional is legally duty-bound to protect any potential victims; this law goes beyond "duty to warn" and requires "duty to protect". Sometimes warning will not be concrete enough.

Suicidal Patients (see also Chapter IV-7 on Suicide)
Suicide can be divided into Active and Passive behaviors.

ACTIVE Suicidal Behavior

(see chapter IV-7)

Some patients just think about suicide as a general "way out" of all the stress but have no current plans or—even better—feel that is against their religion. They feel bad enough that they cannot think about feeling better right now but preserve functioning that tells them that psychiatric treatment will probably be helpful. These people have a "**passive death wish**".

Some people are actually planning a possible suicide if things get even worse. They may have amassed many months of sleeping pills, bought a gun, or figured how they can drive off a cliff without hurting anybody else. Although they have not done anything yet, these patients are of concern. These people have **suicidal ideation** (ideas about usable methods for suicide). Some might be treated as outpatients as long as they have extensive family support. If they have several high-risk factors, they will be placed in a psychiatric bed against their will. Some of these patients may agree to a voluntary admission, but the disadvantage of a voluntary admission is that they can sign themselves out voluntarily—which may not coincide with the psychiatrist's treatment plan.

Some people have done something potentially dangerous to see how much their body can tolerate in preparation for the real suicide attempt. These are patients who are brought into the emergency room (ER) either by the police against their will or voluntarily by ambulance. This is usually some sort of self-injury that they thought would be fatal or they are testing how much harm they need to do in order to succeed at suicide. These self injuries can range anywhere from taking eight aspirin pills to a whole months supply of all their heart and diabetes pills or even a two months supply of sleeping pills. These patients have made a **suicide gesture**. In most cases, they will be admitted to a psychiatric ward. Occasionally women (or men) do this in a dramatic way to get the attention of their significant others. If the significant other comes to the ER expressing positive sentiments toward the patient and the patient feels that her goal has been achieved and if she renounces her gesture, then she might be released into the care of the significant other (depending on the patient's living situation and other social support circumstances).

Finally, we have bona fide **suicide attempts** that are intentionally and usually lethal but that the patient has somehow managed to survive. I have seen surviving cases of self-inflicted gunshots to the chest and head, self stabbings to the abdomen, slashed wrists, overdoses, and people who have rammed their car into a tree at high speeds or jumped off a high bridge or flung themselves into rush hour traffic—and survived. These people will be admitted to the hospital automatically for three days and it is highly likely that the involuntary stay will be legally extended to fourteen days—or beyond. Many others who employ these same means do succeed at suicide. Thus, these are very serious cases.

PASSIVE Suicidal and PARASUICIDAL Behaviors (see Chapter IV-7)

These kinds of risky behavior are often unnoticed by friends and family, but sometimes detected by doctors. These behaviors occur when the patient secretly decides to allow himself to die. Examples include the diabetic who overeats sugar, the renal patient on dialysis who "overdoses" on potassium-rich foods, or patients with cancer or AIDS who willfully and knowingly stop taking the drugs that keep them alive and that keep the disease under control.

ACCIDENTAL Suicidal Behaviors

People who are thrill-seekers or exhibitionists often engage in quite dangerous pastimes. They are well aware of the riskiness in their behaviors, but feel invincible. These people may relish an adrenalin rush or are really desperate for money. Their antics usually go beyond parachuting and bungee-jumping. These people apparently have no real desire to kill themselves (or do they....?). We had such a case in Cleveland of a bridge-jumping thrill-seeker brought in by the police. The bridge-jumper had made no suicide attempt but had displayed really bad judgment or poor impulse control.

See also Chapter IV-7 on Suicide.

Actively Psychotic

These patients are out of contact with reality and must be hospitalized until they are "restored to sanity". Only a psychiatrist can hospitalize and treat patients with this diagnosis. Psychosis can consist of delusions, illusions, hallucinations or mania. **Delusions** are described as a fixed false belief. Some men have jealous delusions about their wives and believe that the wives are having sex with many other men and all the time. Some people think that the government is out to get them. **Illusions** occur when a person sees or hears something real but gives it a different meaning. Hearing a random noise outside and thinking that it is some form of significant communication: this has some basis in reality but is misinterpreted by the patient. **Hallucinations** occur when there is no real noise at all but the patient hears it anyway. This has no basis in reality and this is really psychotic. **Mania** occurs when a patient is really hyperactive or over-stimulated for many days or weeks or even months. Drug-Addicts who act manic are not necessarily manic at all. There are other psychotic symptoms, too. (See chapters IV-1, IV-4)

"Gravely Disabled"

The gravely disabled may have homes or be homeless. In either case, their homes and/ or lives are in a mess in the opinion of most people. People who still have homes may not be managing them very well. This is often the case in severe cases of dementia. These kinds of cases are often aired on the local news when we see that the Health Department or similar agency has been receiving neighbors' complaints about the general squalor of a house and the news blurb shows county officials entering a home that is extremely filthy, cluttered, and unlivable. We had one dementia patient in whom the brain deterioration had apparently started out by affecting his sense of smell which he had lost: he was brought in covered in feces and had to be interviewed outdoors by the doctor and nurse. He was totally unaware of any of this, not by smell, touch, or other senses. These people are gravely disabled and unable to care for themselves. The other option is to have Adult Services or the local police go to their homes for regular safety checks.

Apart from people with brain disorders, severely psychotic patients are usually gravely disabled as well as psychotic (they have two criteria for emergency treatment).

Other cases are those of the homeless. Who are these homeless street people and what is wrong with them? Psychiatric consensus is that about two-thirds have end-stage alcoholism and/or drug addiction ("living under the bridge"),and about one-third are severely psychotic. Finally, there are a few homeless who are actually regular citizens who have become homeless for a brief time period but who are able on their own or with some assistance to make arrangements to go to battered women's shelters, the Salvation Army, etc. This last type of homeless person *is not* gravely disabled whereas the end-stage alcoholics are probably-possibly gravely disabled and the chronic and persistently severely psychotic patients are definitely gravely disabled.

Table VII-3   Who are the Homeless?

Homeless Population	account for __?__% homeless	Is the person Gravely Disabled? Does he have any psychiatric emergency*?
Alcoholics and Drug Addicts	≈ 65 %	~~usually not-/-sometimes~~ *Only if he is having D.T.'s or other psychiatric emergency* — or a medical emergency **
Psychotic	≈ 32 %	~yes~***
Unfortunate poor ("normal" citizens)	≈ 3 %	~no~

* any psychiatric emergency: suicidal, homicidal, psychotic, gravely disabled
**medical emergencies can be common: ascites, bleeding throat, epileptic seizures, heart disease
***besides having a psychiatric emergency, these patients may well have very poor health requiring urgent medical attention (due to "deferred maintenance"): out-of-control diabetes or blood pressure, various infections, malnutrition, and so on

What happens when the end-stage alcoholics end up in the Hospital Emergency Room? If they desire to stop drinking or drugging, it may be possible to find them a bed in a Recovery House or Halfway House. In most cases they do not desire this, and the main reason for the trip to the ER is that they were drunk or high and yelling at the police and wandering around in traffic either because of being in a state of intoxication or in withdrawal—during these two phases of addiction they are prone to bizarre behavior. While in the ER, if they are in withdrawal, they will receive medication to make them feel better (Librium and Thiamine for example); or, if they are intoxicated, then they might "sleep it off" in the ER and then be released after a maximum stay of 23 hours. Statutory law forbids staying in the ER for more than 24 hours, the reason being that if they are sick to that degree, then they should be admitted upstairs to a hospital bed. If their withdrawal symptoms worsen to the point of nearing D.T.'s (delirium tremens) during which they have visual hallucinations (seeing "pink elephants"), then they are automatically admitted to a medical bed in the hospital (not necessarily a psychiatric bed). D.T.'s are both a medical and a psychiatric emergency. Otherwise, they can be released. In most cases, they are not interested in going to any controlled environment. If they are otherwise not psychotic or suicidal or homicidal (the other three criteria for psychiatric emergency), they might indeed be released back onto their own recognizance after treatment for their withdrawal or intoxication symptoms. Alcoholism and drug-addiction are no longer treated as if the patient had a primary psychiatric illness—these are compulsive addiction problems that can only be cured by the patient's own heart-felt desire to be sober. Nobody can will or force alcoholics to get sober—only themselves. (see chapter VI-1 on Alcoholism)

"You can lead a horse to water but you can't make it drink."

What happens to the severely and persistently chronic mentally ill psychotic patients? They are almost always admitted to a psychiatric hospital whether they want it or not. Besides having a psychiatric emergency they often have untreated medical problems, the number and severity of which increase with age. Psychotic patients are not able to organize themselves to make doctor appointments, obtain prescription medicine, and follow through on health initiatives. They lack the planning skills and motivation. Psychotic homeless patients meet two of the criteria for admission: psychotic and gravely disabled: in an extended sense they are a danger to themselves, although may not be actively suicidal by their own statements.

How do psychiatrists know the difference between the three types of people? By experience and by interview. This difference is determined during the psychiatric interview, which is a fairly involved process in some cases. A second ER visit for the same symptoms (in any medical specialty including psychiatry) both within 48 hours is usually an automatic admission whether voluntarily or involuntarily.

These four criteria for determining psychiatric emergencies are based on statutory law (laws made by State legislatures) and the terminology might differ slightly from State to State; however, the intentions of the criteria are generally the same throughout the country. Commonly the patient will be kept in the hospital for 72 hours or "three business days" or "three working days". In California this is literally for exactly seventy-two clock-hours whereas in some States (Ohio, for example) three business days refers to three business days of the Probate Court which does not meet on any State or federal holiday. The unfortunate but foreseeable result in Ohio means that a person admitted Thursday evening before Labor Day might not have his probate hearing until sometime on the Wednesday after Labor

Day. In severe cases, the psychiatrist may petition the court to keep the patient longer and involuntarily, for fourteen days. The California court not infrequently does not agree with the psychiatrist and lets the patients out after only a three day stay—all too often with dire consequences since the courts' decisions are based only on legal codes and tend to reject the medical input. The Ohio courts seem more likely to defer to the psychiatrists' requests and judgment.

Entering a Psychiatric Ward

Patients

This is what to expect if you are admitted to a psychiatric hospital. You will be led onto the Unit and nurses will ask a lot of questions related to your medical history, your reason for coming to the hospital, and list of medications. Nurses will check your belongings for pills, drugs, cords, "sharps" such as razor blades, needles, etc. Hospitals try to make the rooms "suicide-proof" so it will look Spartan and you will not be given metal cutlery or single-edge razor blades. Perhaps the male nurses will shave you—each Unit has adapted to all of these precautions. The windows will be barred or with shatter-proof glass, there will be no places to hang anything. There will be a central nursing station, a combination dining room/TV room probably as patients may be encouraged to be out in conspicuous locations and not isolated to rooms. Locked Units will probably have a "seclusion room" which is suicide-proof, with sound deadening (for screaming and cursing), padded walls (in case of head-banging and pummeling staff), and a central bed for "restraining" patients who are extremely violent. If you are restrained in one of the States with liberal laws, then the rules of restraint will be humane and patient-oriented. There are very rarely any "episodes" involving staff and patients in psychiatric hospitals, such as "dalliance" or punitive physical abuse. When these are uncovered, it is sensational and makes national news (at least in the psychiatric gazettes). However, there may occasionally be serious wounds inflicted on staff as well as patient-to-patient misbehaviors and "liaisons". Smoking rules will depend upon the regulations of that Unit and its hospital as well as on the State laws. Most hospitals do not allow smoking inside the unit because of OSHA laws to protect hospital staff from second-hand smoke. Everything that you do, touch, see, feel, and hear will be designed to be calmative and risk-free.

Visitors

You will notice that the unit has big powerful locking doors and that entry and exit is highly controlled due to escape precautions. Visiting hours may be short. Some family members may be barred from visiting due to fear of agitating the patient. Otherwise, you will find it as described above and hopefully not a depressing experience: remember that you are unable to provide this service in your home and that jail is probably not going to be therapeutic, either.

Hospital Stays and Discharges

Voluntary patients usually stay until the patient and doctor reach some mutual agreement concerning the stability of the patient. Voluntary patients usually want to stay as long as possible, although this is not always the case and depends on circumstances. Voluntary patients are usually discharged back home and have regular out-patient visits with a local out-patient psychiatrist. The first visits occur very frequently, and then the frequency can be decreased.

Most involuntary patients detest the hospital and are angry about being detained there. They cannot wait to leave. But they need to stay in the hospital until they are stable. They can be committed against their will for a few days and if they are still unstable, they can be kept an additional intermediate period of time (about two weeks). If they have committed a crime, then they will be on a "police-hold". This means that when the patient is psychiatrically stable, the police will come and take him into the judicial system. These involuntary patients are not so eager to leave. Rarely, we will have patients nowadays who are still not stable and need to be kept for many months. They need to be sent to a long-term care center, which usually means a State hospital. The elderly in this situation may be sent to a locked unit in a specialized nursing home. All of these placements are involuntary and are processed in the court system.

Usually, dementia patients are sent to a regular nursing home after they are stabilized.

Historical Anecdote

In England under the Common Law, suicide was a felony because of the purely practical fact that a person's premature death denied the Crown of all that potential future yearly tax money: that is why the Crown was legally able to confiscate summarily all of the suicide's properties.

▶QUESTION

Q: Who determines whether a patient is having a psychiatric emergency?

A: The duly appointed authorities based on the laws of that State. In Ohio, this can be the sheriff or medical doctors. In California each County appoints mental health personnel who have passed a specific test regarding involuntarily admissions. And these staff are given a license that looks like a driver's license.

VIII.) CONCLUSION

Whence Psychiatry?

Psychiatry has prehistoric roots—not as a separate treatment, but rather as the evolution from and refinement of a greater treatment. Prehistoric man is believed to have had shamans who functioned as spiritual, surgical, and medical healers as well as forecasters, preventionists, soothsayers, and astrologers (depending upon the size of the clan or tribe). From this one shamanistic profession have come hundreds of modern specialists, among which we find contemporary psychiatry as unique.

Where is Psychiatry Now?

One of the largest medical groups in California out-sourced its Psychiatry Department in 2008.

Remember that California is said to be the "bellwether" of the country.

Is Psychiatry becoming less relevant? This is a partial answer: I see a number of patients who come in every three to four months or every six months for refills. Some of these refills could be granted by a nurse practitioner or a family doctor (as if the primary care doctors were not already overwhelmed).

The County systems here are overwhelmed with more patients, fewer resources, and financial constraints.

Is Psychiatry really necessary for everyone? Where in the world is there any country with such a large percentage of psychiatrists? Psychiatry was originally established to provide custodial care for the severely insane. So is it necessary to see a psychiatrist for job-related stress or the everyday stresses that are caused by living in Los Angeles? Probably not, unless we need a few days off work with a doctor's excuse. Why can't employers provide more sick time? General psychiatrists are not necessarily "occupational psychiatrists". When stressed-out employees come to psychiatrists to get time off work, there is no set standard for how to treat this—stress leave treatment varies widely among psychiatrists from a few days to a few months.

We have a highly mobile society in which most people move several times, sometimes far away from family and friends. This creates loneliness and rupture of traditions. We also have a very heterogeneous population in which there is not a sense of total belonging or of

"We-ness" as in Japan or small countries. How often is a therapist a substitute friend for the geographically or culturally isolated?

The information regarding diagnosis and treatment in this book may become a dwindling art and a luxury service reserved for the well-heeled and well-insured.

Internet Psychiatry: A lot of patients and concerned family members turn to the Internet and do research on line, investigate their parents' new prescriptions, and even order prescriptions for themselves from overseas.

Modern Psychiatry is certainly changing now. It has been changing a lot since the 1980's. Internal Medicine and Surgery have not changed much: still the same diagnoses and same treatment approach. But this is not true of Psychiatry: shamans to priests to astrologers to neurologists to psychoanalysts and then to "black-&-white" movie psychiatry to the present system which is in much flux.

Whither Psychiatry?

Where do we go from here? At least two probable answers: Biogenetic psychiatry and tele-psychiatry. Future treatments will rely heavily on new biochemical assays and genetic documentations. New treatments may be injectables or focused magnetic waves. Biology will be a major feature. Psychiatrists will oversee these injections and will chart various biometric changes (in the brain). Telemedicine is also a likely answer. Tele-psychiatry, more concisely. The future of technologic societies will rely more and more upon the Internet and other interactive communications. Future patients will use telemedicine and tele-health more and more. (telemedicine is delivery of medical care via Internet whereas tele-health includes preventive medicine and other health-related e-activities). Why? Because Telepsychiatry is easy, cheap, efficient, convenient, farsighted, and can be done in the comfort of the patient's own home. It is easy for the doctor also who will need to do less traveling (hence have more time to "see" patients) and can even make late-night consultations from his own home. It is cheaper because it saves travel-time and reduces the cost of travel (gasoline). New technologies in the pipeline will also allow electronic remote readings of patients' prescription drug blood levels—if the levels are to low or too high, then the nurse consultant will send you an e-order to change the dosage of that drug. Telepsychiatry is farsighted because it gives us a working treatment template in case of a catastrophic epidemic (pandemic) or major bio-terrorism. Telemedicine may well become the routine care of the future.

Tele-psychiatry has already had very limited use for some time in Kansas for prison and hospice visits. Currently these are some of the treatments that we could give: computerized psychological testing (MMPI, TOVA). Some county agencies are working to develop tele-psychiatry access for people in remote locations.

Why?

Because people are social creatures and need to feel connected to others, even if only telemetrically. Nonetheless, psychiatry as we know it, will probably change a great deal in the near future.

►Take home points:
They are all good as drugs but can be bad as poisons
The PDR is like a phonebook—it is not a textbook of pharmacology!
The patient who treats himself has a fool for a doctor (the converse, by the way, is also true).

Little by little
Go day by day
Or hour to hour
We're on our way!

This is not a
Dress Rehearsal—
This is really your Life!

...keep on doing the same things
and you'll keep on
getting the same results...

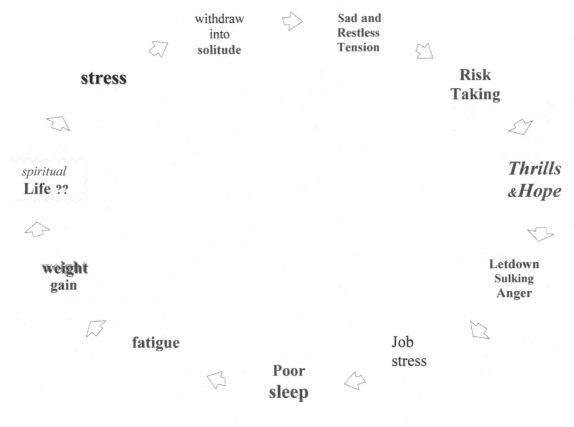

withdraw
into
solitude

Sad and
Restless
Tension

stress

Risk
Taking

spiritual
Life ??

Thrills
&Hope

weight
gain

Letdown
Sulking
Anger

fatigue

Job
stress

Poor
sleep

Epilog

Is it all in my head?"
"Yes, in your head and between your ears".
Try to take charge of your emotions.
Taking medications can be a part of taking charge.
Therapy is definitely a part of taking charge.

Is it all in your head? Yes and No:
None of the physical world is inside your head; however,
Your perceptions of the whole world are.
Learn to meditate and you can change your perceptions of the world
And in so doing you can effect a change in the way you see the world.
Abolish the negative thoughts.
Foster the positive thoughts.
So go to it!
Have at it!

X.) REFERENCES

Numbers in superscript interspersed within the chapters refer to these reference numbers:

1. DSM-IV-TR. (the Fourth Diagnostic and Statistical Manual Text Revision). American Psychiatric Association (APA).

2. The Pharmacologic Basis of Therapeutics, Goodman and Gilman's. 9th edition.

3. Comprehensive Textbook of Psychiatry / VI. 6th edition. Kaplan and Sadock.

4. Handbook of Drug Therapy in Psychiatry. Bernstein, Jerold.

5. Essential Psychopharmacology. Stahl, Stephen.

6. The Cytochrome P450 System: Drug Interaction Principles for Medical Practice. Cozza, Kelly MD, and Armstrong, Scott MD.

7. Relapse Traps: How to Avoid the 12 Most Common Pitfalls in Recovery. Rogers, Ronald L., and McMillin, Chandler Scott.

8. "Big Book" of Alcoholics Anonymous. 3rd edition.

9. Basic and Clinical Pharmacology. 7th edition. Katzung, Bertram.

10. Harrison's Principles of Internal Medicine. 14th edition.

11. Dorland's Illustrated Medical Dictionary. 25th edition.

12. Elements of Chordate Anatomy. Weichert, Charles K. 3rd edition (source for mammal brains in "Brain" chapter)

13. Physician's Desk Reference 2007. 61st edition. (main source of pregnancy ratings)

14. How Alanon works for families and friends of Alcoholics. Alanon literature.

15. personal conversations with pharmaceutical representatives

16. received wisdom from supervising psychiatrists during residency training

17. Apoptosis: neuronal death by design. Stahl, Stephen. J. Clin. Psych.58(5) 183-5.

18. Webster's New World Dictionary, 2nd college edition.

19. Addiction Genetics (review) by Jan Marie Werblin www.treatment-centers.net/addiction-genetics

20. Lighting up the Brain. Gero Miesenböck. Scientific American, Oct. 2008, pp52-59. www.SciAm.com

21. Black's Law Dictionary. Fifth edition.

22. Surplus or Shortage? Unraveling the Physician Supply Conundrum. Rosenblatt, Roger, and Lishner, Denise. Western J of Medicine. Jan. 1991, 154, 1.

23. Bernstein, Jerrold G. Handbook of Drug Therapy in Psychiatry. 3rd ed.

24. New College Latin & English Dictionary. Traupman, John C. PhD. 1995.

25. Tondo, L MD; Albert, MJ MD; Baldessarini, Ross MD. J. Clin. Psychiatry 67Z:4, April 2006; pp. 517-523.

26. Hollander E, Wong CM. Journal of Clinical Psychiatry 56(suppl.4), 3-6,1995.

27. Pocket Oxford Classical Greek Dictionary. 2002.

28. Resnick, Phillip J MD. Clinical assessment of malingered mental illness (seminar).

29. Bipolar Disorder. Keck Paul , Dewan Naakesh, Nasrallah Henry. Supplement to Current Psychiatry. Feb. 2005.

30. Advances in Neurology. September 9, 2006. CME LLC.

31. Pain Clinic. Vol. 2 No. 2. April 2000.

32. Zivin Justin. Understanding Clinical Trials. Sci. Am. April 2000.

33. Burt Vivien K. Depression in Women. CNS News. April 2000.

34. Female Endocrine System. Primary Psychiatry. Vol.7 No.4 April 2000.

35. Ericson A, Källén B, Wilholm B-E. Delivery Outcome after the use of antidepressants in early pregnancy. Eur. J Clin Pharmacology (1999) 55:503-508.

36. Effects of Valproate Acid on Fetuses, Neonates, and Nursing Infants. Psychiatric Annals 30:4 April 2000.

37. Effects of Carbamazepine on Fetuses, Neonates, and Nursing Infants. Psychiatric Annals 30:5 May 2000.

38. Dominguez Roberto, Blackman Karl E, Lugo, Susana. Demographics, Prevalence, and clinical features of the Schizo-Obsessive Subtype of Schizophrenia. CNS Spectrums. Vol4-Number 12. Dec. 1999.

39. Baaré William F C et al. Volumes of Brain Structures in Twins Discordant for Schizophrenia. Arch. Gen. Psychiatry/Vol. 58, Jan. 2001.

40. Stompe Thomas, Ritter Kristina, Schanda Hans. Catatonia as a subtype of Schizophrenia. Psychiatric Annals 37:1 Jan 2007.

41. Seeman Mary. All Psychosis is Not Schizophrenia... Clinical Schizophrenia. Oct. 2007.

42. Iacobini Marco. Face to Face: the Neural Basis of Social Mirroring and Empathy. Psychiatric Annals 37:4 April 2007.

43. Viamontes George, Beitman Bernard. Mapping the Unconscious in the Brain. Psychiatric Annals 37:4. April 2007

44. Beitman Bernard, Viamontes George. Unconscious Role-induction: Implications for Psychotherapy. Psychiatric Annals 37:4 April 2007.

45. Epidemiology, Psychopharmacology, and Neurobiology of Compulsive Sexual Behavior. CNS Spectrums Vol 5 No 1 Jan 2000.

46. Gabbard Glen. Unconscious Enactments in Psychotherapy.

47. Quan Stuart, Zee Phyllis. A Sleep Review of Systems. Geriatrics Mar 2004, Vol 59 No 3.

48. Blinder Barton. The Autobiographical Self: who we know and who we are. Psychiatric Annals 37:4 April 2007.

49. Lindenmayer Jean-Pierre, Cosgrove Victoria. Pharmacologic Treatment Strategies for Schizophrenia. Primary Psychiatry, Nov 2002.

50. Addington Jean PhD. Diagnosis and Assessment of Individuals Prodromal for Schizophrenia. CNS Spectrums Vol 9 No 8 Aug 2004.

51. Medical Aspects of Human Sexuality. pp 31-48. May 2001.

52. Maletzky Barry. Gender Identity Disorder. Primary Psychiatry June 2000.

53. Walsh Eric. Quality of Life and the treatment of Gender Identity Disorder. Primary Psychiatry June 2000

54. Gregory Robert. Evaluation of Readiness for Gender Reassignment. Primary Psychiatry June 2000

55. Boverman Joshua, Loomis Anna. Cross-Sex Hormone Treatment in Transsexualism.. Primary Psychiatry June 2000.

56. Buysse Daniel, Germain Anne, Moul Douglas. Diagnosis, Epidemiology, and Consequences of Insomnia. Primary Psychiatry Aug 2005.

57. Role of Serotonin in Mediating the Effects of Atypical Antipsychotic Drugs. CME Monograph, suppl. To Psychiatric Times. Sept 1999.

58. Barbey Jean, Roose Steven. SSRI Safety in Overdose. J Clin Psychiatry 1998;59(suppl 15)

59. Armstrong Scott, Cozza Kelly, Sandson Neil. Six Patterns of Drug-Drug Interactions. Psychosomatics 44:3 May-June 2003.

60. Canas Fernando. SSRI Discontinuation Syndrome. Primary Psychiatry Aug 2000.

61. PTSD (various articles). Psychiatric Annals Nov 2005.

62. Daniels John. Traumatic Brain Injury. Current Psychiatry Vol5 No 5 May 2006.

63. Social Brain (various articles). Psychiatric Annals 35:10 Oct 2005.

64. Serotonin: the First Decade. J Clin Psychiatry Vol 17 Monograph 3, 1999.

65. Markowitz Paul. Chapter 23 Pharmacotherapy. Handbook of Personality Disorders. Livesly John, ed. 2001.

66. MAOI's (various articles) Psychiatric Annals 31:6 June 2001.

67. Breitbart William, Yesne Alici-Evcimen. Why off-label antipsychotics remain first-choice drugs for delirium. Current Psychiatry Vol 6 No10 Oct 2007.

68. Kelly Peter, Waltz Lynn. Will CATIE-D change dementia treatment? Current Psychiatry Vol 5 No 12 Dec 2006.

69. Circadian Rhythms (various articles) CNS Spectrums Vol 6 No 6 June 2001.

70. Medically Unexplained Symptoms (various articles). Psychiatric Annals April 2005.

71. Trémeau Fabien, Citrome Leslie. Antipsychotics for patients without psychosis? Current Psychiatry Vol 5 No 12 Dec 2006.

72. Harvey Anne, Preskorn Sheldon. Cytochrome P450 Enzymes. J Clin Psychopharmacology Vol 16 No 4 Aug 1996.

73. Smith Michael W. Herbal Remedies in Psychiatric Practice. NIMH Research Center on the psychobiology of ethnicity; Harbor UCLA Medical Ctr, UCLA School of Medicine. Seminar

74. Shapiro David. Neurotic Styles.

75. Texas Algorithm. Texas Dept. of State Health Services.

76. Merikangas, KR et al. "Lifetime and 12-month Prevalence of Bipolar Spectrum Disorder in the National Comorbidity Survey Replication" *Arch. Gen. Psych.* 2007; 64: 543-52.

77. Gordis Leon. Epidemiology, 4th ed.

78. www.medicinenet.com

Page numbers in *italics* refer to illustrations.
Medications are listed under branded names; see cross
reference lists on pages 294–298 for generic names.

C

caffeine/caffeine derivatives, 377, 378–79, *519*

calcium, *373*, 593–94, *594*

California, psychiatry in, 630–31, 633

calorie counting, 438, 440

Campral, 469, 471

Canada, medications available from, 324

cancer, 531–32, 581

Captagon, 325

carbonate form, of Lithium, 373

cardiac dysfunction, as medication side effect, 300, 304, 314, 320, 332–33, 337, 346, 425

cascade function, *93*, 93, 95

casual referrals, 129–30

CATScans, 82

Celexa

    about, 273, 279, *310*, 342, 344–45, 357

    addictiveness/dependence risk, 71

    examples of use, 219, *331*, 348, *349–50*, 387

    pregnancy drug category, *518–19*

    side effects, 584

cerebrum, 84

Chantix, 63, 424

cheese reaction, 321

chemical cascades, in brain, 93, *93*, 95

chemical dependence. *See* addiction; habituation, to medications

"chemical imbalance," 96, 325–27, *326*

chemical treatments. *See* herbs/herbal therapies; medications

child abuse, 42, 504, 607

child/adolescent psychiatrists, 32

Child Protective Services, 468

children/infants, 145. *See also* malformation risks, of medications; teenagers

    of alcoholics, 468

    dosing considerations, 347–48, *347*

    emancipated minors, 144–45

chronic conditions, 49, 291–92, 397–99

chronic pain, 528–43

    overview, 528–29, 542–43

    causes/sources of, 531

    dosage considerations, 539–40

    duration of, 528–33

    pain thresholds and, 534–37, 538

    patient types, *542*

    treatment, 350, 532–33, 537–40

    types of, 530–34, *535–36*

cigarette use, 427, 446, 458, 460, 470, 475, 520. *See also* nicotine

cirrhosis, 456–57

citrate form, of Lithium, 373

civil rights, 121, 601–2, 623

"clean" drugs, 357

Cleaner role, in dysfunctional families, 494, *496*

clinical psychologists, 8, 31

clinical trials. *See* drug research/testing

clinicians, defined, 8

Clozaril

    about, 272, 301–2

    pregnancy drug category, 517, *518*, 523

    side effects, 62, *63*, 64, 419, 421–23, *422–23*

    as treatment of last resort, 293

C-L psychiatry, 32–33, 598

cluster headaches, 374

co-addictions, 458

cocaine, 71, *309*, 324–25, *435*, 455, 456

codeine, 426, *519*

codependence, 463–64, 480–86, *481*

Cogentin, 153, 393–94, *519*

Cognex, 555

cold medicines. *See* allergy/cold medications

commission, acts of, 233, 249–50

common law, English, 632

common major side effects, defined, 447

common minor side effects, defined, 442, 447

communication

    between doctors and families, 145–46

    between doctors and patients. *see* doctor-patient relationships; History of Present Illness (HOPI)

compassionate use, 64

Compazine, 301, *519*

competence, 144–45

compliance/non-compliance, 40, 47–48, 617–19, 621

compulsion

    addiction issues, 452, 456–57, 478

    criminal behavior and, 614–15

    defined, 568

    vs. impulsivity, 565–70, *566–67*

    lying and, 573–74

    scale of, 571

    treatment, *569–70*

exaltation, *201*
Excessive Daytime Sleepiness (EDS), 397
exercise, 152, 404, 438
expressed emotionality, 492–93
extended care facilities. *See* nursing homes
external stressors, 130–33
extra-societal isolation, 572

F

factitious patients, 48, 540–41, *542*
failure to diagnose, legal implications, 605
fainting spells, 260
Famciclovir, *519*
family members. *See also* dysfunctional families; genetics
    addiction and, 451–52, 463–64, 477–78
    borderline personality disorder and, 227
    codependence, 463, 480–86
    of elderly patients, 557, 611–12
    hierarchies among, 489
    of HIV/AIDS patients, 578
    hospital visits by, 631–32
    nature/nurture and, 503–4, *503*
    in patient history gathering, 145–47
    therapy session participation, 51–52
    treatment perspective, 144–48
    violent behavior in, 610–11
Fanapt, 219, 272
FAS, 520
fatality. *See* death
fat-burning drugs, 437–38
favorite child role, in dysfunctional families, 493
FDA. *See* Food and Drug Administration (FDA)
feeding tubes, 550
fee schedules, 38
Fenisec, 437
Fentanyl, 70, 456, 462
Fetal Alcohol Syndrome (FAS), 520
fetishes, 590
FGA medications. *See* First Generation Anti-psychotic (FGA) medications
fight or flight response, 312
Fioricet, 71
First Amendment rights. *See* civil rights
First Generation Anti-psychotic (FGA) medications, 272, 299–301, 557, 585

5-hydroxy-tryptamine. *See* serotonin (5-HT)
fixed false beliefs. *See* delusions
Flagyl, 462
flat affect, 101
Flexeril, 426, *519*, 532
folie-à-deux, 160
Food and Drug Administration (FDA)
    generic medications, 407
    labeling rules, 62
    on off-label prescribing, 289
    on package inserts, 442–43
    pregnancy drug categories, 517–21, *518–19, 520–21*, 526–27, *527*
    regulatory role, 60–62, 65, 284–93
food sensitivities, 256. *See also* eating disorders
forebrain, 84–87, *85–86*
forensic psychiatry, 33, 603–4, 610, 612
France, research studies from, 514
fraud, 48
free-standing hospitals, 622
Freud, Sigmund, 88
frontal lobe dementia, 551
functional illness, in brain, 84
functional pain, 534, 538, *542*

G

GABA
    about, 95, 268, 269, 274, 378, 382
    addictiveness/dependence risk, 433, 461
Gabitril, 393
GAD. *See* generalized anxiety disorder (GAD)
galantamine, 379
GBH, 420, 455
gender. *See also* men's issues; pregnancy, psychiatric medications and; sex/sexual function
    in ADD, 317–18
    addiction issues and, 452
    age of onset and, 176
    in bipolar disorder treatment, 257–58
    in borderline personality disorder, 224, 227–28
    in codependent relationships, 480–82
    in depression, 196–97
    misogyny, 590
    suicide and, 236, 242, *245*
    weight changes and, 333–34
general hospitals, 622

Xyrem, 64, 420, 455
Xyzal, 280

Y
Yohimbine, 377, 589

Z
Zantac, 346, *519*
Zeitgeber, *398*, 403, 404
Zoloft
    about, 273, *310*, 342, 344–45, 368
    addictiveness/dependence risk, 71
    examples of use, 262, *331*, 348, *349–51*, 387,
      408, 556, 558
    off-label use, 527, 586
    pregnancy drug category, *518–19*, 519
    side effects, 150, 584
Zydis, 272
Zyprexa
    about, 272, 302–3, 338–39, 369
    examples of use, 208, 219, 304, 322, 340, 572
    pregnancy drug category, *519*
    side effects, 440, 585
Zyrtec, 280
Zyvox, 321